STROKE MADE SIMPLE

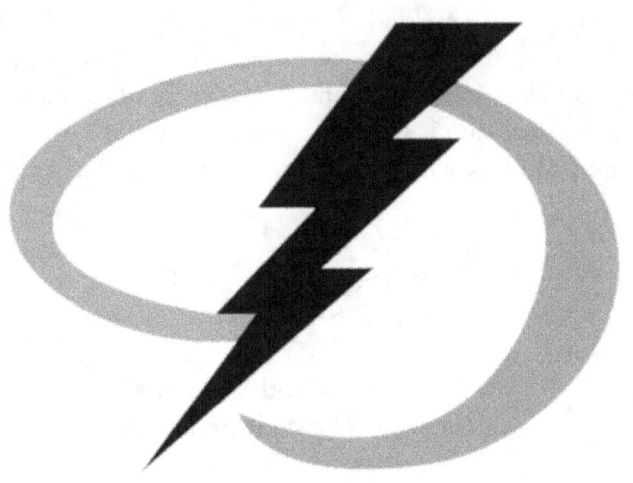

Nasser Razack, MD, JD

Stroke Made Simple
Copyright © 2018 Razack Intellectual Properties, LLC
All rights reserved.

No part of this book may be reproduced by any means, nor transmitted, nor translated into machine language, without the written permission of the publisher.

Condition of Sale

This book is sold subject to the condition that it shall not, by way of trade or otherwise, be lent, re-sold, hired out, or otherwise circulated in any form of binding or cover other than that in which it is published and without a similar condition, including this condition being imposed on the subsequent purchaser.

Disclaimer

Stroke is an ever-changing field. The author and editors of *Stroke Made Simple* have made every effort to provide information that is accurate and complete as of the date of publication. However, in view of the rapid changes occurring in medical science as well as the possibility of human error, this text may contain technical inaccuracies, typographical or other errors. It is the responsibility of the treating physician who relies on experience and knowledge about the patient to determine the best treatment for the patient. The information contained herein is provided "as is" and without warranty of any kind. The contributors to this book, including Raztec Publishing Inc., disclaim responsibility for any errors, omissions, or results obtained from the use of information contained herein. Likewise, they make no representation and assume no responsibility for the accuracy of information contained within this book, and such information is subject to change without notice. You are encouraged to confirm any information contained within this book with other sources and review all information regarding the medical diagnosis and treatment of stroke.

ISBN-10: 1-9877-4013-0
ISBN-13: 978-1-98774-013-4

Visit us on the World Wide Web:
http://www.StrokeMadeSimple.com

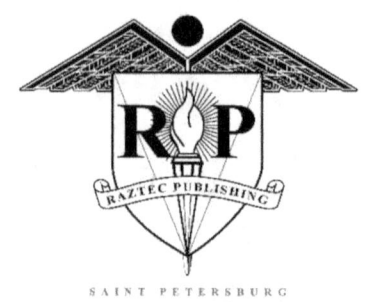

SAINT PETERSBURG

This book is dedicated to my father,
Mohamed S. Razack, M.D.
— the best teacher I ever had.

Contents

FOREWORD vii

INTRODUCTION 1

CHAPTER 1: Stroke 3

CHAPTER 2: The Neuron 7

CHAPTER 3: The Brain 11

CHAPTER 4: Cerebrovascular Anatomy 23

CHAPTER 5: Ischemic Stroke 35

CHAPTER 6: Hemorrhagic Stroke 49

CHAPTER 7: Cerebral Aneurysms 61

CHAPTER 8: The Vasculopathies 77

CHAPTER 9: Cerebrovascular Malformations 85

CHAPTER 10: Cerebral Venous Stroke 93

CHAPTER 11: Cerebellar Stroke 101

CHAPTER 12: Thalamic Stroke 115

CHAPTER 13: Brainstem Stroke 123

CHAPTER 14: Stroke and Vision 137

CHAPTER 15: Basilar Artery Occlusion 145

CHAPTER 16: Anterior Circulation Stroke 149

CHAPTER 17: Transient Ischemic Attack (TIA) 165

CHAPTER 18: Platelets, Stents, and Stroke 171

CHAPTER 19: Stroke Mimics 181

CHAPTER 20: NIHSS 187

CHAPTER 21: Stroke Imaging 197

CHAPTER 22: Contrast-Induced Nephropathy 217

CHAPTER 23: IV TPA 223

CHAPTER 24: Wake-Up Stroke 237

CHAPTER 25: Endovascular Treatment 243

CHAPTER 26: Collateral Circulation 263

CHAPTER 27: Prehospital Stroke Assessment 273

CHAPTER 28: Hospital-Based Stroke Assessment. 291

CHAPTER 29: Stroke Efficiency 315

CHAPTER 30: Stroke Communication. 327

CHAPTER 31: Summary 329

APPENDIX A: Mnemonics. 357

APPENDIX B: Abbreviations. 391

INDEX. 393

Foreword

I vividly remember my first interaction with Dr. Razack. At that time, I was covering an emergency department in Naples, Florida. I called him to discuss a stroke case. His advice pertaining to the case was amazingly simple. After many other interactions, I asked Dr. Razack if he could review his approach to stroke. I and many of my colleagues could not believe how much we learned about stroke and more importantly, how simple its treatment could be. When listening to Dr. Razack speak, it's quite clear that he thinks of stroke differently from most other physicians. His simplistic approach makes a great deal of sense without really sacrificing the ability to manage this complex disease.

Stroke is a tremendous problem. It affects almost 800,000 people in the United States annually. This means that every 40 seconds, someone within the United States suffers a stroke. Stroke is also the leading cause of disability and ranks fifth among the top 10 leading causes of death in the U.S. While stroke is typically considered a subspecialist physician issue, every emergency department physician must deal with it. Furthermore, the enormous magnitude of stroke patients means that every discipline of medicine will encounter this life-threatening condition from a preventive, treatment, or rehabilitation standpoint.

The diagnosis and treatment of stroke continues to evolve, particularly with the advent of major advances in endovascular treatment. Due to its superiority over intravenous tissue plasminogen activator alone for patients with large vessel acute ischemic stroke, endovascular treatment (mechanical thrombectomy) has become the standard of care. This means large-scale changes within hospitals must be implemented to adequately care for a large population of stroke patients. Fortunately, as Dr. Razack has demonstrated, these changes can be made economically and most hospitals can independently care for their own stroke patients. While the management of acute ischemic stroke may appear complex, Dr. Razack has proven that it doesn't have to be.

Many textbooks within this field are highly specialized and contain voluminous content. While comprehensive in scope, this book is purposely intended to be limited in depth in order to provide a simple approach to the diagnosis and management of acute ischemic stroke. *Stroke Made Simple* has been written to provide all healthcare professionals with a concise, practical, and clear reference that can help diagnose and treat acute ischemic stroke. Moreover, this book encompasses a gestalt approach towards stroke management, allowing non-physicians (emergency medical services personnel), non-specialist physicians, and other healthcare professionals to work in a synchronized, efficient manner to rapidly diagnose and treat acute ischemic stroke. I would highly recommend that any individual or healthcare facility which currently provides care for acute ischemic stroke read this wonderful text.

James Roach D.O. FACEP
Chairman, Emergency Department - Cleveland Clinic Florida
Chief Medical Officer/ EMS Medical Director - Broward Sheriff's Office

Introduction

"Everything should be made as simple as possible, but not simpler."
— Albert Einstein

Stroke is a devastating neurological disease and is an enormous diagnostic and treatment challenge. The complexity surrounding the management of stroke is further compounded because it changes on an annual basis. A few years ago, research suggested that endovascular treatment (EVT) for acute ischemic stroke was ineffective. In 2015, however, multiple randomized and controlled trials proved beyond a shadow of a doubt the tremendous benefit of EVT versus intravenous tissue plasminogen activator alone for the treatment of large vessel stroke.

These trials heralded a "Stroke Renaissance" that has led to a paradigm shift in stroke treatment. This includes advancements in neuroimaging to rapidly identify patients with large vessel occlusion (LVO), salvageable brain tissue (ischemic penumbra), and regions of irreparably damaged brain (core infarct). The identification of LVO candidates has been coupled with improvements in workflow, placing major emphasis on rapid treatment. This new philosophy can be summarized as: **FIND THEM FAST AND FIX THEM FAST!**

While many other texts are continually being published, it is often difficult to get a "big picture" view on stroke treatment and its core aspects. The purpose of this book is to emphasize the essential elements in the diagnosis and treatment of stroke. This book has removed the esoteric details and extraneous theories and focuses mainly on the essential elements that form the basis of stroke care. Although this information will be presented in a simple and informal style, it should not be assumed that this was done while sacrificing essential components of stroke management. This book was purposely organized to make the subject matter related to stroke easier to read, understand, retain, and most importantly, *apply*. This is reflected in the many figures, acronyms, mnemonics, and tables designed specifically to convey stroke-related concepts.

Additionally, the complexity of this material necessitated other elements regarding its presentation. First, important stroke concepts are repeated for reinforcement. Multiple abbreviations for terms will also be employed to retain key concepts. The first time they appear, they will be in parentheses. Thereafter, only the acronym will appear. For example, if the term "middle cerebral artery" (MCA) is used, it will first appear in parentheses, and thereafter, it will appear as "MCA." The end of each chapter will contain an abbreviation list for your convenience. Mnemonics are also used throughout the book's text to encapsulate critical information and related themes. This book contains an appendix of mnemonics which is organized by chapter. Review the mnemonics appendix and reread that portion of the chapter to refresh your memory, if necessary. It is remarkable how efficiently a mnemonic can encapsulate knowledge. The key purpose of this book is to transmit information as efficiently as possible. I've worked to simplify the information in this book, but any questions, suggestions, requests, comments or improvements are always welcome. Please contact me at strokenerd@gmail.com for this or any other communications.

Chapter 1

Stroke

A stroke or "brain attack" occurs when blood flow to the brain is compromised by either an arterial occlusion (ischemic stroke) or an arterial rupture (hemorrhagic stroke). The resultant neurologic symptoms correspond to the region of the brain supplied by one or more cerebral blood vessels. This focal disturbance of blood flow to the brain is not caused by a single disease but results from many different pathophysiologic entities leading to a blood vessel occlusion or rupture. Hippocrates, the father of medicine, first recognized and described stroke over 2,400 years ago. He referred to stroke as *apoplexy* which meant "struck down by violence" in Greek. This is because someone who was in otherwise good health would suddenly suffer a severe stroke deficit or even die. It was assumed that this individual had been "struck down" by a god. Hence, "struck" became "stroke." An old Chinese proverb says, "May you live in interesting times." This is especially relevant to stroke, with discoveries occurring at a breathtaking pace.

Stroke is the second leading cause of death worldwide.[1] Stroke is also the leading cause of disability and ranks fifth among the top 10 leading causes of death in the United States. Each year almost 800,000 Americans suffer a stroke, which means someone in the United States has a stroke every 40 seconds. Most cases (600,000) represent an initial stroke and the remainder consists of recurrent strokes. Stroke results in over $72 billion in annual costs. Due to America's aging population and the association of stroke with age, the incidence of stroke continues to increase, with the total annual cost for stroke projected to rise to approximately $240 billion by 2030. There are seven million stroke survivors in the United States. In one minute, a stroke can kill almost two million brain cells. After an hour, that number reaches 120 million brain cells which is comparable to 3.6 years of normal aging.[2] An average stroke results in the death of approximately 1.2 billion brain cells.[2]

A stroke is caused when blood flow to part of the brain is disrupted either from an occluded (ischemic stroke) or ruptured blood vessel (hemorrhagic stroke) causing intracranial bleeding (Figure 1). Approximately 87% of all strokes are ischemic and 13% are hemorrhagic. Hemorrhagic stroke can be further subdivided into bleeding within the brain (intracerebral hemorrhage) or covering the brain (subarachnoid hemorrhage), accounting for 10% and 3% of all strokes respectively (Figure 2).[3] There are several subtypes of ischemic stroke (Figure 3). These different subtypes and presentations of stroke will be discussed in subsequent chapters. Have you ever heard the expression, "No two sets of fingerprints are the same"? Stroke patients share the same characterization because every stroke patient presents differently, making stroke difficult to treat.

FIGURE 1. Types of Stroke

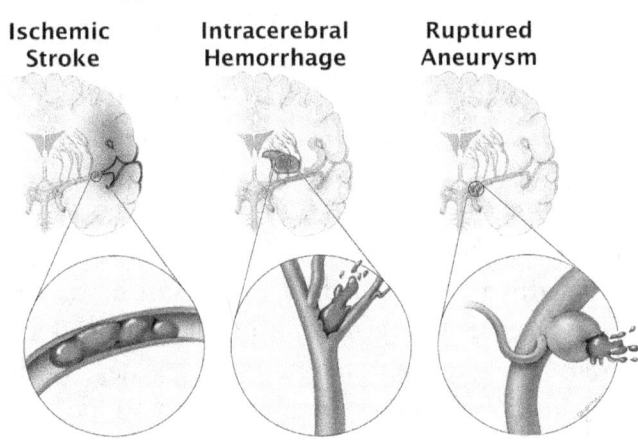

FIGURE 2. Basic Stroke Classification

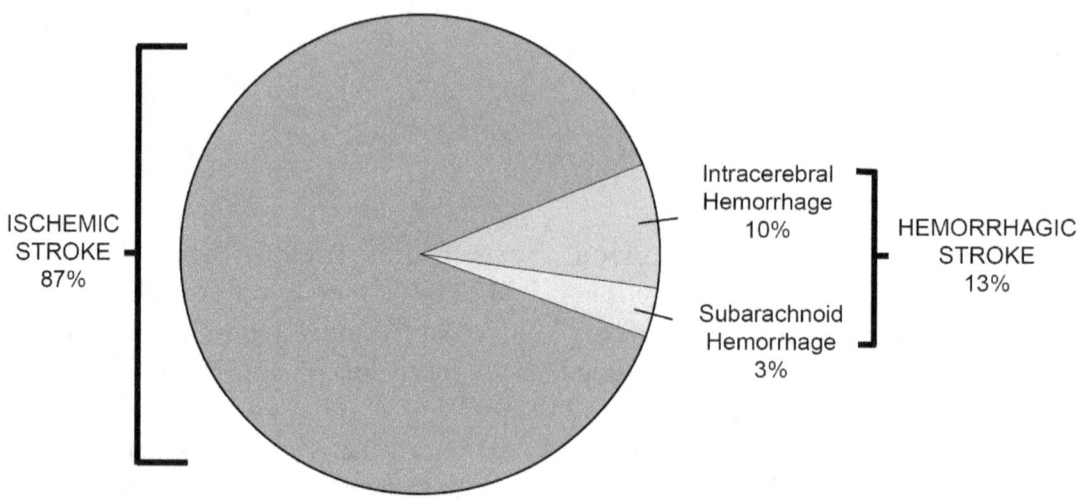

FIGURE 3. Classification of Stroke Subtypes

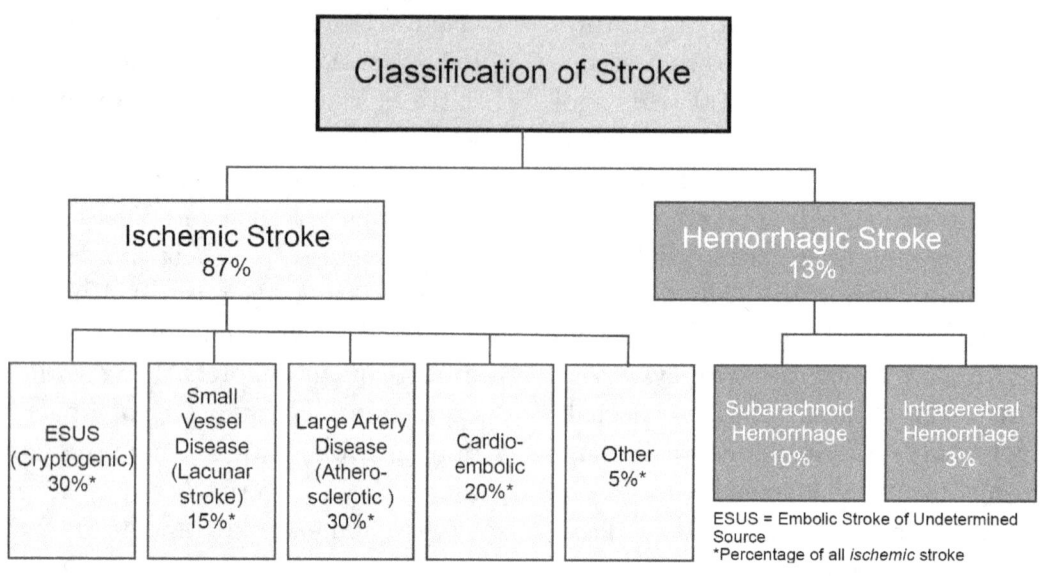

Thanks to the efforts on stroke awareness from societies such as the American Heart Association and the National Stroke Association, stroke has declined from being the third leading cause of death in the United States to just the fifth. In fact, since 1997, the annual per-capita stroke mortality rate in the United States has decreased by 34.3%.[4] While this may sound like wonderful news, the reality is that the number of people who suffer a stroke is stagnant, if not increasing. What's really happening is that we are doing better at keeping stroke victims alive but not reducing the risk or incidence of stroke. So while stroke death numbers are declining, stroke continues to be the leading cause of disability in both the United States and the world as a whole. Elderly patients fear stroke-related disability more than death.[5] These sentiments lead to the inescapable conclusion: *Many people would rather die than lose either the mental or physical functioning of their bodies.*

References

1. Lozano R, Naghavi M, Foreman K, et al. (2012). Global and regional mortality from 235 causes of death for 20 age groups in 1990 and 2010: a systematic analysis for the Global Burden of Disease Study 2010. Lancet, 380, 2095-128.

2. Saver JL. (2006). Time is brain—quantified. *Stroke*, 37(1), 263-66.
3. Mozaffarian D, Benjamin EJ, Go AS, et al. (2015). Heart disease and stroke statistics—2015 update: a report from the American Heart Association. *Circulation*, 131, e29–322.
4. Benjamin EJ, Blaha MJ, Chiuve SE, Cushman M, Das SR, Deo R. (2017). Heart disease and stroke statistics-2017 update: A report from the American heart association. *Circulation*, 135, e146-603.
5. Solomon NA, Glick HA, Russo CJ, Lee J, Schulman KA. (1994). Patient preferences for stroke outcomes. *Stroke*, 25, 1721-5.

Chapter 2

The Neuron

2.1 Introduction

The basic unit of the nervous system is the brain cell or neuron. The brain contains over 100 billion neurons, enabling it to transmit information quickly. Neurons have special properties that make them highly effective at transmitting information. While many different types of neurons exist, every neuron consists of three basic components: **dendrites**, a **cell body**, and the **axon** (Figure 1).

2.2 Neuronal Structure and Function

Dendrites are tree-like extensions surrounding the neuron. They receive information from other neurons and transmit this information to the cell body. An axon is an elongated fiber that extends from the cell body and transmits information from one neuron to the dendrites of another neuron. Located between the axon of one neuron and the dendrites of the next neuron is a gap known as a *synapse* (Figure 1). Neurotransmitters carry signals or transport information across these synapses to other neurons in order to share information with each other. Each neuron can receive and send millions of inputs to and from other neurons. This transmission between neurons allows different parts of the brain to communicate with each other and with the rest of the body.

Despite their special properties, neurons have two significant disadvantages: (1) their enormous sensitivity to oxygen deprivation, and (2) their inability to reproduce or multiply. This is precisely why stroke is such a devastating disease. Stroke results from irreparably damaged, oxygen-deprived brain tissue. An arterial occlusion reduces cerebral perfusion pressure (CPP), causing blood vessels to dilate and increase cerebral blood volume (CBV). Diminished brain perfusion causes two distinct patterns of cerebral blood flow (CBF) resulting in two different degrees of brain tissue injury. Impaired CBF results in one region called an *ischemic penumbra* which typically surrounds a second region referred to as a *core infarct* (Figure 2).[1]

FIGURE 1. The Neuron

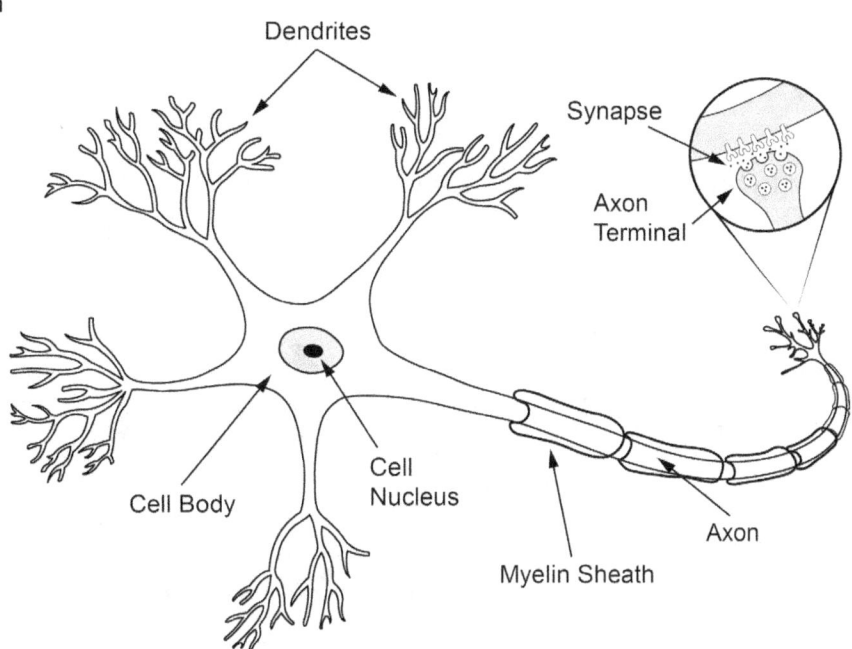

2.3 Core Infarct versus Ischemic Penumbra

A core infarct is caused by two distinct pathophysiologic processes. First, there is a loss of both oxygen and glucose supply secondary to vascular occlusion. Second, without oxygen and nutrients there is a host of cellular changes caused by the inability to produce energy within the cell. This ultimately disintegrates the cell's structures and its membrane in a process referred to as *necrosis*. It is critically important to discern core infarct from ischemic penumbra. Ischemic penumbra refers to threatened but still viable brain tissue, whereas a core infarct is indicative of irreversibly damaged or dead brain tissue. Both conditions are due to reduced blood flow. However, restoration of blood flow to the ischemic penumbra can prevent it from transforming into an irreparably damaged core infarct. This is because the ischemic penumbra is supplied by collateral circulation, but only for a finite period. During this limited time, it is of the utmost importance to restore blood flow to the brain and prevent irreparable brain tissue injury or permanent core infarct.

The ischemic penumbra (zone surrounding the core infarct) still contains viable brain tissue despite impaired blood flow to this region.[2] A core infarct represents irreparably damaged brain tissue and even successful reperfusion will not restore tissue functionality within this area. In contrast to core infarct, an ischemic penumbra can regain functionality if successfully reperfused with oxygen. However, reperfusion of this region is limited by time. During this period, the core infarct continues to expand and destroy what was once salvageable ischemic penumbra (Figure 3).

FIGURE 2. Core Infarct versus Ischemic Penumbra

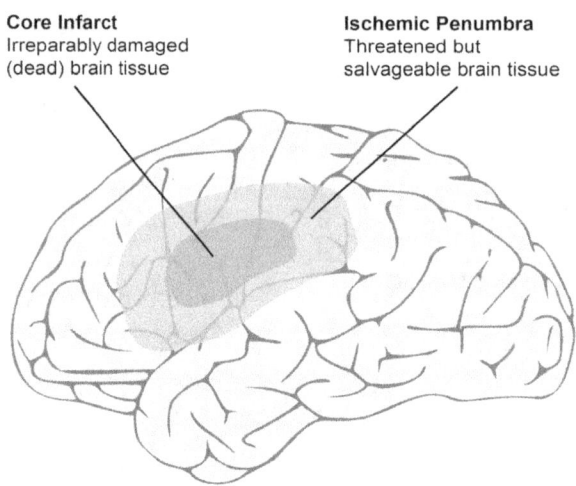

FIGURE 3. Transformation of Ischemic Penumbra into Core Infarct

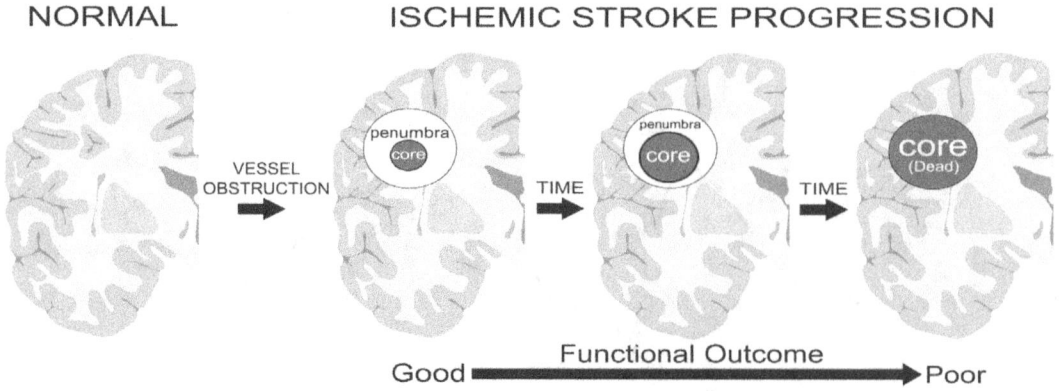

The reason the ischemic penumbra will convert into a core infarct is because blood vessels adjacent to it called *collaterals* can only temporarily supply oxygen to this threatened, but still salvageable, region of brain tissue. So, while the neurons contained within the ischemic penumbra have reduced oxygen supply, the oxygen level is not low enough to kill them. Rather, the ischemic penumbra is maintained in a dynamic state by adjacent collateral vessels and will perish unless sufficient oxygen supply is restored (Figure 2).

2.4 Conclusion

This chapter discussed the functional unit of the brain, the neuron. In addition, it described the concepts of an ischemic penumbra and a core infarct. Ischemic penumbra refers to the loss of functionality due to diminished blood flow, whereas core infarct means irreparable brain tissue death due to loss of blood flow. The goal of all acute ischemic stroke (AIS) treatment is to restore functionality to the penumbra, which is threatened but salvageable brain tissue. Every person has a distinct, individual timeframe during which ischemic penumbra can be preserved.[3] The only method proven to preserve the penumbra is the recanalization of the occluded blood vessel(s) responsible for it.

Abbreviations list

AIS, acute ischemic stroke; CBF, cerebral blood flow; CBV, cerebral blood volume; CPP, cerebral perfusion pressure.

References

1. Goyal M, Menon BK, Derdeyn CP. (2013). Perfusion imaging in acute ischemic stroke: let us improve the science before changing clinical practice. *Radiology*, 266, 16–21.
2. Liu S, Levine SR, Winn HR. (2010). Targeting ischemic penumbra: part I - from pathophysiology to therapeutic strategy. *J Exp Stroke Transl Med.*, 3(1), 47-55.
3. Campbell BC, Christensen S, Tress BM, et al. (2013). EPITHET Investigators, Failure of collateral blood flow is associated with infarct growth in ischemic stroke. *Journal of Cerebral Blood Flow and Metabolism*, 33, 1168–72.

Chapter 3

The Brain

The nervous system is divided into the central nervous system (brain and spinal cord) and the peripheral nervous system (12 pairs of cranial nerves and all the nerves in the body) (Figure 1). The brain and spinal cord are surrounded by three membranes called the *meninges* (Figure 2). The outermost meningeal layer is referred to as the *dura mater* which literally means "tough mother." Beneath the dura mater is the middle meningeal layer called the *arachnoid mater*. Further beneath the arachnoid mater is the innermost meningeal layer, the *pia mater*. The pia mater is also the thinnest meningeal layer. It is directly attached to the surface of the brain and extends into all its sulci. Keep in mind that the meninges literally "pad" the brain, so an easy way to remember the three meningeal layers is by using the mnemonic 'PAD' (Table 1). Lesions within the brain parenchyma beneath the pia mater are termed *intra-axial lesions*. Lesions outside the brain parenchyma are termed *extra-axial lesions* (Figure 3). These include meningeal tumors or meningiomas which are outside of the brain parenchyma and are, therefore, extra-axial lesions (Figure 4). Sometimes all three meningeal layers are collectively referred to as the "dura."

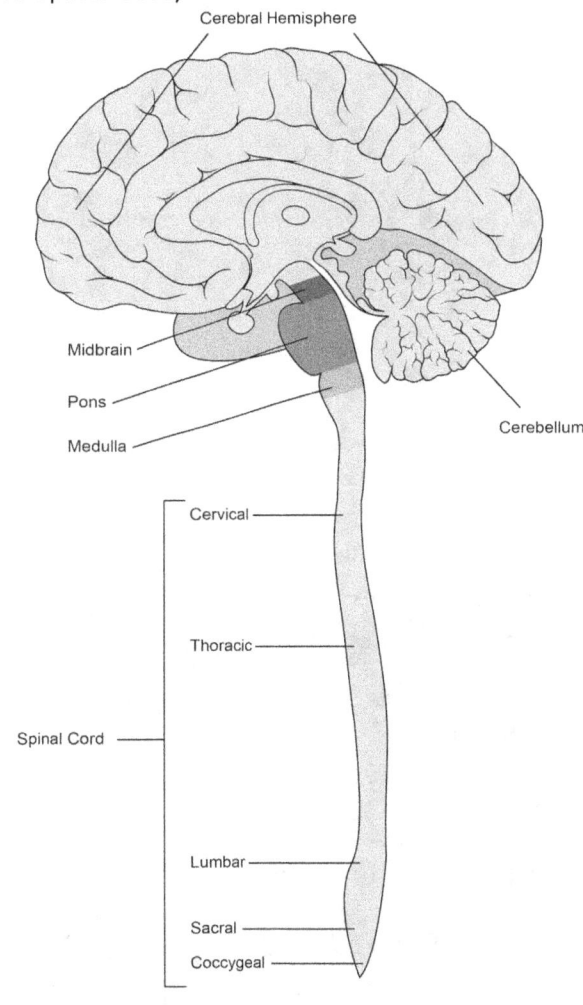

FIGURE 1. The Central Nervous System (The Brain and Spinal Cord)

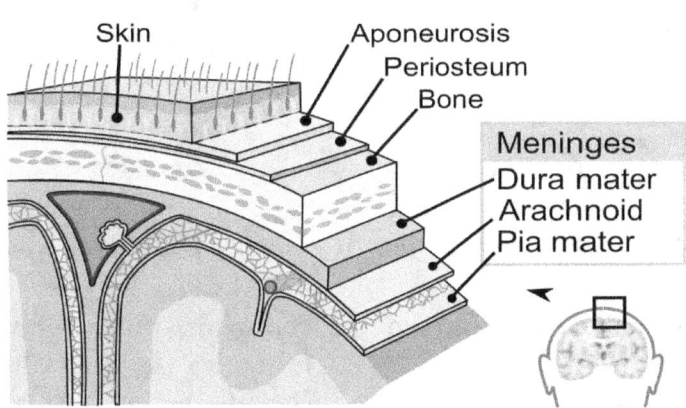

FIGURE 2. The Meninges

TABLE 1. The Meninges: **PAD**

P	Pia Mater
A	Arachnoid Mater
D	Dura Mater

FIGURE 3. Diagram of Extra-Axial Lesion

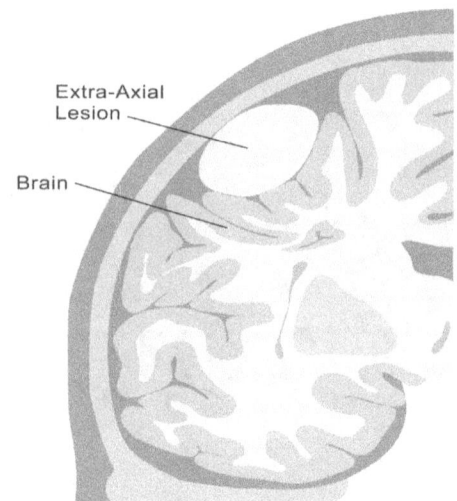

FIGURE 4. Extra-Axial Meningioma

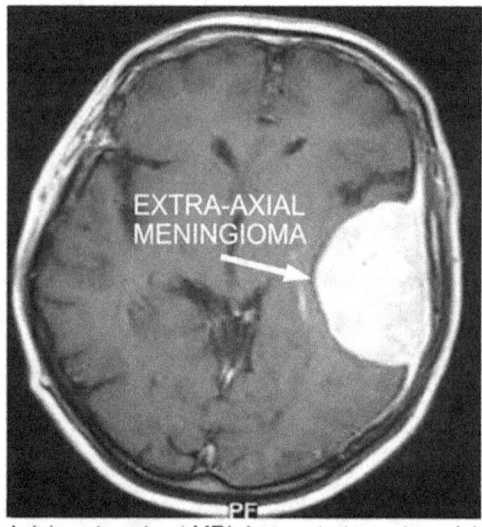

Axial post contrast MRI demonstrates extra-axial meningioma with broad-based dural attachment.

Cerebrospinal fluid (CSF) is produced in cavities within the brain referred to as the *ventricles*. The ventricles are surrounded by brain parenchyma and thus are also considered extra-axial structures. Therefore, the CSF contained within them is also extra-axial in location (Figure 5). CSF is predominantly made by modified ependymal cells located in the choroid plexus of the lateral, third, and fourth ventricles. CSF travels from the lateral ventricles into the third ventricle through the Foramen of Monro, then into the fourth ventricle through the Sylvian Aqueduct (Figure 5). CSF exits the fourth ventricle from the Foramen of Magendie (medially located) and the Foramen of Lushka (laterally located). Intracerebral hemorrhage can interfere with the circulation of CSF within the ventricles, resulting in expansion of the ventricular system or hydrocephalus (Figure 6).

FIGURE 5. The Ventricular System

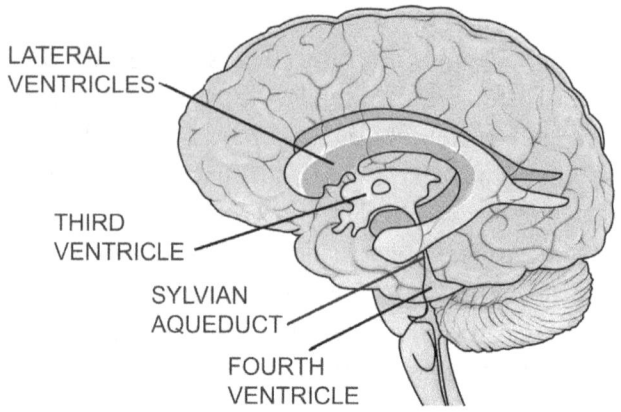

FIGURE 6. Hydrocephalus

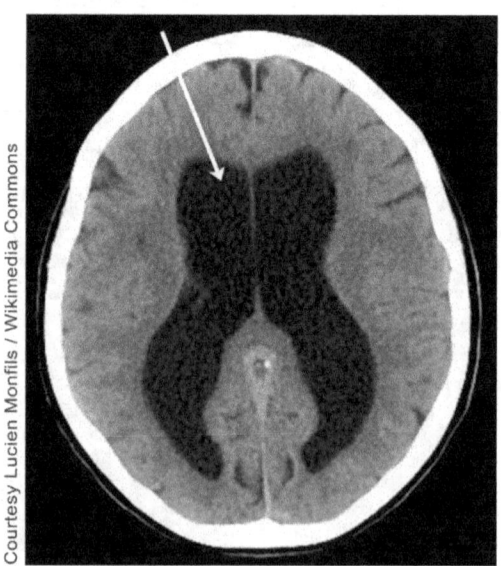

The brain develops from an embryonic basis into five distinct regions: the **telencephalon, diencephalon, mesencephalon, pons and cerebellum**, and the **medulla**. The telencephalon consists of the cerebral hemispheres and the basal ganglia (Figure 7). The diencephalon sits between the cerebral hemispheres and consists of the thalamus and the hypothalamus (Figure 7). The next embryological region of the brain is the mesencephalon or "midbrain" and is located between the diencephalon and the pons (Figure 7). The fourth division of the brain is the pons and cerebellum. The last division of the brain is the medulla oblongata. It forms the lowermost portion of the brainstem and lies between the pons and the spinal cord (Figure 7).

The embryologic distinctions of the brain have little impact regarding stroke treatment. From an anatomic standpoint, the brainstem consists of the midbrain, pons, and medulla. Little emphasis is placed on the fact that the midbrain, pons, and medulla are derived from different embryological precursors. More importantly, from a neurovascular standpoint, the midbrain, pons, and medulla are all supplied by the posterior circulation. Based on this philosophy, our review of neuroanatomy will now proceed from a more practical, anatomic standpoint.

The brain is divided anatomically into four separate lobes by the Sylvian fissure, the central sulcus, and the parieto-occipital fissure (Figure 8). These lobes include the frontal lobe which is anterior to the central sulcus, and the parietal lobe which is located behind it. The temporal lobe is located below the Sylvian fissure. The parieto-occipital fissure separates the parietal lobe superiorly from the occipital lobe inferiorly (Figure 8). Each of these lobes performs specialized functions which can be further delineated by specific regions of the cortex and gyri. The brain can also be divided into *Brodmann areas*, named after the German anatomist who identified them (Figure 9).

FIGURE 7. The Four Embryologic Regions of the Brain

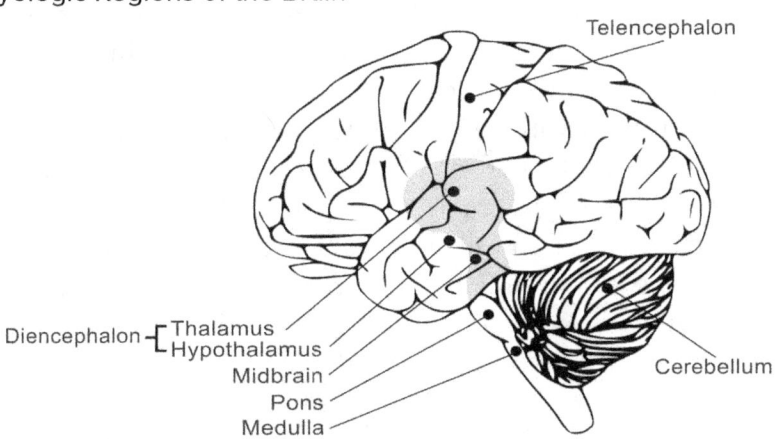

FIGURE 8. The Four Lobes of the Cerebrum

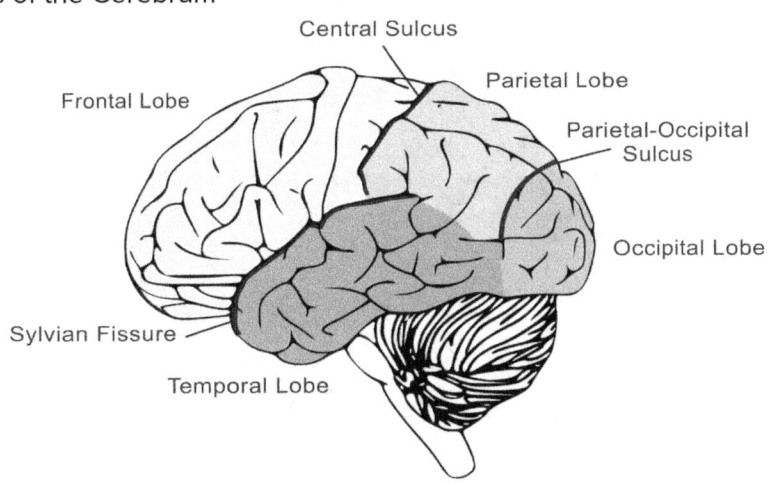

FIGURE 9. Brodmann Cytoarchitectural Labeling

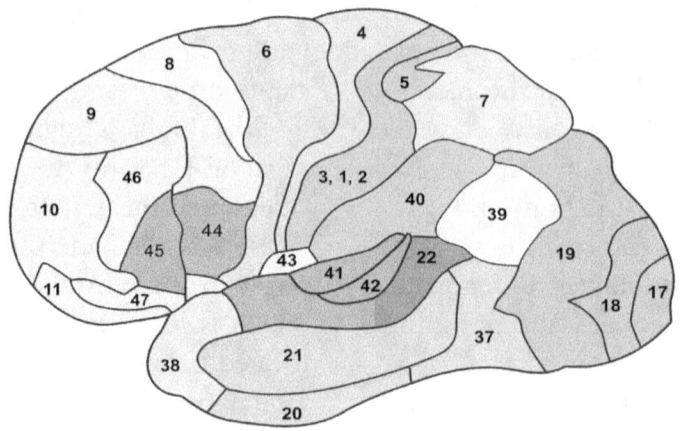

There are specific regions of the brain that are particularly relevant to stroke (Figure 10, Table 2). The frontal eye fields (FEF), which are responsible for initiating and tracking eye movements, are located in the frontal cortex, more specifically in Brodmann area 8. The primary motor cortex, more commonly called the "motor strip," is in the *precentral gyrus* which is located immediately anterior to the *central sulcus* and is the most posterior region of the frontal lobe. It contains the cell bodies of the pyramidal tract and controls voluntary movement. Located immediately behind the central sulcus is the *postcentral gyrus*, the most anterior part of the parietal lobe. This is also called the primary sensory cortex and is responsible for sensation. Broca's Area, which is located within the frontal cortex of the dominant lobe (usually left) of the brain, is responsible for the production of speech. Wernicke's Area is located in the temporal cortex of the dominant lobe (usually left) of the brain and is responsible for language comprehension. Lastly, the primary visual cortex, located within the occipital lobe, is responsible for vision.

Both cerebral hemispheres are separated by a dural fold called the *falx cerebri* (Figures 11 and 12). The cerebellum is separated from the cerebrum by the *tentorium cerebelli* (Figure 13). The tentorium cerebelli is a tent-like dural covering between the occipital lobes and the cerebellum (Figure 13). The supratentorial region of the brain is located above the tentorium cerebelli (both cerebral hemispheres). The infratentorial region of the brain is the region of the brain located below the tentorium cerebelli (Figure 13).

FIGURE 10. Cortical Regions Relevant to Stroke

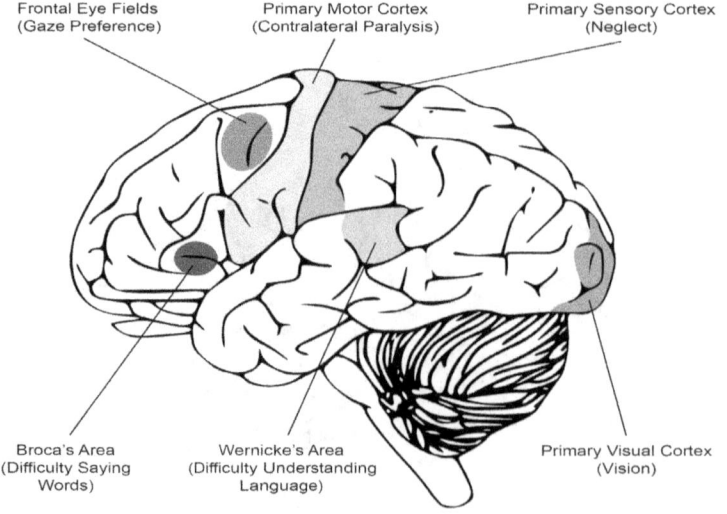

TABLE 2. Cortical Regions Relevant to Stroke

Cortical Structure	Location	Function
Frontal Eye Fields (FEF)	Frontal Lobe	Eye Movement
Primary Motor Cortex	Frontal Lobe	Voluntary Movement
Broca's Area	Frontal Lobe	Production of Speech
Primary Sensory Cortex	Parietal Lobe	Sensation
Wernicke's Area	Temporal Lobe	Language Comprehension
Primary Visual Cortex	Occipital Lobe	Vision

FIGURE 11. The Falx Cerebri

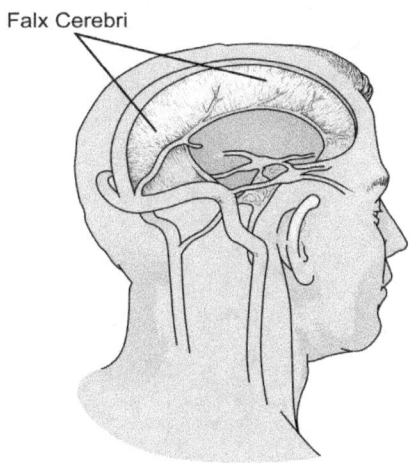

FIGURE 12. The Falx, Sulci, and Gyri

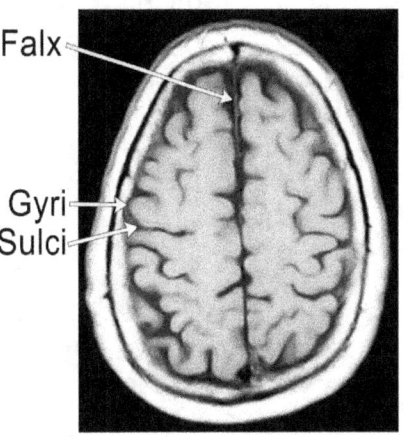

FIGURE 13. Supratentorial Versus Infratentorial

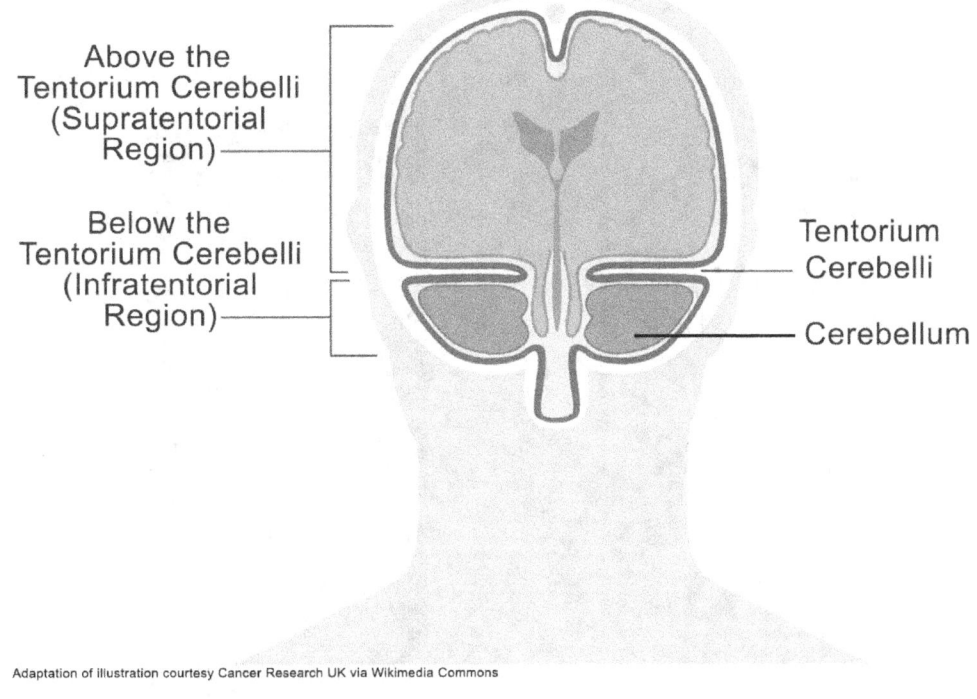

Adaptation of illustration courtesy Cancer Research UK via Wikimedia Commons

Both cerebral hemispheres have surface convolutions called *gyri* (Figure 12). Gyri are separated from each other by shallow indentations called *sulci* (Figure 12). Deeper channels separating gyri are termed "fissures," such as the Sylvian Fissure. Just like individualized fingerprints, no two brains have the same sulcal patterns. In fact, each of the two cerebral hemispheres appear different because they are structurally different. There is a *dominant* cerebral hemisphere (typically the left) which controls language and contralateral motor function. For example, a right-handed person (preferential use of the right hand for skilled movements) is typically left-brain dominant. Incidentally, the left cerebral hemisphere is also dominant in approximately 85% of left-handed individuals.

The surface of both cerebral hemispheres is characterized by an outer gray layer called the *cortex* (Figure 14). Beneath the cortex is the brain's white matter. Neurons extend from the cortex into the white matter. Neuron cell bodies comprise the brain's gray matter and its axons comprise the brain's white matter (Figure 14). Two large regions of white matter within the cerebral hemispheres are called the *centrum semiovale* and the *corona radiata* (Figure 15). The corona radiata is white matter at the level of the ventricular system while the centrum semiovale is white matter superior to that.

FIGURE 14. Gray and White Matter

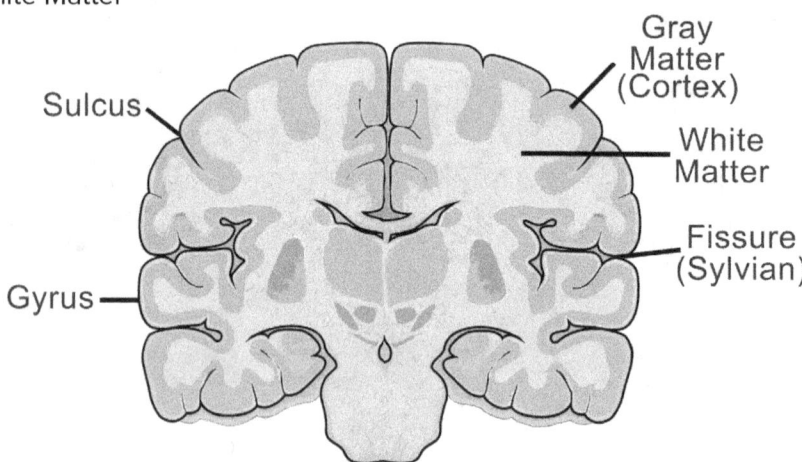

FIGURE 15. The Centrum Semiovale and the Corona Radiata

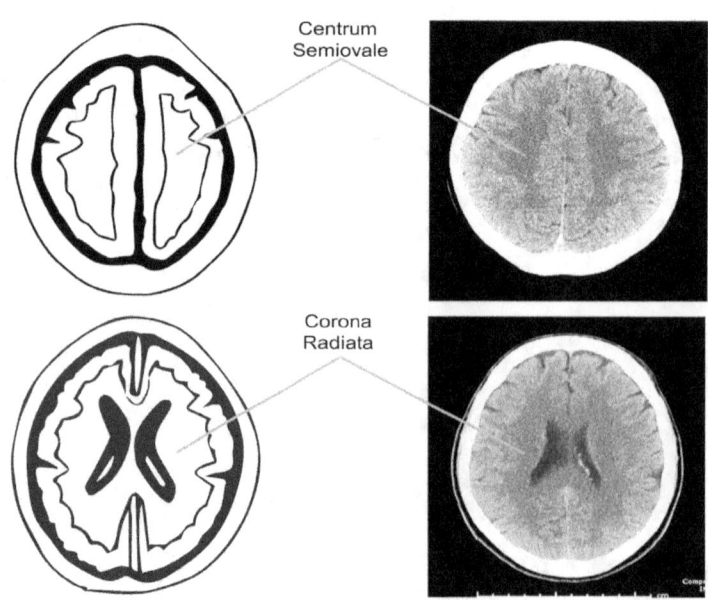

The distinction between gray and white matter is important for several reasons. Vasogenic (interstitial) edema, for instance, more commonly affects the white matter (think VW, vasogenic=white). Cytotoxic (intracellular) edema, on the other hand, involves the cortex or gray matter (cytotoxic=cortex). Exclusive white matter involvement is typically encountered in neoplasms and infection. The combination of cytotoxic edema (gray matter) and vasogenic edema (white matter) is commonly seen in acute ischemic stroke (AIS). This rule is particularly helpful when interpreting brain CTs. An easy way to remember these relationships is with the use of the mnemonic 'VAN CAVES' (Table 3).

White matter (consisting of axons) can connect the cerebral hemispheres to the spinal cord and vice versa. A bundle of axons is called a "tract" which connects one part of the central nervous system to another. Many of these tracts are concentrated into a relatively small structure called the internal capsule. The internal capsule consists of an anterior limb, posterior limb, and genu (Figure 16). Located lateral to the internal capsule is the lentiform nucleus consisting of the globus pallidus and putamen (Figure 16). The basal ganglia consist of the lentiform nucleus plus the caudate (Figure 16).

TABLE 3. Vasogenic and Cytotoxic Edema: **VAN CAVES**

V	Vasogenic
A	Abscess
N	Neoplasm
C	Cytotoxic
A	And
V	Vasogenic
E	Edema
S	Stroke

The corticospinal tract is comprised of a collection of neurons whose cell bodies (gray matter) are in the motor cortex of the frontal lobe, as well as axons (white matter) that exit the cortex and enter the spinal cord to control the majority of voluntary movement (Figure 17). Similarly, a corticobulbar tract is a collection of neurons from the cortex to the brainstem (or bulb) (Figure 17). In this manner, neurons whose cell bodies are found in the cortex (gray matter) transmit information to the rest of the body through their axons (white matter).

FIGURE 16. The Basal Ganglia and Internal Capsule

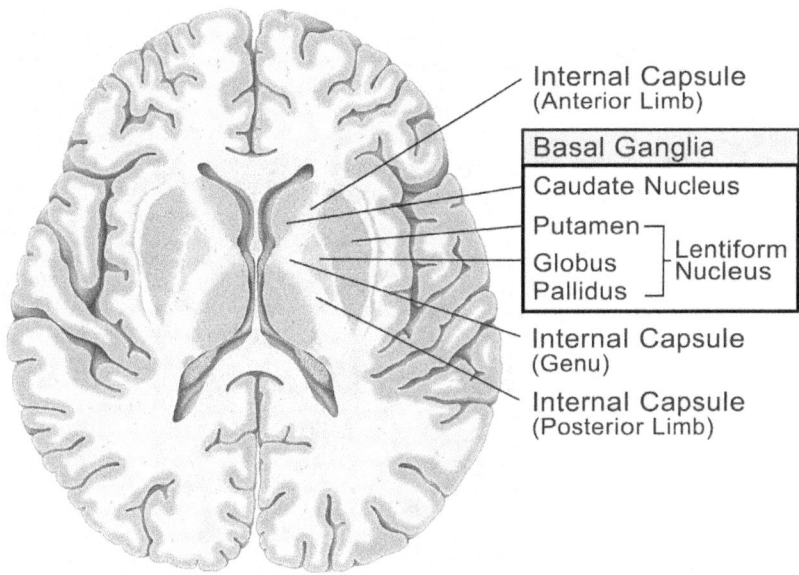

FIGURE 17. Corticospinal and Corticobulbar Tracts

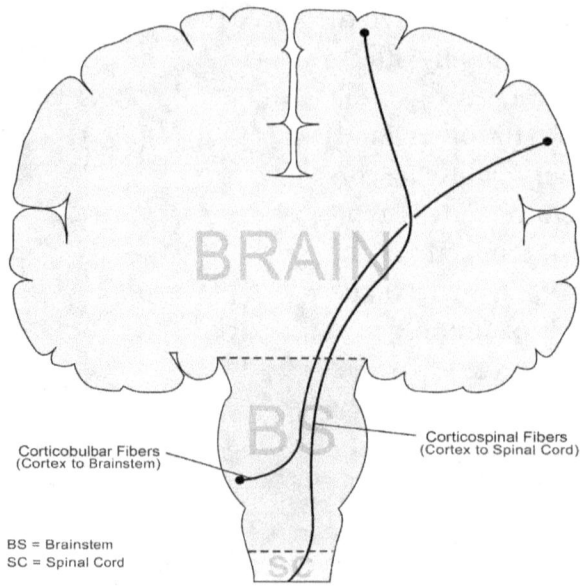

Located between the cerebral hemispheres and the brainstem are the thalami, which relay sensory information from the body to the cortex (Figure 18). The brainstem extends from the base of the brain to the top of the spinal cord and consists of the midbrain, the pons, and the medulla oblongata (Figure 19). The roof of the mesencephalon or midbrain is called the tectum, which consists of four rounded projections called the *corpora quadrigemina* (Figure 19). The upper two structures are referred to as the *superior colliculi* while the lower two are called the *inferior colliculi* (Figure 19).

FIGURE 18. The Thalamus

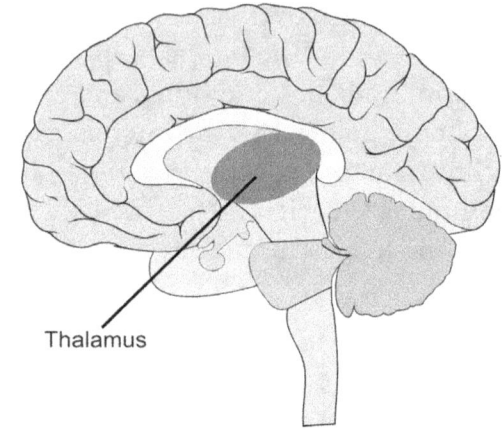

FIGURE 19. The Brainstem

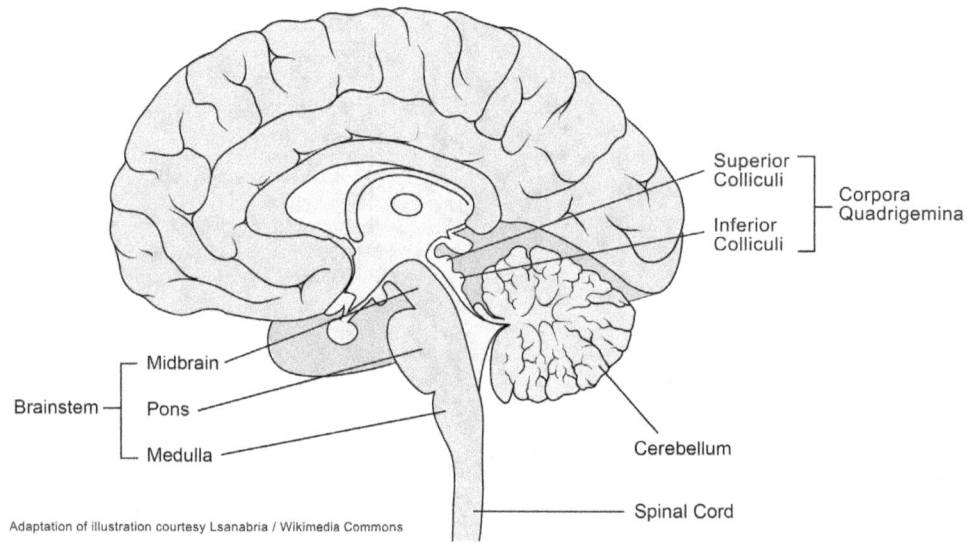

The body of the midbrain or *tegmentum* contains multiple fiber tracts and nuclei including the red nucleus, the oculomotor nucleus, and the trochlear nucleus (Figure 20). The base of the midbrain contains a pair of very large fiber bundles called the *crus cerebri* (basis pedunculi), which are a continuation of the descending fibers from the internal capsule (Figure 20). Located between the body of the midbrain (tegmentum) and the crus cerebri is the *substantia nigra* (Figure 20). Together, the substantia nigra and crus cerebri make up the cerebral peduncle (Figure 20). Damage or mass effect upon the midbrain can lead to unconsciousness, coma and even death.

The pons is located below the midbrain and above the medulla oblongata (Figures 19 and 21). Like the midbrain, the pons contains many ascending and descending fiber tracts. It also includes the trigeminal nuclei (nuclei of CN V), the abducens nuclei (nuclei of CN VI), and the facial nuclei (nuclei of CN VII). The pons also contains the paramedian pontine reticular formation (PPRF) or para-abducens nucleus, which is involved in the coordination of eye movements, particularly horizontal gaze and fast, small movements of both eyes such as scanning a line of print.

FIGURE 20. The Midbrain

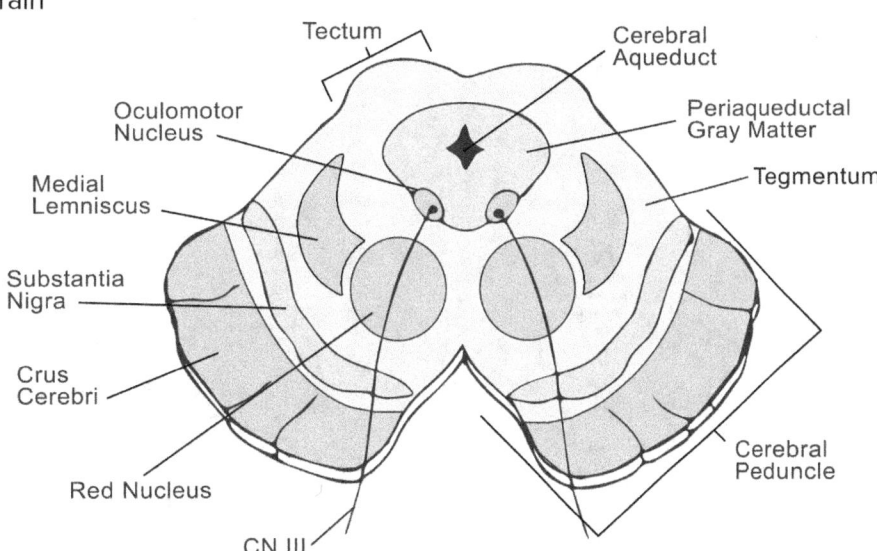

FIGURE 21. The Pons and Cerebellum

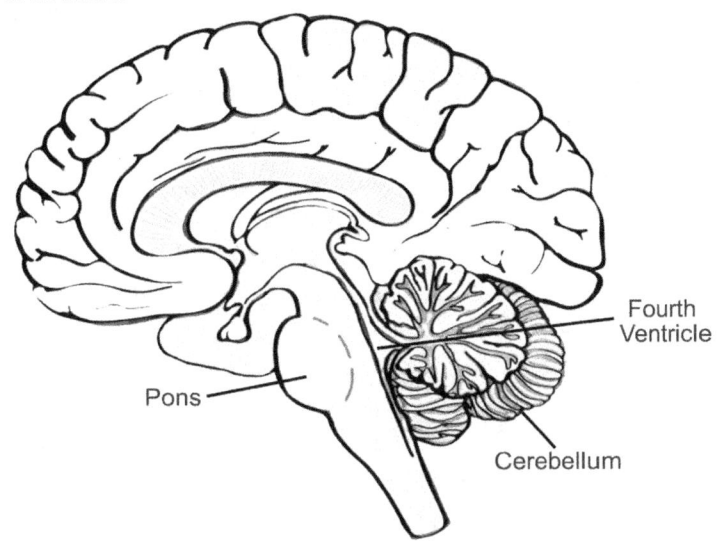

The medulla oblongata is located at the base of the brainstem (Figures 19 and 22). It is the most inferior portion of the brain located superior to the spinal cord and is separated by the spinal cord at the level of the foramen magnum. Like the midbrain and pons, the medulla oblongata also contains fiber tracts and CN nuclei (CN VIII through XII). In addition, the respiratory and cardiac centers are also located within the medulla oblongata. For this reason, any injury affecting the medulla oblongata can result in coma and even death.

The cerebellum is found below the occipital lobes and is separated from the pons anteriorly by the fourth ventricle (Figure 21). The cerebellum is responsible for equilibrium, muscle tone, and coordination. The cerebellum consists of an archicerebellum which is the oldest part of the cerebellum and is responsible for equilibrium (Figure 23). The paleocerebellum consists of the anterior lobe and part of the vermis and is responsible for motor tone (Figures 23 and 24). The neocerebellum is the newest and largest region of the cerebellum and consists of the posterior lobe and most of the vermis (Figure 23). Its prime responsibility is voluntary movement coordination. The cerebellum also contains four important nuclei: (1) **D**entate, (2) **E**mboliform, (3) **F**astigial, and (4) **G**lobose (Figure 24). These cerebellar nuclei can be recalled by remembering a portion of the alphabet - "**D, E, F and G**" (Table 4). The cerebellum also has three white matter tracts which are connected to the brainstem: the superior, middle, and inferior cerebellar peduncles (Figure 25). These are also called the *brachium conjunctivum,* the *brachium pontis,* and the *restiform body*, respectively.

FIGURE 22. The Medulla Oblongata

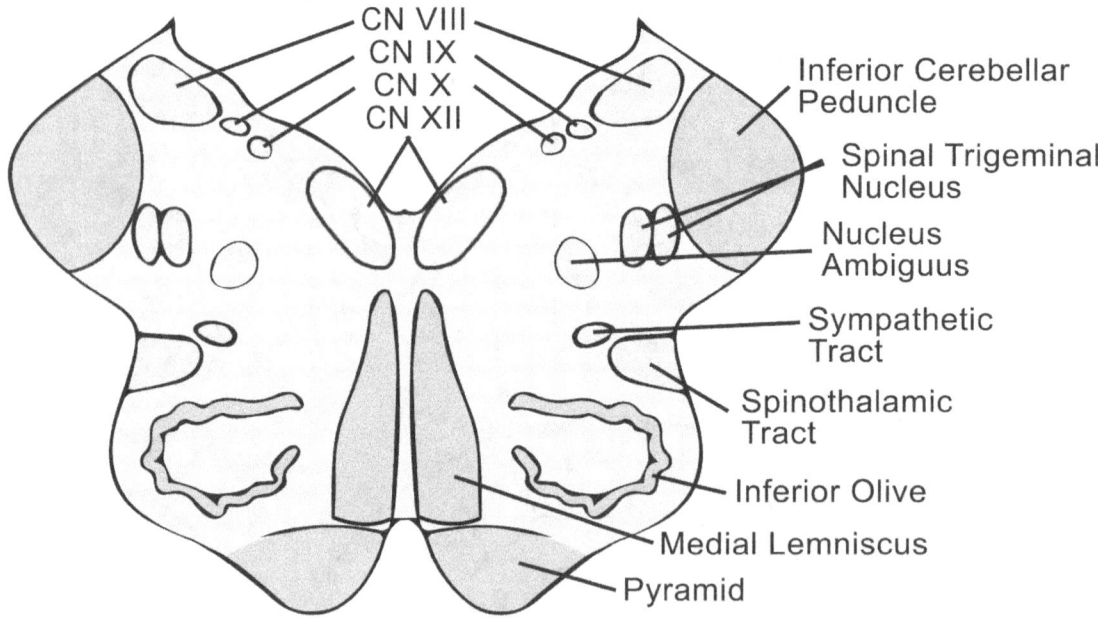

FIGURE 23. The Cerebellar Lobes

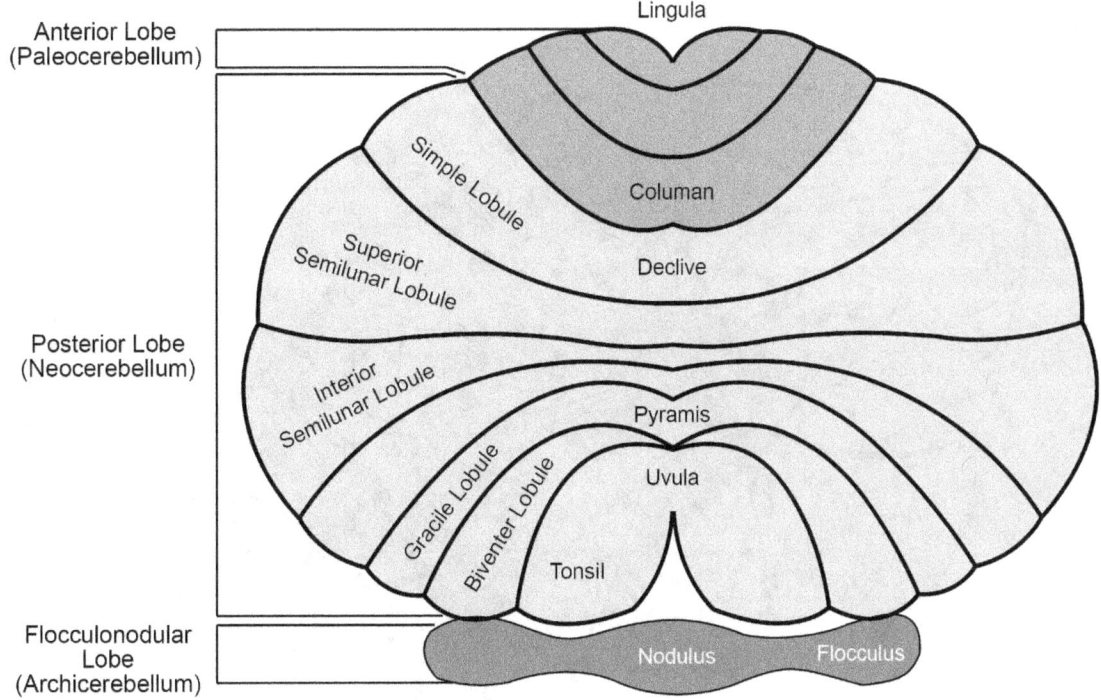

FIGURE 24. The Cerebellar Nuclei

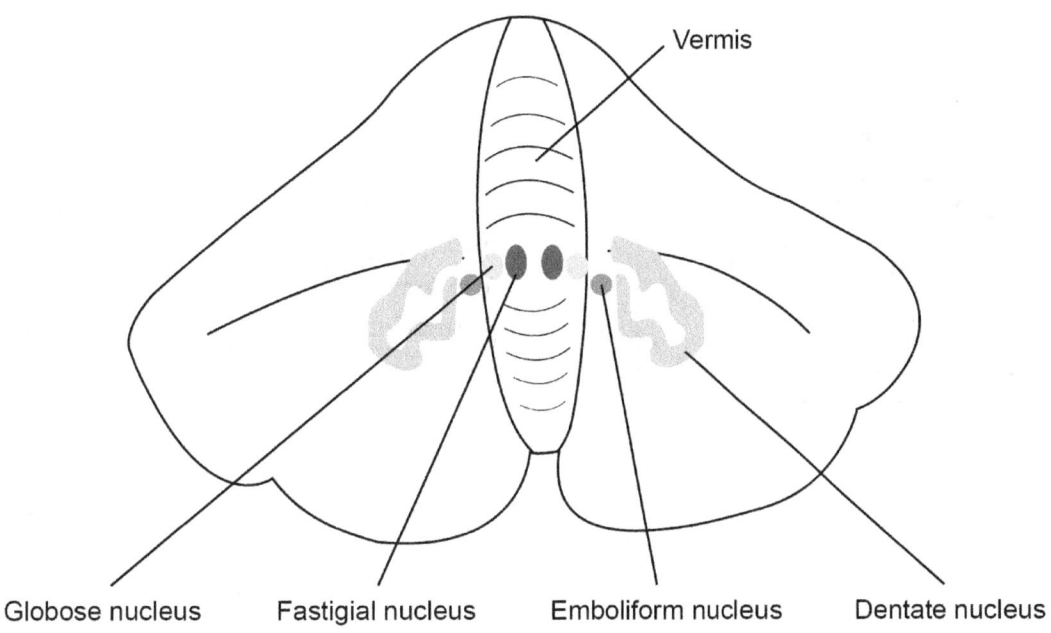

FIGURE 25. The Cerebellar Peduncles

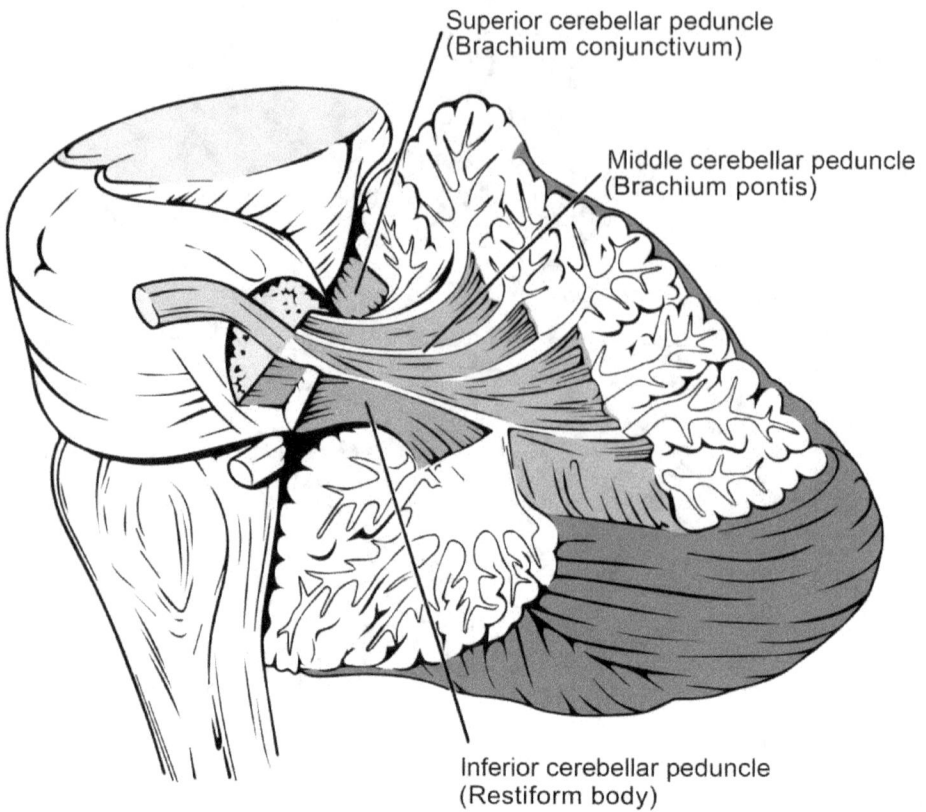

Illustration from Anatomy & Physiology, Connexions Web site, courtesy OpenStax College via Wikimedia Commons

TABLE 4. The Cerebellar Nuclei: **DEFG**

D	Dentate Nucleus
E	Emboliform Nucleus
F	Fastigial Nucleus
G	Globose Nucleus

Abbreviations list

AIS, acute ischemic stroke; CSF, cerebrospinal fluid; CT, computed tomography; FEF, frontal eye fields; PPRF, paramedian pontine reticular formation.

Chapter 4

Cerebrovascular Anatomy

4.1. Introduction

Requisite knowledge of cerebrovascular anatomy is essential for the proper diagnosis and treatment of stroke. Whether interpreting angiography, CT angiography (CTA), or magnetic resonance angiography (MRA), a proper understanding of cerebrovascular anatomy is required for stroke management. While some may consider this to be a Herculean task, the scope of cerebrovascular anatomy needed to manage stroke is relatively defined and straightforward. The purpose of this chapter is to provide a broad but fundamental understanding of cerebrovascular anatomy.

Vascular supply to the brain depends on a pair of vertebral arteries (VAs) and a pair of internal carotid arteries (ICAs). The VAs converge to form the basilar artery (BA). These vessels and the branches that arise from them comprise the *vertebrobasilar system*. This is also referred to as the *posterior circulation* since it supplies the posterior portion of the brain (Figure 1). The ICAs and the branches that arise from them are referred to as the *anterior circulation* because they supply the anterior region of the brain. Before discussing either distribution, we must review their origins, namely the three great vessels of the aortic arch (Figure 2).

FIGURE 1. Anterior and Posterior Intracranial Circulation

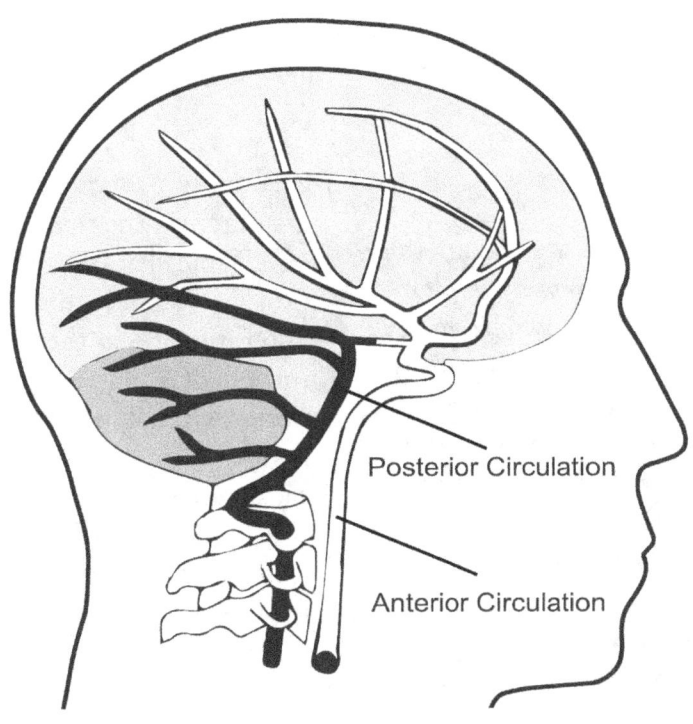

FIGURE 2. The Aortic Arch and the Great Vessels

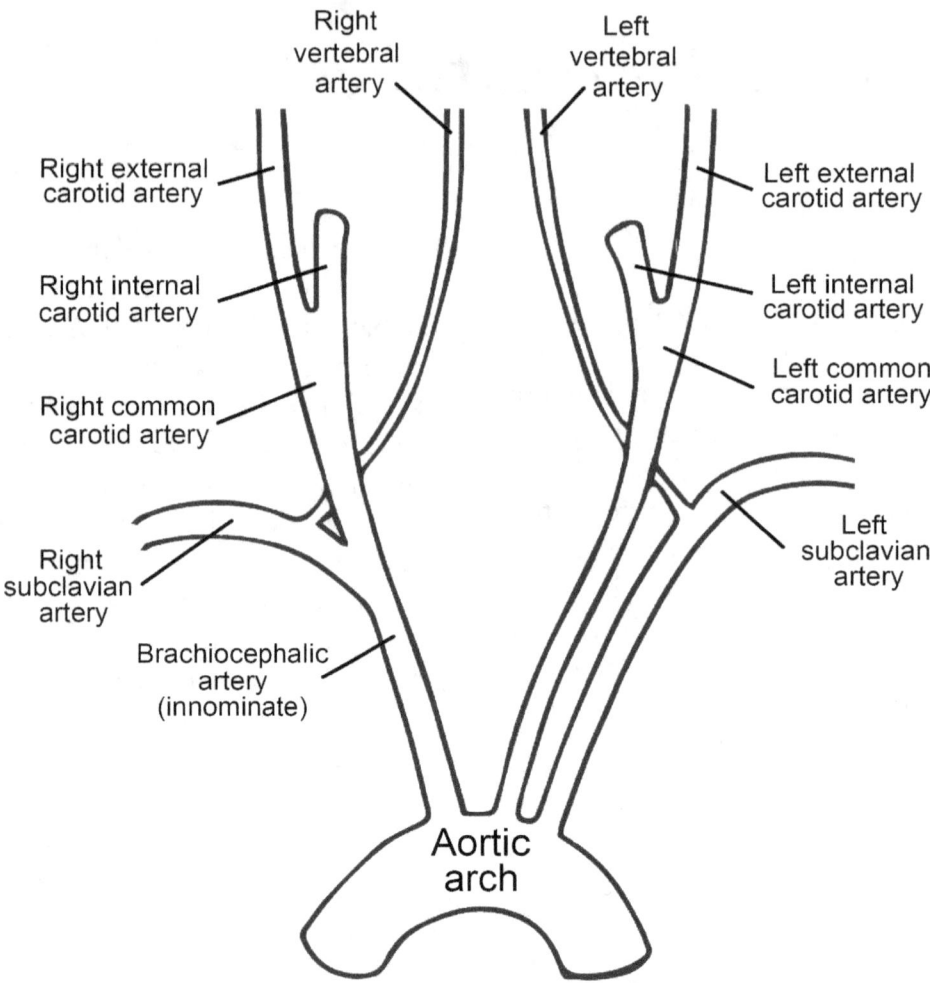

4.2 The Great Vessels

There are three great vessels that arise from the aortic arch. These are the (1) *innominate (brachiocephalic) artery*, (2) *left common carotid artery (CCA)*, and (3) *left subclavian artery* (Figure 2). While variations of this configuration exist, this anatomy is most frequently encountered. The innominate artery bifurcates into the right common carotid artery (CCA) and the right subclavian artery. The right CCA bifurcates at the C3 or C4 vertebral level into the right external carotid artery (ECA) anteromedially, and into the right internal carotid artery (ICA) posterolaterally (Figure 3).

The most proximal, superiorly ascending vessel arising from the right subclavian artery is the right VA. Typically, 70% of patients have a smaller or non-dominant right VA (Figure 2). The left CCA also bifurcates at the C3 or C4 vertebral level into the left ECA anteromedially and into the left ICA posterolaterally (Figure 3). Both ICAs ascend superiorly and form the anterior circulation. The most proximal, superiorly ascending vessel arising from the left subclavian artery is the left VA. Typically, 70% of patients have a larger or dominant left VA (Figure 2). Both VAs ascend superiorly to form the posterior circulation.

FIGURE 3. The Common Carotid Artery Bifurcation

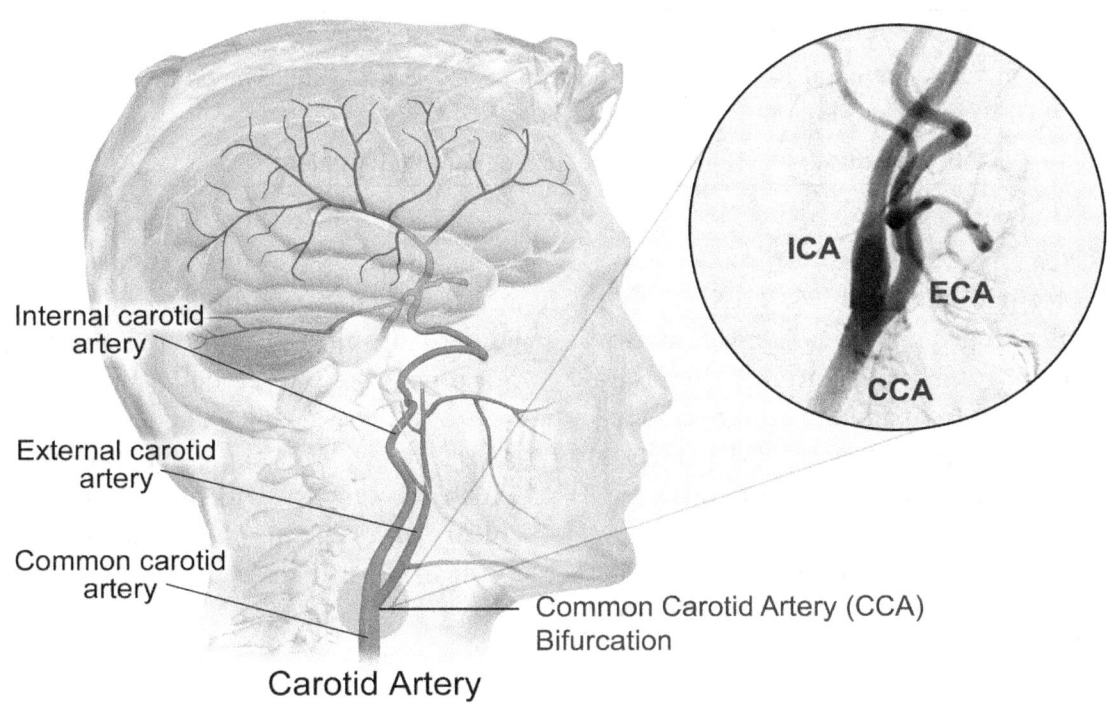

4.3 The Posterior Circulation

Each VA is divided into four segments (Figure 4).[1] The first segment, V1 (preforaminal), extends from the VA origin to the transverse foramen of the C6 vertebral body. The V2 (foraminal) segment is contained within the cervical foramina and extends from the transverse foramen of the C6 vertebral body to the transverse foramen of the C1 vertebral body. The V3 (atlantic or extradural) segment extends from the transverse foramen of the C1 vertebral body to the dura. The V4 (intradural) segment extends from the dura to the confluence of the VAs as they form the BA at the pontomedullary junction (Figures 4, 5 and Table 1).

FIGURE 4. Vertebral Artery Segmental Anatomy

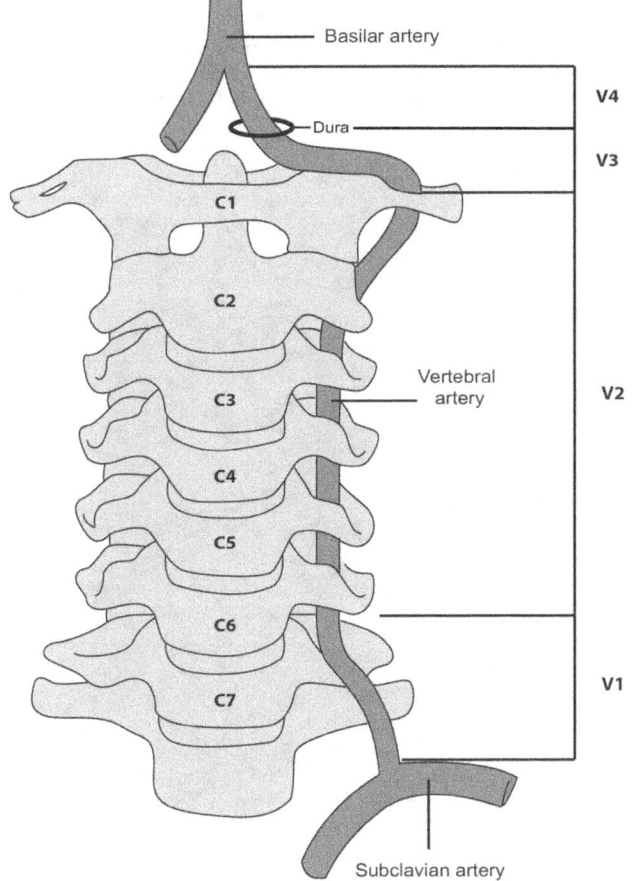

TABLE 1. Vertebral Artery Segmental Anatomy

V1	Preforaminal	Origin to Transverse Foramen C6
V2	Foraminal	Transverse Foramen C6 to Transverse Foramen C1
V3	Extradural	C1 to Dura
V4	Intradural	Dura to Confluence of Vertebral Arteries

Prior to the formation of the BA, each VA (V4 segment) typically gives off a posterior inferior cerebellar artery (PICA) and anterior spinal artery (Figure 5). PICA, as its name implies, supplies the posterior inferior portion of the cerebellum (Figure 6). After the BA is formed, it gives off paired anterior inferior cerebellar arteries (AICA). This vessel has a unique, curlycue pattern because it wraps itself around the seventh and eighth nerve complex (Figure 5). AICA, as its name implies, supplies the anterior and inferior portion of the cerebellum (Figure 6). Arising from AICA (85-100%) or directly off the basilar artery (15%) is the labyrinthine artery (LA), which travels with and supplies the vestibulocochlear nerve (Figure 5). Occlusion of the LA can result in hearing loss.

FIGURE 5. Posterior Circulation

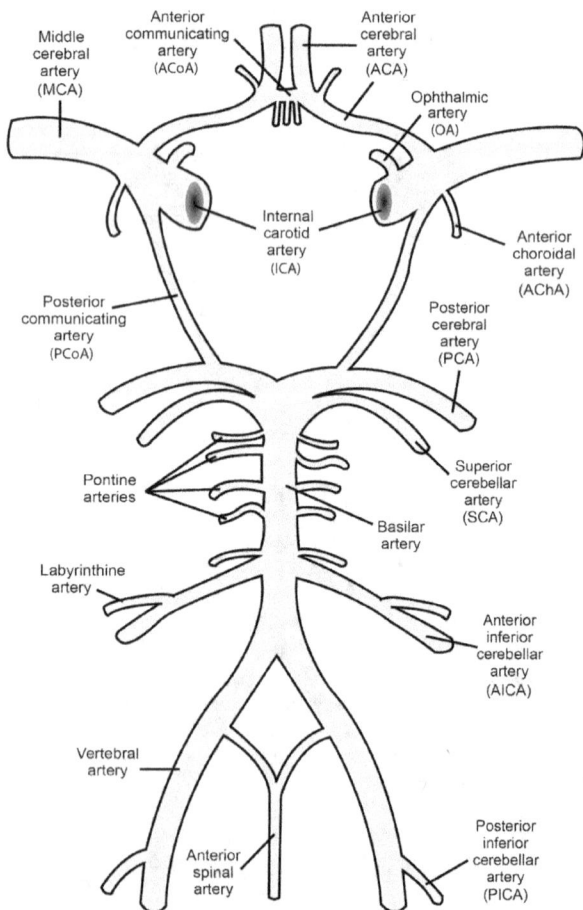
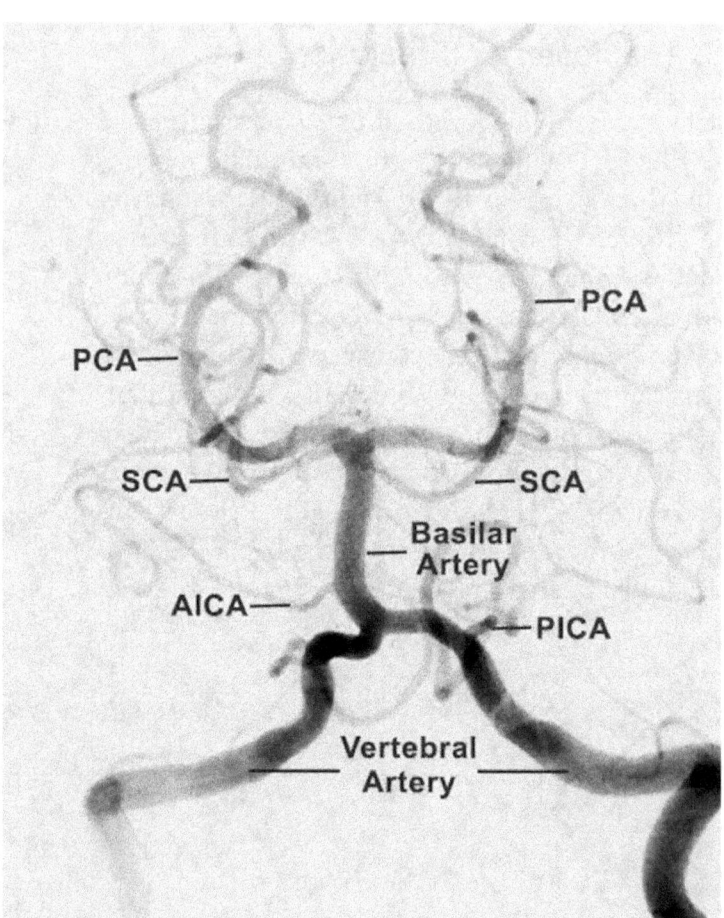

FIGURE 6. Vascular Supply to the Cerebellum

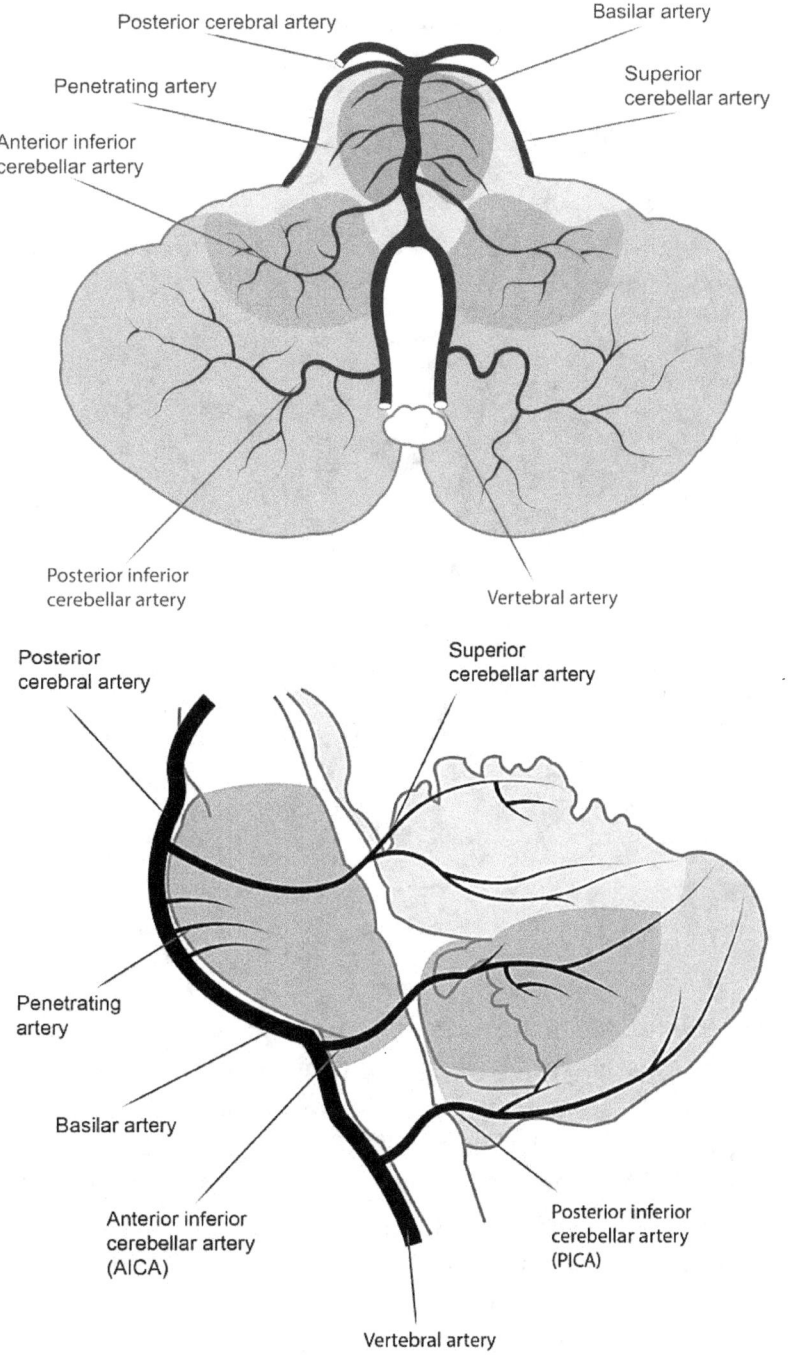

Multiple pontine perforators also arise from the basilar artery (Figure 5). These are typically the size of human hair and thus are too small to be seen on MRA, CTA, or cerebral angiography. The next major vessels which arise from the basilar artery are the paired superior cerebellar arteries (SCA) (Figure 5). The SCA, as its name implies, supplies the superior portion of the cerebellum and the lateral aspects of the pons and midbrain (Figure 6). Finally, the BA terminates into two posterior cerebral arteries (PCA) at the pontomesencephalic junction located at the top of the pons (Figure 5). Cranial nerve III courses between the origin of the PCAs and the SCAs. (Figure 7).

FIGURE 7. Cranial Nerve III Travels Between the Posterior Cerebral Artery and the Superior Cerebellar Artery

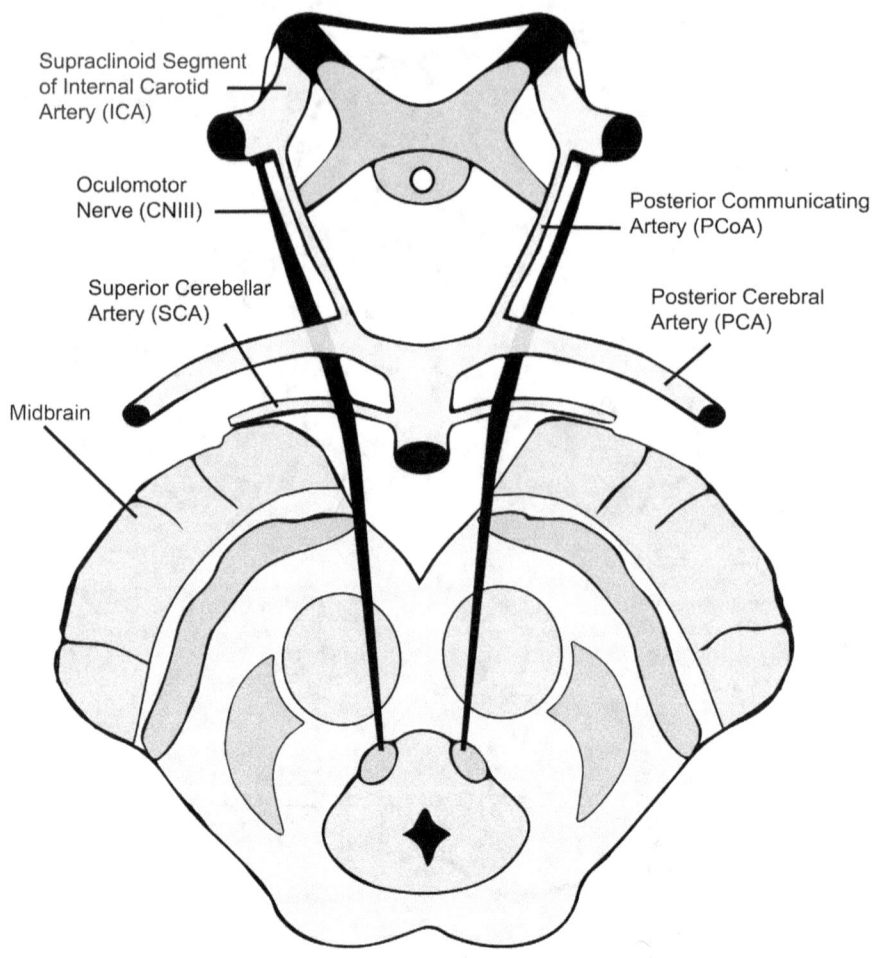

The PCA has four vascular segments. The first segment of the PCA is called the P1 segment. Arising from the distal portion of the P1 segment is the posterior communicating artery (PCoA) (Figure 8). The PCoA connects the PCA, which is part of the posterior circulation, to the supraclinoid segment of the ICA, which is part of the anterior circulation (Figure 8). The PCoA is a "communication" or collateral between the anterior and posterior circulation. This communication or connection is a component of the Circle of Willis (COW), a vascular entity which has three important characteristics (Figure 9). First, less than 20% of the population has a complete COW. Second, because the COW consists of multiple branch points and intracranial aneurysms occur at branch points, it is **a frequent site for intracranial aneurysms** (Figure 10). Third, **the COW serves as an important anastomotic or collateral connection between the anterior and posterior circulation** (Figure 9).

FIGURE 8. The Posterior Communicating Artery (PCoA)

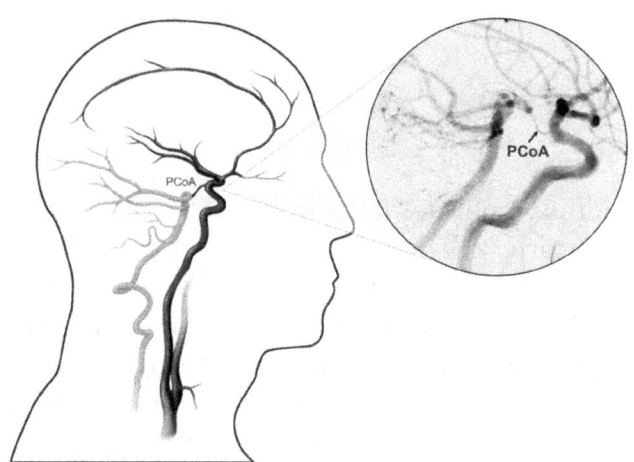

CHAPTER 4: Cerebrovascular Anatomy

FIGURE 9. The Circle of Willis

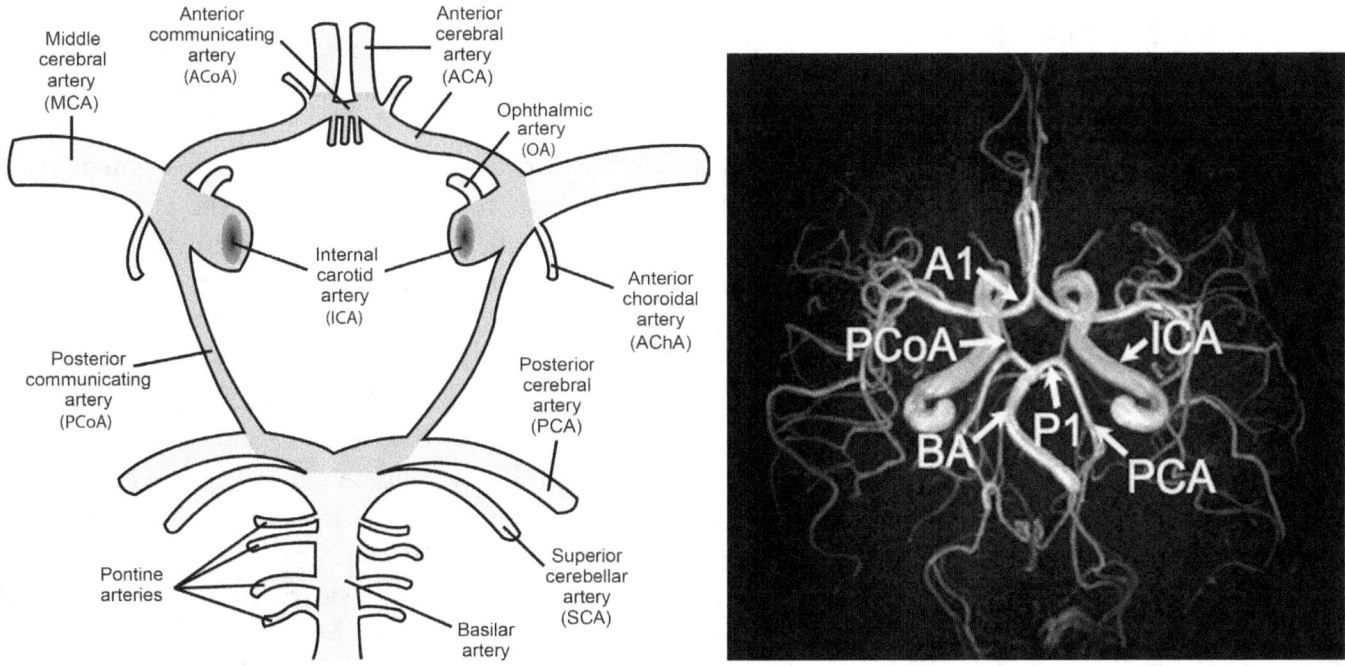

FIGURE 10. The Circle of Willis and Intracranial Aneurysms

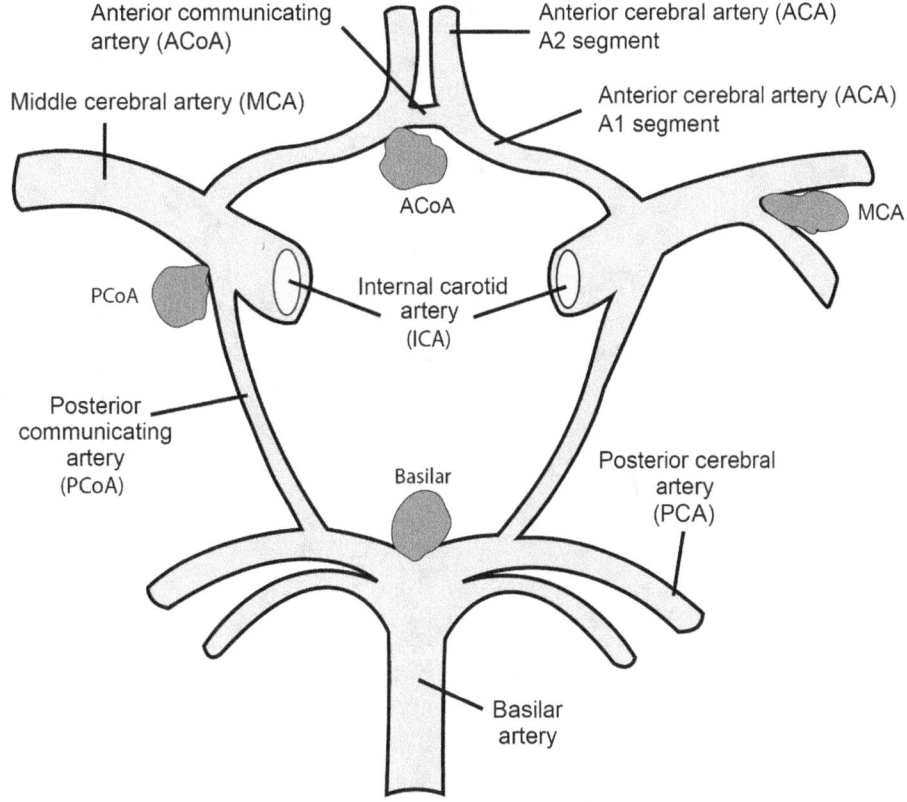

4.4 The Anterior Circulation

4.4.1 Internal Carotid Artery (ICA)

The common carotid artery (CCA) typically bifurcates at the C3 or C4 vertebral level into an ECA anteromedially and an ICA posterolaterally (Figure 3). The ICA has four segments: the *cervical, petrous, cavernous,* and *supraclinoid* segments (Figure 11). The cervical segment begins at the common carotid artery bifurcation and travels through the neck to the skull base. The next segment of the internal carotid artery, the petrous segment, is demarcated proximally and distally by the skull base.

The next two segments (cavernous and supraclinoid) comprise the carotid siphon or genu. Almost every single carotid artery has a carotid siphon or genu, which is best depicted laterally (Figure 11). Arising from the anterior portion of this genu is the ophthalmic artery (OA) (Figure 11). The OA divides the supraclinoid segment superiorly from the cavernous segment inferiorly (Figure 11). Thus, the cavernous segment extends from below the takeoff of the ophthalmic artery to the skull base or petrous segment. It is important to understand that the OA not only separates the supraclinoid segment from the cavernous segment; it also demarcates the intradural contents above the OA from the extradural contents below it (Figure 11). Anything at the level of or above the OA (the supraclinoid segment) is usually contained within the dura and is thus intradural. Everything below the ophthalmic artery (cavernous segment) is located outside of the dura and is thus extradural (Figure 11). To summarize, **the OA separates the supraclinoid segment and intradural contents above from the cavernous segment and extradural contents below.**

FIGURE 11. The 4 Segments of the Internal Carotid Artery

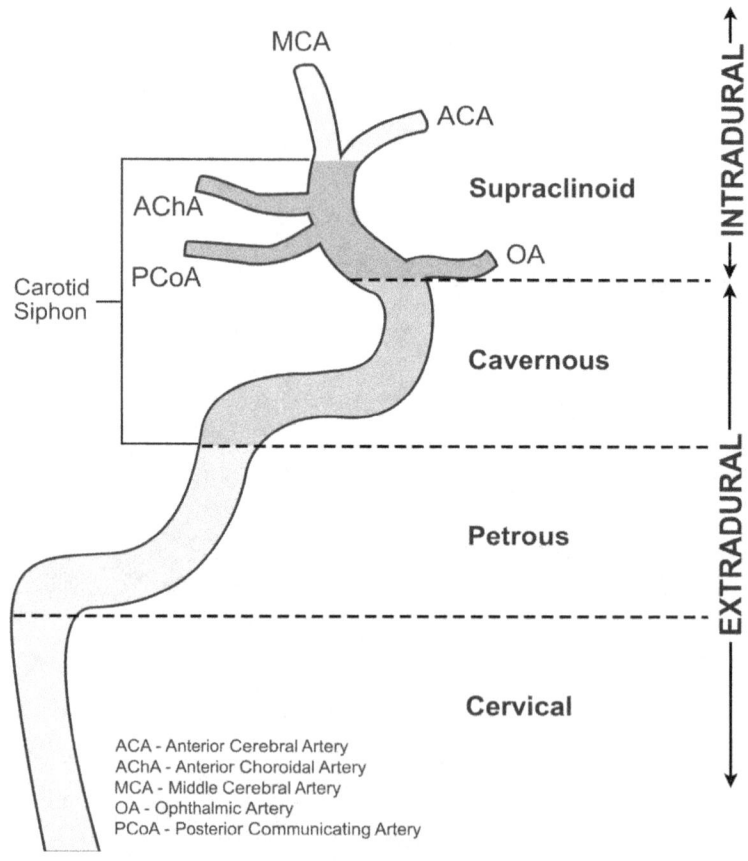

ACA - Anterior Cerebral Artery
AChA - Anterior Choroidal Artery
MCA - Middle Cerebral Artery
OA - Ophthalmic Artery
PCoA - Posterior Communicating Artery

The supraclinoid segment has three major vessels: (1) the *OA*, (2) the *posterior communicating artery* (PCoA), and (3) the *anterior choroidal artery* (AChA) (Figure 11). The supraclinoid segment is the last and most distal segment of the ICA. It terminates into the anterior cerebral artery (ACA) medially and the middle cerebral artery (MCA) laterally. The termination of the supraclinoid segment of the ICA is termed the **ICA bifurcation** or the **carotid terminus** (Figure 12).

FIGURE 12. The Carotid Terminus

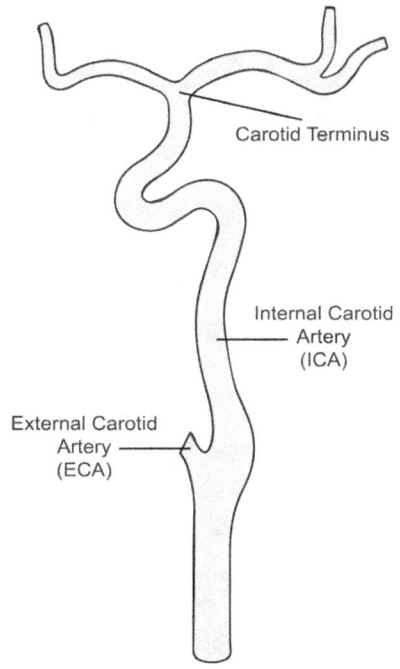

4.4.2 The Anterior Cerebral Artery (ACA)

The ACA arises medially from the bifurcation of the carotid terminus. Its first segment is called the A1 segment (Figure 13). Arising from the A1 segment are multiple medial lenticulostriate arteries which supply the medial portion of the basal ganglia (Figure 13). These medial lenticulostriate arteries are tiny and are termed "end vessels," meaning they have no collateral supply. The distal A1 segment is demarcated by the anterior communicating artery (ACoA) which connects both anterior cerebral arteries (ACAs). The A2 segment is distal to the ACoA. The A2 segment separates into a pericallosal artery and a callosomarginal artery (Figure 14). ACA cortical branches arise from the A2 segment, the pericallosal and callosomarginal arteries (Figure 14). The ACA territory is the most variable intracranial anterior circulation distribution. One common variant is an azygos variant where both A2 segments arise from a single trunk rather than individually (Figure 15). Vascular compromise to this single trunk can result in bilateral hemispheric deficits.

FIGURE 13. The Anterior Cerebral Artery (ACA)

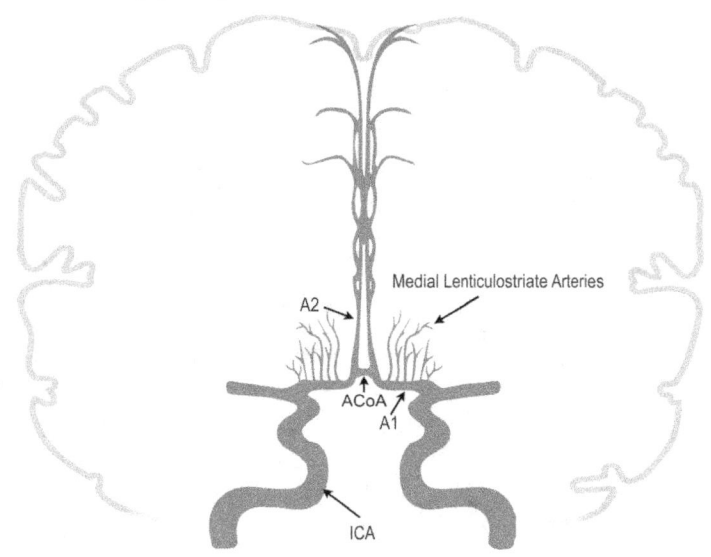

FIGURE 14. The Anterior Cerebral Artery

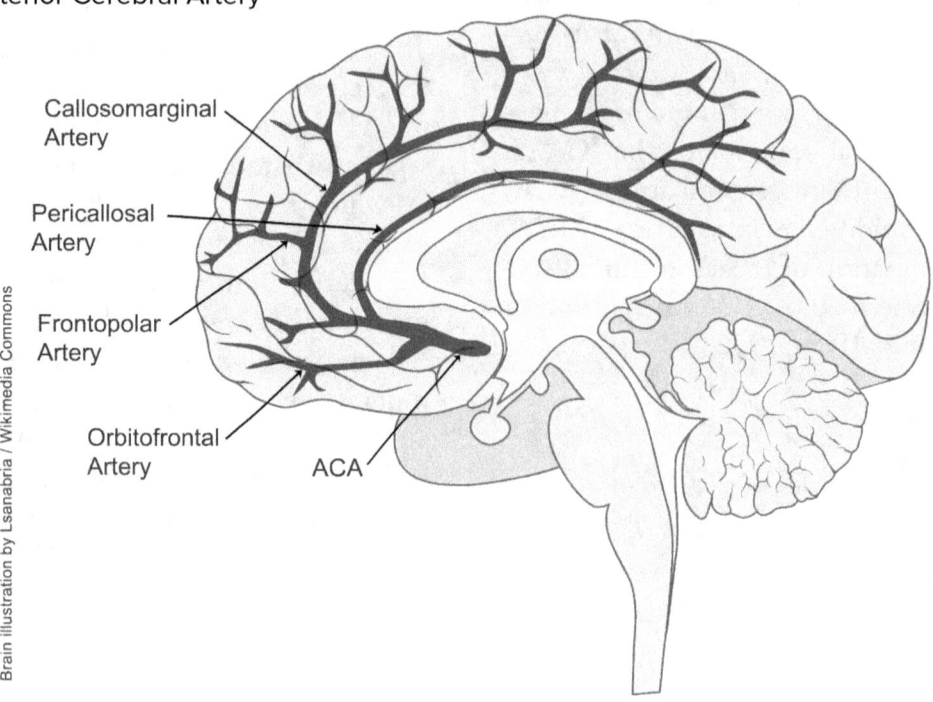

FIGURE 15. Anterior Cerebral Artery (ACA) Azygos Variant

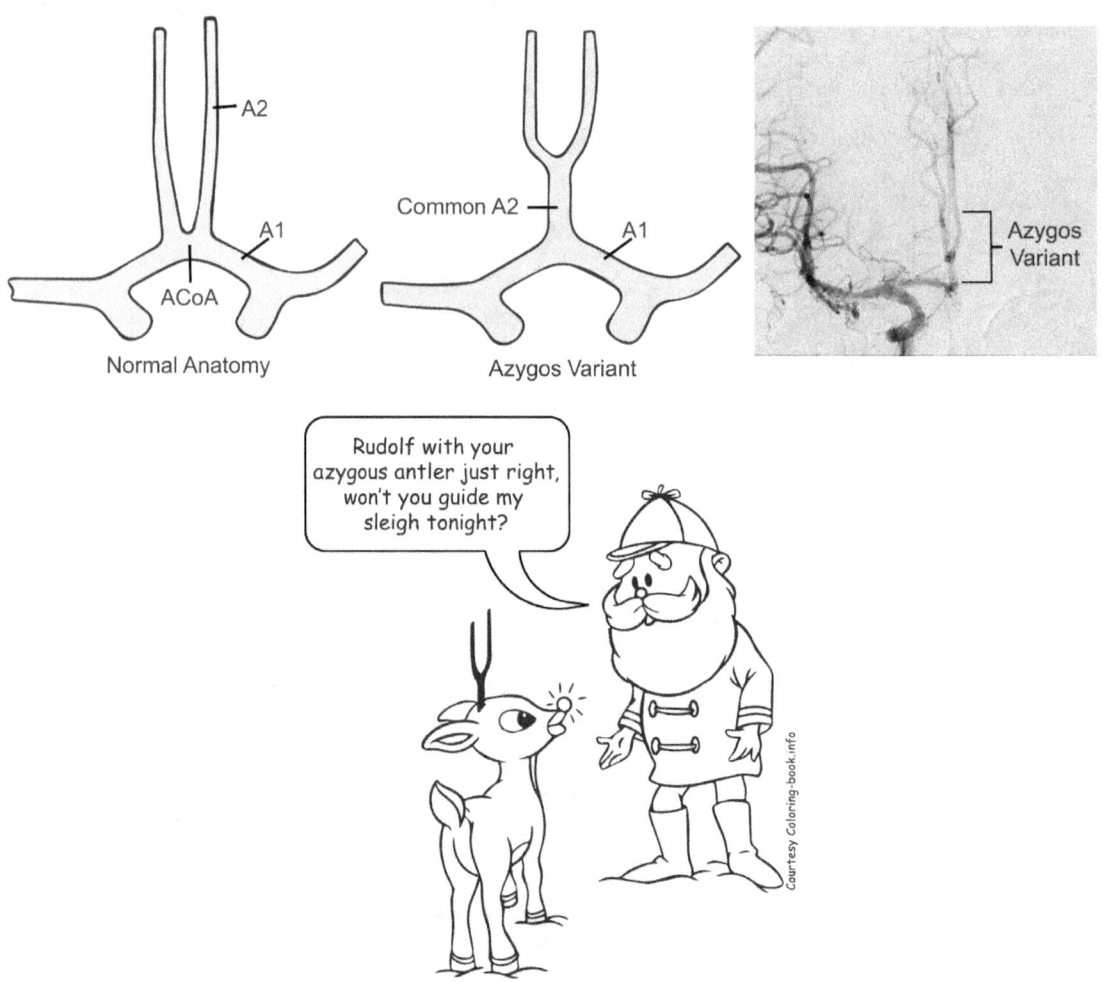

4.4.3 The Middle Cerebral Artery (MCA)

The middle cerebral artery (MCA) arises laterally from the bifurcation of the carotid terminus. The first segment of the middle cerebral artery is the M1 segment (Figures 16 and 17). Arising off the M1 segment are multiple lateral lenticulostriate arteries which supply the lateral portions of the lentiform nucleus (Figures 16 and 17). These lateral lenticulostriate arteries are tiny vessels similar to the medial lenticulostriate arteries. These are also termed "end vessels," which means they have no collateral supply. The M1 segment typically bifurcates into a superior and inferior division which marks the next segment of the middle cerebral artery called the M2 segment (Figures 16 and 17). The M2 or insular segment begins just distal to the last lateral lenticulostriate artery or at the location of a cortical gyrus named the *limen insulae*. These M2 or insular segments lie lateral to the insular cortex as they ascend superiorly. At the top of the Sylvian fissure, they now transition into M3 or opercular branches and then descend along the frontal operculum. As they traverse the cerebral hemisphere, they then transition into M4 or cortical branches (Figures 16 and 17). It is important to distinguish these branches and the major branches of the anterior cerebral artery (Figure 17). The cortical branches of the MCA are related to the regions of the cerebral cortex that they supply (Figure 18).

4.5 Conclusion

This concludes our discussion of cerebrovascular anatomy. In subsequent chapters, more anatomic details will be provided when necessary. Understanding cerebrovascular anatomy is necessary to diagnose and treat stroke. Review the relevant portions of this chapter until this anatomy is fully understood.

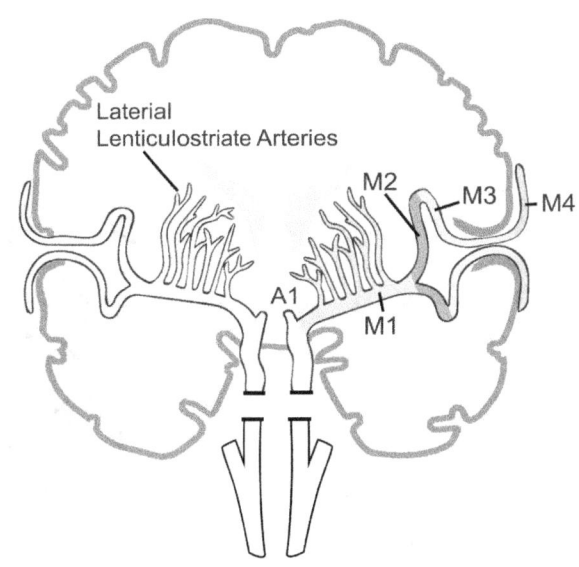

FIGURE 16. The Four Segments of the Middle Cerebral Artery

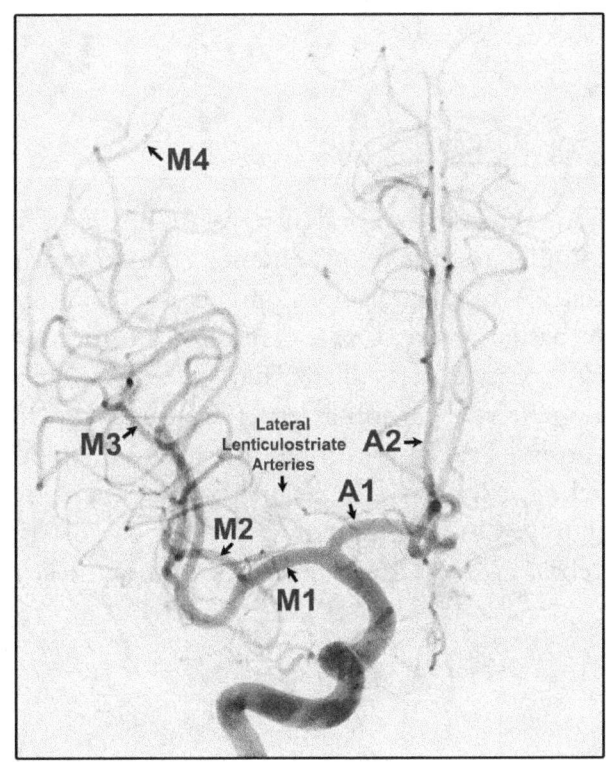

FIGURE 17. Cerebral Angiogram of the Anterior Circulation

FIGURE 18. Middle Cerebral Artery (MCA) Cortical Branches (Lateral View)

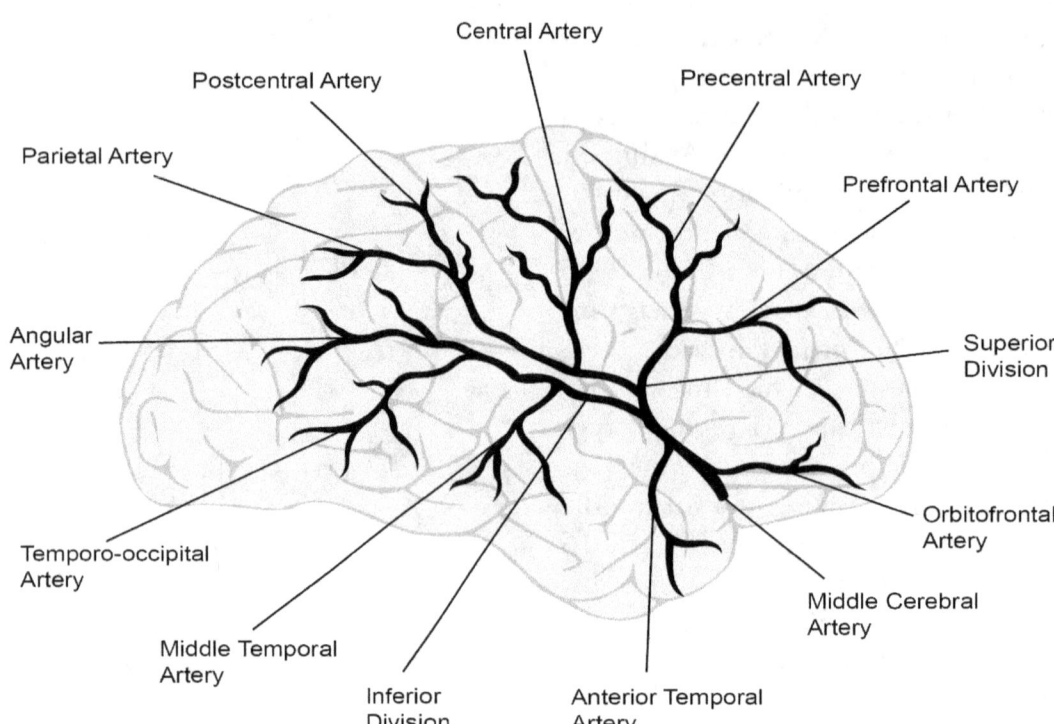

Abbreviations list

ACA, anterior cerebral artery; AChA, anterior choroidal artery; ACoA, anterior communicating artery; AICA, anterior inferior cerebellar artery; BA, basilar artery; CCA, common carotid artery; COW, Circle of Willis; CTA, CT angiography; ECA, external carotid artery; ICA, internal carotid artery; LA, labyrinthine artery; MCA, middle cerebral artery; MRA, magnetic resonance angiography; OA, ophthalmic artery; PCA, posterior cerebral artery; PCoA, posterior communicating artery; PICA, posterior inferior cerebellar artery; SCA, superior cerebellar artery; VA, vertebral artery.

References

1. Fisher CM. (1961). The pathology and pathogenesis of intracerebral hemorrhage. In Fields WS (ed): Pathogenesis and Treatment of Cerebrovascular Disease. Springfield, IL: Charles C Thomas.

Chapter 5

Ischemic Stroke

5.1 Introduction

A stroke is a sudden onset of compromised brain function resulting from either blocked blood flow to a region of the brain (ischemic stroke) or brain hemorrhage (hemorrhagic stroke). Stroke is broadly characterized as either ischemic stroke which accounts for 87% of all stroke or hemorrhagic stroke which represents the remaining 13%. Acute ischemic stroke (AIS) occurs when arterial supply to the brain is occluded (Figure 1). AIS initially consists of a central area of irreparably damaged brain tissue (core infarct), surrounded by a region of threatened brain cells (ischemic penumbra) that may recover provided circulation is reestablished. Hemorrhagic stroke, on the other hand, results from ruptured blood vessels and subsequent brain hemorrhage (Figure 1). The purpose of this chapter is to review the various subtypes and causes of AIS.

5.2 Ischemic Penumbra

Prior to reviewing the different causes of AIS, recall that the paramount goal of all AIS therapy is to preserve the ischemic penumbra by restoring blood flow (Figure 2). Generally, this is a dynamic process during which core infarct increases and ischemic penumbra decreases over time (Figure 3). The only process that will prevent this decay is recanalizing the occluded blood vessel(s) responsible for AIS. The presence and duration of an ischemic penumbra (threatened but salvageable brain tissue) is determined by the collateral circulation which varies on an individual basis.

FIGURE 2. Core Infarct Versus Ischemic Penumbra

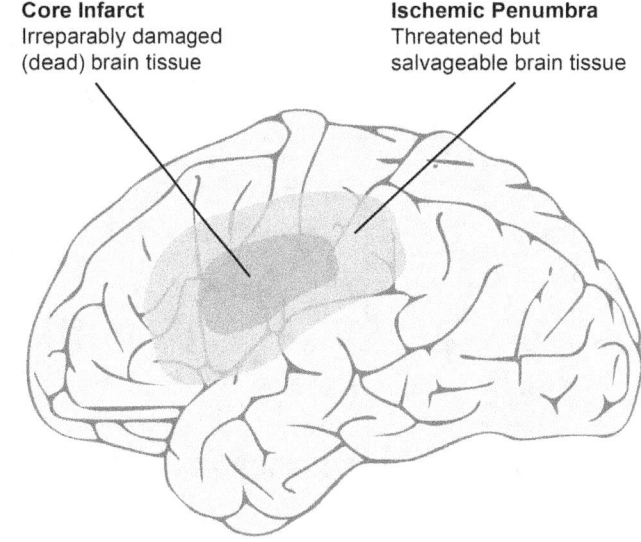

FIGURE 1. Ischemic and Hemorrhagic Stroke

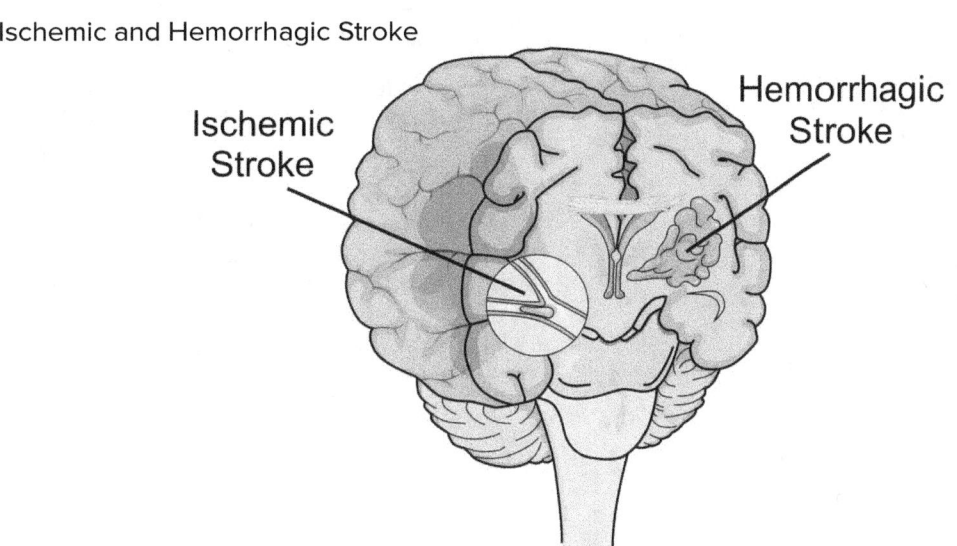

FIGURE 3. Progression of Ischemic Penumbra into Core Infarct

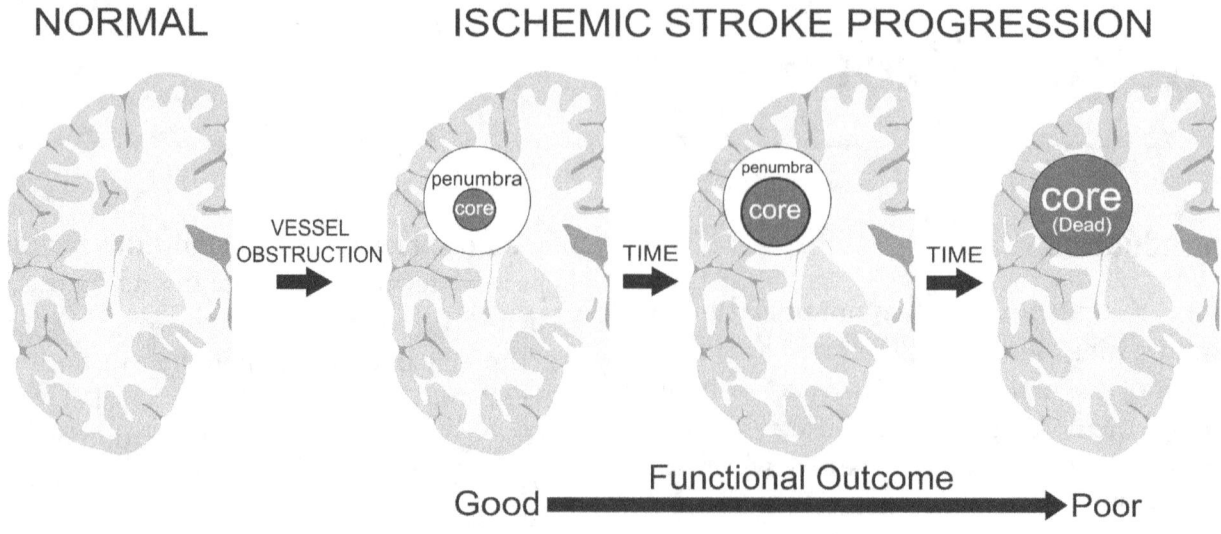

FIGURE 4. Causes of Acute Ischemic Stroke (AIS)

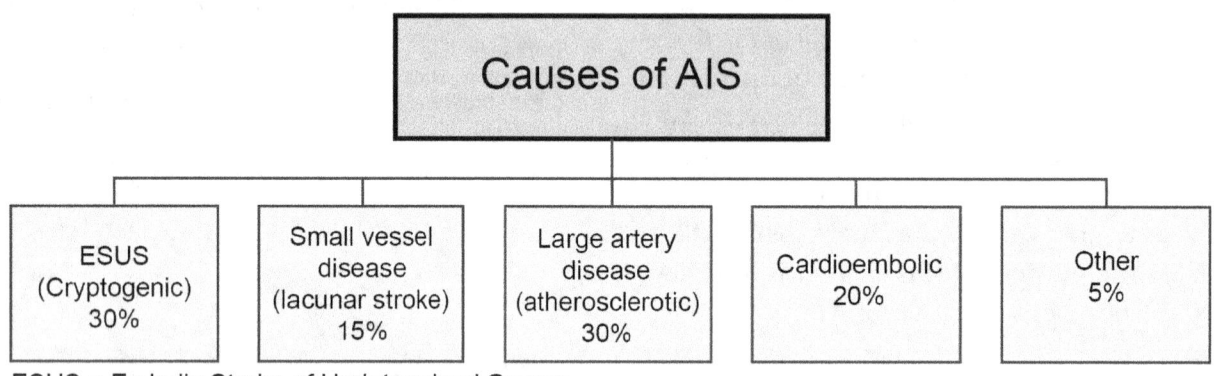

ESUS = Embolic Stroke of Undetermined Source

5.3 Causes of Acute Ischemic Stroke (AIS)

AIS is a heterogeneous disease that is caused by a myriad of underlying pathologic conditions (Figure 4). AIS can be classified according to the underlying cause of the blood vessel occlusion (TOAST criteria).[1] In order of frequency, these classifications include large vessel atherosclerotic disease (30%), embolic strokes of undetermined source (cryptogenic stroke) (30%), cardioembolic stroke (20%), small vessel disease (15%), and other stroke causing conditions (5%) (Table 1, Figure 4 and 5). An easy way to remember the causes of AIS is the mnemonic 'CAUSE' (Table 1).

TABLE 1. Causes of Acute Ischemic Stroke: **CAUSE**

C	Cardioembolic (20%)
A	Atherosclerotic Large Vessel Disease (30%)
U	Undetermined Etiology - ESUS* (30%) (Avoid Cryptogenic Stroke Terminology)
S	Small Vessel Disease or Lacunar Infarct (15%)
E	Everything Else, or Other (5%)

*Embolic Strokes of Undetermined Source

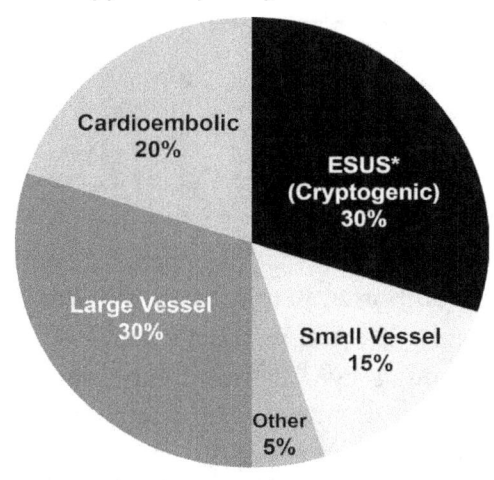

FIGURE 5. Subtype Frequency of AIS

*Embolic Stroke of Undetermined Source

In addition to the underlying pathophysiology responsible for AIS, both the anatomic region of the brain and its arterial territory must be considered. Usually, this evaluation is aided by neuroimaging. For example, the administration of IV TPA cannot be performed without a brain CT. For that matter, as will be discussed in subsequent chapters, endovascular treatment (EVT) generally requires confirmation of a large vessel occlusion (LVO) and viable brain tissue (ischemic penumbra) by neuroimaging.

5.4 Embolic Versus Thrombotic

AIS is generally caused by occluded blood vessels that supply oxygen to the brain. However, this definition can be further distinguished by the origin of the blood clot. That is, does the clot occur within the brain's blood vessels or in some other location? In view of this, AIS can be classified as either **embolic** or **thrombotic**. Embolic stroke is caused by a blood clot that travels to the brain from a more proximal location in the body such as the heart (cardioembolic) or a more proximal artery outside the brain (artery-to-artery disease) (Figure 6).

A blood clot that originates outside of the brain is termed an **embolus**. Embolic disease is the most common cause of AIS. For example, most LVO AIS is embolic, caused by clots that travel to the brain from elsewhere. The three greatest sources that produce emboli to the brain include **cardiogenic emboli** (mitral or aortic valves or the left cardiac chambers), **arteriogenic emboli** (proximal cerebral arteries or the aortic arch), and **paradoxical emboli** (venous emboli). An easy way to remember these sources is with the mnemonic 'CAP' (Table 2). In approximately 20 to 30% of presumed embolic stroke, the source of emboli cannot be established. More likely, this source is from cardiac thrombi (within the heart) which leave no residual clot that can be detected by further imaging (transesophageal echocardiography). The left heart is the presumed source when the origin of emboli cannot be determined.

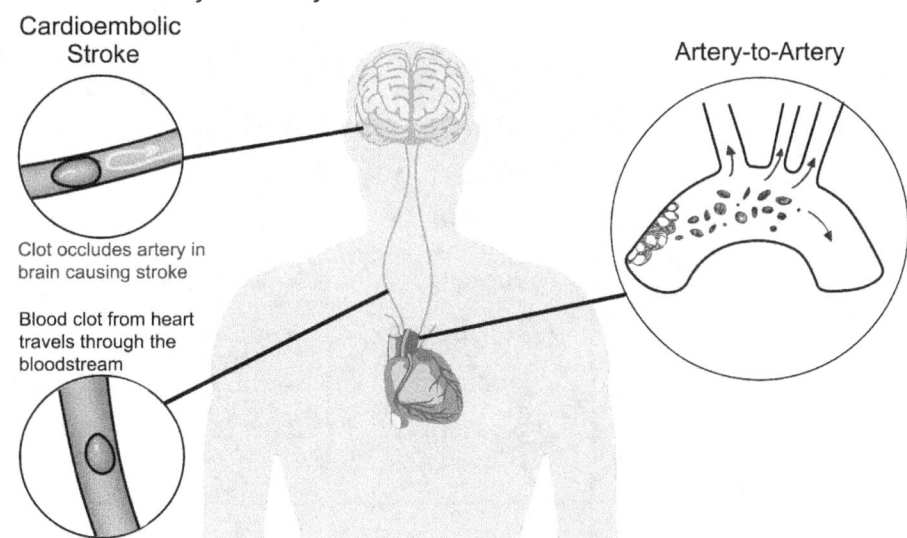

FIGURE 6. Cardioembolic and Artery-to-Artery Embolic Stroke

Stroke Made Simple

TABLE 2. Embolic Sources: **CAP**

C	Cardiogenic (mitral or aortic valves or the left cardiac chambers)
A	Arteriogenic (proximal cerebral arteries or the aortic arch)
P	Paradoxical (venous emboli)

Less frequently, ischemic stroke is classified as **thrombotic** stroke caused by a blood clot from the brain's blood vessels. A thrombotic stroke occurs when a blood clot, called a *thrombus*, is formed within the brain's own blood vessel(s) and remains attached to its place of origin. Most small vessel disease is thrombotic, caused by a clot within the brain's own blood vessels. The terms embolus and thrombus are often confused and misused, which is why proper stroke management requires a clear understanding of stroke vocabulary (Box 1). When evaluating AIS, one should consider several factors such as the source of the clot (embolic versus thrombotic), pathophysiology, the location of the brain affected, arterial territory, and relevant neuroimaging. All these factors should comprise an effective stroke plan when assessing AIS. An easy way to remember the components of this plan is the mnemonic 'S-PLAN' (Table 3).

BOX 1. Embolic Versus Thrombotic Clot

Embolic = **E**lsewhere
THrombotic = Wi**TH**in **TH**e Brain

TABLE 3. Ischemic Stroke Plan: S-PLAN

S	Source (embolic or thrombotic)
P	Pathophysiology (etiology)
L	Location (of brain affected)
A	Artery (arterial territory involved)
N	Neuroimaging

Source	Pathophysiology	Location	Artery	Neuroimaging
• Embolic • Thrombotic	**C**: Cardioembolic (20%) **A**: Atherosclerotic large vessel disease (30%) **U**: Undetermined etiology - ESUS (30%) **S**: Small vessel disease or lacunar infarct (15%) **E**: Everything else or other (5%)	• Frontal • Parietal • Temporal • Occipital • Cerebellar • Thalamic • Brainstem	• ICA • MCA • ACA • Vertebral • Basilar • PICA • ACA • SCA	• CT • CTA • CTP • MRI • MRA • Angio

5.5 Small Vessel Disease

Small vessel disease involves small perforating arteries that arise from larger vessels such as the lateral lenticulostriate arteries (arising from the MCA) or pontine perforators (arising from the BA) (Figure 7). Small vessel disease is more often caused by thrombotic (local, within the brain's own blood vessels) occlusions. This type of stroke typically occurs in deeper regions of the brain and brainstem. Small vessel disease represents approximately 15% of all AIS (Figures 4 and 5).

The great majority of small vessel thrombosis or **lacunar stroke** is related to hypertension but other risk factors include diabetes, aging, smoking, and hyperlipidemia. An easy way to remember these risk factors is the mnemonic 'DASH' (Table 4). Specific lacunar syndromes exist and these include pure motor or pure sensory symptoms, ataxic hemiparesis, dysarthria–clumsy hand syndrome, and simple unilateral sensorimotor deficits. An easy way to remember these lacunar symptoms is the mnemonic 'PADS' (Table 5). Lacunar infarcts can be classified by their vascular distribution (anterior versus posterior circulation), but they're better categorized by understanding their pathology. This is because anterior or posterior circulation lacunar infarcts can present with the same symptoms even though they occur in different regions of the brain. For this reason, a brief description of the more commonly encountered lacunar infarcts will be described in this chapter instead of dedicated chapters addressing the anterior and posterior circulation.

FIGURE 7. Lateral Lenticulostriate Arteries Arising from Middle Cerebral Arteries (MCA)

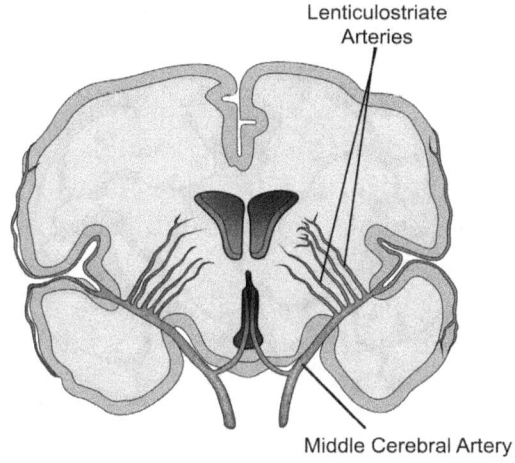

TABLE 4. Small Vessel Disease Risk Factors: **DASH**

D	Diabetes
A	Aging
S	Smoking
H	Hypertension or Hyperlipidemia

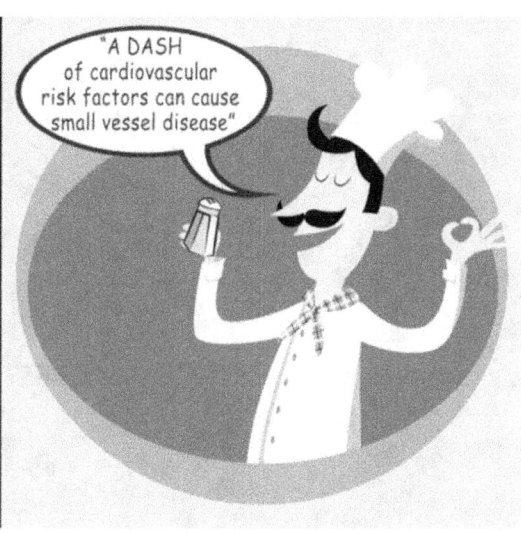

TABLE 5. Lacunar Syndromes: PADS

P	Pure Motor or Pure Sensory Symptoms
A	Ataxic Hemiparesis
D	Dysarthria – Clumsy Hand Syndrome
S	Simple Unilateral Sensorimotor Deficits

Pure motor hemiplegia is the most common lacunar syndrome (33%-50%) presenting with hemiparesis or hemiplegia of the contralateral face, arm, and leg. This is typically caused by a lateral lenticulostriate artery occlusion supplying the posterior limb of the internal capsule and less commonly by a pontine perforator occlusion. This lacunar syndrome (pure motor hemiplegia) can occur in different regions in the brain that are supplied by different arterial territories. This is because the lacunar infarct that causes motor weakness can affect any portion of the motor pathway (corticospinal tract) as it courses through the brain or brainstem (Figure 8).

Ataxic hemiparesis (10%) is caused by a pontine perforator occlusion supplying the pontocerebellar fibers located in the ventral pons and presents as mild hemiparesis with marked ipsilateral limb ataxia. A pure sensory stroke (7%) usually involves the ventral posterolateral (VPL) nucleus of the thalamus supplied by the thalamogeniculate artery. This lacunar syndrome presents with transient numbness, tingling, pain, and burning in the contralateral face and arms. Dysarthria-clumsy hand syndrome (6%) can involve the dorsal pons, the internal capsule, or deep white matter supplied by pontine perforators or lateral lenticulostriate arteries, respectively. Again, **the same deficits can occur in different regions of the brain supplied by different arterial territories, so long as the same pathway is affected.** This lacunar syndrome presents with dysarthria due to weakness of the ipsilateral face and tongue associated with a contralateral clumsy hand. Hand clumsiness is most pronounced when the patient is writing. Simple unilateral sensorimotor deficits (20%) present with hemiparesis or hemiplegia with contralateral sensory impairment. This can involve a lenticulostriate artery supplying the internal capsule or a thalamic perforator. The different lacunar syndromes are summarized in Table 6.

FIGURE 8. Pure Motor Hemiplegia Lacunar Syndrome

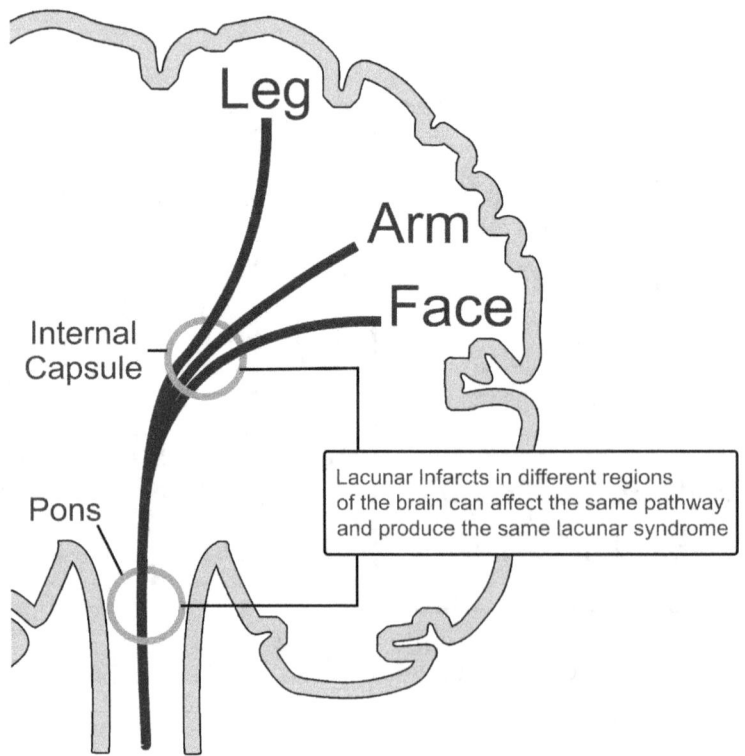

Lacunar Infarcts in different regions of the brain can affect the same pathway and produce the same lacunar syndrome

TABLE 6. The Lacunar Syndromes

Syndrome	Arterial Territory	Brain Location	Symptoms
Pure Motor Hemiparesis	Lenticulostriate/ Pontine Perforator	Internal Capsule, Pons	Contralateral Weakness
Ataxic Hemiparesis	Pontine Perforators	Ventral Pons	Hemiparesis with Prominent Ataxia
Pure Sensory	Thalamogeniculate Artery	VPL Nucleus, Thalamus	Contralateral Sensory Loss
Dysarthria/ Clumsy Hand	Lenticulostriate/ Pontine Perforator	Internal Capsule, Pons	Dysarthria and Hand Clumsiness
Mixed Motor/ Sensory	Lenticulostriate/ Thalamic Perforator	Internal Capsule, Thalamus	Hemiparesis and Contralateral Sensory Impairment

5.6 Atherosclerotic, Large Vessel Disease

Atherosclerotic, large vessel disease involves larger vessels such as the ICA, the proximal MCA, the proximal ACA, and the vertebral or basilar arteries (Figure 9). The mnemonic 'BAMBI' serves to help remember the large vessels of the brain (Table 7). LVO AIS typically involves the cortical and subcortical regions of the brain. Atherosclerotic large vessel disease can cause AIS by one of two mechanisms. First, local plaque can rupture into an arterial lumen leading to acute occlusion and thrombosis. LVO AIS may also result from embolism originating in the heart, aorta, or carotid arteries. LVO AIS is more often the result of this latter mechanism—embolic disease with an embolus traveling to the brain from a more proximal source in the body such as the heart (cardioembolic) or a more proximal artery (artery to artery disease). It is particularly important to identify LVO AIS because it accounts for nearly all AIS death, 90% of its societal cost, and 80% of poor functional outcome. For this reason, LVO AIS requires our utmost attention. Arterial supply to specific regions of the brain will be discussed in subsequent chapters, but a synopsis is provided in Table 8. Distinct from small vessel lacunar infarcts, LVO AIS typically presents with multiple cortical symptoms. An easy way to remember cortical symptoms associated with LVO AIS is the mnemonic 'MANGO™' (Table 9).

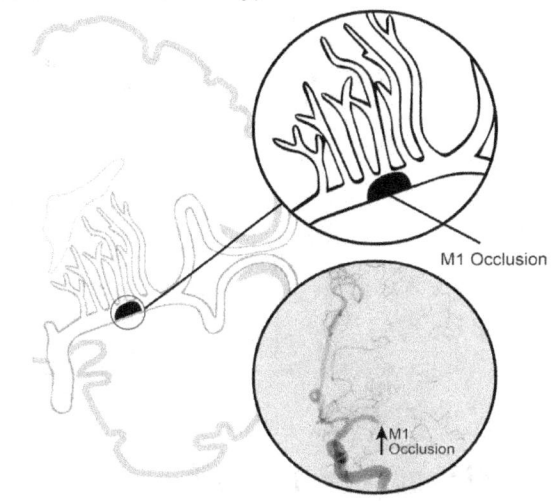

FIGURE 9. Atherosclerotic, Large Vessel Disease (Middle Cerebral Artery)

TABLE 7. Large Vessels of the Brain: **BAMBI**

B	Basilar Artery
A	Anterior Cerebral Artery
M	Middle Cerebral Artery
B	Both Vertebral Arteries
I	Internal Carotid Artery

TABLE 8. Arterial Supply to the Brain

Artery	Anatomy	Deficits
Left MCA	Left frontal/parietal cortex and subcortical structures	Right motor/sensory deficits, face > arm > leg weakness, aphasia, left gaze preference, right visual field cut
Right MCA	Right frontal/parietal cortex and subcortical structures	Left motor/sensory deficits, neglect, right gaze preference, face > arm > leg weakness, agnosia, apraxia, visual field cut
Left ACA	Left frontal and parasagittal areas	Leg > arm weakness, behavioral changes
Right ACA	Right frontal and parasagittal areas	Leg > arm weakness, behavioral changes
Brainstem	Midbrain, pons, medulla and cerebellum	bilateral motor deficits, ataxia/dysmetria, vertigo/nausea/vomiting, coma/altered mentation, ophthalmoplegia
PCA	Occipital cortex, medial temporal lobes, thalamus, upper midbrain	Visual field cut, motor/sensory loss, oculomotor problems, gaze problems, 3rd nerve deficits

ACA = anterior cerebral artery; MCA = middle cerebral artery; PCA = posterior cerebral artery

TABLE 9. Cortical Symptoms Associated with Large Vessel Occlusion: **MANGO**™

Large Vessel Occlusion (Screening Mnemonic): "**MANGO**™"

M	Motor Weakness
A	Aphasia Expressive (name 2 objects) Receptive (follow 2 commands)
N	Neglect Unable to feel both sides at the same time, or Unable to identify own arm, or Ignoring one side
G	Gaze Preference, Inability to Track or Double Vision
O	Optic Field Cut or New Blindness

5.7 Cardioembolic Disease

Cardiogenic emboli account for 20% of AIS and typically involve a cortical distribution. These emboli are usually comprised of red thrombi which form from areas of blood stasis and are termed "red" clots. This is because clotting proteins form a polymer mesh lattice containing platelets and red blood cells which yield a red appearance (Figure 10). Anticoagulant drugs such as heparin and Coumadin® prevent cardioembolic stroke by blocking the formation of clotting proteins that make up red thrombi. These clots typically form in the heart in the setting of abnormal heart rhythm. There are many sources of cardioembolic stroke but atrial fibrillation is by far the most common cause (Figure 11).[2] Cardiogenic emboli also result from damaged heart muscle. Cardiac infarction can cause stasis of blood and clot formation. Approximately 8% of AIS is caused by a recent heart attack. An easy way to recall the salient features of cardioembolic disease is the mnemonic 'CARDIAC' (Table 10).

FIGURE 10. Red Clot

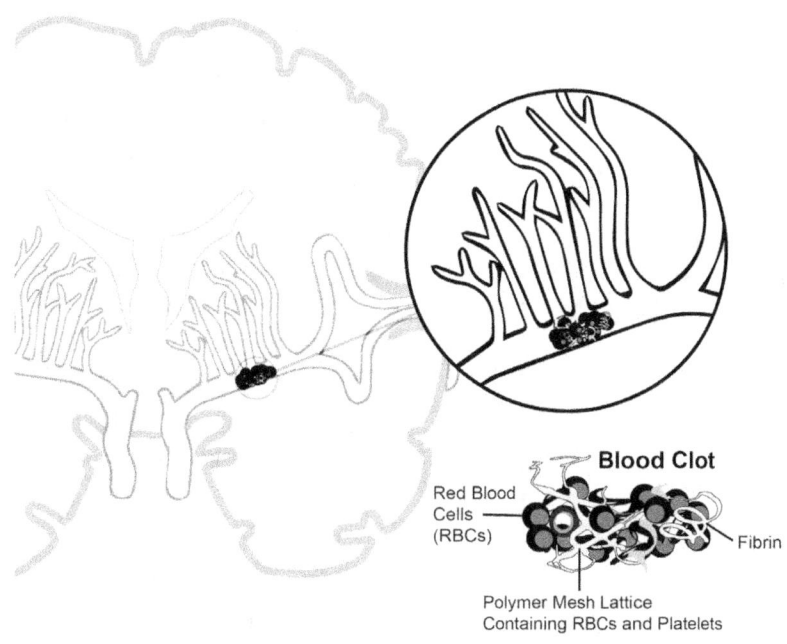

FIGURE 11. Sources of Cardioembolic Stroke

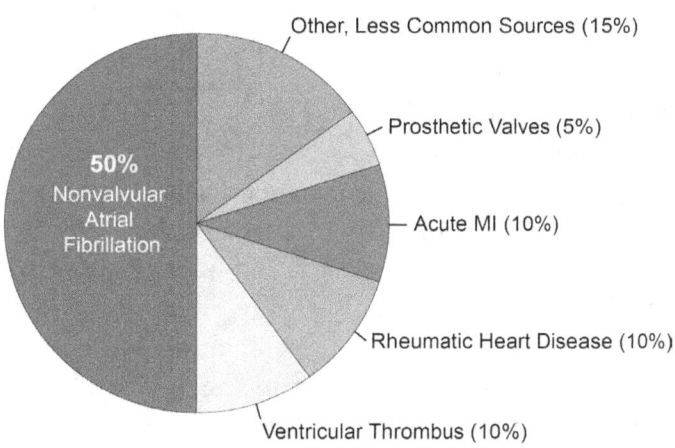

TABLE 10. Features of Cardiogenic Emboli: **CARDIAC**

C	Cardiogenic Emboli
A	Anticoagulants (i.e., Coumadin®)
R	Red Thrombus (RBCs and Platelets)
D	Disrupted Heart Rhythm or Damaged Muscle
I	Infarct (Cardiac) = Stasis = Clot Formation
A	AFib Most Common
C	Cortical Distribution

Cardiac sources of emboli are divided into *major* and *minor* risk categories. Minor risk sources have a low probability of being responsible for an initial or recurrent stroke. Major risk categories, on the other hand, present a high suspicion that either an initial or recurrent stroke is associated with a cardioembolic mechanism. Stroke caused by these high-risk categories is largely preventable, making both primary and secondary preventive efforts essential. Major risk factors for cardiac emboli include atrial fibrillation, atrial flutter, prosthetic valves, infective endocarditis, nonbacterial thrombotic (marantic) endocarditis, left ventricular thrombi associated with prothrombotic states, ischemic heart disease, acute myocardial infarction, left ventricular akinesis or aneurysm, nonischemic cardiomyopathies, and atrial myxoma. The mnemonic 'NAIL PAMELA' is a way to remember these major risk sources of cardioembolic stroke (Table 11).

TABLE 11. Major Risk Sources of Cardioembolic Stroke: **NAIL PAMELA**

N	Nonischemic Cardiomyopathies
A	Atrial Fibrillation and Flutter
I	Ischemic Heart Disease
L	Left Ventricular Thrombi Associated With Prothrombotic States
P	Prosthetic Valves
A	Acute Myocardial Infarction
M	Marantic Endocarditis
E	Endocarditis – Infective
L	Left Ventricular Akinesis or Aneurysm
A	Atrial Myxoma

5.8 Embolic Strokes of Undetermined Source (ESUS)

Cryptogenic (of unknown cause) ischemic stroke is defined as a "brain infarction that is not attributable to a source of definite cardioembolism, large artery atherosclerosis or small artery disease despite extensive vascular, cardiac and serologic evaluation."[1] This definition was derived from the TOAST Trial published in 1993.[1] However, there have been tremendous advances in both imaging techniques and the understanding of stroke pathophysiology since that time. Both advances have heralded a reassessment of cryptogenic stroke. There is now persuasive evidence that the pathophysiology of most cryptogenic stroke is thromboembolic. These thrombi are believed to develop from embolic sources such as cardiac (cardioembolic), venous (paradoxical embolism), and arterial (arteriogenic aortic arch and extracranial arteries) sources (Table 2).

The diagnostic and therapeutic mystery of cryptogenic stroke is compounded by the fact that it represents approximately 30% of all AIS. For this reason, a more proactive, clinically useful, and positively defined term to facilitate the understanding of these types of stroke has been advocated—*embolic strokes of undetermined source* (**ESUS**). This is a paradigm shift from the vague, negatively defined term of cryptogenic stroke. The underlying premise is that ESUS is a **thromboembolic disease resulting from cardiac abnormalities or other sources** instead of a diagnosis of exclusion when no underlying cause can be determined. ESUS is defined as *a non-lacunar stroke lacking either proximal arterial stenosis or cardioembolic sources.* These criteria can easily be remembered by the mnemonic 'NONE' (Table 12). Since ESUS are presumptively caused by thromboembolic phenomenon and these emboli are mainly comprised of red thrombus, anticoagulants can likely prevent secondary stroke more effectively than antiplatelet therapy.

TABLE 12. Embolic Stroke of Undetermined Source (ESUS): **NONE**

N	Non-lacunar Stroke
O	Open Arteries (Less Than 50% Stenosis)
N	No Major Risk Cardioembolic Source
E	ESUS (Embolic Stroke of Undetermined Source)

Emerging data continues to link thromboembolic causing cardiac abnormalities with ESUS.[3] One possible strategy for stroke prevention in ESUS patients is to improve the detection of clinically silent atrial fibrillation. Both the Cryptogenic Stroke and Underlying AF (CRYSTAL-AF) and the 30-Day Cardiac Event Monitor Belt for Recording AF After a Cerebral Ischemic Event (EMBRACE) Trials demonstrated the benefits of implantable devices and prolonged ambulatory monitoring in detecting AFib.[4,5] While most ESUS cases are related to unrecognized paroxysmal atrial fibrillation, other pathophysiologic mechanisms exist. These include atrial high rate episodes, heart failure, silent myocardial infarction, patent foramen ovale, hypercoagulable states, aortic arch atherosclerotic plaque, or non-stenotic atherosclerotic plaque within the extracranial or intracranial arteries. ESUS can also be determined by specific biomarkers such as brain natriuretic peptide (BNP), N-terminal proBNP (NT-proBNP), and D-dimer. For example, recent studies have demonstrated elevated levels of BNP and NT-proBNP in ESUS patients with these values independent of other clinical factors.[6] Furthermore, acutely elevated levels of NT-proBNP greater than 750 pg/mL in ESUS may be related to an occult cardioembolic mechanism.[7] Biomarker analysis may also aid in other non-cardiogenic causes of ESUS. For example, elevated D-dimer levels following the diagnosis of stroke may indicate a hypercoagulable state secondary to occult malignancy.[8]

5.8.1 Diagnosis of ESUS

ESUS is a diagnosis of exclusion which requires ruling out other major risk cardioembolic sources, extracranial atherosclerotic occlusive disease, and lacunar stroke. Hart et al. proposed a stepwise approach to aid in the diagnosis of ESUS.[9] First, one must confirm the diagnosis of ischemic stroke (i.e., exclude a stroke mimic) by CT or MRI imaging and exclude the presence of a lacunar infarct. Second, major risk cardioembolic sources must also be excluded with ECG, Holter monitoring (to exclude atrial fibrillation), and echocardiography (to exclude intraventricular thrombus). Next, vascular imaging must be performed to exclude hemodynamically significant or occlusive extracranial atherosclerotic disease. Finally, infrequent causes of stroke such as moyamoya disease, migrainous headaches, arteritis, reversible cerebrovascular vasoconstriction syndrome, etc., must also be excluded.

Aortic arch and atheromatous disease is an underdiagnosed thromboembolic mechanism for AIS.[10] Typically, this is evaluated with transesophageal echocardiography. However, CT angiography which is frequently used in AIS evaluation can also be utilized. It is currently not performed on a routine basis but including the aorta and even the left ventricle (to exclude intraventricular thrombus) should be considered since both of these structures could easily be included in current AIS CTA protocols.[11]

Embolic composition currently determines the use of anticoagulants or antiplatelet agents. For example, platelets tend to aggregate on regions of irregular plaque (referred to as a white thrombus due to their appearance) and platelet aggregation is diminished by aspirin and other antiplatelet agents. That is why white clot (platelet-rich), arterial origin embolism is believed to be more responsive to antiplatelet therapy whereas red clot (fibrin-rich), venous, or stasis (cardiac chamber) precipitated embolism is typically responsive to anticoagulants (Table 13). However, the distinctions between antiplatelet-responsive white clot and anticoagulant-responsive red clot are not absolute. For example, the ESPRIT Trial investigated 1,068 patients with non-cardioembolic ischemic stroke.[12] They found no difference in recurrent stroke rate among patients randomly allocated to oral vitamin K antagonists versus aspirin demonstrating that anticoagulants can reduce thrombotic events in the arterial circulation. Because ESUS consists of several subgroups with multiple potential overlap and embolic sources, anticoagulation may serve as a therapeutic strategy to address both white and red clot for secondary stroke prevention.

The leading priority for ESUS treatment is secondary stroke prevention. However, there are no well-established guidelines for secondary stroke prevention in this patient population. The American Heart Association/American Stroke Association and the American College of Chest Physicians recommend antiplatelet agents for non-cardioembolic ischemic strokes. However, a post-hoc analysis of a subset of participants in the Warfarin vs. Aspirin for Recurrent Stroke Study (WARSS) suggests anticoagulation with warfarin was associated with one-third fewer recurrent strokes than cryptogenic stroke patients with an embolic appearance taking aspirin alone.[13]

TABLE 13. White Versus Red Clot

Clot Type	Clot Consistency	Clot Origin	Treatment
White Clot	Platelet Rich	Arterial	Antiplatelet
Red Clot	Fibrin Rich	Venous or Stasis	Anticoagulant

Despite this data, the role of anticoagulation in ESUS or cryptogenic stroke has yet to be determined. No randomized trials have been performed to determine antithrombotic prophylaxis for ESUS. So how do we deal with ESUS or cryptogenic stroke? First, the antiquated terminology of "cryptogenic stroke" must be abandoned. Next, the more progressive term "embolic strokes of undetermined source" (ESUS) must be embraced. Hospital systems should educate their staff with this new terminology and have an order set specifically designed for ESUS patients. To aid with this process, remember the mnemonic 'HAPPY MEDUSA' (Table 14).

5.8.2 Hypercoagulable Abnormalities

One cause of ESUS is hypercoagulable abnormalities (Table 14). Hypercoagulable related AIS reflects hematologic abnormalities that lead to thrombosis within the cerebral vasculature. These include resistance to activated protein C (factor V Leiden mutation), deficiencies in proteins C&S, antithrombin III deficiencies, erythrocyte disorders (sickle cell disease and polycythemia vera), hyperhomocystinemia, prothrombin gene mutation, thrombotic thrombocytopenic purpura (TTP), autoantibody syndromes, and a single lipoprotein, lipoprotein (a). These blood dyscrasias have two unique characteristics. First, these patients are usually younger. Second, they do not have vascular risk factors typically associated with AIS patients. AIS patients with these blood dyscrasias are estimated to account for approximate 4% of the ischemic stroke population.[14,15] An easy way to remember blood dyscrasias associated with AIS is the mnemonic 'GREAT SHAPE' (Table 15).

TABLE 14. Embolic Strokes of Undetermined Source (ESUS): **HAPPY MEDUSA**

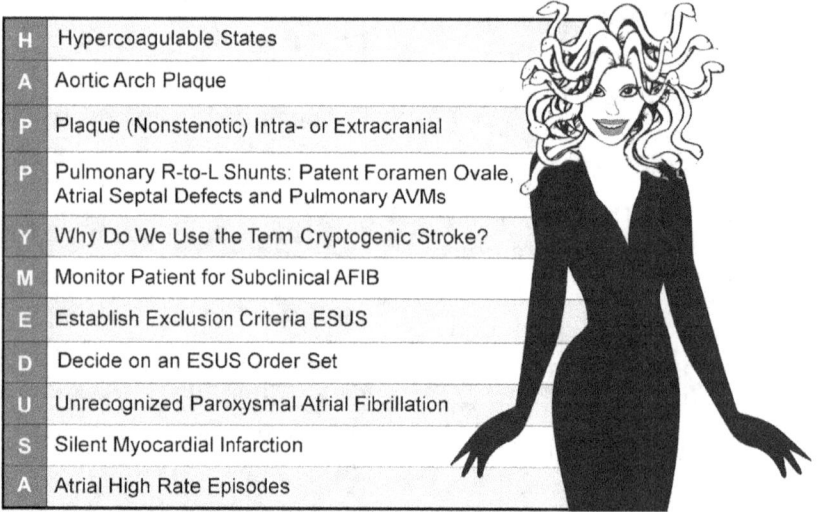

H	Hypercoagulable States
A	Aortic Arch Plaque
P	Plaque (Nonstenotic) Intra- or Extracranial
P	Pulmonary R-to-L Shunts: Patent Foramen Ovale, Atrial Septal Defects and Pulmonary AVMs
Y	Why Do We Use the Term Cryptogenic Stroke?
M	Monitor Patient for Subclinical AFIB
E	Establish Exclusion Criteria ESUS
D	Decide on an ESUS Order Set
U	Unrecognized Paroxysmal Atrial Fibrillation
S	Silent Myocardial Infarction
A	Atrial High Rate Episodes

TABLE 15. AIS Associated Blood Dyscrasias: **GREAT SHAPE**

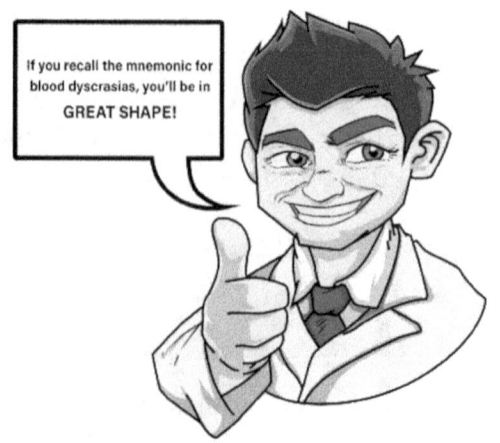

G	Gene Mutation – Prothrombin
R	Resistance to Activated Protein C (Mutation In Factor V Leiden)
E	Erythrocyte Disorder - Sickle Cell Disease
A	Anti-Thrombin III Deficiency
T	Thrombotic Thrombocytopenic Purpura (TTP)
S	Single Lipoprotein, Lipoprotein (A)
H	Hyperhomocystinemia
A	Autoantibody Syndromes
P	Proteins C and S Deficiencies
E	Erythrocyte Disorder - Polycythemia Vera

If you recall the mnemonic for blood dyscrasias, you'll be in GREAT SHAPE!

5.9 Everything Else

This category includes unusual causes of AIS. These different etiologies typically occur in patients without classic risk factors for cerebrovascular disease. Sometimes, AIS may be the manifestation of another disease process such as vasculitis associated with connective tissue disorders (systemic lupus erythematosus), infections (endocarditis), or cancer. Other unusual causes include arterial dissection, aortic dissection, moyamoya disease, migrainous headaches, arteritis, reversible cerebrovascular vasoconstriction syndrome, etc. While this category only accounts for 5% of AIS, recognize that two entities within it (**suspected infectious endocarditis and suspected aortic dissection**) are contraindications to the administration of IV TPA.

5.10 Summary

AIS is a heterogeneous disease with multiple different underlying pathologic conditions. The purpose of this chapter was to review these different etiologies and provide simple learning tools to assist in this process. The quintessential goal of all AIS treatment is to restore blood flow to the brain. In order to accomplish this goal, one must understand the causes of AIS. This chapter also introduced mnemonics for these causes as well as a stroke plan (S-PLAN). Always consider the components of this plan when evaluating stroke. These components will help decipher the complexity of AIS.

Abbreviations list

AIS, acute ischemic stroke; BNP, brain natriuretic peptide; ESUS, embolic strokes of undetermined source; EVT, endovascular treatment; LVO, large vessel occlusion; NT-proBNP, N-terminal proBNP; S-PLAN, stroke plan; TTP, thrombotic thrombocytopenic purpura; VPL, ventral posterolateral.

References

1. Adams HP, Bendixen BH, Kappelle LJ, Biller J, Love BB, Gordon DL, and Marsh EE. (1993). Classification of subtype of acute ischemic stroke. Definitions for use in a multicenter clinical trial. TOAST. Trial of Org 10172 in Acute Stroke Treatment. Stroke, 24, 35-41.
2. Kamel H, Okin PM, Elkind MSV, and Iadecola C. (2016). Atrial Fibrillation and Mechanisms of Stroke. *Stroke*, 47, 895-900.
3. Choe WC, Passman RS, Brachmann J, et al. (2015). A Comparison of Atrial Fibrillation Monitoring Strategies After Cryptogenic Stroke (from the Cryptogenic Stroke and Underlying AF Trial). *Am J Cardiol*, 116(6), 889–93.
4. Sanna T, et al. (2014). Cryptogenic Stroke and Underlying Atrial Fibrillation. *N Engl J Med*, 370, 2478-86.
5. Gladstone DJ, et al. (2014) Atrial Fibrillation in Patients with Cryptogenic Stroke. *N Engl J Med*, 370, 2467-77.
6. Llombart V, Antolin-Fontes A, Bustamante A, et al. (2015). B-type natriuretic peptides help in cardioembolic stroke diagnosis: pooled data meta-analysis. *Stroke*, 46(5), 1187–95.
7. Longstreth WT, Jr, Kronmal RA, Thompson JL, et al. (2013). Amino terminal pro-B-type natriuretic peptide, secondary stroke prevention, and choice of antithrombotic therapy. *Stroke*, 44(3), 714–9.
8. Kim SJ, Park JH, Lee MJ, et al. (2012). Clues to occult cancer in patients with ischemic stroke. *PLoS One*, 7(9), e44959.
9. Hart, RG, et.al. (2014) Embolic strokes of undetermined source: the case for a new clinical construct. *The Lancet Neurol*, 13(4), 429-38.
10. Macleod MR, Amarenco P, Davis SM, Donnan GA. (2004). Atheroma of the aortic arch: an important and poorly recognised factor in the aetiology of stroke. *Lancet Neurol*, 3, 408–14.
11. Furtado AD, Adraktas DD, Brasic N, Cheng SC, Ordovas K, Smith WS, Lewin MR, Chun K, Chien JD, Schaeffer S, Wintermark M. (2010). The Triple Rule-Out for Acute Ischemic Stroke: Imaging the Brain, Carotid Arteries, Aorta, and Heart. *Amer Jrnal of Neuroradiol*, Aug, 31(7), 1290-96.
12. Halkes PH, van Gijn J, Kappelle LJ, Koudstaal PJ, Algra A. (2007). Medium intensity oral

anticoagulants versus aspirin after cerebral ischaemia of arterial origin (ESPRIT): a randomised controlled trial. *Lancet Neurol*, Feb, 6(2):115-24.
13. Sacco RL, Prabhakaran S, Thompson JL, et al. (2006). Comparison of warfarin versus aspirin for the prevention of recurrent stroke or death: subgroup analyses from the Warfarin-Aspirin Recurrent Stroke Study. *Cerebrovasc Dis,* 22(1), 4–12.
14. Hart RG, Kanter MC. (1990). Hematologic disorders and ischemic stroke. A selective review. *Stroke,* Aug, 21(8), 1111-21.
15. Martinez HR, Rangel-Guerra RA, Marfil LJ. (1993). Ischemic stroke due to deficiency of coagulation inhibitors. Report of 10 young adults. *Stroke*, Jan, 24(1), 19-25.

Hemorrhagic Stroke

6.1 Introduction

Stroke can be classified as ischemic (87%) or hemorrhagic (13%) (Figure 1). Acute ischemic stroke (AIS) can be further subcategorized into large vessel atherosclerotic disease (30%), embolic strokes of undetermined source (ESUS) (30%), cardioembolic stroke (20%), small vessel disease (15%), and other stroke causing conditions (5%) (Figure 2). An easy way to remember AIS etiologies is with the mnemonic 'CAUSE' (Table 1).

TABLE 1. Etiologies of Acute Ischemic Stroke: **CAUSE**

C	Cardioembolic (20%)	
A	Atherosclerotic Large Vessel Disease (30%)	
U	Undetermined Etiology - ESUS* (30%) (Avoid Cryptogenic Stroke Terminology)	
S	Small Vessel Disease or Lacunar Infarct (15%)	
E	Everything Else, or Other (5%)	

*Embolic Strokes of Undetermined Source

Hemorrhagic stroke can be further sub-classified into intracerebral hemorrhage (ICH) which occurs within the brain, and subarachnoid hemorrhage (SAH) which occurs in the subarachnoid space surrounding the brain (Figure 3). Both ICH and SAH are forms of intracranial hemorrhage; however, intracranial hemorrhage (within the skull) is not the same as intracerebral hemorrhage (ICH), which is hemorrhage within the brain parenchyma. Hemorrhagic stroke accounts for 13% of stroke, with ICH comprising 10% and SAH accounting for the remaining 3% (Figure 4). Hemorrhagic stroke results from both ruptured blood vessels within (ICH) or covering (SAH) the brain.

FIGURE 1. Ischemic and Hemorrhagic Stroke

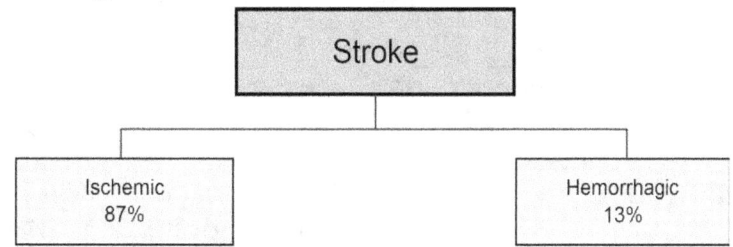

FIGURE 2. Subtypes of Acute Ischemic Stroke (AIS)

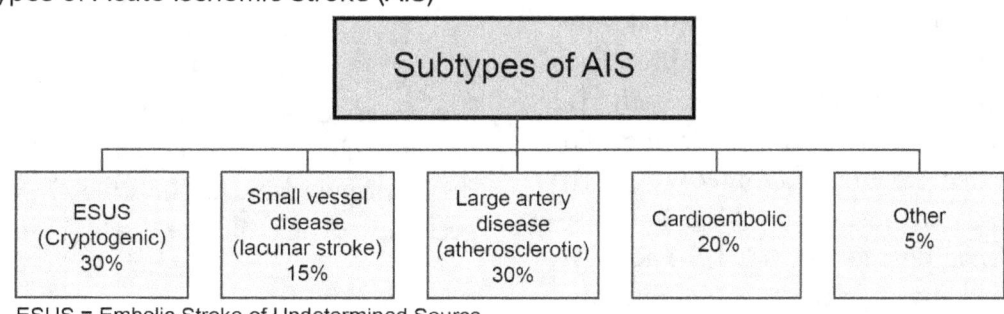

ESUS = Embolic Stroke of Undetermined Source

FIGURE 3. Intracerebral Hemorrhage (ICH) and Subarachnoid Hemorrhage (SAH)

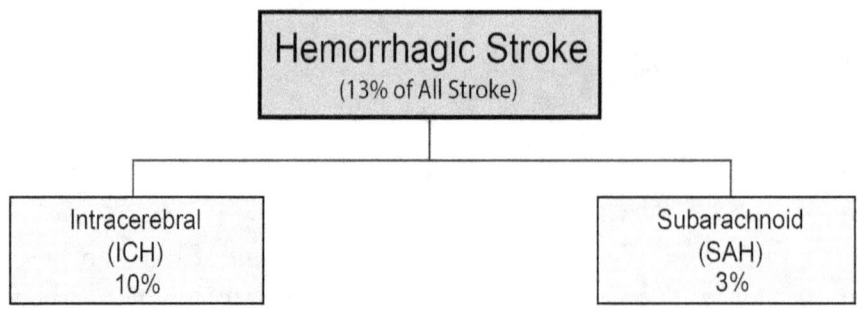

FIGURE 4. Subtypes of Hemorrhagic Stroke

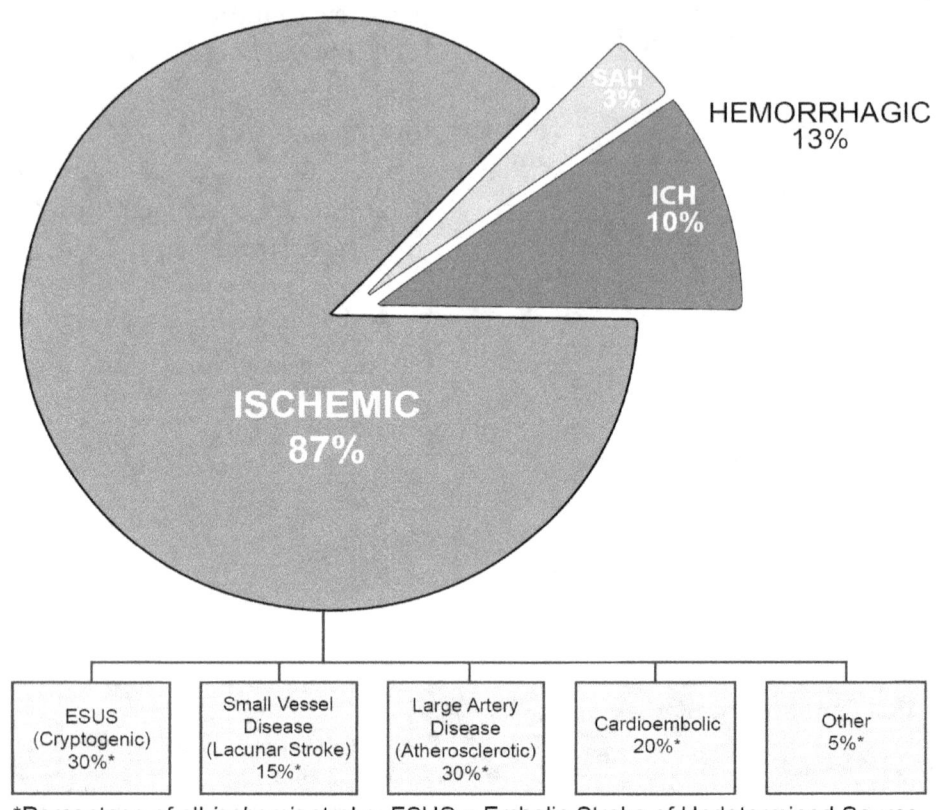

*Percentage of all *ischemic* stroke; ESUS = Embolic Stroke of Undetermined Source

6.2 Intracerebral Hemorrhage

While there are many causes of non-traumatic ICH (within the brain), most are related to hypertensive hemorrhage (HH) and cerebral amyloid angiopathy (CAA) (Box 1). In addition to causing overt intracerebral hemorrhage, both HH and CAA can cause small, perivascular hemosiderin deposits called cerebral microbleeds (CMBs) which appear as dark lesions on MRI hemosiderin-sensitive imaging sequences. HH and CAA are characterized by CMBs and parenchymal hemorrhage that occur in different regions of the brain, with HH occurring in deeper regions, and CAA CMBs or parenchymal hemorrhage occurring in more superficial, lobar locations (Figure 5). HH is representative of an acquired disease related to long-standing hypertension affecting the brain's deeper, small penetrating arteries. On the other hand, CAA is characterized by amyloid deposition within the superficially located meningeal and cortical blood vessels (Figure 6).

BOX 1. Causes of Intracranial Hemorrhage

Subarachnoid (SAH)	• Aneurysm • Perimesencephalic Venous • Vasculitis • Mycotic • Cerebral Vein Thrombosis • Arteriovenous Malformation (AVM)
Intracerebral (ICH)	• Hypertension • Amyloid Angiopathy • Cardioembolic • Non-Cardiogenic Embolization • Vascular Tumors • Anticoagulent Therapy • Thrombolytic Therapy • Vasculitis • Bleeding Disorders

FIGURE 5. Intracerebral Hemorrhage (ICH) and Cerebral Microbleeds (CMBs): Hypertensive Hemorrhage (HH) and Cerebral Amyloid Angiopathy (CAA) Distribution

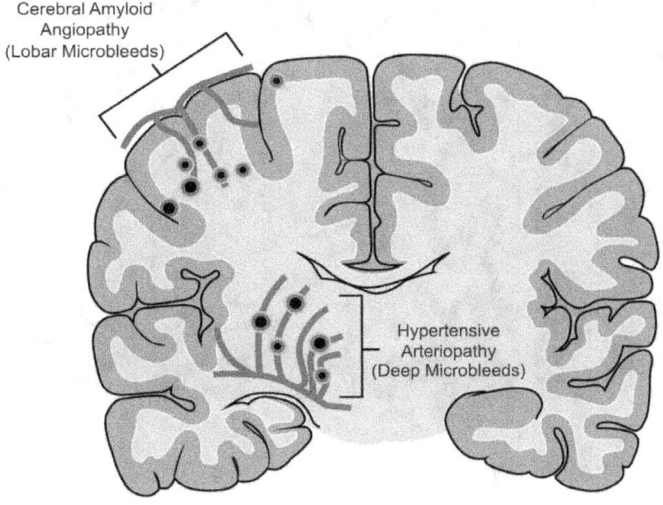

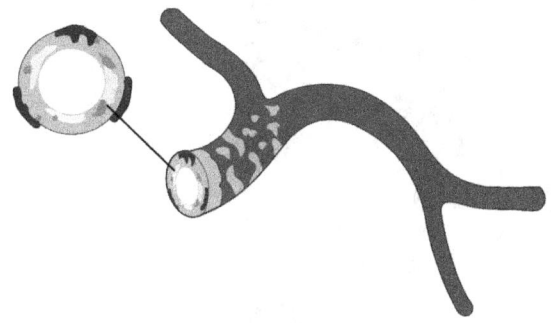

FIGURE 6. Cerebral Amyloid Angiopathy (CAA) Characterized by Vascular Amyloid Deposition

6.3 Cerebral Amyloid Angiopathy

Lobar hemorrhage is most commonly caused by CAA, a degenerative vascular disorder. CAA weakens vascular integrity causing lobar ICH. Because CAA is a chronic degenerative disease, it is more prevalent in the elderly. The plaque that forms within these vessel walls is the same plaque associated with Alzheimer's disease, but CAA is not the same disease. Since CAA is more prone to develop in the elderly, CAA should be considered in elderly patients with superficial, lobar hemorrhages. In addition to causing frank hemorrhage, CAA can cause microbleeds in superficially located intracerebral blood vessels. Thus, both CAA related microbleeds and lobar hemorrhages involve superficially located meningeal and cortical blood vessels. Microbleeds appear as a dark signal on gradient echo MRI images.(Figure 7).

6.4 Hypertensive Hemorrhage

HH can be caused by long-standing hypertension affecting small penetrating arteries. The underlying pathophysiology for hypertensive angiopathy includes Charcot-Bouchard micro-aneurysms, arteriosclerosis, and fibrohylinosis. In contradistinction to CAA (which affects more superficial brain blood vessels), hypertensive angiopathy is characterized by cerebral microbleeds that are located in deep brain structures such as the basal ganglia and the thalamus (Figures 8, 9 and 10). Hemorrhagic stroke caused by hypertension (in order of frequency) occurs in the basal ganglia (80%), the pons (10%), and the cerebellum (10%) (Figure 10). Again, in contradistinction to CAA lobar bleeds, HH involves deeper regions within the brain rather than superficial locations.

FIGURE 7. Superficial Distribution of Cerebral Amyloid Angiopathy (CAA)

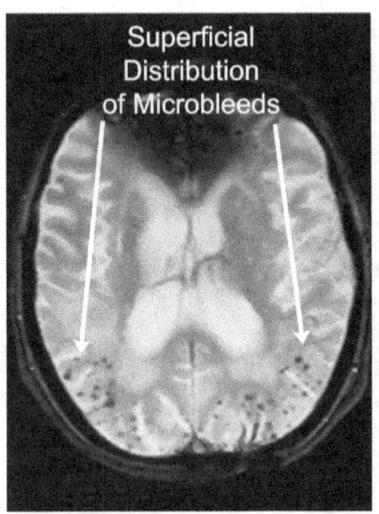
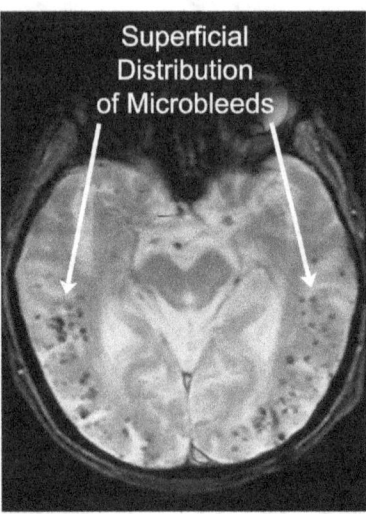
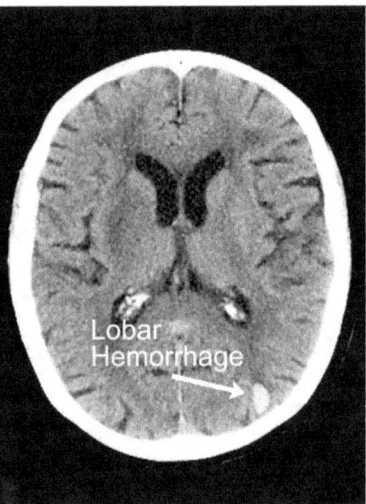

FIGURE 8. Central or Deep Distribution of Hypertensive Hemorrhage (HH)

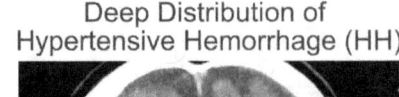
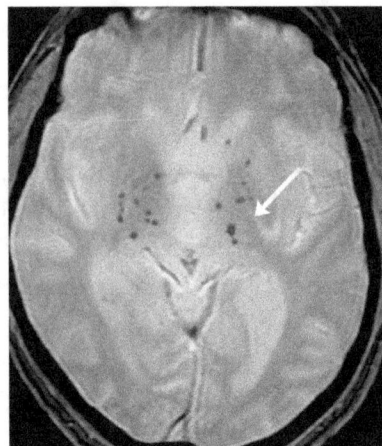
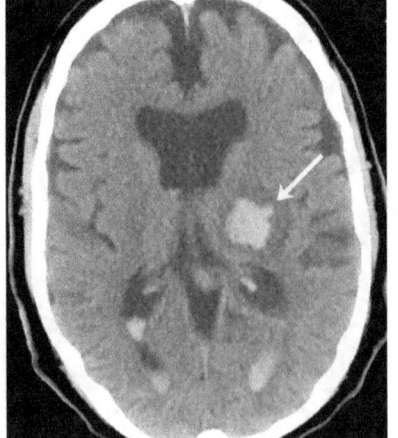

FIGURE 9. Superficial and Deep Location of Intracerebral Hemorrhage (ICH)

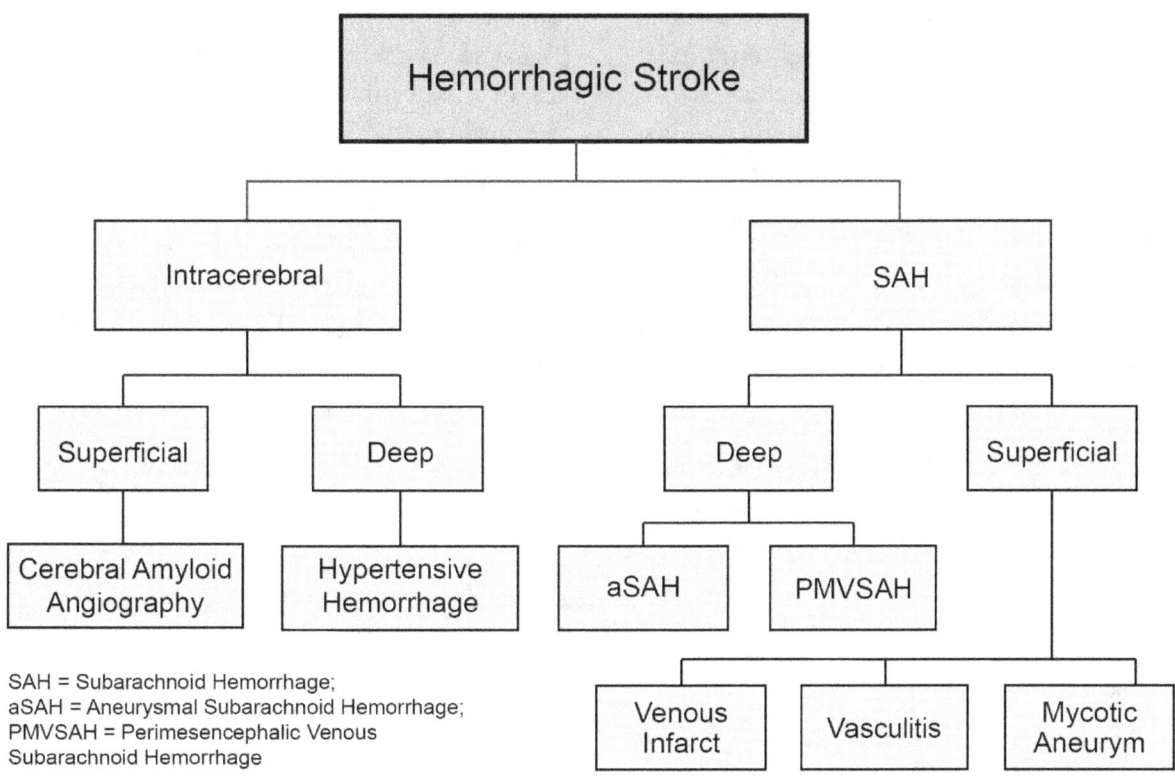

SAH = Subarachnoid Hemorrhage;
aSAH = Aneurysmal Subarachnoid Hemorrhage;
PMVSAH = Perimesencephalic Venous Subarachnoid Hemorrhage

FIGURE 10. Location and Frequency of Hypertensive Hemorrhage

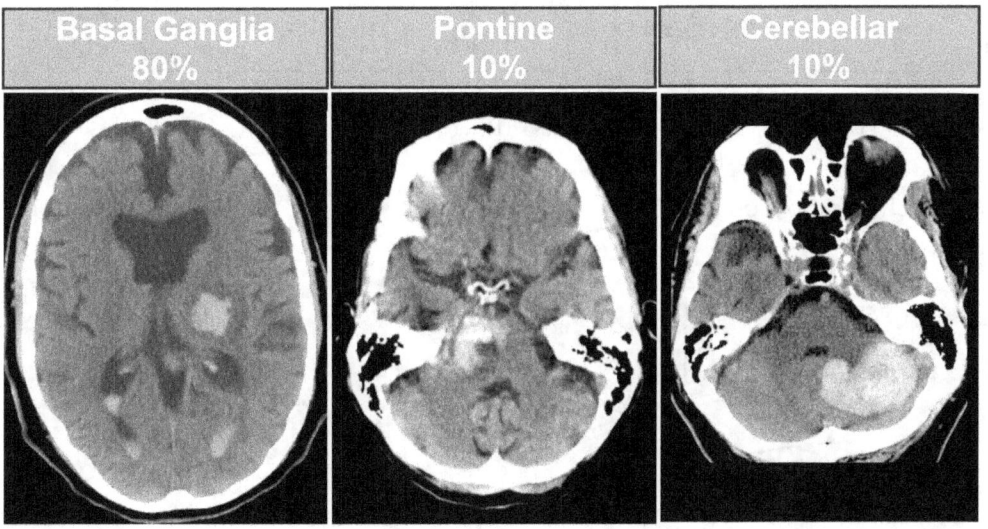

6.5 Subarachnoid Hemorrhage

Subarachnoid hemorrhage (SAH) is hemorrhage within the subarachnoid space. The most common cause of subarachnoid hemorrhage is trauma. However, this discussion pertains to non-traumatic causes of SAH including intracranial ruptured aneurysms, mycotic aneurysms, non-aneurysmal causes of SAH like perimesencephalic venous subarachnoid hemorrhage (PMVSAH), and vasculitis. A more indepth discussion pertaining to intracranial aneurysms is provided in Chapter 7 (Cerebral Aneurysms).

SAH can also be divided into central (deep) and superficial locations (Figure 11). Recall from Chapter 3 that three meningeal layers cover the brain. The subarachnoid space is located between the arachnoid mater (the middle meningeal layer) and the pia mater (the innermost meningeal layer). The subarachnoid space houses extra-axial arteries and veins. Therefore, hemorrhage from ruptured aneurysms, perimesencephalic veins, vasculitis, mycotic aneurysms, and venous infarct will be located within the subarachnoid space (Figure 12).

SAH can have a central or superficial distribution depending on its etiology. An aneurysm is a focal bulging or outpouching of a weakened arterial wall (Figure 13). Most brain aneurysms are located within the Circle of Willis (Figure 14). Because of their central location, ruptured brain aneurysms typically have a central distribution of SAH (Figure 15). PMVSAH is typically caused by ruptured veins within the posterior fossa. It also has a central distribution of SAH and is often confused with aneurysmal SAH (aSAH) (Figure 16). Because PMVSAH involves the posterior fossa, it can be confused with a ruptured basilar tip aneurysm.

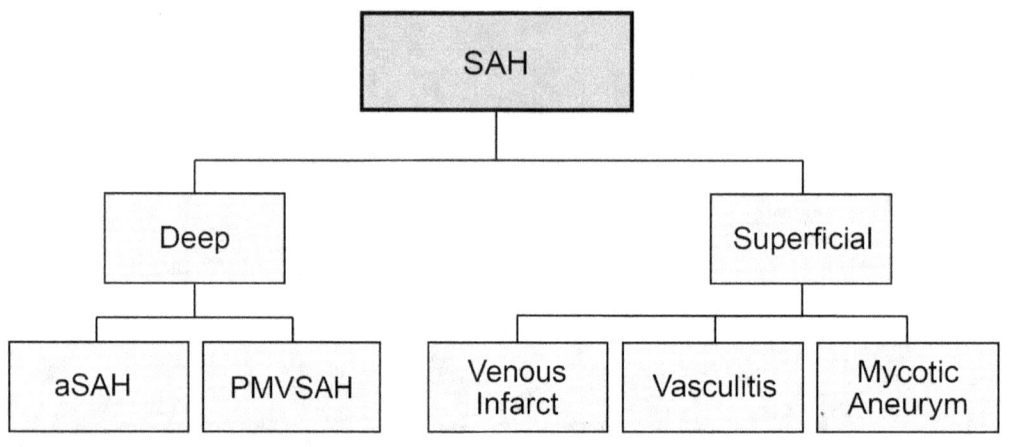

FIGURE 11. Subarachnoid Hemorrhage (SAH) Distribution Patterns

SAH = Subarachnoid Hemorrhage; aSAH = Aneurysmal Subarachnoid Hemorrhage; PMVSAH = Perimesencephalic Venous Subarachnoid Hemorrhage

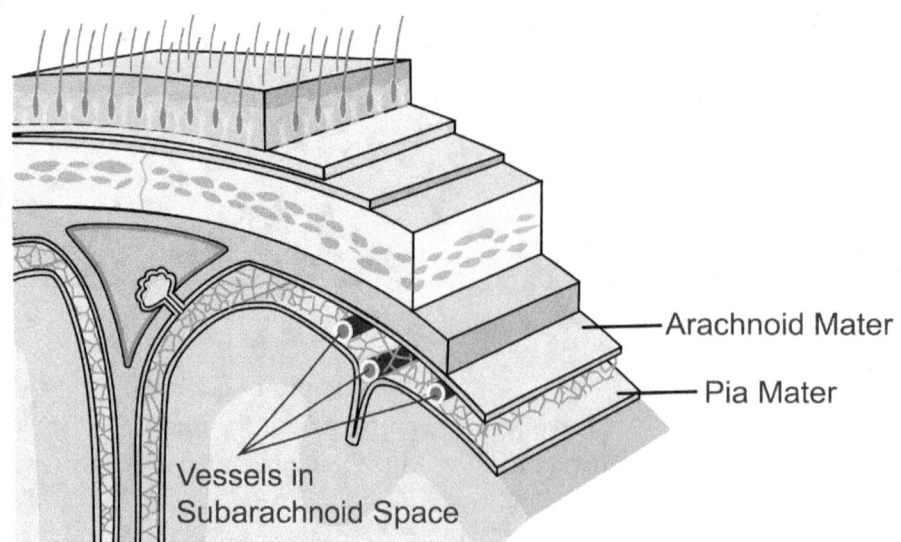

FIGURE 12. The Subarachnoid Space

FIGURE 13. Intracranial Aneurysm

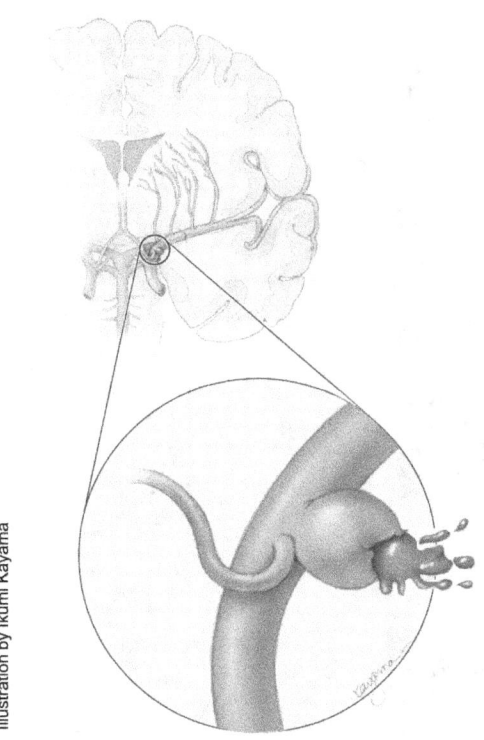

FIGURE 14. The Circle of Willis (COW) and Intracranial Aneurysms

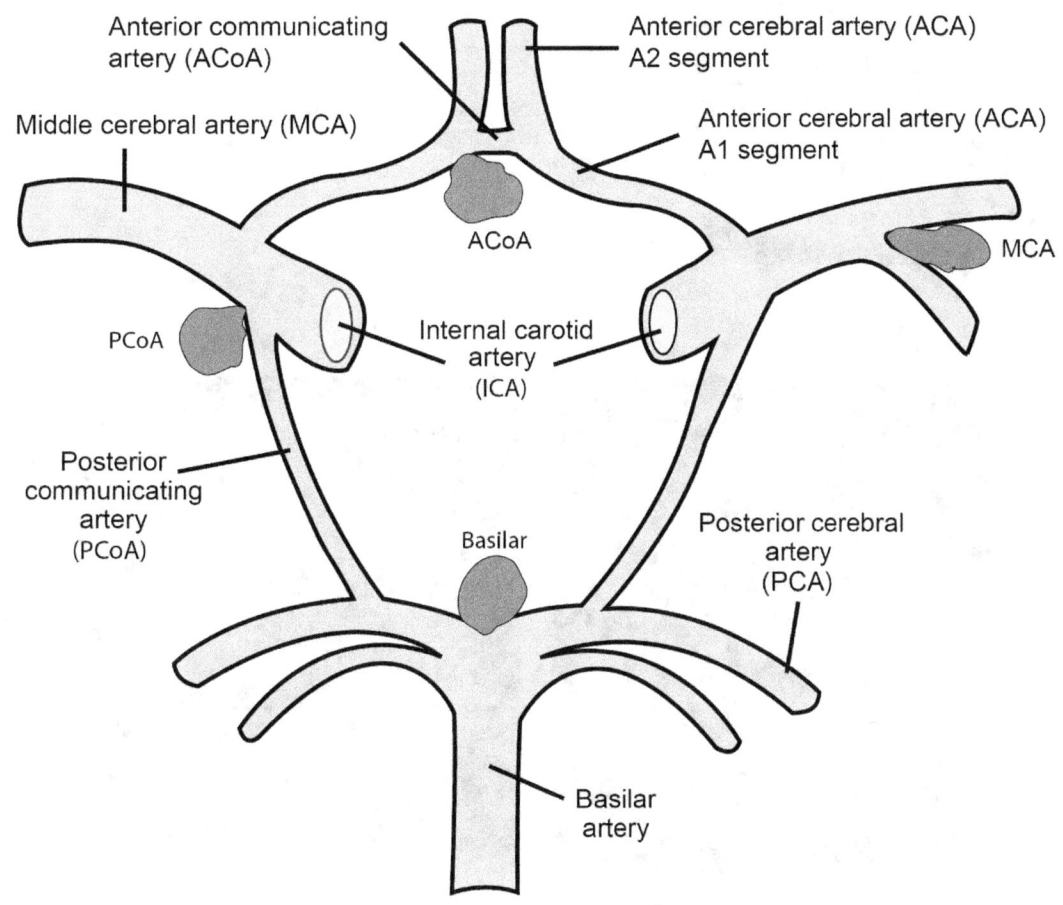

FIGURE 15. Central Distribution of Aneurysmal Subarachnoid Hemorrhage (aSAH)

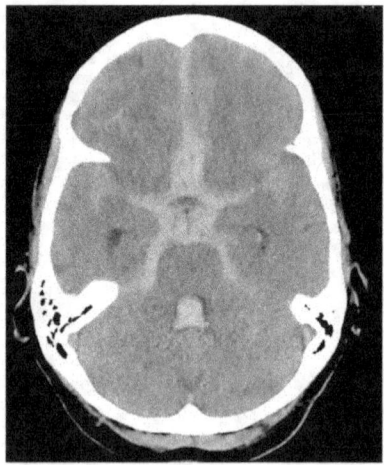

aSAH

FIGURE 16. Perimesencephalic Venous Subarachnoid Hemorrhage (PMVSAH)

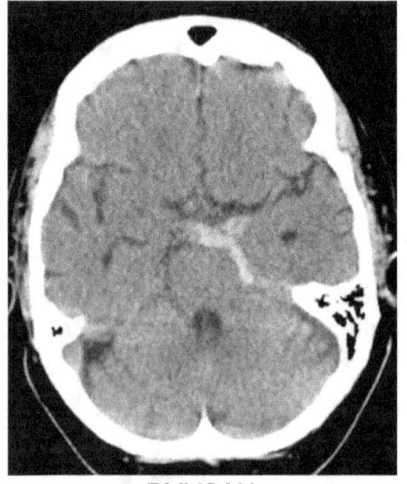

PMVSAH

There are three important neuroimaging clues that can distinguish PMVSAH from aSAH (Figure 15 and 16). First, perimesencephalic veins are located adjacent to and contained within the prepontine and ambient cistern (Figure 17). SAH that is predominantly located within the prepontine and ambient cisterns raises the diagnosis of venous PMVSAH. Second, because PMVSAH has lower venous pressure than arterial aSAH, PMVSAH will often be lateralized to one side of the pons or midbrain. Lastly and for the same reason, PMVSAH rarely extends into the sylvian fissures while aSAH (higher arterial pressure) typically extends into the sylvian fissures (Figure 18). Also, look for the aneurysm within the region of the subarachnoid hemorrhage (Figure 19). Like aSAH, PMVSAH is identified in a central location. A cerebral angiogram or CTA is still recommended to confirm the diagnosis of PMVSAH and exclude the diagnosis of aSAH. PMVSAH has an excellent prognosis with much better outcomes than aSAH.

FIGURE 17. Cisternal Anatomy

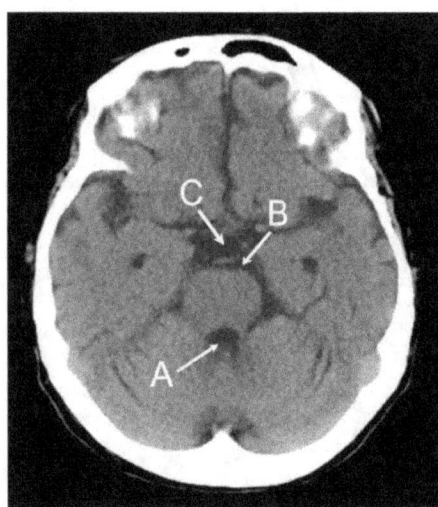
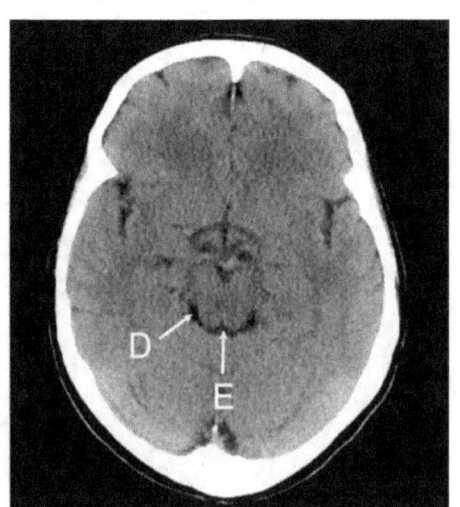

Normal cisterns and fourth ventricle. A) Fourth ventricle B) Prepontine cistern C) Suprasellar cistern D) Right ambient cistern E) Quadrigimenal cistern

FIGURE 18. Perimesencephalic Venous SAH (PMVSAH) vs. Aneurysmal SAH (aSAH)

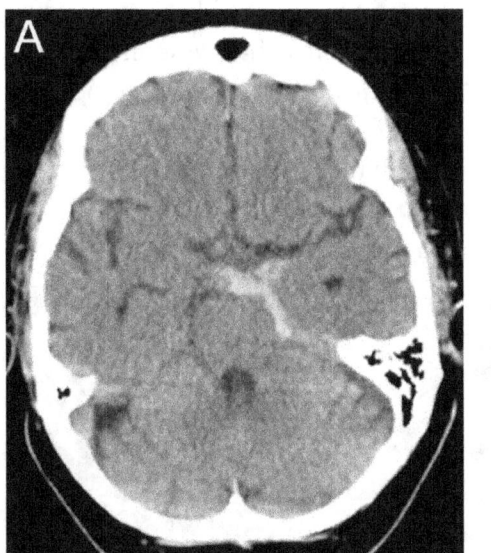 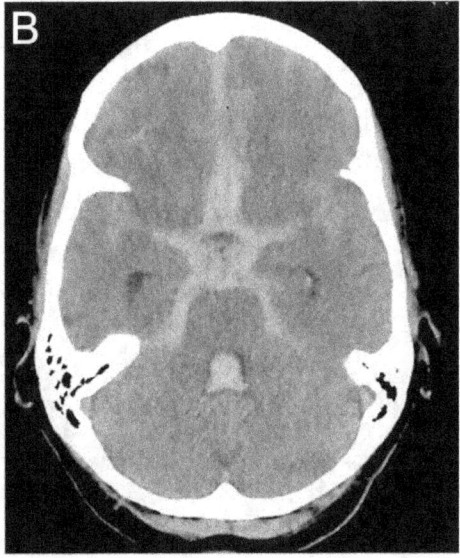

(A). PMVSAH predominantly within the prepontine and ambient cistern, lateralized to one side of the pons and does not extend into the Sylvian fissures as seen in a SAH (B).

FIGURE 19. Basilar Tip Aneurysm Lumen Identified Within Subarachnoid Hemorrhage (SAH)

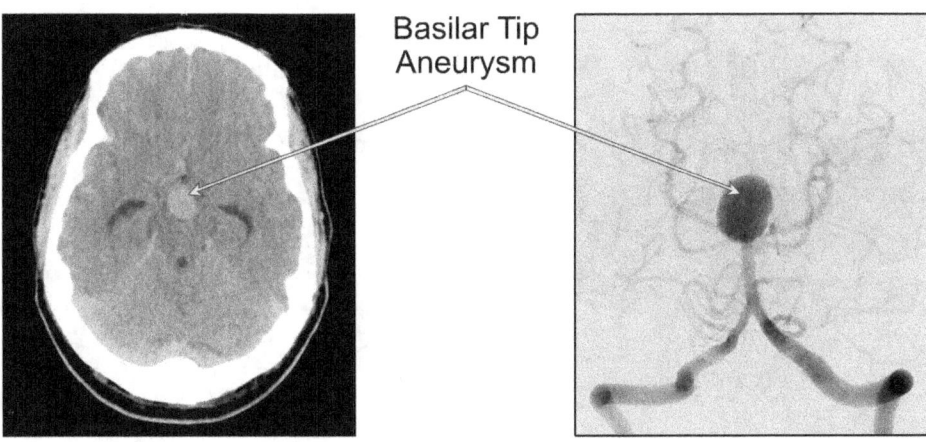

Vasculitis or inflammation of brain arteries can be associated with viral or bacterial infections and autoimmune diseases such as systemic lupus erythematosus. Despite its etiology, vasculitis typically involves medium and small size vessels that are superficially located. When vessels within the brain are affected by vasculitis, they typically have a "sausage link" pattern angiographic appearance. This pattern tends to have smoother, more fusiform regions of narrowing and dilation compared to the discrete plaque morphology identified with atherosclerotic disease (Figure 20). Because the walls of these superficially located blood vessels are weakened, they can bleed and cause a *superficially* located SAH pattern (Figure 20).

Another entity that can affect superficial vessels and cause a superficial appearance of SAH is a mycotic aneurysm or microbial arteritis. A mycotic aneurysm arises from an infection that involves a blood vessel in the brain. For example, a mycotic aneurysm can be a complication of hematogenous spread of a bacterial infection. Mycotic aneurysms are distinct from saccular, intracranial aneurysms that were discussed earlier. Saccular intracranial aneurysms arise from arteries located more centrally around the Circle of Willis, whereas mycotic aneurysms tend to involve smaller, more superficially located vessels. Furthermore, intracranial aneurysms arise from arterial bifurcations like those within the Circle of Willis. Mycotic aneurysms, on the other hand, are caused by an infection of the arterial wall rather than hemodynamic stress. They tend to involve more distal, superficial arteries and need not be located at arterial bifurcations (Figure 21). Due to their superficial location, ruptured mycotic aneurysms, just like vasculitis, tend to have a more superficial SAH pattern typically identified within the convexities of the brain (Figure 22). Another entity that can present with a superficial SAH pattern is a venous infarct.

FIGURE 20. Vasculitis "Sausage-Link" Vascular Pattern and Superficial SAH Distribution

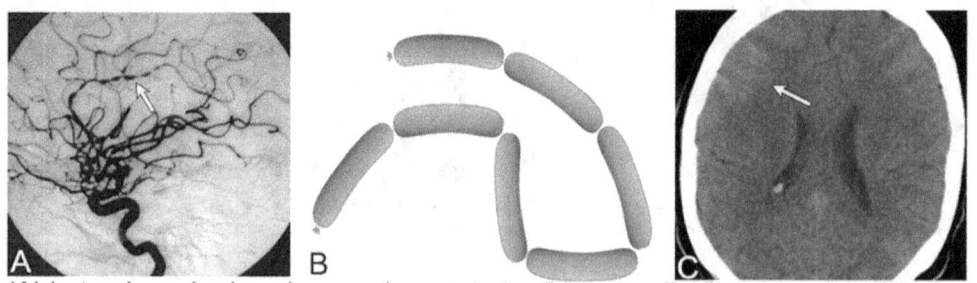

(A) Lateral cerebral angiogram demonstrates "sausage link" appearance (B) of vasculitis. (C) Axial CT demonstrates superficial subarachnoid hemorrhage (SAH) characteristic of vasculitis.

FIGURE 21. Mycotic Aneurysm

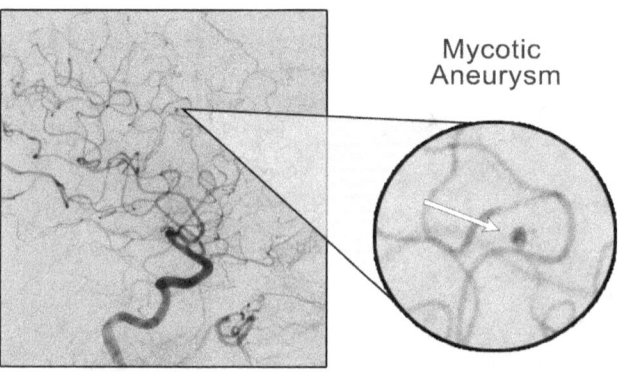

FIGURE 22. Superficial Subarachnoid Hemorrhage Pattern of Mycotic Aneurysm

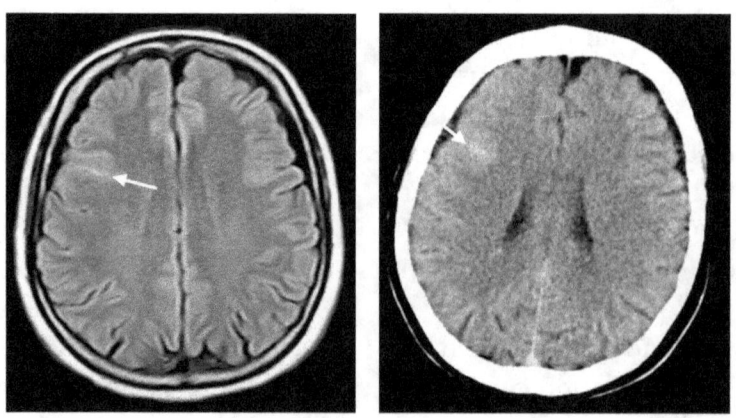

6.6 Intracerebral Hemorrhage (ICH) Score

The intracerebral hemorrhage (ICH) score is a clinical grading scale based upon the evaluation of the Glasgow Coma Scale (GCS) score, ICH volume, presence of intraventricular hemorrhage (IVH), age, and infratentorial origin.[1] The ICH score stratifies intracerebral hemorrhage risk and predicts 30-day mortality (Table 2). The ICH score also serves as a standardized and consistent clinical grading scale for ICH, improving communication and management between clinicians.

6.7 Summary

This concludes the discussion of hemorrhagic stroke. Every AIS patient receives a noncontrast brain CT and about 10% of them will have intracranial hemorrhage. Intracranial hemorrhage will typically involve the brain parenchyma (ICH) or its surface (SAH). Remember, intracranial hemorrhage (within the skull) is not the same as ICH (hemorrhage within the brain parenchyma). ICH in a superficial distribution suggests CAA whereas a more central or deep distribution indicates hypertensive hemorrhage. Similarly, SAH can also present with a central or superficial distribution. Typically, ruptured intracranial aneurysms and PMVSAH tend to involve vascular structures located centrally within the brain, resulting in a central distribution of SAH. Entities involving more superficial arteries such as vasculitis, mycotic aneurysms, and venous infarcts tend to have a more superficial SAH pattern. The ability to discern a parenchymal and subarachnoid hemorrhage based upon a superficial or central distribution will greatly aid in determining the etiology of intracranial hemorrhage (Figure 23).

TABLE 2. The Intracerebral Hemorrhage (ICH) Score

Variables		Score
GCS	3 to 4	2
	5 to 12	1
	13 to 15	0
ICH VOL	≥30 cm3	1
	<30 cm3	0
IV Extension	Present	1
	Absent	0
Infratentorial Origin	Yes	1
	No	0
Age	≥80	1
	<80	0

Source: Hemphill, J. C., Bonovich, D. C., Besmertis, L., Manley, G. T., Johnston, S. C., & Tuhrim, S. (2001). The ICH Score: A Simple, Reliable Grading Scale for Intracerebral Hemorrhage Editorial Comment: A Simple, Reliable Grading Scale for Intracerebral Hemorrhage. Stroke, 32(4), 891-897. doi:10.1161/01.str.32.4.891

FIGURE 23. Superficial and Deep Location of Intracranial Hemorrhage (ICH)

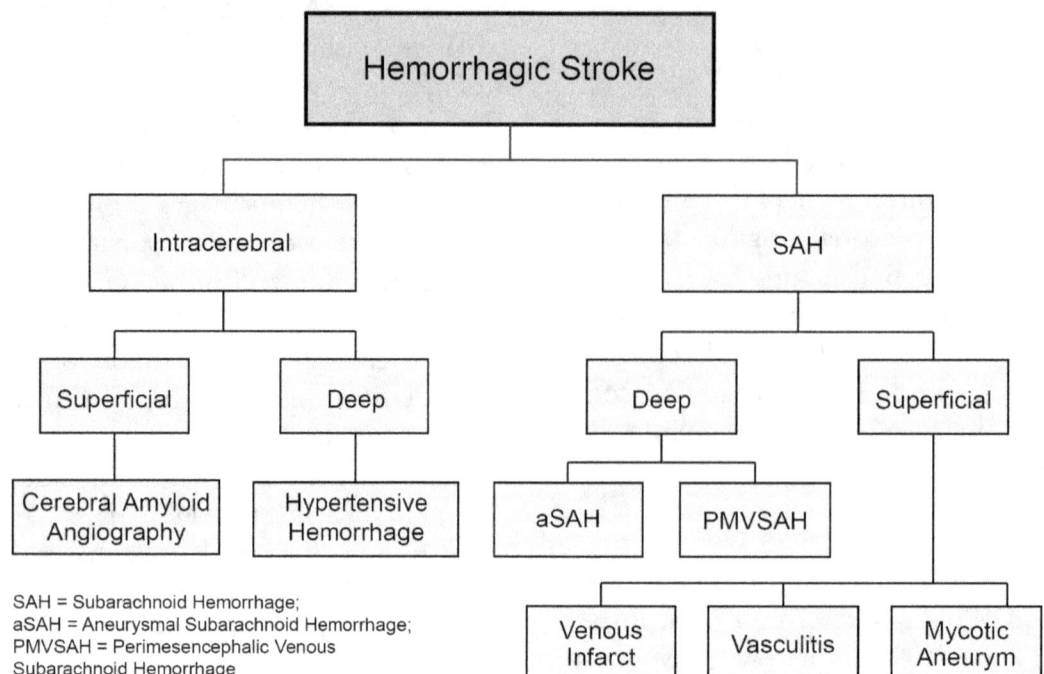

Abbreviations list

AIS, acute ischemic stroke; aSAH, aneurysmal SAH; CAA, cerebral amyloid angiopathy; ESUS, embolic strokes of undetermined source; GCS, Glasgow Coma Scale; HH, hypertensive hemorrhage; ICH, intracerebral hemorrhage; IVH, intraventricular hemorrhage; PMVSAH, perimesencephalic venous subarachnoid hemorrhage; SAH, subarachnoid hemorrhage.

References

1. Hemphill JC 3rd, Bonovich DC, Besmertis L, Manley GT, Johnston SC. (2001), The ICH score: a simple, reliable grading scale for intracerebral hemorrhage. *Stroke*. Apr., 32(4), 891-7.

Chapter 7

Cerebral Aneurysms

7.1 Introduction

Subarachnoid hemorrhage caused by ruptured intracranial aneurysms represents a form of hemorrhagic stroke. However, prior to discussing aneurysmal subarachnoid hemorrhage (aSAH), a brief description of intracranial aneurysms is required. Saccular intracranial aneurysms are focal expansions or outpouchings of cerebral arteries (Figure 1). Intracranial aneurysms are commonly referred to as "berry" aneurysms because they usually have a berry-like shape. Aneurysms typically occur at arterial branch points, particularly around the Circle of Willis (Figure 2). Approximately 10 million to 12 million Americans have intracranial aneurysms.[1,2] However, an estimated 50%-80% of all aneurysms are small and do not rupture during a person's lifetime.[3] Intracranial aneurysms are believed to arise from a combination of prolonged hemodynamic stress and alterations in flow, which eventually form an aneurysmal lumen and are thus considered to be sporadic acquired lesions. Conditions associated with intracranial aneurysms include polycystic kidney disease, fibromuscular dysplasia, Marfan syndrome, Ehlers-Danlos syndrome, and arteriovenous malformations of the brain.

FIGURE 1. Intracranial Aneurysm

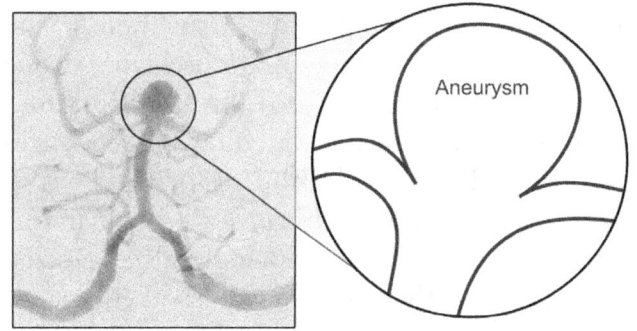

FIGURE 2. Circle of Willis

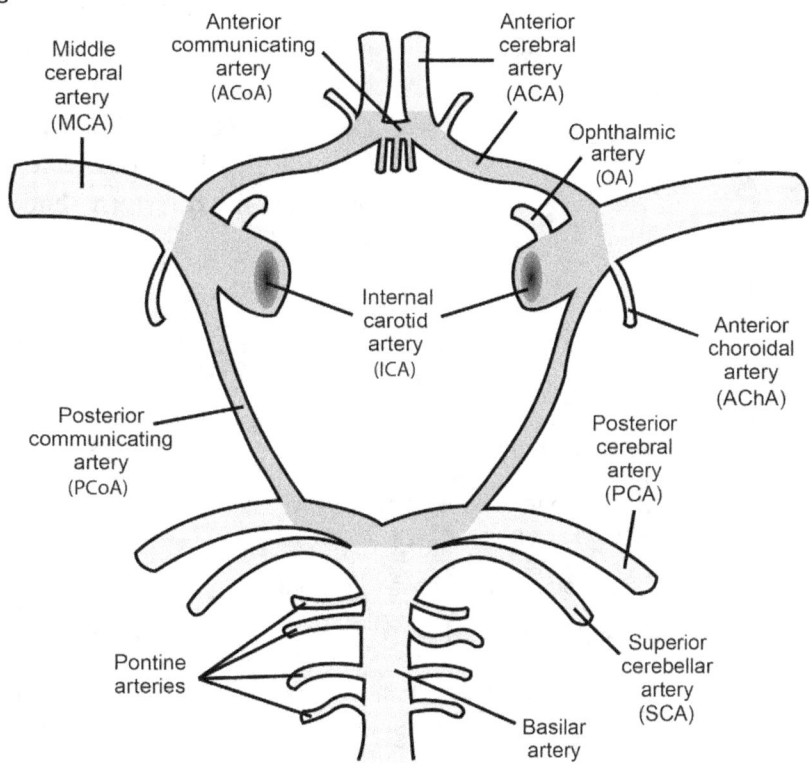

7.2 Ruptured Intracranial Aneurysms

A ruptured intracranial aneurysm causes SAH, a form of hemorrhagic stroke. As discussed in Chapter 6 (Hemorrhagic Stroke), aSAH represents approximately 3% of all stroke cases. Intracranial saccular aneurysms are the most common cause of *non-traumatic* SAH. The incidence of ruptured aneurysms and SAH in the United States is one case per 10,000 persons, resulting in 27,000 cases of aSAH annually.[4] The peak incidence occurs in patients 55-60 years old and SAH is twice as common in women as men.[5,6] This form of hemorrhagic stroke is particularly concerning because it has a 30-day mortality rate of 45%, with 30% of survivors suffering moderate to severe disability.[7,8]

Patients with aSAH typically present with a sudden and severe headache, often described as the "worst headache of my life." Usually, headache is an uncommon presentation for ischemic stroke (except for dissection-related stroke). Ruptured brain aneurysms have devastating consequences dictated by the **Rule of Thirds**: One-third of patients will die before reaching the hospital, another third will have permanent neurological deficits, and only half of the last third will have minimal or no permanent disability (Figure 3).[9]

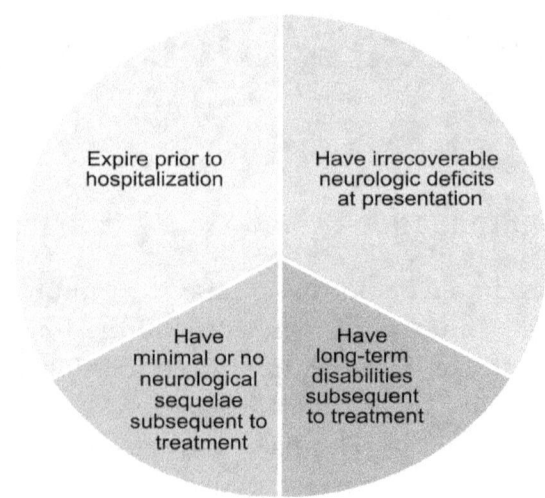

FIGURE 3. Aneurysmal Subarachnoid Hemorrhage (aSAH) Rule of Thirds

7.3 Clinical Assessment of Aneurysmal Subarachnoid Hemorrhage (aSAH)

The clinical presentation of aSAH is related to the volume of hemorrhage within the subarachnoid space irritating the surrounding meninges, as well as its degree of mass effect. This clinical severity is described to be the strongest predictor of functional outcome and can be quickly determined by implementing the Hunt-Hess grading scale (Table 1).[10] Poor-grade aSAH (Hunt-Hess ≥ 4) patients have mortality rates of greater than 70%. Most ruptured intracranial aneurysms have a central distribution of SAH in the suprasellar cistern because this is where the Circle of Willis is located (Figure 4). The suprasellar cistern is a cerebrospinal fluid-filled cistern that contains the Circle of Willis (Figure 5).

TABLE 1. The Hunt-Hess Scale

Grade	Clinical Features	Mortality Outcome
I	Asymptomatic or mild headache	11
II	Moderate to severe headache, or with oculomotor palsy	26
III	Confused, drowsy, or mild focal signs	37
IV	Stupor (localizes pain)	71
V	Coma (posturing or no motor response)	100

Source: Hunt, William E., and Robert M. Hess. "Surgical Risk as Related to Time of Intervention in the Repair of Intracranial Aneurysms." *Journal of Neurosurgery* 28.1 (1968): 14-20.

FIGURE 4. Aneurysms and the Circle of Willis

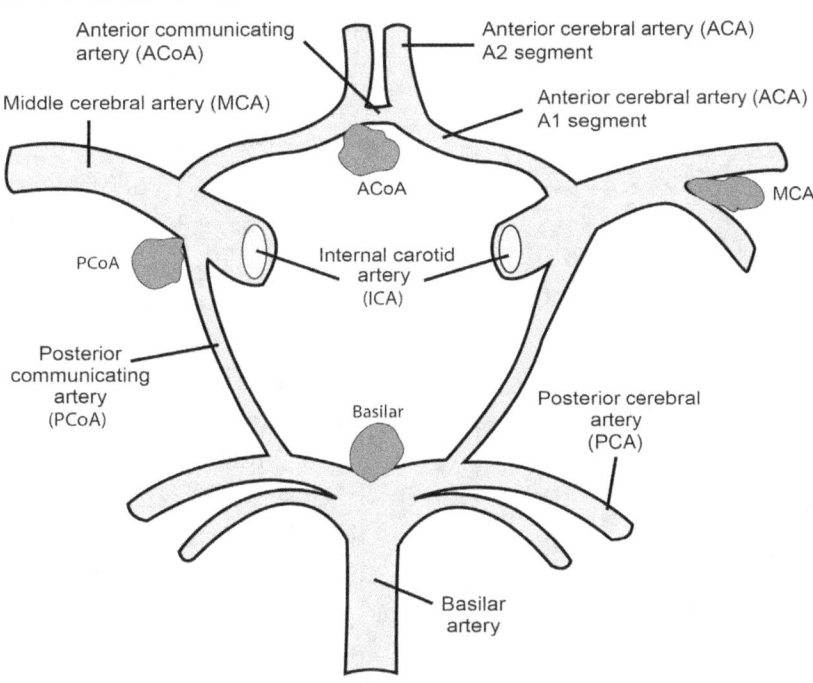

FIGURE 5. Normal Cisternal Anatomy

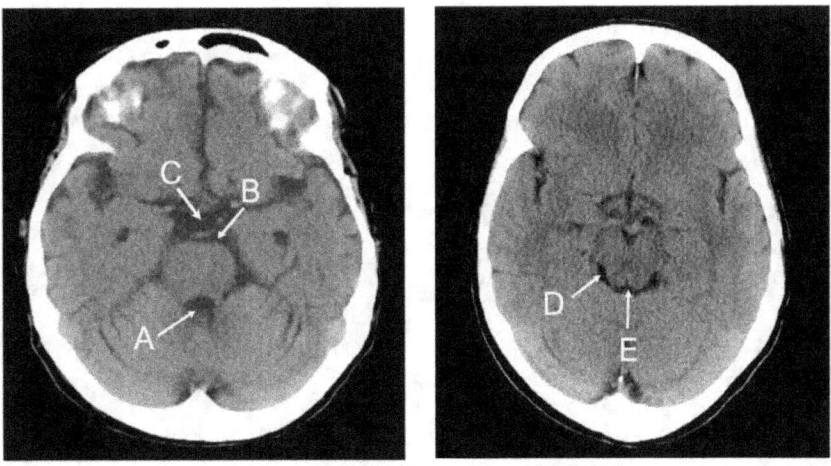

Normal cisterns and fourth ventricle. A) Fourth ventricle B) Prepontine cistern C) Suprasellar cistern D) Right ambient cistern E) Quadrigimenal cistern

The Fisher scale can grade the CT appearance of SAH with higher scores predictive of developing symptomatic cerebral vasospasm (Table 2).[11] The mortality rate of aSAH and any form of intracranial hemorrhage can be predicted by the Intracranial Hemorrhage (ICH) Score which is calculated based on several factors: the Glasgow Coma Scale, intracranial hemorrhage volume, the presence or absence of intraventricular extension, infratentorial location, and age (Table 3).

TABLE 2. The Fisher Scale

Points	Description
0	Unruptured
1	No blood detected
2	Diffuse or vertical layers <1mm thick
3	Clot and/or vertical layer >1mm thick
4	Intracerebral or intraventricular clot

TABLE 3. The Intracranial Hemorrhage (ICH) Score

Variables		Score
GCS	3 to 4	2
	5 to 12	1
	13 to 15	0
ICH VOL	≥30 cm3	1
	<30 cm3	0
IV Extension	Present	1
	Absent	0
Infratentorial Origin	Yes	1
	No	0
Age	≥80	1
	<80	0

Source: Hemphill, J. C., Bonovich, D. C., Besmertis, L., Manley, G. T., Johnston, S. C., & Tuhrim, S. (2001). The ICH Score: A Simple, Reliable Grading Scale for Intracerebral Hemorrhage Editorial Comment: A Simple, Reliable Grading Scale for Intracerebral Hemorrhage. *Stroke*, 32(4), 891-897. doi:10.1161/01.str.32.4.891

7.4 CSF Analysis

In addition to imaging studies, lumbar puncture and cerebral spinal fluid (CSF) analysis can also diagnose SAH. Typically, lumbar puncture should be performed six hours after symptom onset to ensure blood cells from the CSF have reached the lumbar region. Four separate sterile tubes are required for analysis, specifically looking for red blood cell (RBC) count in all four tubes.

A consistently high RBC count in all four tubes and xanthrochromia are indicative of subarachnoid hemorrhage. Degraded RBC products within CSF result in a yellowish discoloration of the CSF termed *xanthrochromia*. This is detected by spectrophotometric analysis which has a specificity of 97%, compared to visual inspection which has a specificity of only 29%.[12] Xanthochromia is present in nearly 100% of all cases of SAH after 12 hours and still remains in 70% at three weeks.[13] A traumatic tap initially contains no xanthochromia (but can be present in subsequent lumbar punctures from an initial traumatic tap). Therefore, any blood-tinged lumbar puncture performed after 12 hours without xanthrochromia that is confirmed by spectro-photometric analysis should be considered traumatic, unless proven otherwise.

Consistently high RBC counts in all four CSF collection tubes are also indicative of SAH. In contrast, a traumatic tap would contain many RBCs in the first CSF collection tube and far less in the fourth tube. A CSF analysis with a high number of RBCs in all four collection tubes and xanthrochromia is consistent with SAH until proven otherwise (Table 4). **To effectively test for SAH, four CSF collection tubes are always necessary.** CSF analysis is particularly useful in patients who arrive at the hospital and are evaluated days after symptom onset. In these cases, a brain CT scan will have diminished sensitivity because, over time, blood products can disperse within the CSF.

TABLE 4. Subarachnoid Hemorrhage (SAH) Versus Traumatic Lumbar Puncture

Analysis	SAH	Traumatic Lumbar Puncture
RBC - 4 tubes	Same RBCs	Diminishing RBCs
Supernatant post-centrifuge	Xanthochromic	Clear

RBC = Red Blood Cell

7.5 Imaging

When dealing with *acute* SAH, brain CT is a very sensitive modality with some studies reporting a 100% sensitivity within five days of symptom onset. Brain CT also has an overall sensitivity of 99.7% and a specificity of 100%.[14] In fact, a recent study concluded that CSF analysis had no additional value in patients presenting with acute headaches and a normal head CT within six hours of symptom onset.[15] The authors could effectively diagnose all patients with aneurysmal and perimesencephalic SAH by brain CT alone. However, it is this author's opinion that due to the enormous consequences of a "missed" brain aneurysm, patients presenting with classic signs of aSAH and a negative brain CT should still receive a lumbar puncture for CSF analysis.

CT angiography (CTA) has several advantages over digital subtraction angiography (DSA) for the detection of ruptured intracranial aneurysms.

These include its noninvasive nature, increased availability, lower risk, easier access, and shorter time requirements for unstable patients.[16] However, CTA still has **one critical flaw** in that its sensitivity continues to be less than 90% for the detection of aneurysms less than 3 mm in size.[17] As stated earlier, due to the enormous consequences of a "missed" brain aneurysm, patients presenting with a CT appearance of aSAH pattern and a negative CTA should still receive a cerebral angiogram.

Brain CT and CTA are typically more sensitive in detecting aSAH and ruptured intracranial aneurysms compared to MRI and MRA, with one important exception: MRI has a greater sensitivity (91%-100%) than CT in the detection of SAH **five days after** symptom onset utilizing gradient echo sequencing (Figure 6).[18] MRI can also determine non-aneurysmal sources of SAH such as cavernous malformations, dural sinus venous thrombosis, and spinal cord vascular malformations.

Cerebral angiography remains the gold standard for the detection of ruptured intracranial aneurysms, particularly smaller ones. Now commonly used in clinical practice, 3D rotational angiography is the optimal diagnostic method. Cerebral angiography has greater sensitivity (90.9%) for the detection of intracranial aneurysms less than 3 mm than either CTA or MRA.[19]

It is minimally invasive and associated with less than 1% risk of systemic or neurologic complications. There is, however, a 2.6% risk of aneurysm re-rupture during a cerebral angiogram performed six hours after the initial SAH.[20] Unsecured ruptured intracranial aneurysms have a short-term rebleed rate of 4% within the first 24 hours and a 1% to 1.5% rate thereafter for each day the aneurysm is not secured. Longer-term rebleed rates for nonsecured intracranial aneurysms approach 50% in six months and then drop to approximately 3% per year thereafter. Fifty percent of unsecured ruptured aneurysm patients who rebleed will expire.[21]

7.6 Clinical Concerns Regarding Ruptured Intracranial Aneurysms

After the diagnosis of a ruptured intracranial aneurysm has been confirmed, there are several clinical concerns that must be addressed. First, hypertension must be controlled (systolic blood pressure less than 130) to prevent re-rupture. The American Heart and Stroke Associations have endorsed the use of nicardipine, labetalol, and esmolol, but cautioned against the use of nitro-prusside which can raise intracranial pressure.[22] A more recent study has also concluded that nicardipine was superior to labetalol for aSAH blood pressure control.[23]

FIGURE 6. Subarachnoid Hemorrhage Detected by Gradient Echo and FLAIR Sequencing

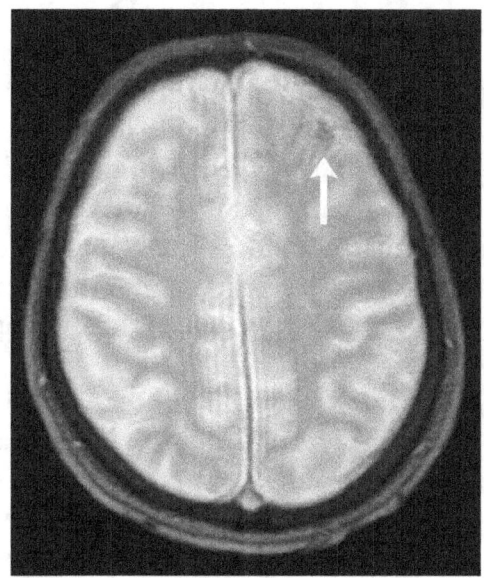
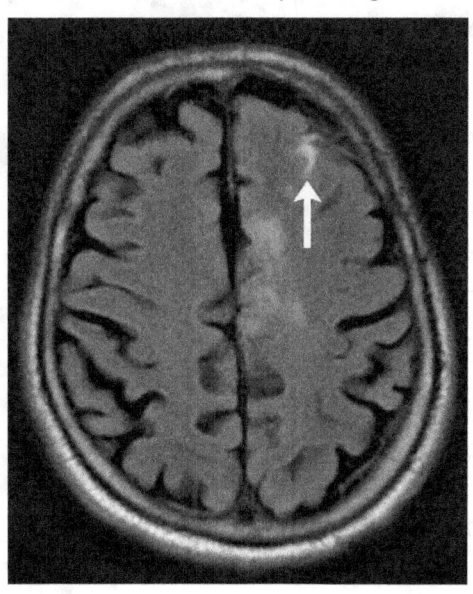

Mass effect and hydrocephalus are also clinical concerns related to ruptured intracranial aneurysms. Hydrocephalus develops in about 15-20% of aneurysmal SAH patients and approximately 40% of these patients will become symptomatic (Figure 7).[6] Hydrocephalus usually results from the obstruction of CSF through the ventricular system by SAH. Factors that raise its probability include poor clinical grade, increased SAH on noncontrast brain CT, and increased age. Symptomatic hydrocephalus requires an external ventricular drain (EVD) to reduce intracranial pressure and prevent brainstem herniation.[24] Aneurysmal SAH seizure prophylaxis with antiepileptic drugs is controversial, and as such, their long-term use should be reserved in high risk patients (intra-parenchymal hematomas, cerebral infarct, and hydrocephalus), noting that prolonged phenytoin prophylaxis is associated with worse outcome.[25-28]

FIGURE 7. Hydrocephalus

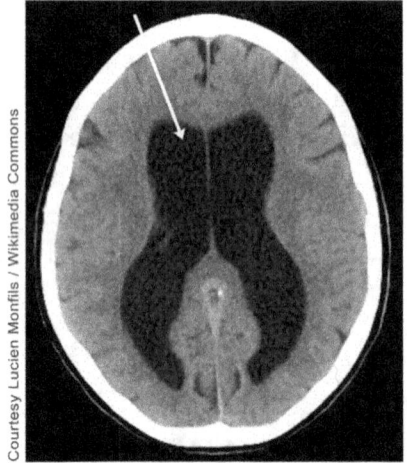

Aneurysmal SAH can be associated with cardiac changes theorized to result from increased central sympathetic activity. This transient increase in sympathetic nervous activity can induce myocardial damage known as "neurogenic stunned myocardium," which may be caused by free radicals or transient calcium overload.[29] Both mechanisms are believed to diminish the response of heart contractile filaments to calcium. This is manifested by electrocardiographic changes, elevation in cardiac enzymes, and left ventricular dysfunction.[30] Thus, neurogenic stunned myocardium is unrelated to coronary artery disease and must be distinguished from the latter since it is a reversible form of cardiac failure. Due to diminished cardiac output and restrictions on hyperdynamic and hypervolemic therapy, there is a high association of delayed cerebral vasospasm. Patients with these conditions are not considered good open surgical candidates and endovascular therapy is recommended. Patient management is largely supportive, with some case reports acknowledging the use of inotropes such as dobutamine and milrinone, as well as intra-aortic balloon pumps in extreme cases.

Abnormalities of salt and water balance are also commonly encountered with aSAH patients. Diabetes insipidus (DI) occurs in approximately 15% of aSAH cases and can be associated with a worse prognosis and increased mortality.[31] DI and resultant hypovolemia may exacerbate vasospasm and worsen aSAH patient outcome. It is essential to ensure adequate fluid replacement to maintain blood volume and, therefore, pressure. The diagnosis of diabetes insipidus is determined by a plasma sodium greater than 145 mmol/liter in the presence of dilute urine (osmolality <300 mOsm/kg) and polyuria (>300ml/h for two consecutive hours or >3 liters/d) as proposed by Seckl et al.[32]

Hyponatremia (sodium level of <135mEq/L) is the most common electrolyte imbalance encountered in aSAH patients, with prevalence values ranging from 30 to 56 percent.[31,33-34] Hyponatremia, which is more common with hydrocephalus and poor clinical grade patients, is an independent risk factor for poor outcome.[31,35] In fact, hyponatremic aSAH patients are 15 times more likely to have a poor outcome.[31,35] There is no significant difference in the incidence of hyponatremia and anatomic location of the ruptured aneurysm, or whether the cerebral aneurysm was treated with open surgical clipping versus endovascular coiling.[36] The poor outcome associated with hyponatremia in aSAH patients necessitates vigilance, timely detection, and appropriate management of this disorder.

The syndrome of inappropriate antidiuretic hormone (SIADH) or cerebral salt wasting (CSW) syndrome are two conditions usually responsible for hyponatremia in aSAH patients. Regardless of the cause, hyponatremia in aSAH patients is associated with a prolonged hospital course, increased morbidity, and increased risk of vasospasm.[34] SIADH, the excessive secretion of antidiuretic hormone, is caused by hypothalamic stimulation causing water reabsorption in the distal convoluted tubule of the kidney, which results in fluid retention and dilutional hyponatremia. On the other hand, CSW is characterized by normal antidiuretic hormone levels but results from urinary sodium excretion causing hyponatremia. Thus, SIADH patients tend to be euvolemic or hypervolemic, while CSW patients are more likely to be hypovolemic. An easy way to remember this is that SIADH (hypervolemic) has more letters than CSW (Box 1).

BOX 1. SIADH Versus CSW

SIADH	More letters	Hypervolemic
CSW	Less letters	Hypovolemic

SIADH - Syndrome of Inappropriate Antidiuretic Hormone
CSW - Cerebral Salt Wasting

Yet, these two conditions are difficult to discern in clinical practice based on this "volume approach" to hyponatremia. In addition, while this approach has been utilized for decades, it is often misleading and inaccurate. For example, central venous pressure (CVP) is considered one of the most reliable and accurate assessments of a patient's volume status. Hypovolemia is considered to be reliably diagnosed when CVP is diminished while hypervolemia leads to an elevated CVP. However, CVP is a poor marker of cardiac filling pressure.[37] The basis of this distinction between hypovolemia and hypervolemia is believed to be critical due to the opposing therapeutic goals of SIADH and CSW: to provide salt and water to a volume-depleted CSW patient and to restrict water in a waterloaded SIADH patient.

However, there are several reasons not to implement fluid restriction when treating an SIADH aSAH patient. First, it is well-known that a significant portion of hyponatremic aSAH patients are incorrectly diagnosed with SIADH, when in fact they have CSW.[38-40] Water restriction in patients who have been incorrectly diagnosed with SIADH (when they actually have CSW) increases both morbidity and mortality rates in aSAH patients.[41-43] Cerebral edema, vasospasm, and subsequent cerebral infarction are also serious concerns in aSAH patients. For these reasons, volume infusion of hypertonic saline will always be favored and is considered routine practice.[44] Fluid restriction in the treatment of hyponatremia in aSAH patients is related to an increased incidence of delayed cerebral ischemia.[35,45] Furthermore, the use of fluid restriction in aSAH patients is associated with an increased risk of cerebral vasospasm.[43,46] Also, while SIADH can be treated by restricting fluid to less than 500 ml/day, many aSAH patients receive enteral tube feeding resulting in fluid intakes of 1 - 2 L daily.

At this point, some readers may still be insistent that they can differentiate SIADH from CSW (even though both conditions, for the reasons stated above, will be treated with hypertonic saline). Fractional excretion of urate can be utilized to differentiate SIADH from CSW. This is determined by dividing the ratio of urine to plasma urate by the ratio of urine to plasma creatinine and multiplying this by 100. In SIADH, correction of hyponatremia will normalize the fractional excretion of urate to 4%-11%, whereas it will be persistently increased to >11% in CSW. So how does one correct hyponatremia to determine the fractional excretion of urate and find out whether the patient has SIADH or CSW? The same way we treat either SIADH or CSW, namely with the administration of hypertonic saline.

Remember, SIADH associated with aSAH in critically ill patients should mandate treatment with hypertonic saline. Water restriction is too slow, may exasperate vasospasm and can be the wrong treatment in patients commonly misdiagnosed with SIADH. Essentially, the treatment for SIADH and CSW is the same: **salt**. Thus, the use of hypertonic saline can be used to treat both SIADH and CSW (being mindful that rapid correction of hyponatremia can lead to osmotic demyelination and fluid overload) (Figure 8). Alternatively, insufficient or delayed correction of hyponatremia can result in cerebral edema, seizures, or even death. Therefore, to reliably diagnose and differentiate SIADH from CSW, hypertonic saline is utilized. By the same token, both conditions can be treated in precisely the same manner.

Cerebral vasospasm is yet another major source of morbidity and mortality in aSAH patients. Blood products associated with aSAH induce an inflammatory reaction which can result in cerebral vasospasm. The risk of cerebral vasospasm increases with the degree of subarachnoid hemorrhage (see the Fisher scale discussed earlier) and is a potential threat for 4 to 21 days after SAH.[47] Cerebral vasospasm can be diagnosed with CTA, transcranial Doppler studies (TCDs), and cerebral angiography. Cerebral angiography remains the gold standard for diagnosis of cerebral vasospasm. However, CTA also has a high sensitivity for its detection. TCDs are operator dependent but typically, only severe cerebral vasospasm can be reliably determined by this method.[22] While a vast array of proposed vasospasm prevention and treatment methods exists, the medical literature supports the prophylactic use of oral nimodipine and triple-H therapy. Nimodipine is the only FDA approved drug for the treatment of cerebral vasospasm.[48] Nimodipine use (60 mg every four hours for 21 days) is associated with a 34% reduction in cerebral infarction and a 40% reduction in poor outcome.[49]

Currently, the mainstay for medical management of aSAH is triple-H therapy which consists of hypertension, hypervolemia, and hemodilution.[50] However, studies suggest there is no significant difference in the rate of cerebral vasospasm or clinical outcomes utilizing triple-H versus euvolemic therapy.[51] An analysis of the different components of triple-H therapy suggests that hypertension is more effective in increasing cerebral blood flow than either hemodilution or hypervolemia.[52] The current American Heart Association guidelines suggest maintenance of euvolemia for vasospasm prevention and induced hypertension for active cerebral vasospasm patients. Hypervolemia without radiographic evidence of vasospasm is also discouraged.[53] To remember the clinical concerns associated with a subarachnoid hemorrhage, use the mnemonic 'SHAVES' (Table 5).

FIGURE 8. Treatment of Hyponatremia in Aneurysmal Subarachnoid Hemorrhage (aSAH)

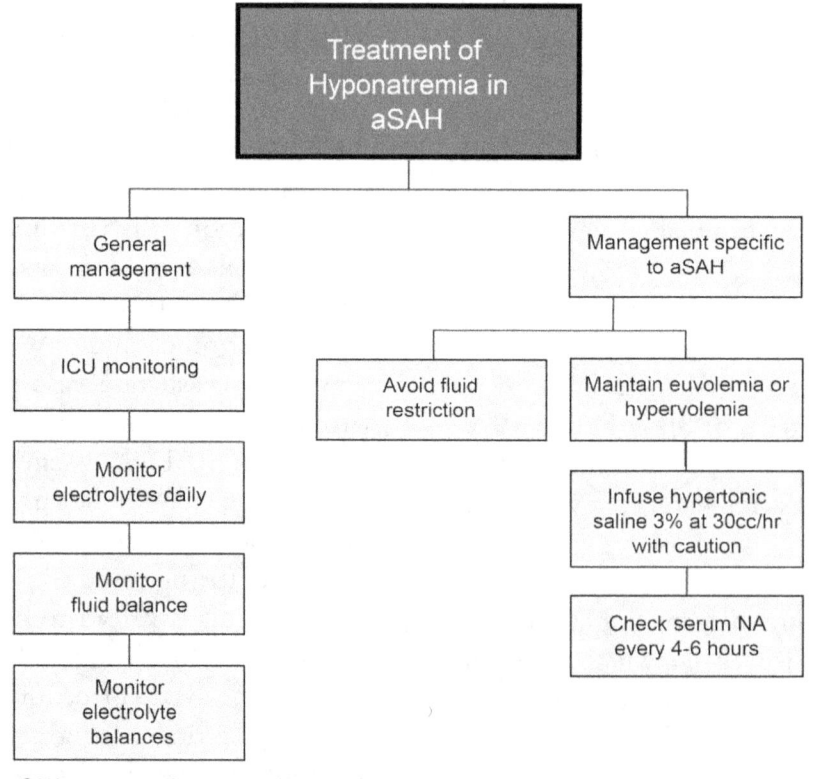

aSAH - aneurysmal subarachnoid hemorrhage

TABLE 5. Aneurysmal SAH Clinical Concerns: **SHAVES**

S	Seizure - No Prolonged Phenytoin Use
H	Hydrocephalus and Mass Effect
A	A Stunned Myocardium
V	Vasospasm; 4-21 Days, Use Nimodipine
E	Elevated Blood Pressure, Use Nicardipine
S	SIADH Versus CSW

7.7 Aneurysm Rupture Risk

Most intracranial aneurysms are unruptured, asymptomatic, and usually found incidentally. However, unruptured aneurysms may occasionally be diagnosed based on symptoms from aneurysmal mass effect causing cranial nerve palsies or other deficits. For example, a posterior communicating artery (PCoA) aneurysm can exert mass effect on the third cranial nerve (CN III) and cause a third nerve palsy. Signs of CN III involvement include deviation of the ipsilateral eye laterally (lateral or divergent strabismus) caused by unopposed action of the lateral rectus muscle, ptosis (drooping of the upper eyelid), mydriasis (dilated pupil), and accommodation paralysis from interruption of the CN III parasympathetic fibers (Figure 9). Symptomatic unruptured intracranial aneurysms should be treated. However, no established protocol exists for the management of unruptured, asymptomatic intracranial aneurysms. This problem is further compounded by anxiety over the 50% mortality rate of a ruptured intracranial aneurysm.

The International Study of Unruptured Intracranial Aneurysms (ISUIA) was a large multicenter, prospective cohort study which examined the behavior of unruptured intracranial aneurysms. It was performed in 60 centers in the United States, Canada, and Europe.[54] In this study, the rates of aneurysm rupture were reported as a five-year cumulative rupture rate based on the size and location of the unruptured aneurysm (Table 6). However, this study has been met with some criticism. For example, according to ISUIA data, patients with small anterior circulation (less than 7 mm) have a rupture rate of zero. However, anyone practicing in this field has treated ruptured aneurysms in the anterior circulation which are less than 7 mm in size. To this point, subsequent studies have shown higher rates of rupture for unruptured intracranial aneurysms than ISUIA.[55, 56]

FIGURE 9. Posterior Communicating Artery Aneurysm and Third Cranial Nerve

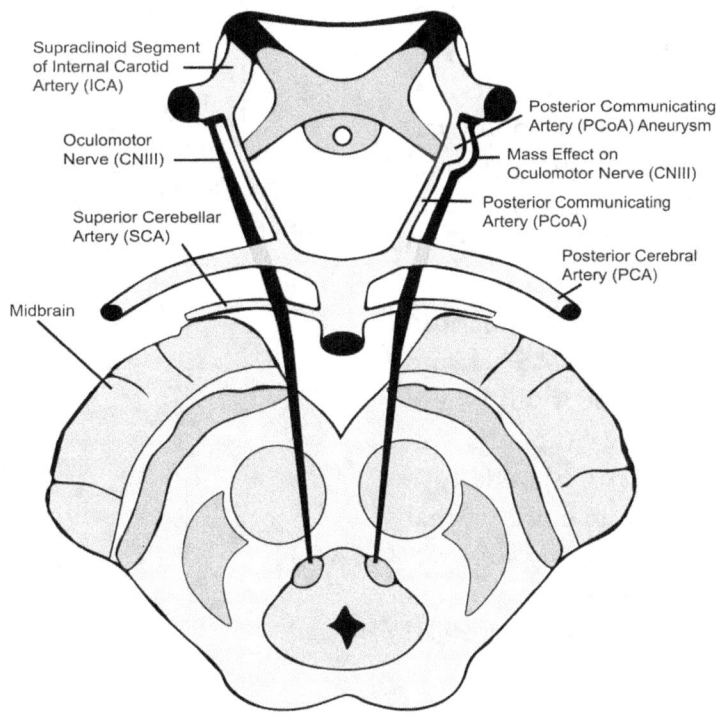

TABLE 6. The International Study of Unruptured Intracranial Aneurysms (ISUIA) and Five-Year Cumulative Rupture Risk

Location	Rupture Rate By Aneurysm Size				
	<7mm		7-12mm	13-24mm	≥25mm
	Group 1	Group 2			
Cavernous carotid artery	0	0	0	3.0%	6.4%
Anterior circulation*	0	1.5%	2.5%	14.5%	40%
Posterior circulation**	2.5%	3.4%	14.5%	18.4%	50%

*Includes anterior cerebral circulation (anterior communicating, middle cerebral artery and internal carotid artery aneurysms).

**Includes posterior cerebral circulation (vertebrobasilar and posterior communicating artery aneurysms).

Source: Wiebers DO, Whisnant JP, Huston J 3rd, et al. Unruptured intracranial aneurysms: natural history, clinical outcome, and risks of surgical and endovascular treatment. Lancet 2003;362(9378):103-110.

So how is this discrepancy resolved? One solution is the development of the PHASES score.[57] The PHASES score was developed after a systematic review and pooled analysis from six prospective cohort studies analyzing aSAH as an outcome in 8,382 participants. The authors of this study prefaced that limitations in current knowledge of the natural history of incidentally encountered, nonruptured, intracranial saccular aneurysms make the risk of rupture difficult to determine. Nonetheless, they developed the PHASES score consisting of six predictors of prognostic outcome: age, presence of hypertension, prior history of subarachnoid hemorrhage, current aneurysm size, aneurysmal location and geographical region. Each one of these variables is assigned a point value, and all are added together to obtain a total risk score (Table 7). The PHASES risk score corresponds to a five-year cumulative risk of aneurysm rupture (Table 8).

For example, a 75-year-old North American man with no hypertension, no previous SAH, and a 9mm middle cerebral artery aneurysm would have a risk score of 1+0+0+0+3+2= 6 points. According to Table 8, this score corresponds to a five-year rupture risk of 1.7%. Note however, that the degree of risk assessed by this scoring system is only valid for the first five years after aneurysm detection. This risk cannot be extrapolated or added over the patient's remaining lifetime.[58]

TABLE 7. The Phases Score

		POINTS
P	Population • North American • European (Other than Finnish) • Japanese • Finnish	0 0 3 5
H	Hypertension • No • Yes	0 1
A	Age • <70 Years • 70 Years	0 1
S	Size of Aneurysm • <7.0 mm • 7.0-9.9 mm • 10.0-19.9 mm • ≥20 mm	0 3 6 10
E	Earlier SAH from Another Aneurysm • No • Yes	0 1
S	Site of Aneurysm • ICA • MCA • ACA/PCoA/Posterior	0 2 4

TABLE 8. PHASES: 5-Year Cumulative Risk of Aneurysm Rupture

PHASES Risk Score	5-Year Cumulative Risk of Aneurysm Rupture
≤2	0.4%
3	0.7%
4	0.9%
5	1.3%
6	1.7%
7	2.4%
8	3.2%
9	4.3%
10	5.3%
11	7.2%
≥12	17.8%

7.8 Cerebral Aneurysm Treatment

There are three treatment options for both ruptured and unruptured intracranial aneurysms: (1) observation (no treatment), (2) open surgical clipping, and (3) minimally invasive endovascular treatment. Determining which option to pursue depends on multiple factors such as the patient's age, existing premorbid conditions, the location of the aneurysm, the aneurysm neck-to-dome ratio, and the experience and competence of hospital staff in its ability to perform these procedures. However, both surgical clipping and endovascular treatment have the same two goals. First, the aneurysm must be disconnected from its parent artery. Second, the patency of the parent artery must be preserved (Figure 10). Anything that compromises the patency of the parent vessel can potentially result in stroke. Whatever treatment option is decided, the risks associated with a particular treatment must be balanced against the risk of aneurysm rupture.[59]

Surgical clipping involves placing a metallic surgical clip (resembling a miniature clothes pin) across the neck of the aneurysm (Figure 10). This clip "pinches" the neck of the aneurysm, thereby disconnecting it from the parent artery (goal 1). By placing the clip on the aneurysm neck, the patency of the parent artery is preserved (goal 2). Open surgical clipping tends to have a higher risk of complications but has lower aneurysm recurrence rates than coil embolization.[60] Intracranial aneurysms can also be treated by a variety of endovascular methods. The oldest and most common method is endovascular coil embolization (Figure 10). If an aneurysm is endovascularly coil embolized, the coiled aneurysm is disconnected from the parent circulation yet the patency of the parent artery is preserved (achieving goals 1 and 2). The endovascular treatment of intracranial aneurysms carries approximately a 5% risk of combined treatment-related fatality and morbidity.[61]

Sometimes, intracranial stents are used to assist coil embolization of wide-necked aneurysms (Figure 11). This is because without a supporting stent, coils can protrude from the lumen of a widenecked aneurysm and enter the parent artery circulation. If this happens, overhanging coil segments can interfere with blood flow in the parent vessel and potentially result in a stroke. For this reason, stent-assisted techniques are employed to maintain coils within the aneurysm lumen, preserving parent artery patency and preventing disruption of parent artery laminar blood flow. Newer *flow diversion* devices are also used for embolization (Figure 12). These stent-like devices (Pipeline® device) are placed across the neck of an aneurysm to divert flow away from the aneurysm lumen, causing it to eventually thrombose.

FIGURE 10. Treatment Options for Intracranial Aneurysms

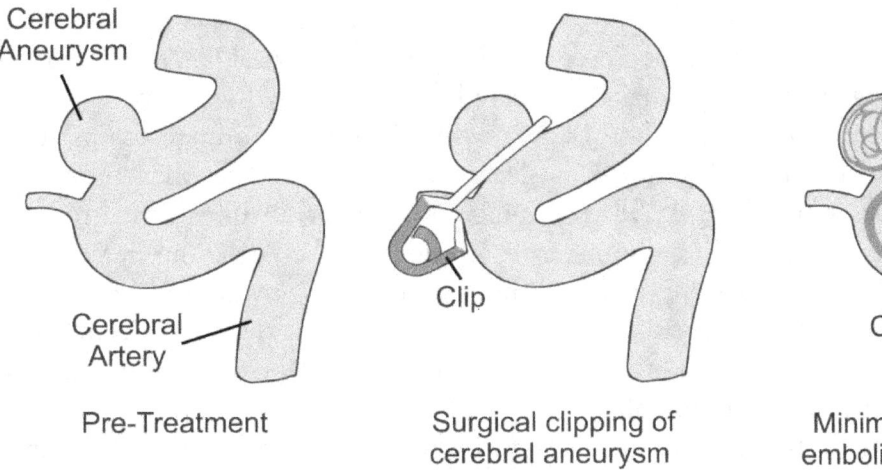

FIGURE 11. Stent Assisted Coil Embolization

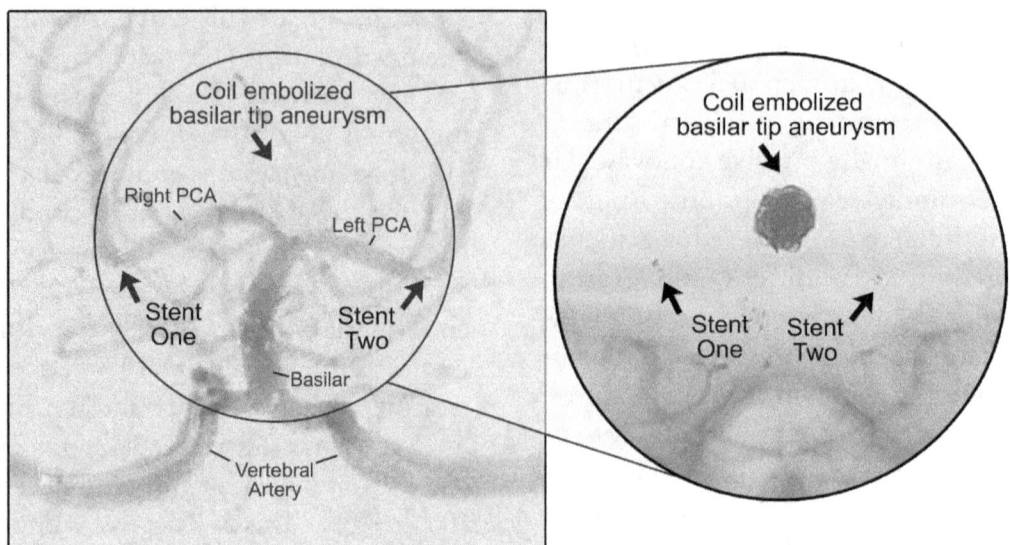

FIGURE 12. Pipeline® Embolization

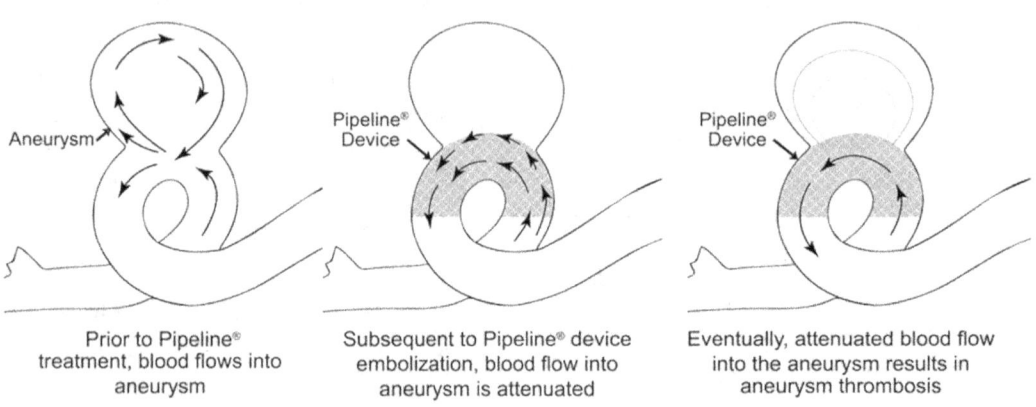

There are multiple considerations when determining which method of aneurysm repair to pursue. Aggressive management is recommended in all ruptured aneurysms absent brain death.[64] The minimally invasive nature of endovascular coil embolization is associated with less physiologic stress compared to open surgical clipping, making this technique the primary treatment method for ruptured intracranial aneurysms.[62] The International Subarachnoid Aneurysm Trial (ISAT) demonstrated that minimally invasive coil embolization of ruptured intracranial aneurysms was safer than open surgical clipping (reduced risk of functional dependency and death).[63] Several other retrospective studies demonstrated that minimally invasive coil embolization of both ruptured and unruptured intracranial aneurysms is safer than open surgical clipping.[64-66]

Based on this data, it seems coil embolization would be the treatment choice for all intracranial aneurysms. However, coil embolization is not without its limitations. Intracranial aneurysms treated with minimally invasive coil embolization have a higher recurrence rate (20.9%-33.6%) when compared to those treated with open surgical clipping (1.5%).[67, 68] While minimally invasive coil embolization may appear safer than open surgical clipping, this higher aneurysm recurrence rate must be considered when deciding treatment. However, the significance of recurrence has yet to be determined because the degree of recurrence does not correlate with the incidence of hemorrhage.

When treating saccular, intracranial aneurysms, the ideal choice would be a method that not only has the low risk of minimally invasive endovascular coil embolization, but also maintains the low recurrence rate of open surgical clipping. Endovascular flow diversion devices may offer such a treatment option. Flow-diverting devices have an increased metallic surface area (30%-50%) and decreased porosity which causes blood flow to be directed away from the aneurysm. These devices also maintain parent vessel and adjacent perforator vessel patency. Over time, this method reconstructs the parent vessel from the inside (endoluminal reconstruction), resulting in endothelialization of the device's interstices rather than endovascular filling of the aneurysm lumen (Figure 12).[69] These devices are deployed as a minimally invasive procedure and thus have a lower complication risk similar to minimally invasive endovascular coil embolization. Additionally, these devices have a lower recurrence rate similar to surgical clipping (Table 9).[70] Flow diversion devices are a great option in the treatment of intracranial aneurysms not only because they have a relatively low procedural risk (similar to minimally invasive endovascular coil embolization), but also because they have a low recurrence rate (similar to open surgical clipping).

TABLE 9. Risk and Recurrence Trends for Surgical Clipping, Coil Embolization and Flow Diversion

	Risk	Recurrence
Open surgical clipping	↑er	↓er
Coil embolization	↓er	↑er
Flow diversion	↓er	↓er

7.9 Conclusion

This chapter reviewed both ruptured and unruptured cerebral aneurysms. A ruptured cerebral aneurysm results in aSAH, a form of hemorrhagic stroke which is associated with very high mortality. Every successful stroke center requires a multidisciplinary team approach, which is certainly relevant for the successful management of aSAH. Aneurysmal SAH patients have very poor probabilities of achieving a good functional outcome. They have devastating presentations which typically involve complex management. A team approach is thus required to optimize every aspect of this horrendous form of hemorrhagic stroke.

Abbreviations list

aSAH, aneurysmal subarachnoid hemorrhage; CN III, third cranial nerve; CSF, cerebral spinal fluid; CSW, cerebral salt wasting; CTA, CT angiography; CVP, central venous pressure; DI, diabetes insipidus; DSA, digital subtraction angiography; EVD, external ventricular drain; ICH, intracranial hemorrhage; PCoA, posterior communicating artery; RBC, red blood cell; SAH, subarachnoid hemorrhage; SIADH, syndrome of inappropriate antidiuretic hormone; TCDs, transcranial Doppler studies.

References

1. Wiebers DO, Whisnant JP, Huston J III, et al. (2003). Unruptured intracranial aneurysms: natural history, clinical outcome, and risks of surgical and endovascular treatment. *Lancet*, 362, 103-10.
2. Schievink WI. (1997). Intracranial aneurysms. *N Engl J Med*, 336, 28-40, Erratum, *N Engl J Med*, 336, 1267.
3. Connolly ES, Solomon RA. (2004). Management of unruptured aneurysms. In: Le Roux PD, Winn HR, Newell DW, eds. *Management of cerebral aneurysms*. Philadelphia: Saunders, 271-85.
4. Wijdicks EF, Kallmes DF, Manno EM, Fulgham JR, Piepgras DG. (2005). Subarachnoid hemorrhage: neurointensive care and aneurysm repair. *Mayo Clin Proc*, 80, 550-59.
5. Stapf C, Mohr JP. (2004). Aneurysms and subarachnoid hemorrhage — epidemiology. In: Le Roux PD, Winn HR, Newell DW, eds. *Management of cerebral aneurysms*. Philadelphia: Saunders, 183-7.
6. Greenberg MS. (2000). SAH and aneurysms. In: Greenberg MS, ed. *Handbook of neurosurgery*. 5th ed. New York: Thieme Medical, 754-803.
7. Bederson JB, Awad IA, Wiebers DO, et al. (2000). Recommendations for the management of patients with unruptured intracranial aneurysms: a statement for healthcare professionals

from the Stroke Council of the American Heart Association. *Stroke*, 31, 2742-50.
8. Johnston SC, Selvin S, Gress DR. (1998). The burden, trends, and demographics of mortality from subarachnoid hemorrhage. *Neurology*, 5:1413-18.
9. Washington CW, Vellimana AK, Zipfel GJ, Dacey RG. (2011). The current surgical management of intracranial aneurysms. *J Neurosurg Sci*, Sep, 55(3), 211-31.
10. Hunt WE, Hess RM. (1968). Surgical risk as related to time of intervention in the repair of intracranial aneurysms. *J Neurosurg*, Jan, 28(1), 14-20.
11. Frontera JA, Claassen J, Schmidt JM, Wartenberg KE, Temes R, Connolly ES Jr. (2006). Prediction of symptomatic vasospasm after subarachnoid hemorrhage: the modified fisher scale. *Neurosurgery*, Jul, 59(1), 21-7.
12. Perry JJ, Sivilotti MLA, Stiell IG, Wells GA, Raymond J, Mortensen M. (2006). Should spectrophotometry be used to identify xanthochromia in the cerebrospinal fluid of alert patients suspected of having subarachnoid hemorrhage? *Stroke*, Oct, 37(10), 2467-72.
13. Vermeulen M, Hasan D, Blijenberg BG, Hijdra A, van Gijn J. (1989). Xanthochromia after subarachnoid haemorrhage needs no revisitation. *J Neurol Neurosurg Psychiatry*, Jul, 52(7), 826-8.
14. Cortnum S, Sørensen P, Jørgensen J. (2010). Determining the sensitivity of computed tomography scanning in early detection of subarachnoid hemorrhage. *Neurosurgery*, May, 66(5), 900-2; discussion, 903.
15. Backes D, Rinkel GJ, Kemperman H, Linn FH, Vergouwen MD.(2012). Time-dependent test characteristics of head computed tomography in patients suspected of nontraumatic subarachnoid hemorrhage. *Stroke*, Aug, 43(8), 2115-9.
16. Hoh BL, Cheung AC, Rabinov JD, Pryor JC, Carter BS, Ogilvy CS. (2004). Results of a prospective protocol of computed tomographic angiography in place of catheter angiography as the only diagnostic and pretreatment planning study for cerebral aneurysms by a combined neurovascular team. *Neurosurgery*, Jun, 54(6), 1329-40; discussion, 1340-2.
17. Treggiari MM. (2011). Hemodynamic management of subarachnoid hemorrhage. *Neurocrit Care*, Sep, 15(2), 329-35.
18. Brown SC, Brew S, Madigan J. (2011). Investigating suspected subarachnoid haemorrhage in adults. *BMJ*, May, 342d2644.
19. Wang H, Li W, He H, Luo L, Chen C, Guo Y. (2013). 320-detector row CT angiography for detection and evaluation of intracranial aneurysms: comparison with conventional digital subtraction angiography. *Clin Radiol*, Jan, 68(1), e15-20.
20. Koenig MA. (2012). Management of delayed cerebral ischemia after subarachnoid hemorrhage. *Continuum*, Minneapolis, Minn, Jun, 18(3), 579-97.
21. Wirth FP. (1986). Surgical treatment of incidental intracranial aneurysms. *Clin Neurosurg*, 33125-35.
22. Bederson JB, Connolly ES Jr, Batjer HH, Dacey RG, Dion JE, Diringer MN. (2009), Guidelines for the management of aneurysmal subarachnoid hemorrhage: a statement for healthcare professionals from a special writing group of the Stroke Council, American Heart Association. *Stroke*, Mar, 40 (3), 994-1025.
23. Woloszyn AV, McAllen KJ, Figueroa BE, DeShane RS, Barletta JF. (2012). Retrospective evaluation of nicardipine versus labetalol for blood pressure control in aneurysmal subarachnoid hemorrhage. *Neurocrit Care*, Jun, 16(3), 376-80.
24. Rajshekhar V, Harbaugh RE. (1992). Results of routine ventriculostomy with external ventricular drainage for acute hydrocephalus following subarachnoid haemorrhage. *Acta Neurochir* (Wien), 115(1–2), 8-14.
25. Sakowitz OW, Raabe A, Vucak D, Kiening KL, Unterberg AW. (2006). Contemporary management of aneurysmal subarachnoid hemorrhage in Germany: results of a survey among 100 neurosurgical departments. *Neurosurgery*, 58, 137–45.
26. Rose FC, Sarner M. (1965). Epilepsy after ruptured intracranial aneurysm. *Br Med J.*, 1, 18-21.
27. Diringer MN. (2009). Management of aneurysmal subarachnoid hemorrhage. *Crit Care Med.*, 37, 432–40.
28. *Neurocrit Care* (2011) 15, 247–56.
29. Bolli R, Marban E. (1999). Molecular and cellular mechanisms of myocardial stunning. *Physiol Rev*, 79, 609–34.
30. Jain R, Deveikis J, Thompson BG. (2004). Management of patients with stunned myocardium

associated with subarachnoid hemorrhage. *AJNR Am J Neuroradiol*, 25, 126-29.

31. Qureshi AI, Suri MF, Sung GY, Straw RN, Yahia AM, Saad M, Guterman LR, Hopkins LN. (2002). Prognostic significance of hypernatremia and hyponatremia among patients with aneurysmal subarachnoid hemorrhage. *Neurosurgery*, 50, 749–55.
32. Seckl JR, Dunger DB, Lightman SL. (1987). Neurohypophyseal peptide function during early postoperative diabetes insipidus. *Brain*, 110, 737–46.
33. Sherlock M, O'Sullivan E, Agha A, Behan LA, Rawluk D, Brennan P, Tormey W, Thompson C.J. (2006). The incidence and pathophysiology of hyponatraemia after subarachnoid haemorrhage. *Clin. Endocrinol*, 64, 250–54.
34. Chandy D, Sy R, Aronow WS, Lee WN, Maguire G, Murali R (2006). Hyponatremia and cerebrovascular spasm in aneurysmal subarachnoid hemorrhage. *Neurol. India*, 54, 273–75.
35. Hasan D, Wijdicks EF, Vermeulen M. (1990). Hyponatremia is associated with cerebral ischemia in patients with aneurysmal subarachnoid hemorrhage. *Ann. Neurol.*, 27, 106–8.
36. Hannon MJ, Behan LA, O'Brien MM, Tormey W, Ball SG, Javadpour M, Sherlock M, Thompson CJ. (2014). Hyponatremia following mild/moderate subarachnoid hemorrhage is due to siadh and glucocorticoid deficiency and not cerebral salt wasting. *J. Clin. Endocrinol. Metab.*, 99, 291–98.
37. Kumar A, Anel R, Bunnell E, Habet K, Zanotti S, Marshall S, Neumann A, Ali A, Cheang M, Kavinsky C, Parrillo JE. (2004). Pulmonary artery occlusion pressure and central venous pressure fail to predict ventricular filling volume, cardiac performance, or the response to volume infusion in normal subjects. *Crit Care Med*, 32, 691–99.
38. Isotani, E, et al. Alterations in plasma concentrations of natriuretic peptides and antidiuretic hormone after subarachnoid hemorrhage. *Stroke*, 25.11, 2198-2203.
39. Betjes, MGH. (2002). Hyponatremia in acute brain disease: the cerebral salt wasting syndrome. Eur J Intern Med. Feb; 13 (1):9-14.
40. Tomida, M, et al. (1998). Plasma concentrations of brain natriuretic peptide in patients with subarachnoid hemorrhage. *Stroke*, 29.8, (1998): 1584-87.
41. Maesaka JK, Miyawaki N, Palaia T, Fishbane S, Durham J. Renal salt wasting without cerebral disease: Value of determining urate in hyponatremia. *Kidney Int.*, 71, 822–26.
42. Gutierrez OM, Lin HY. (2007). *Refractory hyponatremia. Kidney Int.*, 71:79–82.
43. Wijdicks EF, Vermeulen M, Hijdra A, van Gijn J. (1985). Hyponatremia and cerebral Infarction in patients with ruptured intracranial aneurysm: Is fluid restriction harmful? *Ann. Neurol.*, 7, 137–40.
44. Ogden AT, Mayer SA, Connolly ES Jr (2005). Hyperosmolar agents in neurosurgical practice: the evolving role of hypertonic saline. *Neurosurgery*, 57, 207–15; discussion 207–15.
45. Wijdicks EF, Vermeulen M, ten Haaf JA, HA, Bakker WH, van Gijn J. (1985). Volume depletion and natriuresis in patients with a ruptured intracranial aneurysm. *Ann. Neurol.*, 18, 211–16.
46. Tommasino C, Moore S, Todd MM. (1988). Cerebral effects of isovolemic hemodilution with crystalloid or colloid solutions. *Crit. Care Med.*, 16, 862–68.
47. Heros RC, Zervas NT, Varsos V. (1983). Cerebral vasospasm after subarachnoid hemorrhage: an update. *Ann Neurol*, Dec, 14(6), 599-608.
48. Philippon J, Grob R, and Dagreou F. (1986). Prevention of vasospasm in subarachnoid haemorrhage. A controlled study with nimodipine. *Acta Neurochirurgica*, 82(3-4), 110–14.
49. Pickard JD, Murray GD, Illingworth R, et al. (1989). Effect of oral nimodipine on cerebral infarction and outcome after subarachnoid haemorrhage: British aneurysm nimodipine trial. *Brit Medl Jrnl*, 298 (66740, 636–42.
50. Treggiari MM, Walder B, Suter PM, Romand JA. (2003). Systematic review of the prevention of delayed ischemic neurological deficits with hypertension, hypervolemia, and hemodilution therapy following subarachnoid hemorrhage. *Jrnl of Neurosur*, 98 (5), 978–84.
51. Egge A, Waterloo K, Sjøholm H, Solberg T, Ingebrigtsen T, Romner B. (2001). Prophylactic hyperdynamic postoperative fluid therapy after aneurysmal subarachnoid hemorrhage: a clinical, prospective, randomized, controlled study. *Neurosurgery*, 49(30), 593–606.
52. Dankbaar JW, Slooter AJC, Rinkel GJE, Schaaf ICVD. (2010) Effect of different components of triple-H therapy on cerebral perfusion in patients

with aneurysmal subarachnoid haemorrhage: a systematic review. *Critical Care*, 14(1), R23.
53. Connolly ES, Rabinstein AA, Carhuapoma JR, et al. (2101). Guidelines for the management of aneurysmal subarachnoid hemorrhage: a guideline for healthcare professionals from the American heart association/American stroke association. *Stroke*, 43(6), 1711–37.
54. International Study of Unruptured Intracranial Aneurysms Investigators. (2003). Unruptured intracranial aneurysms: natural history, clinical outcome, and risks of surgical and endovascular treatment. *Lancet*, 362, 103–10.
55. Tsutsumi K, Ueki K, Morita A, Kirino T. (2000). Risk of rupture from incidental cerebral aneurysms. *J Neurosurg*, 93, 550-53.
56. Juvela S, Porras M, Poussa K. (2000). Natural history of unruptured intracranial aneurysms: probability of and risk factors for aneurysm rupture. *J Neurosurg*, 93, 379-87.
57. Algra A, Greving JP, Wermer MJH, Brown RD, Morita A, Juvela S, Yonekura M, Rinkel GJE. (2014) Development of the PHASES score for prediction of risk of rupture of intracranial aneurysms: A pooled analysis of six prospective cohort studies. *The Lancet Neurology*, 13 (1), 59-66.
58. Koffijberg H, Buskens E, Algra A, Wermer MJ, Rinkel GJ. (2008). Growth rates of intracranial aneurysms: exploring constancy. *J Neurosurg*, 109, 176–85.
59. Greving JP, Rinkel GJ, Buskens E, Algra A. (2009). Cost-effectiveness of preventive treatment of intracranial aneurysms: new data and uncertainties. *Neurology*, 73, 258–65.
60. Brinjikji W, Rabinstein AA, Nasr DM, Lanzino G, Kallmes DF, Cloft HJ. (2011). Better outcomes with treatment by coiling relative to clipping of unruptured intracranial aneurysms in the United States, 2001–2008. *AJNR Am J Neuroradiol*, 32, 1071–75.
61. Naggara ON, White PM, Guilbert F, Roy D, Weill A, Raymond J. (2010). Endovascular treatment of intracranial unruptured aneurysms: systematic review and meta-analysis of the literature on safety and efficacy. *Radiology*, 256, 887–97.

62. Le Roux PD, Winn HR. (2004). Management of the ruptured aneurysm. In: Le Roux PD, Winn HR, Newell DW, eds. *Management of cerebral aneurysms*. Philadelphia: Saunders, 303-33.
63. Molyneux A, Kerr R, Stratton I, et al. (2002). International Subarachnoid Aneurysm Trial (ISAT) of neurosurgical clipping versus endovascular coiling in 2143 patients with ruptured intracranial aneurysms: a randomised trial. *Lancet*, 360, 1267-74.
64. Johnston SC, Wilson CB, Halbach VV, et al. (2000). Endovascular and surgical treatment of unruptured cerebral aneurysms: comparison of risks. *Ann Neurol*, 48, 11-19.
65. Johnston SC, Zhao S, Dudley RA, Berman MF, Gress DR. (2001). Treatment of unruptured cerebral aneurysms in California. *Stroke*, 32, 597-605.
66. Johnston SC, Dudley RA, Gress DR, Ono L. (1999). Surgical and endovascular treatment of unruptured cerebral aneurysms at university hospitals. *Neurology*, 52, 1799-1805.
67. Raymond J, Guilbert F, Weill A, et al. (2003). Long-term angiographic recurrences after selective endovascular treatment of aneurysms with detachable coils. *Stroke*, 34, 1398-1403.
68. David CA, Vishteh AG, Spetzler RF, Lemole M, Lawton MT, Partovi S. (1999). Late angiographic follow-up review of surgically treated aneurysms. *J Neurosurg*, 91, 396-401.
69. Alderazi YJ, Shastri D, Kass-Hout T, Prestigiacomo CJ, Gandhi CD. (2014). Flow diverters for intracranial aneurysms. *Stroke Res Treat*, 415653.
70. Chalouhi N, Tjoumakaris S, Starke RM, Gonzalez LF, Randazzo C, Hasan D, McMahon JF, Singhal S, Moukarzel LA, Dumont AS, Rosenwasser R, Jabbour P. (2013). Comparison of flow diversion and coiling in large unruptured intracranial saccular aneurysms. *Stroke*, 44, 2150–54.

Chapter 8

The Vasculopathies

8.1 Introduction

A vasculopathy is defined as an arterial wall disease process. This chapter will discuss cerebrovascular vasculopathies related to stroke. While many different vasculopathies are stroke-related, this chapter will briefly describe fibromuscular dysplasia (FMD), arterial dissection, and moyamoya disease. These vasculopathies have a common similarity—**they can account for stroke in younger patients.**

The wall of an artery has three components (Figure 1). The innermost layer is the intima and consists of the endothelium, connective tissue, and an internal elastic membrane or lamina. The internal elastic lamina is an elastic membrane comprising the outermost portion of the intima. The middle arterial layer is the media and consists of involuntary smooth muscle tissue. The outermost layer is the tunica or adventitia or tunica adventitia and consists of an external elastic membrane and strong fibrous tissue. Intracranial arteries lack an external elastic lamina and adventitia. Different vasculopathies affect different components within the arterial wall.

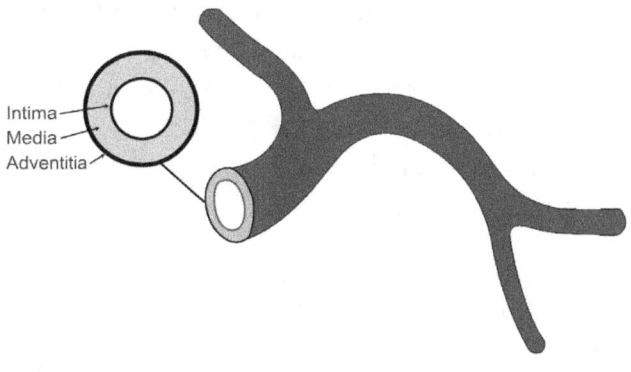

FIGURE 1. The Three Components of an Arterial Wall

8.2 Fibromuscular Dysplasia (FMD)

Fibromuscular dysplasia (FMD) is a nonatherosclerotic, noninflammatory vasculopathy caused by the abnormal cellular growth of fibrous tissue (fibroplasia) within the smooth muscle layer or media of arteries. This abnormal growth can cause arteries to become dilated and narrowed. There are different types of FMD which commonly affect the carotid arteries. The most common type of carotid FMD is the medial type which has a characteristic "string of beads" appearance (Figure 2). Typically, FMD spares the carotid origin and proximal cervical segment.

FIGURE 2. Cervical Carotid Fibromuscular Dysplasia (FMD)

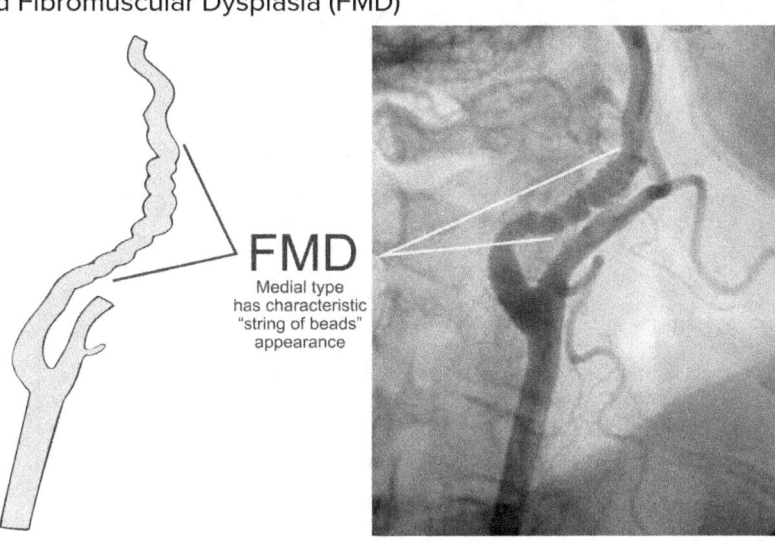

Unlike the other vasculopathies discussed in this chapter, FMD has no unique symptoms and requires advanced imaging for diagnosis. Most patients presenting with fibromuscular dysplasia are women between the ages of 40 and 60. While most patients with FMD are asymptomatic, FMD can contribute to stroke by a variety of mechanisms, particularly in younger patients. These include artery to artery thromboembolism, carotid dissection, and SAH. There is an increased prevalence of brain aneurysms in patients with either cervical or vertebral FMD of about 7%. An easy way to remember how FMD can contribute to stroke is the mnemonic 'SAD' (Table 1).

TABLE 1. Fibromuscular Dysplasia (FMD) Contributory Factors Related to Stroke: **SAD**

S	SAH - Intracranial Aneurysm
A	Artery-to-Artery Thromboembolism
D	Dissection

8.3 Arterial Dissection

Arterial dissection is included in the "other" category that comprises approximately 5% of acute ischemic stroke (AIS) (Figure 3). Arterial dissection of the internal carotid artery is three to five times more common than those involving the vertebral artery.[2] For this reason, the majority of this discussion will pertain to carotid artery dissection (CAD). Most CAD is spontaneous, with the remainder resulting from minor or major cervical trauma.[3] Various pathophysiologic risk factors are associated with CAD but the most compelling are connective tissue abnormalities which may result in vascular wall weakening. One theory suggests an underlying arterial wall abnormality is required for a dissection to occur. For example, one risk factor associated with CAD is an elevated homocysteine level which is associated with arterial weakness.[4] An easy way to remember the common risk factors associated with carotid artery dissection (CAD) is with the mnemonic 'FEMALE' (Table 2). Note however, that unlike FMD which has a higher female predominance, arterial dissection is equally prevalent in men and women. This is just a mnemonic.

FIGURE 3. Subtypes of Ischemic Stroke

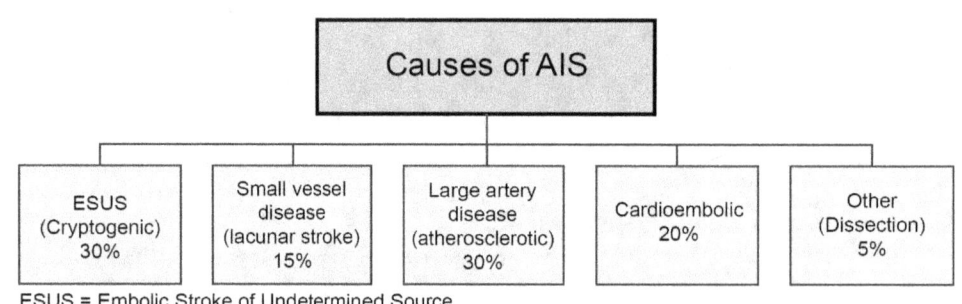

ESUS = Embolic Stroke of Undetermined Source

TABLE 2. Risk Factors Associated with Carotid Artery Dissection: **FEMALE**

F	FMD
E	Ehlers-Danlos Syndrome, Type IV
M	Marfan Syndrome
A	Autosomal Dominant Polycystic Kidney Disease
L	Linked to Elevated Homocysteine
E	Elevated Blood Pressure

Proper understanding of a dissection depends anatomically on which segment of the artery is affected and pathologically on which layer of the arterial wall is involved. As mentioned in Chapter 4 (Cerebrovascular Anatomy), the internal carotid (comprising the anterior circulation) and vertebral (comprising the posterior circulation) arteries both have four segments. The **mobile extracranial portions** of both the ICA and VA are especially susceptible to dissection. CAD typically occurs in the cervical segment, distal to the carotid bulb where the artery is freely mobile and can extend to the skull base or petrous junction. Vertebral artery dissections (VAD) most commonly occur at the entry into the transverse foramen of the C6, V2, and V3 segments.[5] Distal vertebral artery (V3) dissection is related to the VA's extended course around the C1 vertebral body before it enters the dura mater.

Both CAD and VAD can involve damage to the artery's intima, media, or adventitia. The most common form involves a tear in the innermost lining of the artery or intima because this layer is the thinnest and most susceptible to injury. This form of dissection is termed a *subintimal* dissection. Subintimal hematoma occurs when blood enters the space between the intima and outer layers of the vessel, resulting in luminal stenosis (Figure 4). Sometimes a potential space can form within the subintimal region producing a "false" lumen. A subintimal dissection results in a characteristic intimal "flap" associated with these types of dissections. An extracranial internal carotid dissection involves the cervical segment of the artery distal to the carotid bulb and typically does not extend into the petrous portion. Often, a carotid dissection appears as a tapering stenosis just distal to the carotid bulb (Figure 4).

FIGURE 4. Subintimal Dissection

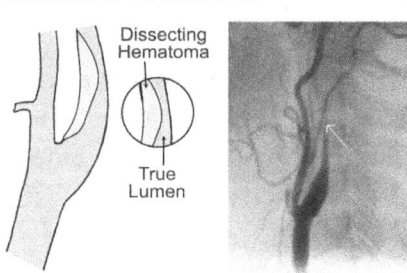

A subadventitial dissection results in hemorrhage between the media and outer wall of an artery and is not associated with a "flap." However, hemorrhage extravasation through an injured adventitial layer can result in a pseudoaneurysm (dissecting aneurysm) (Figure 5). This consequence of CAD is not uncommon, with a recent study reporting that 49% of CAD patients had pseudoaneurysms.[6] **However, as opposed to *subintimal* CAD, this same study demonstrated no patients with *subadventitial* CAD experienced transient ischemic attack or stroke.** Because the cervical segment of the internal carotid artery is innervated with pain sensitive nerve fibers, both forms of dissection (subintimal or subadventitial) may produce neck pain. An easy way to remember the distinguishing characteristics between a subintimal and subadventitial dissection is with the mnemonic 'FLAP' (Table 3). Table 4 also summarizes the relevant distinctions.

FIGURE 5. Left Carotid Artery Dissecting Pseudoaneurysm

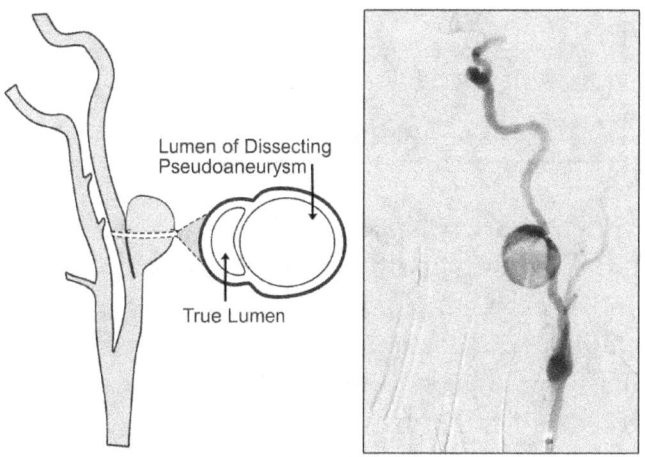

TABLE 3. Arterial Dissection Distinguishing Characteristics: **FLAP**

F	FLAP - Subintimal
L	Luminal Stenosis or Occlusion
A	Arterial Lumen Tapering
P	Pseudoaneurysm - Subadventitial

TABLE 4. Subintimal Versus Subadventitial Dissection Pseudoaneurysm

Dissection Type	Frequency	Arterial Layer	Appearance	Stroke Pathology
Subintimal	Frequent	Intima	Flap	Embolic>Occlusive
Subadventitial	Less Frequent	Adventitia	Pseudoaneurysm	No Stroke

Although carotid artery dissection is responsible for less than 2% of all AIS cases, it accounts for 10%-25% of AIS in young and middle-aged adults.[7] Carotid artery dissection patients can present with a variety of different complaints. However, typical symptoms include contralateral weakness, headache, amaurosis fugax (unilateral transient blindness), miosis, and ptosis (partial Horner syndrome) (Table 5). An easy way to recall these symptoms is with the mnemonic 'WHAM' (Table 5).

TABLE 5. Carotid Artery Dissection Symptoms: **WHAM**

W	Weakness, Contralateral
H	Headache
A	Amarousis Fugax
M	Miosis and Ptosis (Partial Horner Syndrome)

Vertebral artery dissection (VAD) patients commonly present with headache (often occipital) and neck pain. VAD has multiple etiologies including spinal manipulation, minor neck trauma, yoga, hypertension, FMD, female sex, and recent infection. Compared with CAD patients, VAD patients tend to be younger, more commonly present with neck pain, more commonly have SAH, and typically take longer to diagnose.[8] While nearly all VAD is extracranial, about 10% have intracranial extension which carries a higher risk of a dissecting aneurysm, associated SAH, and mortality (Figure 6).[5,9]

VAD can affect any posterior circulation supplied structure. However, most VAD related strokes are associated with involvement of the **posterior inferior cerebellar artery (PICA)** and accompanying **lateral medullary (Wallenberg) syndrome**.

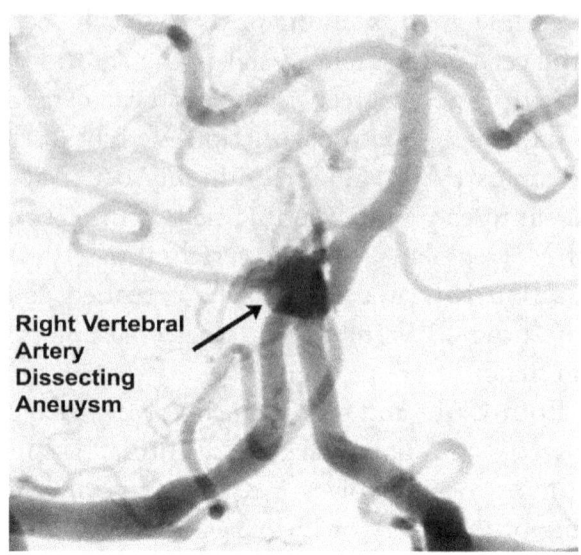

FIGURE 6. Right Vertebral Artery Dissecting Aneurysm

8.4 Arterial Dissection and Stroke

Dissection can affect blood flow to the brain by one of two mechanisms. First, blood flow can be compromised by luminal stenosis from a subintimal hematoma. Second, embolic disease can arise from the dissection site (artery-to-artery embolic disease) (Figure 7). Artery-to-artery embolic disease from dissection site thrombus is the most common pathophysiologic mechanism for dissection-related stroke.[10,11] Transcranial Doppler studies have also demonstrated cerebral microemboli and stroke within the vascular distribution of the dissected vessel.[12] Additionally, recurrent stroke was more common in patients with dissection-related stroke at presentation.[13] These observations have led clinicians to use either antiplatelet drugs or anticoagulants to reduce stroke recurrence rate.[14] However, there is no consensus regarding optimal medical management of internal carotid dissection.[15]

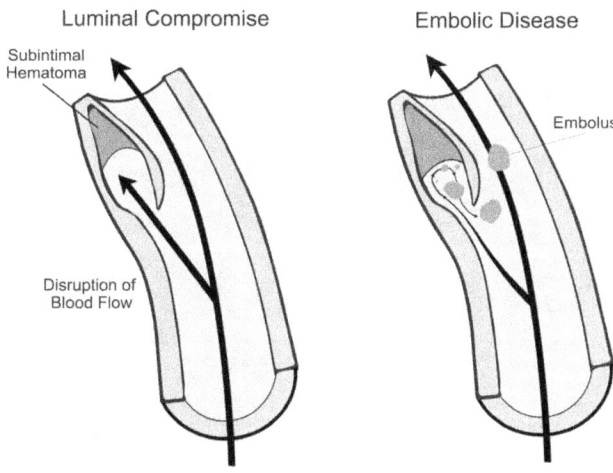

FIGURE 7. Subintimal Dissection Related Luminal Compromise and Embolic Disease

The Cervical Artery Dissection and Stroke Study (CADISS) investigated secondary stroke prevention with either anticoagulation or anti-thrombotic (antiplatelet) treatment in both internal carotid artery and vertebral artery dissections.[16] This study demonstrated a low stroke recurrence and death rate with either treatment option. Stroke occurred in one of 59 patients (2%) treated with antiplatelet drugs and one of 28 patients (4%) treated with anticoagulant drugs. The study concluded that there is no significant difference in efficacy between anticoagulation treatment (heparin or Lovenox® bridging to warfarin) and antiplatelet treatment (aspirin, dipyridamole, or clopidogrel alone or in combination) for recurrent stroke prevention or death. The same findings have been confirmed by another randomized trial and two meta-analyses.[13,17] These studies concluded that the recurrent stroke rate after dissection is extremely low and that there is no difference in recurrent stroke rate between anticoagulation and antiplatelet therapy. While antiplatelet therapy has lower hemorrhagic complications, earlier AHA / ASA guidelines suggest either antiplatelet or anticoagulation regimens as reasonable treatment options for three to six months (class IIa, level B, a weak recommendation). The newer 2018 AHA/ASA stroke guidelines have maintained these recommendations stating: "For patients with AIS and extracranial carotid or vertebral artery dissection, treatment with either antiplatelet or anticoagulant therapy for 3 to 6 months may be reasonable."[18]

If indicated, carotid artery dissections can be effectively managed with carotid stenting. One review reported a 99.1% technical success rate with no procedural-related morbidity.[15] Another study demonstrated carotid artery stenting to be safe and effective in the treatment of carotid dissection.[19] Since antiplatelet therapy is required to perform these endovascular procedures, it is gaining more acceptance as the preferred therapeutic option (compared to anticoagulants) for the prevention of dissection-related stroke recurrence.

8.5 Moyamoya Disease

Moyamoya disease is a progressive vasculopathy which slowly compromises and can eventually occlude the supraclinoid segment of the ICA and the proximal portions of the anterior and middle cerebral arteries (Figure 8). Recall that the internal elastic lamina, the outermost portion of the intima, lies between the intima and the media. Moyamoya disease causes thickening of the intima, as well as irregularities of the internal elastic lamina and media. This process slowly diminishes the luminal diameter of these larger vessels. Small perforating and anastomotic branches surrounding these vessels develop a network of multiple collaterals to "bypass" these larger vessels. The term moyamoya (Japanese for "puff of smoke") describes the angiographic appearance of these collaterals, which is the gold standard for diagnosis (Figure 8).[20] This disease typically occurs at an early age (usually 10 years and under) but should be considered in children and younger patients presenting with stroke symptoms. Typically, patients' symptoms reflect the anatomic territory affected by moyamoya disease. However, adults with this disease can also present with SAH.

FIGURE 8. Moyamoya Disease

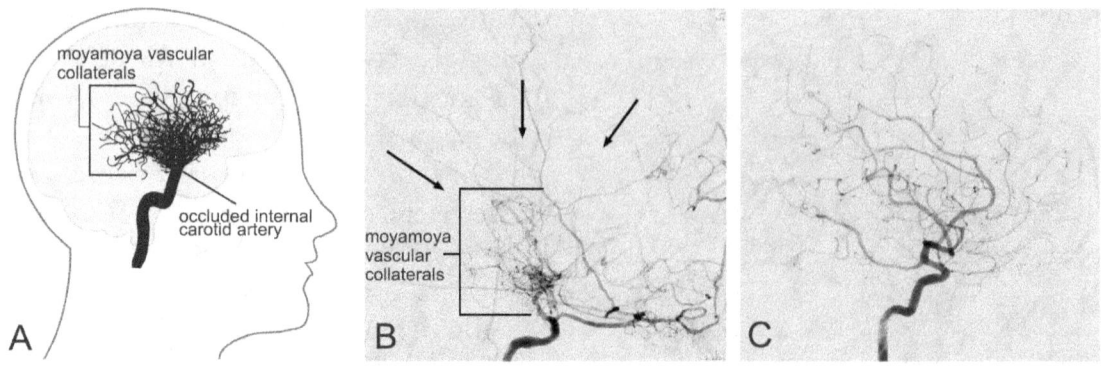

Moyamoya pattern illustrated (A), demonstrated by a lateral cerebral angiogram (B) and compared to normal lateral cerebral angiogram on the right (C). Arrows indicate paucity of large vessels in the moyamoya lateral cerebral angiogram (B) compared to normal cerebral angiogram on the right (C).

8.6 Summary

Fibromuscular dysplasia, arterial dissection, and moyamoya disease are frequently encountered within stroke centers. The first vasculopathy discussed in this chapter was fibromuscular dysplasia (FMD). FMD is not just an acronym for the term fibromuscular dysplasia but is also an ideal mnemonic for the vasculopathies discussed in this chapter (Table 6). In addition, this mnemonic serves as a reminder to consider vasculopathies as a potential cause of stroke in younger patients.

TABLE 6. The Vasculopathies: **FMD**

F	Fibromuscular Dysplasia
M	Moyamoya
D	Dissection

Consider these vasculopathies in younger patients presenting with stroke

Abbreviations list

AIS, acute ischemic stroke; CAD, carotid artery dissection; FMD, fibromuscular dysplasia; PICA, posterior inferior cerebellar artery; VAD, vertebral artery dissection.

References

1. Cloft HJ, Kallmes DF, Kallmes MH, Goldstein JH, Jensen ME, Dion JE. (1998). Prevalence of cerebral aneurysms in patients with fibromuscular dysplasia: a reassessment. *J Neurosurg.*, Mar, 88(3), 436-40.
2. Hart RG, Easton JD. (1983). Dissections of cervical and cerebral arteries. *Neurol Clin*, 1(1), 155–82.
3. Haneline MT, Lewkovich GN. (2005). An analysis of the etiology of cervical artery dissections: 1994 to 2003. *J Manipulative Physiol Ther*, 28(8), 617–22.
4. Rosner A.L. (2004). Spontaneous cervical artery dissections and implications for homocysteine. *J Manipulative Physiol Ther*, 27(2), 124–32.
5. Arnold M, Bousser MG, Fahrni G, Fischer U, Georgiadis D, Gandjour J, et al.(2006). Vertebral artery dissection presenting findings and predictors of outcome. *Stroke,* 37(10), 2499–503.
6. Touze E., Randoux B., Meary E., Arquizan C., Meder JF, Mas J. (2001). Aneurysmal forms of cervical artery dissection: associated factors and outcome. *Stroke*, 32(2), 418–23.
7. Debette S, Leys D. (2009). Cervical artery dissections: predisposing factors, diagnosis, and outcome. *Lancet Neurol*, 8, 668–78.
8. von Babo M, De Marchis GM, Sarikaya H, Stapf C, Buffon F, Fischer U, et al. (2013). Differences and similarities between spontaneous dissections of the internal carotid artery and the vertebra artery. *Stroke*, 44(6), 1537-42
9. Ramgren B, Cronqvist M, Romner B, Brandt L, Holtås S, Larsson EM. (2005). Vertebrobasilar dissection with subarachnoid hemorrhage: a retrospective study of 29 patients. *Neuroradiology*, 47(2), 97–104.

10. Benninger DH, Georgiadis D, Kremer C, Studer A, Nedeltchev K, Baumgartner RW. (2004). Mechanism of ischemic infarct in spontaneous carotid dissection. *Stroke*, 35(2), 482–85.
11. Weimar C, Kraywinkel K, Hagemeister C, et al. (2010). German Stroke Study Collaboration. Recurrent stroke after cervical artery dissection. *J Neurol Neurosurg Psychiatry*, 81, 869–73.
12. Molina CA, Alvarez-Sabin J, Schonewille W, et al. (2000). Cerebral microembolism in acute spontaneous internal artery dissection. *Neurology*, 55, 1738–40.
13. Georgiadis D, Arnold M, von Buedingen HC, et al. (2009). Aspirin vs anticoagulation in carotid artery dissection: a study of 298 patients. *Neurology*, 72, 1810.
14. Menon RK, Markus HS, Norris JW. (2008). Results of a UK questionnaire of diagnosis and treatment in cervical artery dissection. *J Neurol Neurosurg Psychiatry*, 79, 612.
15. Xianjun H, Zhiming Z. (2013). A systematic review of endovascular management of internal carotid artery dissections. *Interv Neurol*, Sep. 1(3-4), 164-70.
16. CADISS trial investigators. (2015). Antiplatelet treatment compared with anticoagulation treatment for cervical artery dissection (CADISS): a randomised trial. *Lancet Neurol*, 14, 361-67.
17. Lyrer P, Engelter S. (2003). Antithrombotic drugs for carotid artery dissection. *Cochrane Database Syst Rev*, 3, CD000255; Lyrer P, Engelter S. (2004). Antithrombotic drugs for carotid artery dissection. *Stroke*, 35, 613–14.
18. Powers WJ, Rabinstein AA, Ackerson T, Adeoye OM, Bambakidis NC, Becker K, Biller J, Brown M, Demaerschalk BM, Hoh B, et al. (2018). Guidelines for the Early Management of Patients With Acute Ischemic Stroke: A Guideline for Healthcare Professionals From the American Heart Association/American Stroke Association. *Stroke,* Jan 24. Epub.
19. Juszkat R, Liebert W, Stanisławska K, et al. (2015) Extracranial Internal Carotid Artery Dissection Treated with Self-expandable Stents: A Single-Centre Experience. *Cardiovasc Intervent Radiol*, Dec., 38 (6), 1451-57.
20. Suzuki J, Takaku A (1969) Cerebrovascular "moyamoya" disease. Disease showing abnormal net-like vessels in base of brain. *Archives of neurology*, 20 (3), 288-99.

Chapter 9

Cerebrovascular Malformations

9.1 Introduction

Cerebrovascular malformations or vascular malformations of the central nervous system are various conditions which can either affect blood vessels or are related to hemorrhage within the brain. The most common types are: (1) arteriovenous malformations (AVM), (2) cavernous malformations (CM), (3) developmental venous anomalies (DVA), and (4) capillary telangiectasias (CT). These entities are commonly encountered in stroke centers. Often, patients are transferred from facilities that either do not recognize these entities or are not equipped to manage them. For example, some of these entities may cause headaches, seizures, strokes, or intracranial hemorrhage. However, others can be incidental findings that do not require further treatment. Either way, it is important to have a basic understanding of these entities, how they present, and, if necessary, how they should be treated.

9.2 Arteriovenous Malformations (AVMs)

Entire textbooks have been dedicated to the discussion of arteriovenous malformations (AVM). However, the purpose of this section is to provide a basic understanding of AVMs. Brain AVMs are typically congenital lesions consisting of a tangled mass of dilated vessels that form an abnormal communication between the arterial and venous system. AVMs have three anatomic components: (1) arterial feeders, (2) a nidus, and (3) venous outflow (Figure 1).

Arterial feeders supply an AVM nidus or tangle of vessels. This nidus does not contain intervening normal brain tissue. Most importantly, the nidus does not contain capillaries which typically dampen arterial blood pressure (Figure 2 and Table 1). For this reason, arterial feeders supply an AVM nidus with high pressure arterial blood, which then enters the draining vein without any intervening capillary bed—that is, high pressure arterial blood travels through the nidus to the venous system without reducing arterial blood pressure. Incidentally, if no nidus is present and arteries directly connect to draining veins, this entity is termed an *arteriovenous fistula* (AVF) rather than an AVM.

FIGURE 1. Arteriovenous Malformation (AVM) Components

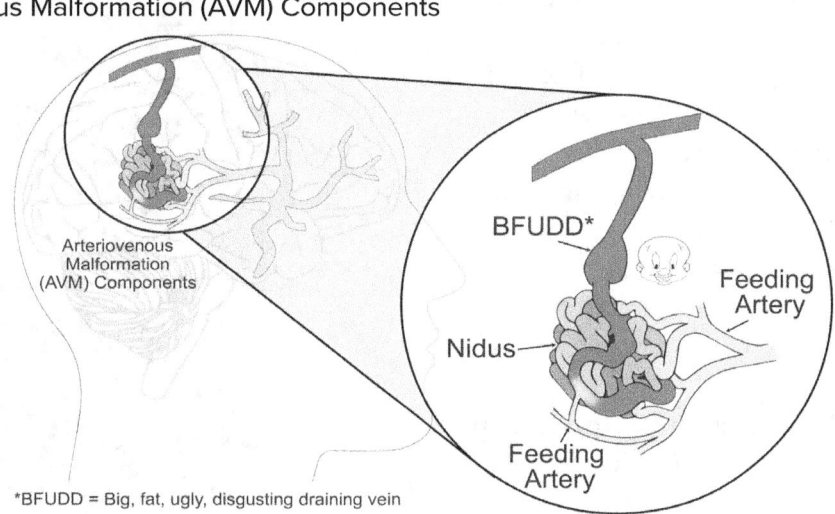

*BFUDD = Big, fat, ugly, disgusting draining vein

FIGURE 2. Normal Capillary Bed and Arteriovenous Malformation (AVM) Nidus

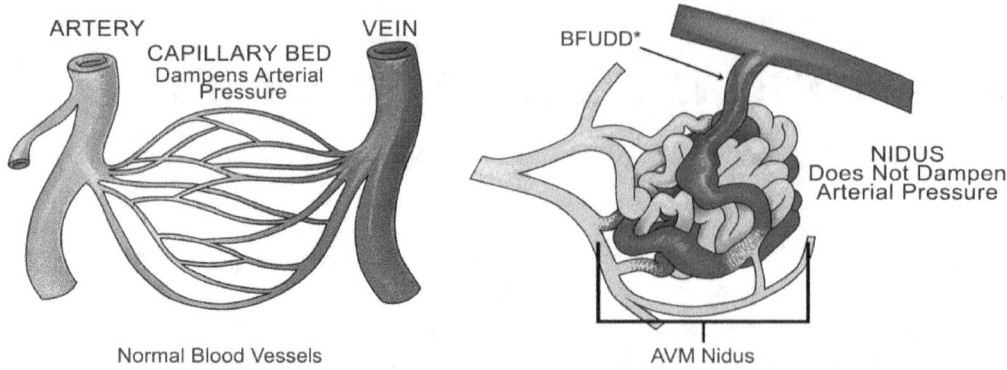

*BFUDD = Big, Fat, Ugly, Disgusting Draining Vein - Receives elevated arterial pressure

TABLE 1. AVM Versus Normal Capillary Bed Characteristics

Structure	Unit	SBP*	Result
AVM	Nidus	No Change	BFUDD**
Normal Capillary Bed	Capillary	Reduced	Normal Draining Vein

*SBP - Systolic Blood Pressure **BFUDD - Big, fat, ugly, disgusting draining vein

An AVM contains a nidus which connects high-flow arterial blood to the venous system. The wall of the artery contains more muscle tissue and is stronger than the wall of the vein. Arteries are built to handle high-pressure arterial blood. However, veins have weaker walls and are designed to maintain low-pressure venous blood. Typically, this is not an issue because arterioles and capillaries dampen high-pressure arterial blood before it enters a draining vein. However, a nidus does not contain an intervening capillary bed and does not dampen high-pressure arterial blood before it enters the draining vein(s). Because venous walls are weaker and not structured to handle high-pressure arterial blood, they tend to expand and weaken. If a vein becomes abnormally dilated, it is called a venous varix (Figure 3). This is not an aneurysm because it is affecting a vein and not an artery (Box 1). Because veins are weaker than arteries, high blood pressure may cause them to rupture. AVMs bleed because they contain weakened, dilated veins that may rupture.

In summary, AVMs have three anatomic components: (1) arterial feeders, (2) a nidus, and (3) a BIG, FAT, UGLY, DISGUSTING, DRAINING VEIN (BFUDD) (Figures 1, 2 and 4).

BOX 1. Aneurysm (Artery) and Varix (Vein) Terminology

Artery = **A**neurysm
Vein = **V**arix

FIGURE 3. Venous Varix Associated with Arteriovenous Malformation

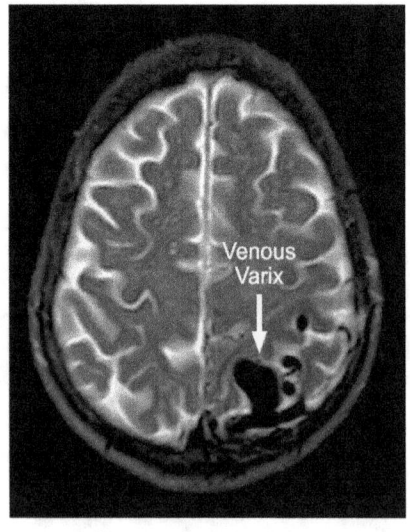

FIGURE 4. Arteriovenous Malformation (AVM) Nidus

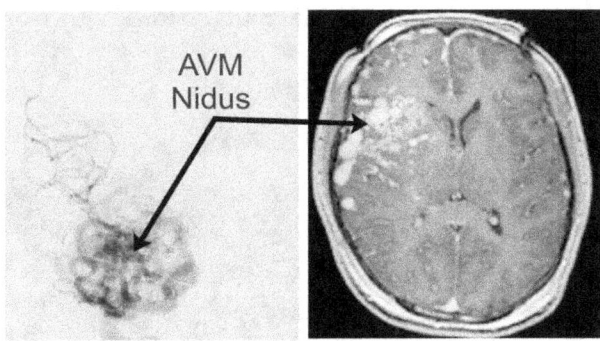

AVMs are the most symptomatic cerebrovascular malformation, with symptoms generally presenting in the second, third, or fourth decade of life. AVMs can present with seizure or spontaneous hemorrhage because of that big, fat, ugly, disgusting, draining (BFUDD) vein. Brain CT is an excellent modality for the detection of cerebral hemorrhage. However, because the underlying anatomic components of AVMs are typically isodense to brain parenchyma, they can be easily overlooked on a noncontrast brain CT. Therefore, contrast-enhanced CT or CTA is preferable. In either case, MRI typically follows CT if an underlying vascular lesion such as an AVM is suspected. MRI demonstrates parenchymal involvement and low signal, serpiginous vessels representing both dilated feeding arteries and big, fat, ugly, disgusting, draining veins (Figure 3). MRA can further supplement MRI by demonstrating the anatomic components of AVMs which again include arterial supply, an intervening nidus, and a big, fat, ugly, disgusting, draining vein (BFUDD) (Figure 5).

While CT and MRI can provide AVM anatomical data, the gold standard is still angiography. Angiography is a dynamic real-time study that demonstrates the anatomic components of an AVM. It can delineate the number of feeding arteries, the size of the AVM nidus, and venous drainage. Angiography can also demonstrate certain features that are believed to increase the risk of AVM hemorrhage, such as intranidal aneurysms and venous stenosis. Approximately 70%-90% of AVMs are supratentorial and 10-15% are infratentorial lesions. The annual risk for initial hemorrhage in patients with an unruptured AVM is approximately 1%.[1] The five-year risk for initial seizure in patients with unruptured AVM is 8%; however, 58% of patients will develop epilepsy after an initial seizure.[1] The ARUBA Trial demonstrated an 80% risk reduction of death and stroke by not intervening on unruptured AVMs.[2] However, the results of the ARUBA Trial do not represent a definitive strategy in the treatment of AVMs, but rather point to a need for better understanding of the risks and benefits of different AVM treatment options. Further randomized control trials are required before any definitive statements regarding the treatment of unruptured brain AVMs can be made.

FIGURE 5. Magnetic Resonance Angiography (MRA) of AVM

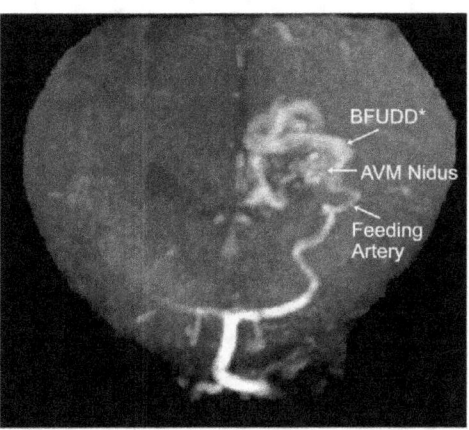

*BFUDD - Big, fat, ugly, disgusting draining vein
AVM - Arteriovenous malformation

The types of AVMs that have been described thus far are termed *pial* or *parenchymal AVMs*. In distinction to pial or parenchymal AVMs, dural arteriovenous fistulas (dAVF) are another type of vascular malformation. These are theorized to be acquired lesions that can result from trauma, surgery, or thrombosis of an adjacent venous sinus. These entities consist of a direct arterial to venous connection with no intervening nidus (Figure 6). Another vascular malformation worth noting is the **vein of Galen** aneurysmal malformation. Like AVMs, these entities do not have intervening capillaries between the arterial and venous connection (Figure 7). These present during early childhood with features of a left-to-right shunt and high output cardiac failure.

FIGURE 6. Dural Arteriovenous Fistula (dAVF)

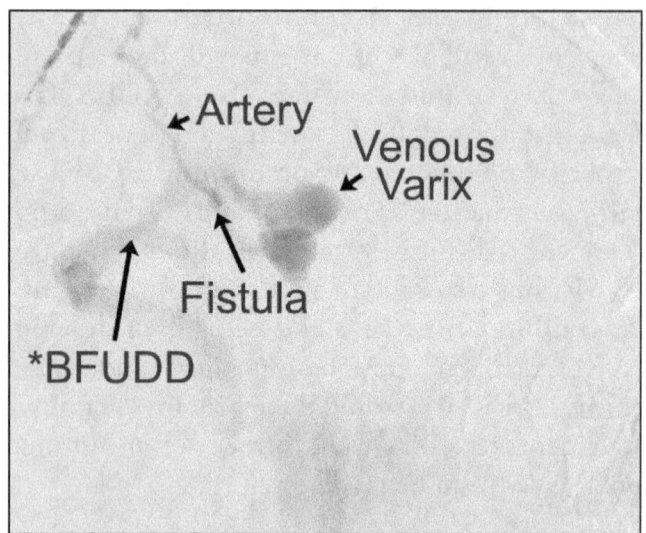

*BFUDD - Big, fat, ugly, disgusting draining vein

FIGURE 7. Vein of Galen Malformation

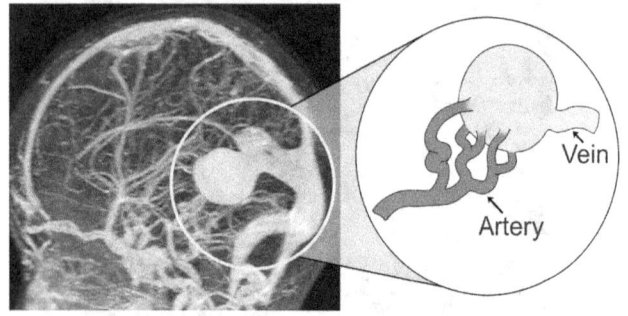

9.3 Cavernous Malformations (CMs)

Cavernous malformations (also called *angiomas* or *cavernous hemangiomas* or *cavernomas*) are discrete, well-circumscribed, multilobulated lesions that contain blood-filled cysts in various stages of evolution. Essentially, these entities are berry-like lesions that contain multiple endothelial-lined sinusoidal spaces with no intervening normal neural tissue (Figure 8). Often, these sinusoidal spaces are characterized by various stages of hemorrhage. Essentially, when one of the sinusoidal spaces bleeds, it coats the entire cavernous malformation with blood. Immune cells then digest these blood components but leave behind iron. This iron then coats each of these little sinusoids, leaving behind "iron deposition." Think of each of the sinusoids resembling an M&M—but instead of being candy-coated, they are coated with iron.

FIGURE 8. Cavernous Malformation

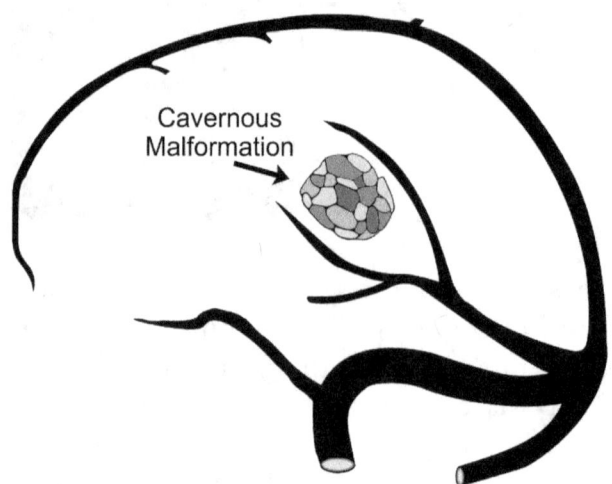

Because the different sinusoids in these berry-like lesions have different stages of hemorrhage, they present with heterogeneous signal on T1-weighted images (Figure 9). Due to iron deposition from repetitive bleeds, they typically have a dark band of hemosiderin on T2-weighted images (Figure 9). Furthermore, this iron deposition results in "blooming" artifact gradient echo images (Figure 9).

Like AVMs, cavernous malformations do not contain normal neuronal tissue and are more frequently (80% of the time) located supratentorially. Most of the time, these are benign entities with no surrounding edema. However, if one of these sinusoidal spaces bleeds significantly, parenchymal hemorrhage can result. In addition, the location of these entities is important. For example, cavernous malformations located in an eloquent region of the brain with even a small bleed can have devastating consequences. The risk of bleeding from cavernous malformations is 0.1% per year. However, a condition called *familial cavernous angioma syndrome* (autosomal dominant) can increase the risk of hemorrhage from cavernous malformations to 1% annually.

FIGURE 9. Cavernous Malformation and Surrounding Iron Deposition

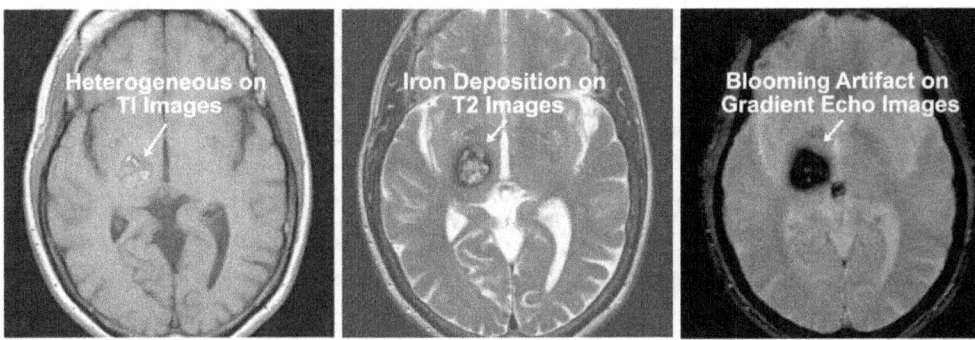

FIGURE 10. Developmental Venous Anomaly (DVA)

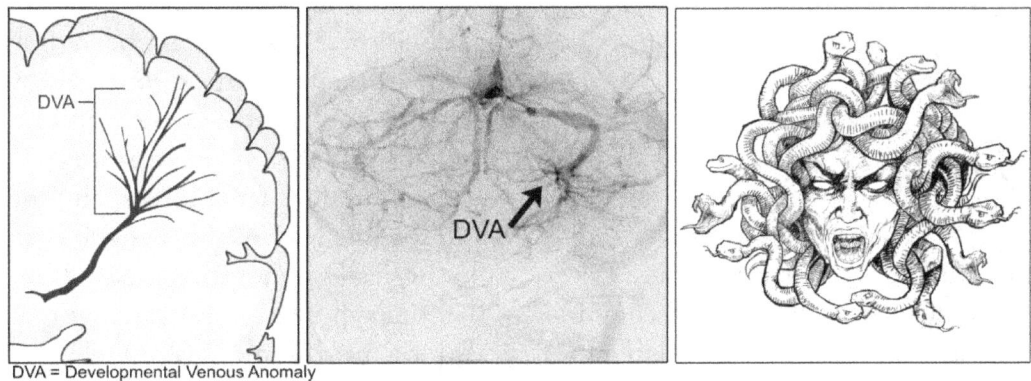

DVA = Developmental Venous Anomaly

9.4 Developmental Venous Anomalies (DVAs)

Developmental venous anomalies (previously referred to as *venous angiomas*) are radially arranged, dilated medullary (white matter) veins that converge into an enlarged transcortical or subependymomal draining vein (Figure 10). This cerebrovascular malformation represents an anatomic variant, which is why the term *developmental venous anomaly* (DVA) is preferred over the term *venous angioma*. DVAs are usually solitary lesions. So, what are "radially arranged dilated draining medullary veins"?

We have all heard of Medusa from Greek mythology (Figure 10). Her hair was replaced by snakes and her glance turned mortal men into stone. The "radially arranged dilated draining medullary veins" found in developmental venous anomalies have been described as having a "head of Medusa" or "caput Medusa" appearance (like the snakes on Medusa's head). They converge into a larger vein which looks like the head of Medusa (Figure 10).

Unlike AVMs and cavernous malformations, normal brain tissue is identified between these radially arranged draining veins. They are typically found in deep cerebral or cerebellar white matter. They are often periventricular in location and are most commonly found adjacent to the frontal horn of the lateral ventricle. They are also commonly found within the cerebellum. Angiographically, DVAs have a classic "caput medusa" appearance with radially arranged draining veins converging into a single larger vein (Figure 11).

FIGURE 11. Angiographic Appearance of Developmental Venous Anomaly (DVA)

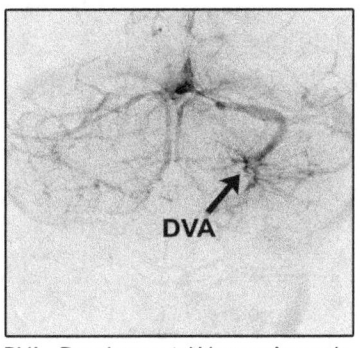

DVA - Developmental Venous Anomaly

On non-enhanced brain CT, they are typically unnoticeable. However, on contrast CT, there appear as a stellate tangle of vessels which resemble the snakes on Medusa's head. These typically drain into a sharply defined transcortical vein which resembles the head of Medusa. These same characteristics are seen on MRI with strong enhancement. When these are solitary lesions, there is little bleeding risk. However, 30% of developmental venous anomalies are associated with cavernous malformations which increase hemorrhagic risk. Additionally, hemorrhage associated with the coexistence of DVAs and cavernous malformations is most often caused by the cavernous malformation rather than the DVA.

9.5 Capillary Telangiectasias

Capillary telangiectasias are small regions of abnormally dilated capillaries within the brain. Like developmental venous anomalies, they contain normal intervening neural tissue. Although capillary telangiectasias are commonly found vascular malformations, they are rarely symptomatic. They are usually found in the pons and have faint contrast enhancement and dark signal on gradient echo images (Figure 12). Consider a capillary telangiectasia when a MRI has normal T1 and T2 signal within the pons but contains faint enhancement. Often, these are clinically silent. However, like DVAs, they may coexist with cavernous malformations. If they do, just like DVAs, there is an increased risk of bleeding. This risk of hemorrhage, however, is likely due to the cavernous malformation rather than the capillary telangiectasia.

9.6 Conclusion

That concludes the short and sweet synopsis of cerebrovascular malformations. Remember, the two lesions that are most commonly symptomatic include **AVMs** and **cavernous malformations**. Both malformations do not contain normal intervening neuronal tissue and instead contain a nidus and sinusoidal lesions, respectively. For this reason, these lesions can be removed surgically when necessary. The two cerebrovascular malformations that are most commonly found incidentally are **DVAs** and **capillary telangiectasias**. Both contain normal intervening neuronal tissue and for this reason, these entities typically cannot be surgically removed. An easy way to remember the four types of cerebrovascular malformations is with the mnemonic '**ABCD**' (Table 2). These four entities are also summarized in Table 3.

TABLE 2. Cerebrovascular Malformations: **ABCD**

A	AVMs
B	Berry-like Lesions - Cavernous Malformations
C	Capillary Telangiectasias
D	Developmental Venous Anomalies

FIGURE 12. Pontine Capillary Telangiectasia

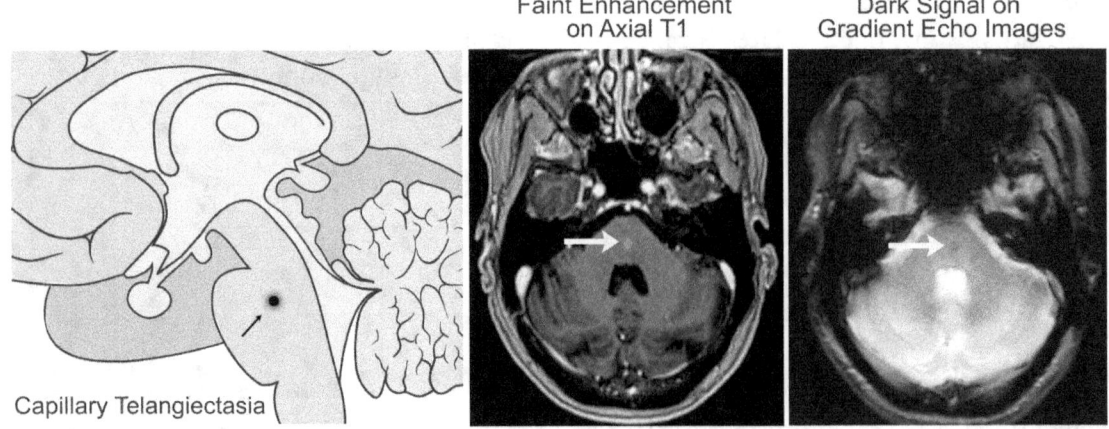

TABLE 3. Cerebrovascular Malformation (CVM) Characteristics

CVM	SYMPTOMATIC?	CONTAINS BRAIN?	REMEMBER
AVMs	YES	NO	BFUDD*
CM	YES	NO	IRON COATING
DVA	NO**	YES	MEDUSA
CT	NO**	YES	IRON POOLING

AVM - Arteriovenous Malformation; CM - Cavernous Malformation; DVA - Developmental Venous Anomaly; CT - Capillary Telangiectasia

*BFUDD - Big, fat, ugly, disgusting, draining vein
**Both developmental venous anomalies and capillary telangiectasias can be associated with cavernous malformations which can result in symptomatic hemorrhage.

Abbreviations list

AVM, arteriovenous malformation; BFUDD, big, fat, ugly, disgusting, draining vein; CM, cavernous malformation; CT, capillary telangiectasias; CVM, cerebrovascular malformation; dAVF, dural arteriovenous fistulas; DVA, developmental venous anomaly; MRA, magnetic resonance angiography.

References

1. Derdeyn CP, Zipfel GJ, Albuquerque FC, Cooke DL, Feldmann E, Sheehan JP, Torner JC. (2017). Management of Brain Arteriovenous Malformations: A Scientific Statement for Healthcare Professionals From the American Heart Association/American Stroke Association. American Heart Association Stroke Council. *Stroke,* Aug, 48(8), e200-e224.
2. International Stroke Conference (ICS). (2016). Abstract LB11. Presented February 18, 2016.

Chapter 10

Cerebral Venous Stroke

10.1 Introduction

Cerebral venous thrombosis (CVT) is caused by acute thrombosis in a superficially located dural venous sinus or deep brain venous structure. Dural sinuses are venous structures found between the periosteal (adherent to the calvarium) and meningeal layers of the dura mater (Figure 1). This superficial venous system and a deeper venous system are responsible for the brain's venous drainage. CVT is a rare but serious condition affecting two to seven persons per million annually.[1] CVT or venous stroke accounts for only 0.5%-1% of all stroke.[2] Unlike arterial strokes, CVT typically affects the younger population, with higher incidence among women. With adequate treatment, CVT has a good prognosis. However, the lack of prompt diagnosis and treatment can lead to devastating consequences. To make matters worse, venous stroke has a large degree of variability in both its clinical presentation and imaging manifestations.

10.2 Superficial and Deep Cerebral Venous Drainage

There are two regions of venous drainage: **superficial** and **deep**. Most CVT (85%) occurs in the superficial system and approximately 10% takes place in the deep system. Just like arterial stroke, knowledge of cerebral venous anatomy is essential for CVT evaluation. This is because just like arterial stroke, symptoms associated with CVT are related to the areas of the brain affected by venous thrombosis (Figure 2). For example, CVT involving the deep venous system can cause venous infarction of the basal ganglion and other subcortical structures such as the thalamus.

FIGURE 1. The Dural Sinuses

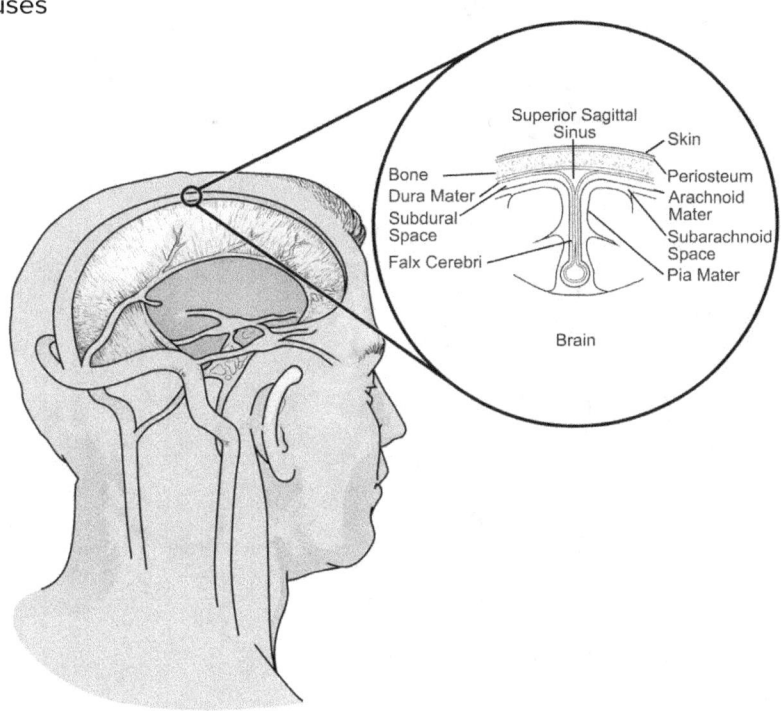

The superficial venous drainage from the cerebral cortex travels via superficial cerebral veins which drain into the superior sagittal sinus (Figure 3). The most prominent superior cerebral vein is termed the **vein of Trolard**. More inferiorly located superficial cerebral veins called inferior cerebral veins drain into the transverse sinus. The most prominent inferior cerebral vein is termed the **vein of Labbe**. To help remember this, keep in mind that 'T' is for top or 'Trolard' and 'L' is for lower or 'Labbe' (Box 1). The transverse sinuses then drain into the sigmoid sinus which drains into the internal jugular vein of the neck.

BOX 1. Superficial Cortical Venous Drainage

| **T**rolard = **T**op |
| **L**abbe = **L**ower |

Deeper venous drainage from the center of the brain drains into the inferior sagittal sinus and the vein of Galen, both of which join to form the straight sinus (Figure 4). Note that the superior sagittal sinus, both transverse sinuses, and the straight sinus connect at one location called the *confluence of sinuses*. Anteriorly, surrounding the cavernous segment of the internal carotid artery is another dural venous sinus called the **cavernous sinus.** In addition to encasing the cavernous segment of the internal carotid artery, it also contains cranial nerves III, IV, V1 and V2 (Figure 5). The cavernous sinus drains posteriorly through the superior and inferior petrosal sinuses. The superior petrosal sinus drains into the transverse sinus, while the inferior petrosal sinus drains into the internal jugular vein (Figure 3).

FIGURE 2. Distributions of Intracranial Venous Drainage

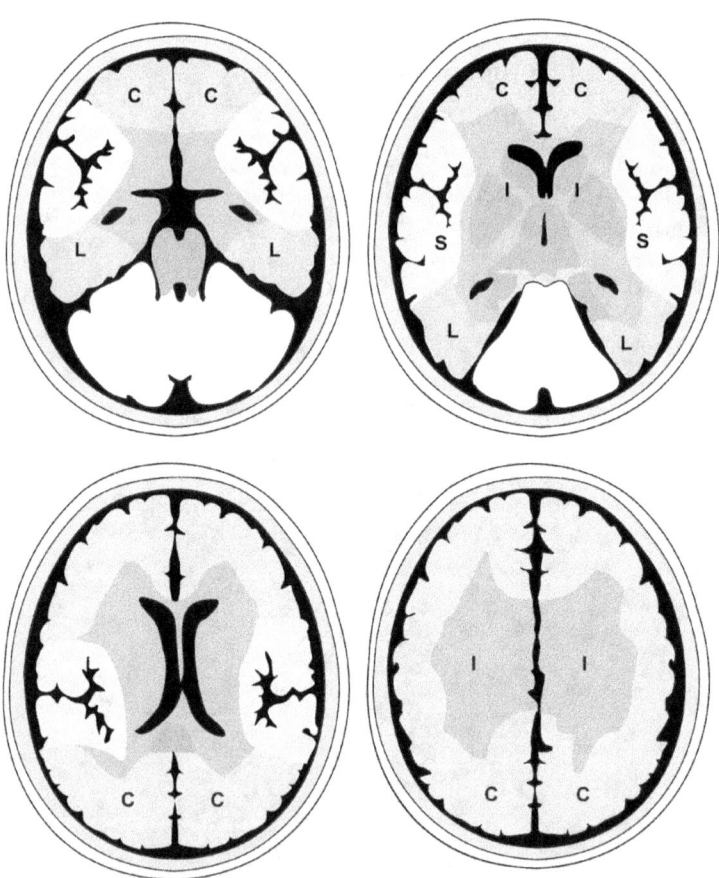

C = Cortical Veins (Drain into Superior Sagittal Sinus)
I = Internal Cerebral Veins
L = Vein of Labbe
S = Sphenoparietal Sinus (Drain into Cavernous Sinus)

FIGURE 3. The Cerebral Venous Circulation

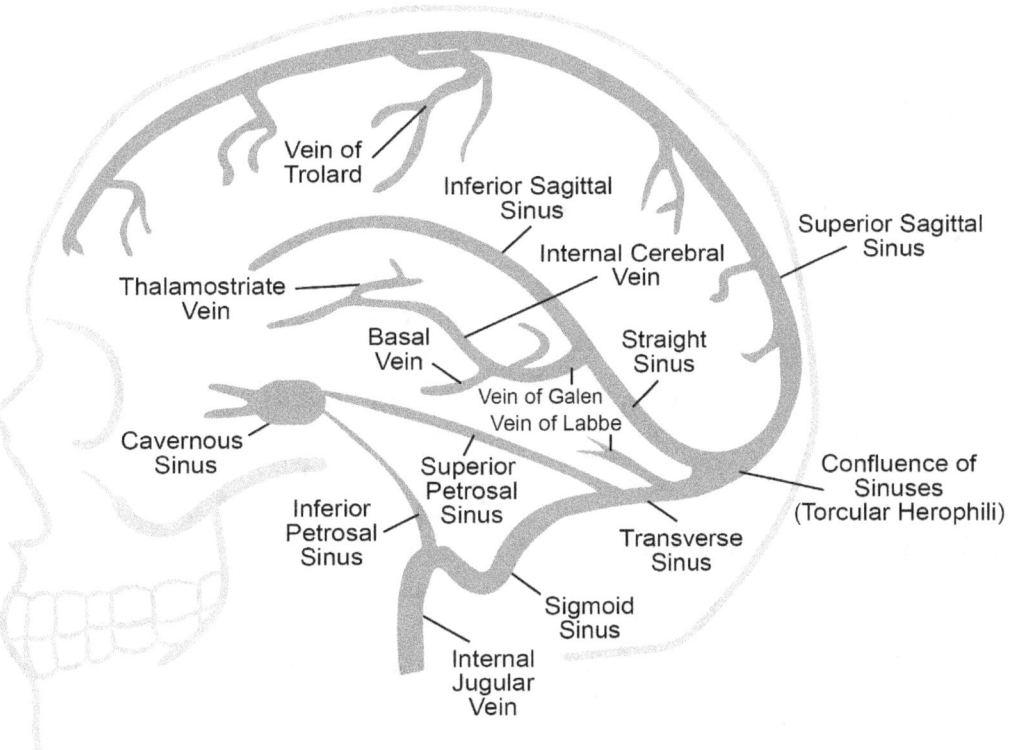

FIGURE 4. Deep Venous Drainage

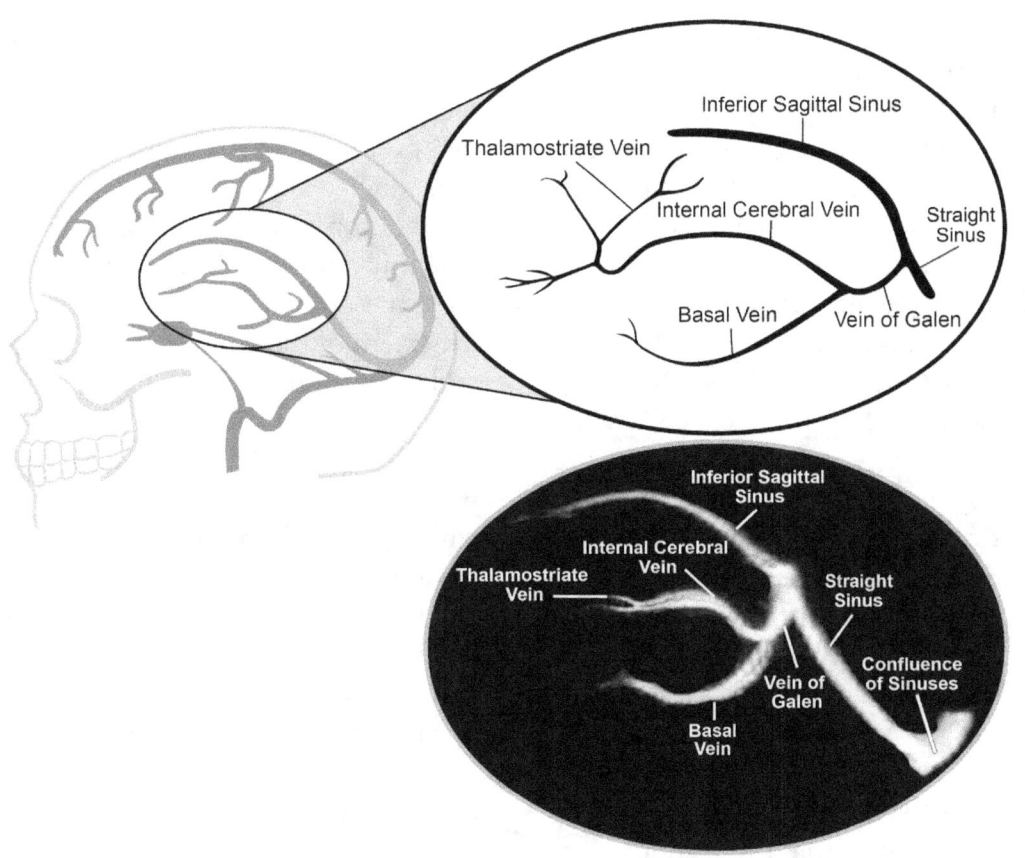

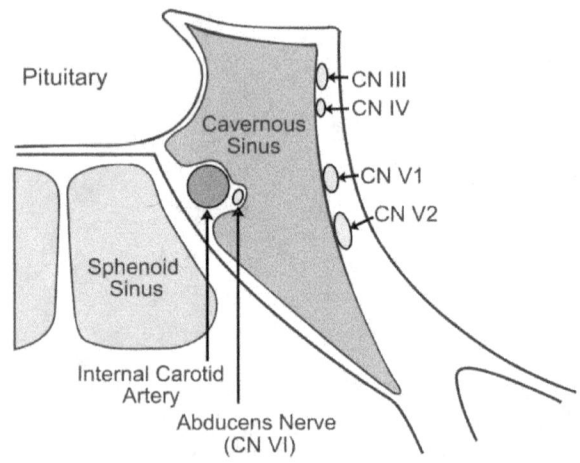

FIGURE 5. The Cavernous Sinus and Contained Structures

10.3 Cerebral Venous Hemorrhage

Dural venous sinuses differ from other blood vessels in the body in that they lack a full set of vessel layers. The walls of dural venous sinuses consist of dura mater lined with endothelium. They are thin, fragile, and valveless structures deficient of smooth muscle. Arteries deliver blood into the brain while veins facilitate its removal. Think of blood flow entering the brain from arteries just like water entering the sink from a faucet. Using this analogy, blood exiting intracranial veins is similar to a drain removing water from a sink. When the drain in the sink becomes obstructed, water flowing from a faucet will fill the sink and eventually overflow—that is, the flow of water from the faucet into the sink and its drainage are obstructed.

When cerebral veins are obstructed, this leads to the obstruction of venous drainage and stagnation of arterial flow. Furthermore, obstructed intracranial veins lead to elevated venous pressure which prevents flow of blood into brain tissue, causing cytotoxic and vasogenic edema. Once venous pressure rises above arterial inflow pressure, oxygen can no longer be transported to the brain, resulting in a venous infarct. In addition, the walls of cerebral veins are weaker than arteries. If the cerebral veins cannot contain this elevated pressure, they can rupture and cause subarachnoid or parenchymal hemorrhage.

Thrombotic occlusion of the venous system is associated with infection, dehydration, malignancy, coagulation disorders, smoking, pregnancy, puerperium, and birth control pill use. The diagnosis of CVT is dependent upon clinical presentation, clinical laboratory studies, and imaging confirmation. Symptoms are either related to increased intracranial pressure secondary to impaired venous drainage or focal brain injury from venous ischemia and/or hemorrhage. Headache (resulting from increased intracranial pressure) is the most common presenting CVT-related symptom. Recall that unless related to an arterial dissection, headaches are typically not a presenting symptom among arterial ischemic stroke patients. Another symptom that distinguishes CVT from arterial ischemic stroke patients is generalized seizures which occur in approximately 40% of CVT patients.

10.4 Cerebral Venous Work-Up

Patients with suspected CVT should receive routine blood work to exclude processes that can cause CVT. These processes include hypercoagulation, infection, or inflammation. For example, leukocytosis may indicate an infectious process. While CVT does not cause specific CSF abnormalities, 80% of patients have elevated opening pressures with lumbar puncture.[3] D-dimer, a product of fibrin degradation, can also aid in the workup of CVT patients but cannot provide a definitive diagnosis. Kosinski et al. demonstrated that D-dimer levels positively correlated with the extent of thrombosis and negatively correlated with symptom duration in CVT patients.[4] Thus, patients with subacute or chronic symptoms are more likely to have negative D-dimer levels than patients with acute symptoms. Further, patients with less clot burden have a higher probability of having a false negative D-dimer test result. Kosinski et al. further demonstrated D-dimer levels greater than 500 mcg/L had a sensitivity of 97.1% with a negative predictive value of 99.6% and a specificity of 91.2% with a positive predictive value of 55.7%. However, there are two critical things to remember about D-dimer analysis. First, D-dimer positivity does not confirm the diagnosis of CVT, and second, it cannot definitively exclude the diagnosis of CVT. **Imaging studies are required to either definitively confirm or exclude the diagnosis of CVT.**

10.5 Cerebral Venous Imaging

Since most CVT patients present with nonspecific neurologic signs, the first imaging study obtained is a noncontrast brain CT. CT findings in CVT patients are variable and sometimes, a hyperdense sinus might be the only sign of a thrombosed dural sinus (Figure 6). Approximately 30 to 40% of patients with CVT present with intracranial hemorrhage (Figure 7).[5,6] However, fewer than 1% of CVT patients present with subarachnoid hemorrhage (SAH) (Figure 7).[7] CVT SAH can be distinguished from aneurysmal subarachnoid hemorrhage (aSAH) both clinically and radiographically. CVT headaches are typically described as diffuse, which gradually progress in severity over time. Most CVT patients do not present with "the worst headache of my life" symptom as do aSAH patients. Additionally, CVT SAH is typically identified in the convexity (superficial) as opposed to the central distribution of aSAH surrounding the circle of Willis (Figure 8). While there are no specific brain parenchymal changes, hemorrhage and edema may be identified on CT or MRI studies as secondary signs of CVT. The better way to diagnose CVT is to look for direct signs of venous occlusion. This requires a radiologic study that outlines the dural sinuses with contrast. CT or MR venography will demonstrate a filling defect within the suspected sinus if occluded and are excellent studies to visualize the dural venous sinuses (Figure 9). Additionally, cerebral angiography can also visualize the dural venous sinuses during the venous phase.

FIGURE 6. Hyperdense Superior Sagittal Sinus on Noncontrast Brain CT

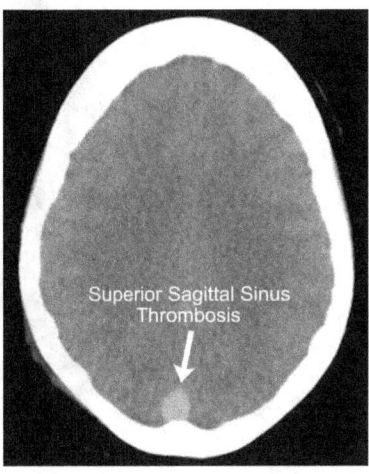

FIGURE 7. Subarachnoid and Parenchymal Venous Hemorrhage Secondary to Venous Infarct

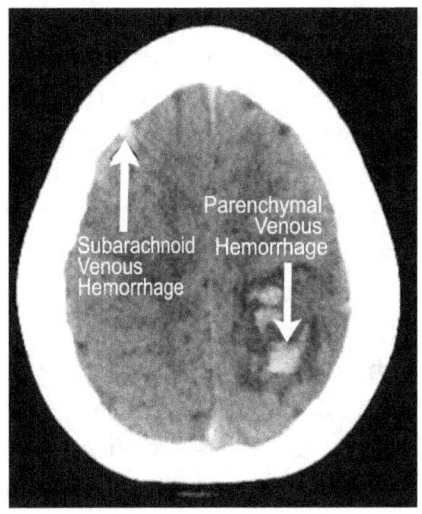

FIGURE 8. Superficial Subarachnoid Hemorrhage Associated with Intracranial Venous Infarct

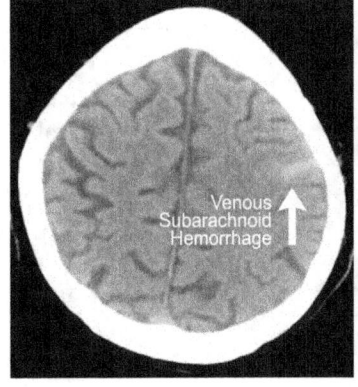 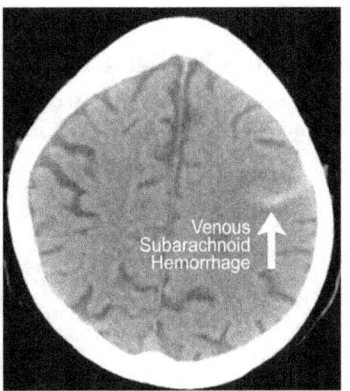

FIGURE 9. MRA Demonstrating Superior Sagittal Sinus Thrombosis

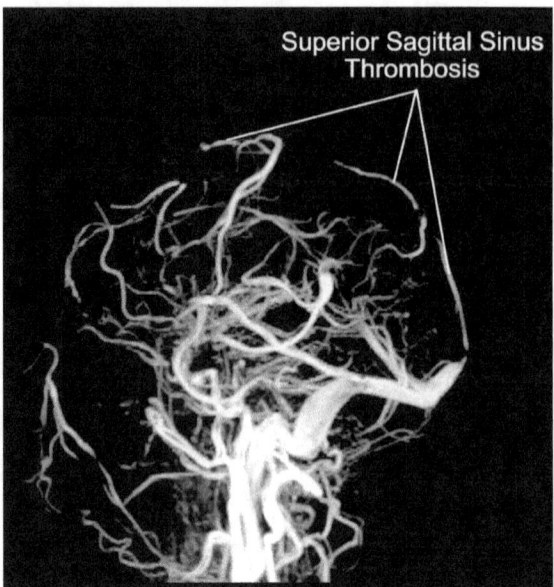

10.6 Cerebral Venous Treatment

Anticoagulation with low molecular weight heparin or unfractionated heparin is the first line of treatment for cerebral venous thrombosis and infarct. This treatment is recommended even if venous thrombosis is associated with parenchymal hemorrhage. While parenchymal hemorrhage associated with venous infarct worsens outcome, it does not increase the risk of new or the progression of existing hemorrhage after anticoagulation.[8] Thus, the use of systemic anticoagulation as an initial therapy for CVT patients is supported even with the presence of intracranial hemorrhage.[9] Multiple other studies have confirmed anticoagulation can be used safely for CVT treatment with the presence of intracranial hemorrhage.[10,11]

10.7 Conclusion

CVT is a relatively uncommon form of stroke (0.5%) and often presents as a diagnostic dilemma because patients typically present with a headache rather than focal neurologic symptoms. CVT is a rare but potentially devastating type of stroke that most commonly affects young adult women. This chapter reviewed cerebral venous anatomy, CVT risk factors, presentation, work up, and treatment.

It's important to recognize this potentially devastating stroke variant because its proper diagnosis and subsequent management can result in excellent outcomes.

Abbreviations list

aSAH, aneurysmal subarachnoid hemorrhage; CVT, cerebral venous thrombosis; SAH, subarachnoid hemorrhage.

References

1. Leach J L, Fortuna, R B, Jones, B V, et al. (2006). Imaging of cerebral venous thrombosis: current techniques, spectrum of findings, and diagnostic pitfalls. *Radiographics*, 26, Suppl 1, S19-41.
2. Stam J. (2005). Thrombosis of the cerebral veins and sinuses. *N Engl J Med*, 352, 1791–98.
3. Ferro JM, Canhão P, Stam J, Bousser MG, Barinagarrementeria F. (2004). ISCVT Investigators.. Prognosis of cerebral vein and dural sinus thrombosis: reults of the International Study on Cerebral Vein and Dural Sinus Thrombosis (ISCVT), *Stroke*, 35, 664–70.
4. Kosinski CM, Mull M, Schwarz M, Koch B, Biniek R, Schläfer J, Milkereit E, Willmes K, Schiefer J. (2004). Do normal D-dimer levels reliably exclude cerebral sinus thrombosis? *Stroke*, 35, 2820–25.

5. Wasay M, Bakshi R, Bobustuc G, Kojan S, Sheikh Z, Dai A, Cheema Z. (2008). Cerebral venous thrombosis: analysis of a multicenter cohort from the United States. *J Stroke Cerebrovasc Dis*, 17, 49-54.
6. Girot M, Ferro JM, Canhão P, Stam J, Bousser MG, Barinagarrementeria F, Leys D. (2007). ISCVT Investigators. Predictors of outcome in patients with cerebral venous thrombosis and intracerebral hemorrhage. *Stroke,* 38, 337–42.
7. Oppenheim C, Domigo V, Gauvrit JY, Lamy C, Mackowiak-Cordoliani MA, Pruvo JP, Méder JF. (2005) Subarachnoid hemorrhage as the initial presentation of dural sinus thrombosis. *AJNR Am J Neuroradiol*, 26, 614–17.
8. Ferro J M, Canhao P. (2014). Cerebral venous sinus thrombosis: Update on diagnosis and management. *Curr Cardiol Rep,* 16(9), 523.
9. Medel R, Monteith SJ, Crowley RW, Dumont AS. (2009). A review of therapeutic strategies for the management of cerebral venous sinus thrombosis. *Neurosurg Focus*, Nov. 27, 5, E6.
10. Einhaupl KM, Villringer A, Meister W, et al. (1991). Heparin treatment in sinus venous thrombosis. *Lancet*, Sep 7, 338(8767), 597-600.
11. de Bruijn SF, Stam J, Vandenbroucke JP. (1998). Increased risk of cerebral venous sinus thrombosis with third-generation oral contraceptives. Cerebral Venous Sinus Thrombosis Study Group. *Lancet*, May 9, 351(9113), 1404.

Chapter 11

Cerebellar Stroke

11.1 Introduction

This is the first of five chapters that will discuss posterior circulation stroke. Posterior circulation stroke accounts for approximately 20% of all ischemic stroke.[1] Posterior circulation stroke is defined as stroke involving the vertebrobasilar system. The term *vertebrobasilar insufficiency* (VBI) encompasses all transient ischemic (TIA) syndromes of the posterior circulation but often is inappropriately used to describe posterior circulation ischemic stroke. *Vertebrobasilar atherothrombotic disease* (VBATD) is the more appropriate term for both transient and permanent ischemic insults involving the posterior circulation.

Stroke deficits are determined by the region of the brain affected, its functionality and its arterial territory. The posterior circulation supplies the thalamus, brainstem, occipital lobe, cerebellum, inferior temporal lobe, and medial occipital lobe. Thus, posterior circulation stroke can produce a variety of clinical features because of the various regions of the brain supplied. Furthermore, some of these regions such as the thalamus and brainstem contain densely packed neural pathways and cranial nerves. This further complicates the understanding of posterior circulation stroke. Succinctly put, the spectrum for posterior circulation ischemic disease is massive.

Fortunately, most posterior circulation stroke can be understood by correlating deficits with the relevant vascular anatomy and region of the brain affected. Unfortunately, however, posterior circulation supplied brain structures can be complex. Due to the voluminous material related to the posterior circulation, the next four chapters will concentrate on four distinct regions of the brain: the **thalamus, brainstem, cerebellum** and **occipital lobe.** This discussion begins with the cerebellum.

11.2 Cerebellar Anatomy

The cerebellum is located below the occipital lobes and is separated from the pons anteriorly by the fourth ventricle (Figure 1). The cerebellum has two hemispheres which are connected by the cerebellar vermis (Figure 2). The cerebellum has multiple functions but is predominantly involved with the coordination of voluntary movement. It is not responsible for the initiation of movement, and for this reason, a cerebellar infarct does not present with paralysis. Instead, cerebellar stroke results in uncoordinated, slow, clumsy, and tremulous movements. The cerebellum receives a great deal of information related to the positional state of muscles and joints, the equilibrium state of the body, and what impulses are being sent from the motor cortex throughout the body. The cerebellum interprets this information through feedback pathways and, in this manner, regulates voluntary movement.

FIGURE 1. The Cerebellum

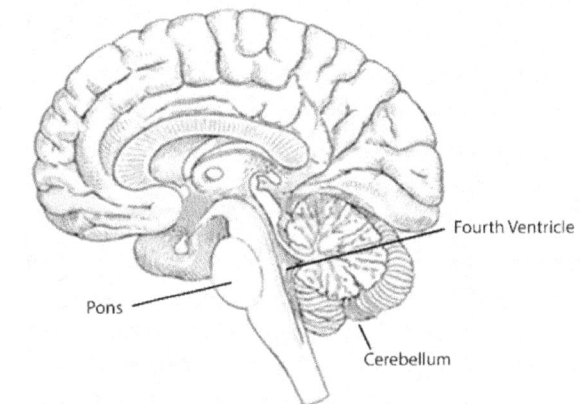

FIGURE 2. The Cerebellar Vermis

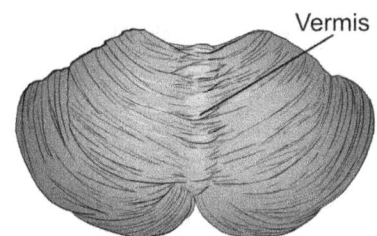

To do this, the cerebellum is connected to the brainstem by three sets of white matter tracts called the cerebellar peduncles. From top to bottom, the brainstem consists of the midbrain, pons, and medulla (Figure 3). The superior cerebellar peduncle connects the cerebellum to the midbrain which comprises the top of the brainstem (Figure 4). The middle cerebellar peduncle connects the cerebellum to the middle of the brainstem or pons. The superior cerebellar peduncle transmits information from the cerebellum to the cerebrum, while the middle cerebellar peduncle transmits information from the cerebrum to the cerebellum. The inferior cerebellar peduncle connects the cerebellum to the bottom of the brainstem, the medulla oblongata, and the spinal cord. The inferior cerebellar peduncle contains both incoming vestibular and proprioceptive fibers as well as outgoing motor fibers. Essentially, the inferior cerebellar peduncle receives vestibular and proprioceptive information from parts of the body such as the arm, then interprets this information and sends out signals in conjunction with motor signals from the cerebrum to help coordinate movement. *The main purpose of the cerebellum is to coordinate movement.*

11.3 Cerebellar Stroke Symptoms

Cerebellar stroke is uncommon and accounts for 2% of all ischemic stroke (AIS). Yet, it is still important to recognize this form of stroke and its potential complications.[2] Cerebellar stroke can present with diverse and variable symptoms, the most common of which include headache, dizziness, nausea, vomiting, and vertigo. These diverse and nonspecific symptoms can cause cerebellar stroke to be mistaken for more benign conditions.[3] However, while less than 50% of cerebellar infarct can present with nausea and vomiting and even more with dizziness (75%), **90% of patients have localizing signs such as truncal and appendicular ataxia, nystagmus, and dysarthria.**[4]

FIGURE 3. The Brainstem

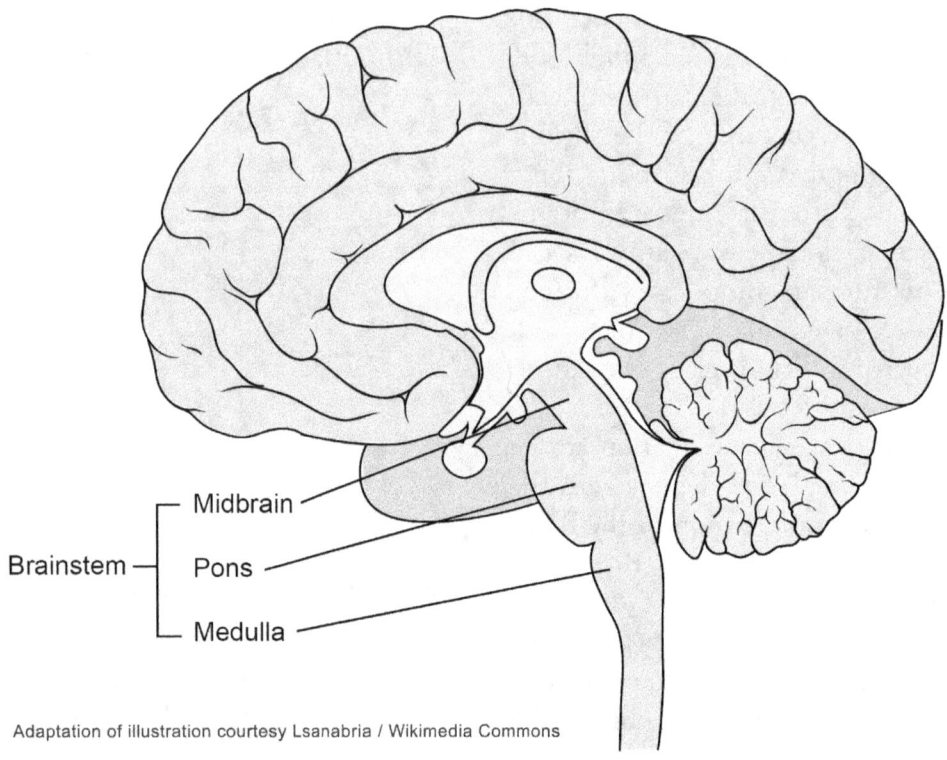

Adaptation of illustration courtesy Lsanabria / Wikimedia Commons

FIGURE 4. The Cerebellar Peduncles

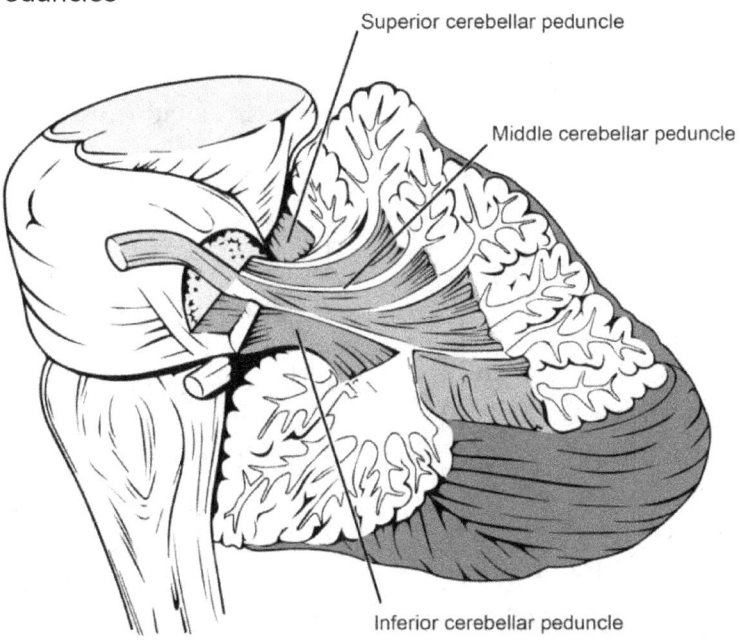

Cerebellar motor symptoms are usually ipsilateral. There are several other characteristic ipsilateral deficits produced by cerebellar stroke such as dysmetria, adiadochkinesia, asynergia, intention tremor, gait abnormalities, vertigo, dysphonia, hypotonia, and nystagmus. An easy way to remember cerebellar stroke symptoms is with the mnemonic 'DARK NIGHT DIVA' (Table 1). Altered mental status may indicate a large cerebellar infarction, with the level of consciousness after stroke onset being predictive of poor clinical outcome.[5]

TABLE 1. Cerebellar Stroke Symptoms: **DARK NIGHT DIVA**

D	**Dysmetria** - inability to judge distance and stop movement at a chosen point	
A	**Ataxia** - uncoordinated movement	
R	**Relaxed Muscles** - hypotonia (floppy and weak muscles)	
K	**Kinesia** - Dysdiadochokinesis, inability to perform rapidly alternating movements (i.e. pronation and supination of hands) Dysrhythmokinesis, disorder of the rhythm of rapidly alternating movements	
N	**Nystagmus**	
I	**Intention Tremor** - during movement and not at rest	
G	**Gait Abnormality** (one form of ataxia)	
H	**Headache**	
T	**Tipsy** - vertigo, falls to injured side	
D	**Dysphonia** - slurred explosive speech	
I	**Ipsilateral Motor Symptoms**	
V	**Vomiting** and nausea	
A	**Asynergia** - loss of motor coordination, jerky movements	

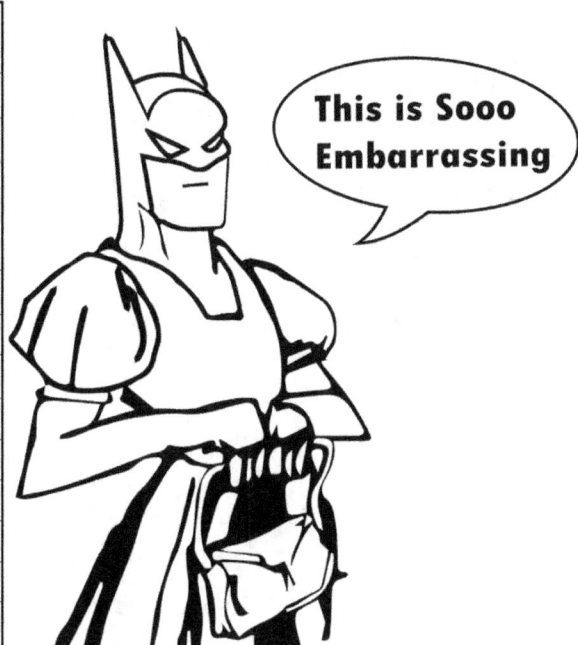

11.4 Cerebellar Exam

So how does one assess for cerebellar disease and run through this laundry list of cerebellar deficits? The five principal signs of cerebellar dysfunction include **gait, ataxia, tremor, ocular motor abnormalities**, and **relaxed muscles or hypotonia** (Table 2).[6] These can be quickly assessed. During examination, assess for nystagmus by having the patient track the examiner's fingers. Also, hold one hand directly in front of the patient and the other 45° away from this position. Ask the patient to shift gaze from one hand to the other and check the eyes for overshooting of the target. Have the patient take a deep breath, then say "ahhh" as long as possible while checking the expiratory muscles and vocal cords. Next have the patient say "la, la, la" as long as possible to check for rapid alternating movements of the tongue.

TABLE 2. The Five Principal Signs of Cerebellar Dysfunction: **GATOR**

G	Gait
A	Ataxia
T	Tremor
O	Oculomotor Abnormalities
R	Relaxed Muscles or Hypotonia

Next, examine the arms or upper extremities. Check for rapid alternating movements with each hand using the thigh-slapping test. Test finger-nose-finger alternating movements by having the patient touch the tip of your index finger with the tip of their index finger. Then have the patient touch their nose with the tip of their index finger. Have the patient perform this as rapidly as possible. Dysdiadochokinesis refers to the impaired ability to perform rapid alternating movements (i.e. diadochokinesia). Next, have the patient use their fingers to tap out a tune and check for abnormalities in timing and finger motion. Dysrhythmokinesis is a disorder of the rhythm of rapid alternating movements.

Lastly, examine the lower extremities. Have the patient stand at rest. Cerebellar dysfunction results in the patient constantly shifting and often unable to stand without support. Next, assess gait. Bilateral cerebellar disease results in an abnormal gait resembling drunkenness or insobriety. Unilateral cerebellar disease results in deviation to the side of the lesion, likely due to hypotonia. Have the patient walk a straight-line heel-to-toe. This is one of the most sensitive tests of cerebellar vermis function. Next, have the patient tap their left knee gently with their right heel. Observe abnormalities in force and rhythm. Finally, have the patient place their right heel on top of the left knee and slide it down the shin to the left foot. Check to ensure the heel stays exactly on top of the shin and take note of coarse side-to-side tremors.

So how can someone possibly memorize these symptoms and this examination? Just remember two mnemonics. The first is 'HAL' and the second is 'GATOR,' which was discussed earlier (Box 1). Combined, this mnemonic becomes 'HAL-A-GATOR.'

BOX 1. Cerebellar Examination: **HAL**

H: Head	Nystagmus Overshooting of eyes "Ahhh" "La, La, La"
A: Arms (Upper Extremities)	Thigh slapping Finger to nose Tap a tune
L: Lower Extremities	Stand at rest Gait Heel to toe Heel to knee Heel to shin

11.5 Cerebellar Vascular Anatomy

As discussed earlier, the vascular supply to the cerebellum comes from three sets of arteries: the posterior inferior cerebellar artery (PICA), anterior inferior cerebellar artery (AICA) and superior cerebellar artery (SCA) (Figure 5). Recall that two paired vertebral arteries form the basilar artery at the pontomedullary junction. Before they do, PICA typically arises from each vertebral artery. Anterior spinal arteries typically also rise from the vertebral arteries before they form the basilar artery. After the basilar artery is formed, paired AICAs and SCAs arise from it. These three sets of paired vessels (PICA, AICA, and SCA) are the predominant vascular supply to the cerebellum (Figure 5). PICA supplies the posterior, inferior cerebellum, and inferior cerebellar peduncle. AICA supplies the anterior, inferior cerebellum, and middle cerebellar peduncle. SCA supplies the superior cerebellum and superior cerebellar peduncle (Figure 6).

In addition to the inferior cerebellum, the PICA also supplies the lateral medulla. The medial medulla is supplied by the anterior spinal artery which arises from the vertebral artery. The medulla is the most inferior component of the brainstem and will be discussed shortly. **PICA infarcts are the most common vascular distribution responsible for cerebellar infarcts**. The labyrinthine artery (LA) arises from AICA (85-100%) or directly off the basilar artery (15%) and supplies the vestibulocochlear nerve (Figure 5). Occlusion of the LA can result in hearing loss. In addition to supplying the anterior portion of the inferior cerebellum, the AICA also supplies the facial (VII) and vestibulocochlear (VIII) nerves. Besides supplying the superior portion of the cerebellum, the SCA also supplies most of the cerebellar cortex (Table 3). Infarcts in this distribution present with gait and limb ataxia, dysarthria, and horizontal nystagmus.

FIGURE 5. The Posterior Circulation

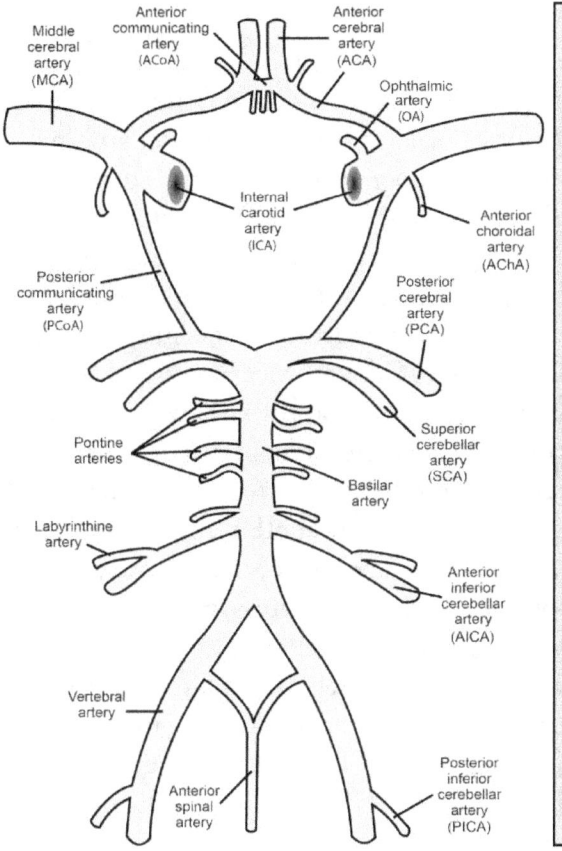
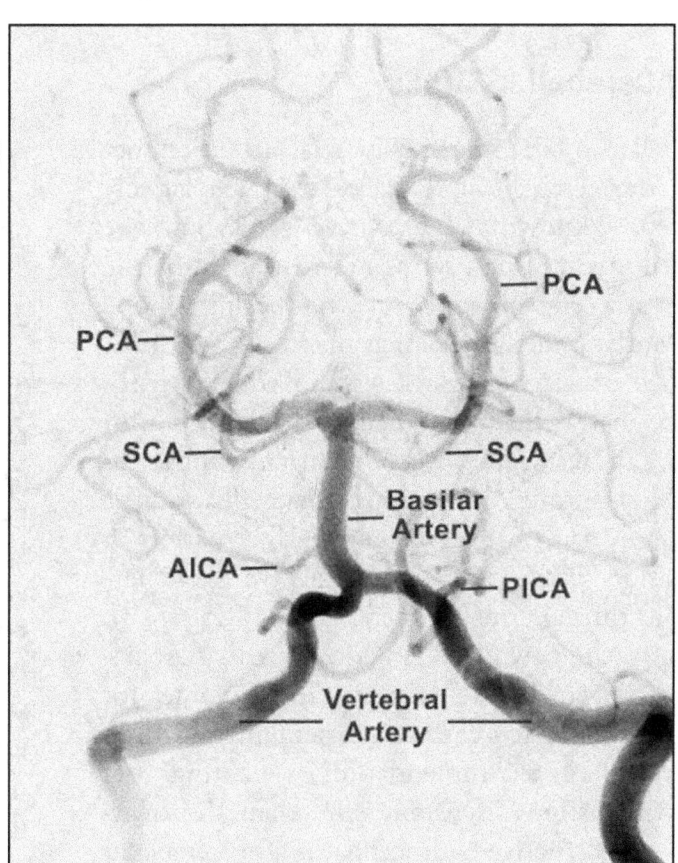

FIGURE 6. Vascular Supply to the Cerebellum

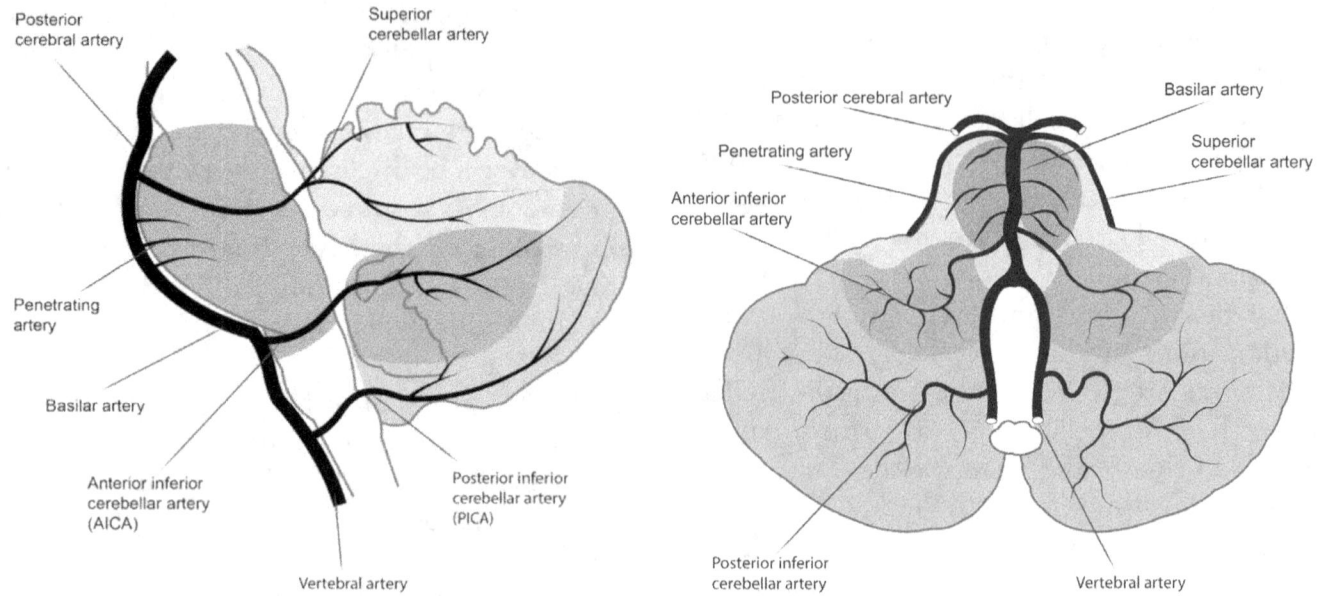

TABLE 3. Vascular Supply to the Cerebellum

Vessel	Structure
PICA	Posterior, Inferior Cerebellum and Inferior Cerebellar Peduncle
AICA	Anterior, Inferior Cerebellum and Middle Cerebellar Peduncle
SCA	Superior Cerebellum, Superior Cerebellar Peduncle and Cortex

11.6 Cerebellar Stroke

Cerebellar infarct requires special attention because the cerebellum is enclosed in a relatively tight space known as the *posterior fossa*. Both the cerebellum and brain stem are constrained by the tentorium cerebelli superiorly, the occipital bone posteriorly, and the foramen magnum inferiorly. Cerebellar infarct can cause cerebral edema which, when constrained in the tightly spaced posterior fossa, can result in fourth ventricular obstruction leading to hydrocephalus. Mass effect on the brainstem can cause transtentorial herniation or herniation of the cerebellar tonsils (tonsillar herniation) through the foramen magnum (Figure 7). Recently, the new 2018 American Heart Association/American Stroke Association Guidelines for acute ischemic stroke management revised their current 2014 recommendation by stating that "Ventriculostomy is recommended in the treatment of obstructive hydrocephalus after cerebellar infarct. Concomitant or subsequent decompressive craniectomy may or may not be necessary on the basis of factors such as infarct size, neurologic condition, degree of brainstem compression and effectiveness of medical management."[7]

Cerebellar infarction represents approximately 2% of all acute ischemic stroke.[8] While cerebellar stroke can result from an occlusion of the SCA, AICA, or PICA and have a myriad of brainstem related symptoms, approximately 10% of patients can present with isolated vertigo without other neurologic deficits. **In this population, 96% of these infarcts (cerebellar infarcts that present with vertigo exclusively) are caused by an occlusion of the posterior inferior cerebellar artery (PICA).** Patients who present with isolated vertigo due to cerebellar infarction pose a significant diagnostic challenge to emergency department physicians because it is this form of stroke that is frequently misdiagnosed and commonly results in disability.[9]

FIGURE 7. Transtentorial and Tonsillar Herniation

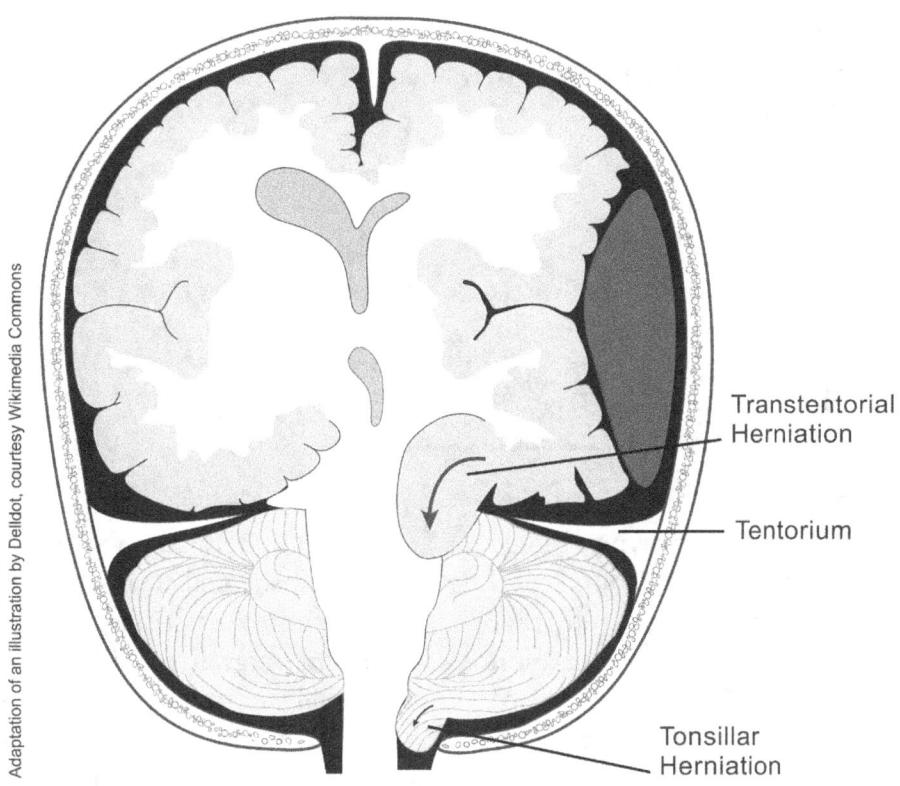

11.7 Cerebellar Stroke Versus Benign Vertigo

Cerebellar stroke in patients who only present with vertigo pose an enormous diagnostic challenge. Each year, over four million Americans visit the emergency department for dizziness or vertigo. Vertigo is a medical condition wherein patients feel as if they or the objects surrounding them are spinning or moving in the absence of any movement. This can be caused by pathology within the ear, the brain, or the nerve pathways that connect them. The emergency department evaluation of vertigo is complex. While most patients who present with isolated vertigo have benign disorders, up to 3% can have cerebellar infarcts.[10] Worse, 35% of these patients having a cerebellar stroke are not diagnosed at all.[9] This section will discuss the work up of vertigo and how to determine if it is benign or representative of an underlying cerebellar infarct.

Fortunately, there are some historical and physical clues that may aid the diagnosis of cerebellar infarct. First, stroke occurs suddenly with immediate onset of symptoms. Second, vascular risk factors are found in most patients who have cerebellar infarcts. Next, patients with cerebellar infarcts tend to have severe ataxia. One study demonstrated 71% of cerebellar infarct patients with isolated vertigo could not walk without support.[4] Finally, 56% of patients with cerebellar infarcts have direction-changing nystagmus.[4] An easy way to remember these deficits that indicate cerebellar infarction is with the mnemonic 'DIVAS' (Table 4). It is important to remember these deficits because when recognized together, they increase the detection sensitivity of cerebellar infarct. For example, the inability to walk without support and direction-changing nystagmus are important symptoms because in most cases no other findings of brainstem infarct are present. In fact, **at least one of these two signs were identified in 84% of cerebellar infarct patients who presented with isolated vertigo.**[4]

TABLE 4. Clues to Cerebellar Infarction: **DIVAS**

D	Direction Changing Nystagmus
I	Inability to Walk
V	Vascular Risk Factors
A	Ataxia, Severe
S	Sudden Immediate Symptoms

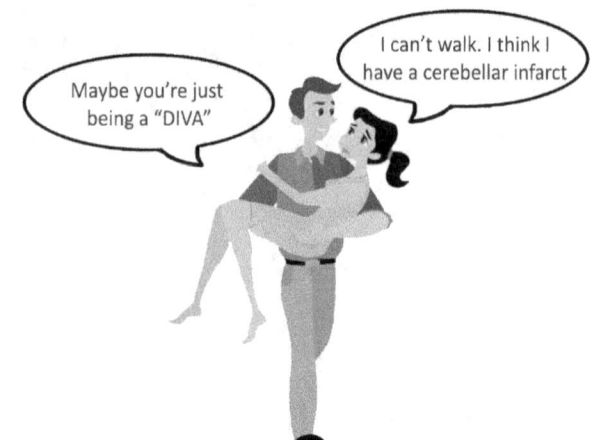

While these clues are helpful, proper neurologic examination is essential in distinguishing cerebellar stroke from benign vertigo. One study that examined cases of missed cerebellar infarction demonstrated no documentation of a standard neurologic examination or gait.[9] To properly evaluate a patient with vertigo, the examiner must know the benign causes of vertigo, how they differ from cerebellar stroke, and what neurologic exams can distinguish these conditions. The four most common benign vertigo syndromes are: **benign paroxysmal positional vertigo (BPPV)**, **Ménière's disease**, **migrainous vertigo**, and **vestibular neuritis** (Table 5).[11]

Benign paroxysmal positional vertigo (BPPV), vestibular neuritis, Ménière's disease and migrainous vertigo have different histories and symptomatic presentations. BPPV is characterized by intense symptoms that typically last less than a minute and are triggered by change in position (typically vertical head movement). However, every form of vertigo can be exasperated by position. Vestibular neuritis, on the other hand, typically presents with hours or days of ongoing and continuous vertigo and spontaneous nystagmus. Ménière's disease patients present with simultaneous vertigo and cochlear symptoms such as hearing loss, tinnitus, or aural fullness. Except when hearing loss presents as total ipsilateral deafness, vertigo with hearing loss indicates a peripheral disorder. A history of recurrent migraines with associated vertigo and a normal neurologic exam is the typical presentation of migrainous vertigo. Some studies rank migrainous vertigo as the second most common cause of vertigo experienced in clinical practice.[11]

Different neurologic tests are utilized to test BPPV and vestibular neuritis. Again, these forms of vertigo present differently. Patients who present with **short** episodes (30-60 seconds) of vertigo triggered by head movement and **no spontaneous** nystagmus are suspected of having BPPV and should be examined with the Dix-Hallpike exam. Patients presenting with **longer** episodes (hours or days) of ongoing and continuous vertigo and **spontaneous** nystagmus are suspected of having vestibular neuritis and should be examined with the HINTS exam (Table 6). The HINTS exam is an acronym for the three tests used to assess vestibular neuritis. These include **H**ead **I**mpulse, **N**ystagmus, and **T**est of **S**kew. Studies have demonstrated high inter-evaluator reliability between emergency department physicians and specialists when performing these examinations.[12]

TABLE 5. Benign Causes of Vertigo

Peripheral Causes of Vertigo	Central Causes of Vertigo
Benign Paroxysmal Positional Vertigo	Migrainous Vertigo
Ménière's Disease	
Vestibular Neuritis	

TABLE 6. Benign Paroxysmal Positional Vertigo (BPPV) and Vestibular Neuritis

Vertigo Cause	Symptoms	Exam
BPPV	Intense, less than 1 minute symptoms Positional exacerbation	Dix-Hallpike
Vestibular Neuritis	Hours or days of continuous vertigo Positional exacerbation	HINTS

11.7.1 Benign Paroxysmal Positional Vertigo (BPPV)

The Dix-Hallpike exam is performed in patients suspected of having BPPV, those with short episodes (30-60 seconds) of vertigo triggered by head movement, and no spontaneous nystagmus (Figure 8). To perform this maneuver, the patient should be seated with legs flat and arms crossed over the chest. Turn the patient's head 45° towards the examiner and stabilize the head with both hands. Check for nystagmus with the head turned toward the examiner. Then quickly lower the patient backwards so that the head is extended approximately 20 to 30° below the exam table. To do this, the patient's head must extend below the end of the exam table. If the patient has benign paroxysmal positional vertigo, a delayed vertigo will manifest and nystagmus will appear in approximately 20 to 30 seconds. After sitting the patient up, see if the nystagmus has resolved. Now repeat the exam with the patient's head positioned in the opposite direction. Be careful to perform this maneuver on both sides and make sure the patient continues to keep their eyes open during this exam. Torsional or vertical nystagmus on the Dix-Hallpike test is indicative of an otolith in the posterior semicircular canal, which is the most common form of BPPV.[13] Episodic and positional symptoms can differentiate negative Dix-Hallpike test patients from those with posterior circulation infarction. Patients who lack these symptoms and have a negative Dix-Hallpike test require further evaluation for cerebellar stroke.

FIGURE 8. The Dix-Hallpike Maneuver

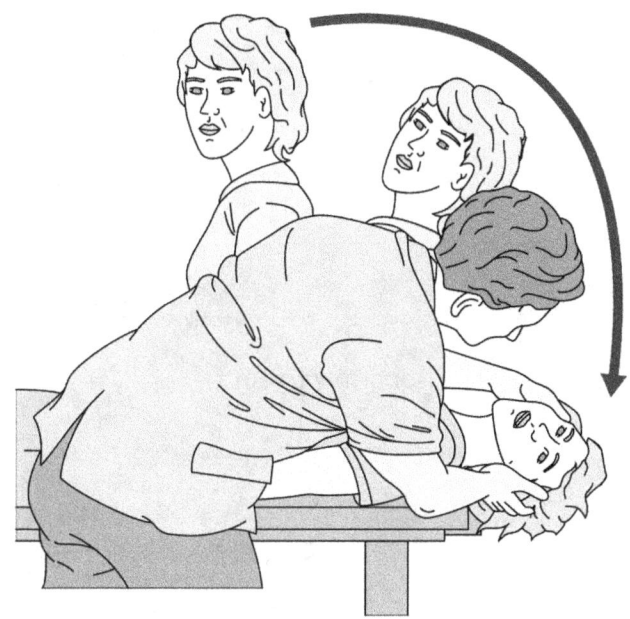

11.7.2 Vestibular Neuritis

Vestibular neuritis typically presents with a gradual onset of persistent and ongoing vertigo, associated with positional exacerbation lasting hours or days with spontaneous nystagmus. Limb coordination determined by finger-to-nose and heel-to-shin exams is typically preserved. Vestibular neuritis is currently considered to be caused by viral etiology.[14] The HINTS exam can reliably diagnose vestibular neuritis, thereby excluding stroke. Again, the three components of the HINTS exam are (1) **H**ead **I**mpulse Test, (2) **N**ystagmus, and (3) **T**est of (Vertical) **S**kew (Table 7).

TABLE 7. The Three Components of the HINTS Exam

H I	**H**ead **I**mpulse Test
N	**N**ystagmus
T S	**T**est of (Vertical) **S**kew

The Head Impulse test is abnormal if the patient has vestibular neuritis (Figure 9). This abnormal finding is good because a positive head impulse test indicates the patient has vestibular neuritis, not a stroke. This examination tests the vestibular-ocular reflex which allows the eyes to focus while the head is moving. When this reflex is interrupted, the eyes experience a lag which is an indication of peripheral vertigo that could be caused by vestibular neuritis. To perform this test, hold onto the patient's head with both hands and have the patient fixate on your nose with their eyes. Move the patient's head back and forth slowly in a relaxed fashion and then briskly to the center, looking for an abnormal catch-up saccade (Figure 9). Again, an abnormal Head Impulse Test is good because this demonstrates the patient has vestibular neuritis (a nerve problem), not a stroke. When evaluated in emergency department populations, a positive head impulse test was 100% sensitive for the detection of peripheral disorder causing vertigo.[15] A negative head impulse test correlated to a 91-96% rate of patients with cerebellar infarction.[4, 15]

FIGURE 9. The Head Impulse Test

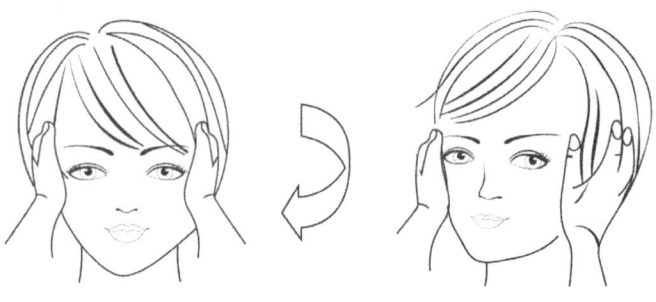

Normal Exam

Patient focused on examiner's nose

After sharp turn to the patient's right, patient remains focused on examiner's nose

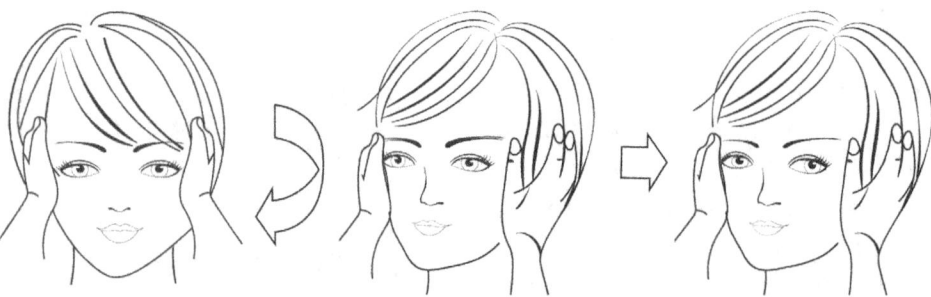

Abnormal Exam

Patient focused on examiner's nose

After sharp turn to the patient's right, patient's gaze remains forward and not on examiner

Patient's gaze returns back to examiner (corrected saccades)

Test of (Vertical) Skew is performed by placing the examiner's hand or a visual shield over the patient's eye and moving it to cover the patient's other eye. While doing this, the examiner should look for any vertical movement in the uncovered eye (Figure 10). Any abnormal vertical skew deviation of the patient's uncovered eye is worrisome for stroke. Nystagmus is assessed with primary and lateral gaze by asking the patient to look to the left and the right. Nystagmus that is unidirectional (meaning the direction of nystagmus will not change despite which direction the patient looks) is suggestive of vestibular neuritis and not stroke. However, unidirectional nystagmus has been identified in 46% of patients with cerebral infarction, so this is not a reliable finding that can confirm peripheral vertigo and exclude a cerebellar infarct.[4] Alternatively, **bidirectional (directional changing) nystagmus is indicative of stroke until proven otherwise**. Thus, vertical nystagmus as assessed by the Test of (Vertical) Skew or bidirectional or direction changing nystagmus is concerning for cerebellar stroke.

FIGURE 10. The Test of (Vertical) Skew

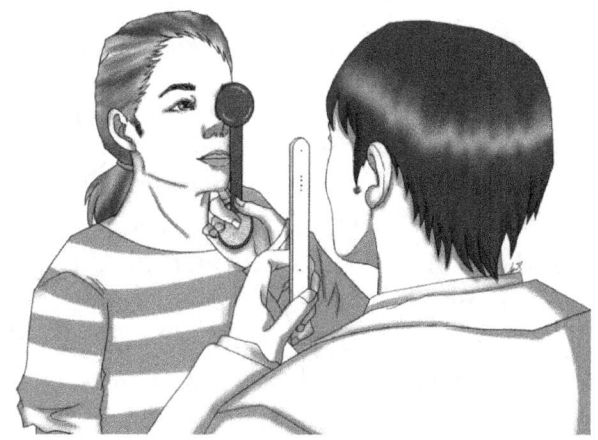

Vestibular neuritis is diagnosed only if all three components of the HINTS exam confirm such. That is, there must be an abnormal head impulse test, unidirectional nystagmus, and no vertical skew. **All three components of the HINTS must be present to make this diagnosis**. Stroke should be suspected if any of the following exist: (1) bidirectional nystagmus, (2) abnormal test of skew, **OR** (3) a **normal** head impulse test. Remember the HINTS exam should only be performed on patients with hours or days of continuous vertigo and spontaneous nystagmus.

In addition to neurologic examination, don't forget the stroke plan (S-PLAN) (Table 8). Always remember neuroimaging. In this regard, evidence-based recommendations for neuroimaging for vertiginous patients have not yet been established. However, indications for neuroimaging for vestibulopathic patients include the inability to walk, direction changing nystagmus, and any focal neurologic deficit. An easy way to remember these indications is with the mnemonic 'IDA' (Table 9). On this matter, diffusion-weighted magnetic resonance imaging (DWI) with magnetic resonance angiography (MRA) is the clear-cut study to identify cerebellar infarct. Computed tomography (CT) and MRI are both excellent studies for the identification of hemorrhagic stroke.[16] However, MRI is clearly superior to CT for the detection of ischemic stroke as it has an 83% sensitivity compared to CT which only has 26%.[17]

History, presentation, neurologic evaluation, and/or neuroimaging that is suggestive of cerebellar infarct place these patients in three distinct therapeutic windows. Each of these therapeutic windows requires specific neurologic management. For patients who present less than 4.5 hours since onset, IV TPA should be considered and large vessel occlusion (LVO) should be excluded with CTA. Patients presenting between 4.5 and 24 hours since onset should have LVO excluded with CTA. The suspicion of a LVO prompts neurointerventional consultation. Finally, patients presenting more than 24 hours from symptom onset likely would not benefit from either IV TPA or endovascular treatment (EVT) and secondary stroke prevention should be considered.

TABLE 9. Indications for Neuroimaging for Vertigo: **IDA**

I	Inability to Walk Without Support
D	Direction-Changing Nystagmus
A	Any Focal Neurologic Deficit

TABLE 8. The Stroke Plan: **S-PLAN**

S	Source (embolic or thrombotic)
P	Pathophysiology (etiology)
L	Location (of brain affected)
A	Artery (arterial territory involved)
N	Neuroimaging

<u>S</u>ource	<u>P</u>atho-physiology	<u>L</u>ocation	<u>A</u>rtery	<u>N</u>euro-imaging
• Embolic • Thrombotic	**C**: Cardioembolic (20%) **A**: Atherosclerotic large vessel disease (30%) **U**: Undetermined etiology - ESUS (30%) **S**: Small vessel disease or lacunar infarct (15%) **E**: Everything else or other (5%)	• Frontal • Parietal • Temporal • Occipital • Cerebellar • Thalamic • Brainstem	• ICA • MCA • ACA • Vertebral • Basilar • PICA • ACA • SCA	• CT • CTA • CTP • MRI • MRA • Angio

11.8 Summary

Cerebellar infarction represents approximately 2% of all acute ischemic stroke and can present with only vertigo.[18] It is very difficult to diagnose cerebellar stroke whose only deficit is vertigo. However, most cases of cerebellar infarction also present with either direction-changing nystagmus or the inability to walk without support.[4] The neurologic examination techniques discussed in this chapter can further aid in differentiating benign peripheral vertigo from central vertigo related to a cerebellar infarct (Figure 11). Lastly, always remember the stroke plan (Table 8) and include neuroimaging when appropriate (Table 9).

Abbreviations list

AICA, anterior inferior cerebellar artery; BPPV, benign paroxysmal positional vertigo; CT, computed tomography; DWI, diffusion-weighted imaging; EVT, endovascular treatment; LA, labyrinthine artery; LVO, large vessel occlusion; MRA, magnetic resonance angiography; PICA, posterior inferior cerebellar artery; SCA, superior cerebellar artery; S-PLAN, stroke plan; VBATD, vertebrobasilar atherothrombotic disease; VBI, vertebrobasilar insufficiency.

FIGURE 11. Vertigo Algorithm

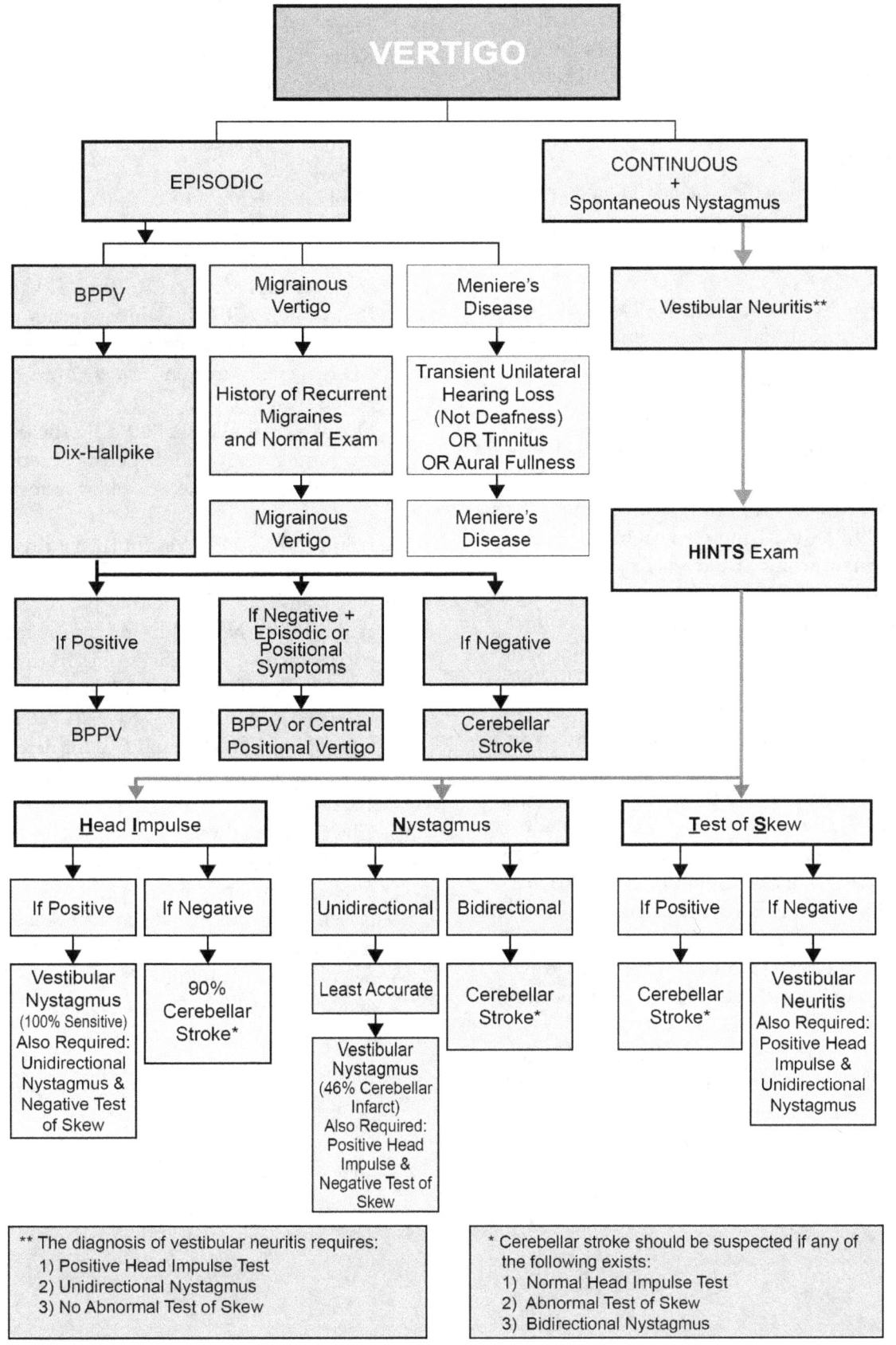

References

1. Gulli G, Marquardt L, Rothwell PM, Markus HS. (2013). Stroke risk after posterior circulation stroke/transient ischemic attack and its relationship to site of vertebrobasilar stenosis pooled data analysis from prospective studies. *Stroke*, 44(3), 598–60410.
2. Cano LM, Cardona P, Quesada H, et al. (2012). Cerebellar infarction: prognosis and complications of vascular territories. *Neurologia*, 27, 330-35.
3. Edlow JA, Newman-Toker DE, Savitz SI. (2008). Diagnosis and initial management of cerebellar infarction. *Lancet Neurol*, 7, 951-64.
4. Lee H, Sohn SI, Cho YW, Lee SR, Ahn BH, Park BR, et al. (2006). Cerebellar infarction presenting isolated vertigo: frequency and vascular topographical patterns. *Neurology*, 67, 1178–83.
5. Jauss M, Krieger D, Hornig C, Schramm J, Busse O. (1999). Surgical and medical management of patients with massive cerebellar infarctions: results of the German-Austrian Cerebellar Infarction Study. *J Neurol*, 246, 257–64.
6. Walker HK. (1990). The Cerebellum. In: Walker HK, Hall WD, Hurst JW, editors. *Clinical Methods: The History, Physical, and Laboratory Examinations*. 3rd edition. Boston: Butterworths, Ch 69. Available from: https://www.ncbi.nlm.nih.gov/books/NBK392/.
7. Powers WJ, Rabinstein AA, Ackerson T, Adeoye OM, Bambakidis NC, Becker K, Biller J, Brown M, Demaerschalk BM, Hoh B, et al. (2018). Guidelines for the Early Management of Patients With Acute Ischemic Stroke: A Guideline for Healthcare Professionals From the American Heart Association/American Stroke Association. *Stroke,* Jan 24.
8. Tohgi H, Takahashi S, Chiba K, et al. (1993). Cerebellar infarction. Clinical and neuroimaging analysis in 293 patients. The Tohoku Cerebellar Infarction Study Group. *Stroke*, 24, 1697–1701.
9. Savitz SI, Caplan LR, Edlow JA. (2007). Pitfalls in the diagnosis of cerebellar infarction. *Acad Emerg Med*, 14, 63–8.
10. Kerber KA, Brown DL, Lisabeth LD, et al. (2006). Stroke among patients with dizziness, vertigo, and imbalance in the emergency department: a population-based study. *Stroke*, 37, 2484–87.
11. Neuhauser HK. (2007). Epidemiology of vertigo. *Curr Opin Neurol*, 20, 40-6.
12. Vanni S, Nazerian P, Casati C, Moroni F, Risso M, Ottaviani M, Pecci R, Pepe G, Vannucchi P, Grifoni S. (2015). Can emergency physicians accurately and reliably assess acute vertigo in the emergency department? *Emerg Med Australas*, Apr, 27(2), 126-31.
13. Dix MR, Hallpike CS. (1952). The pathology, symptomatology and diagnosis of certain common disorders of the vestibular system. *Proc R Soc Med*, 45, 341-54.
14. Baloh RW. (2003). Vestibular neuritis. *N Engl J Med*, 348, 1027–32.
15. Newman-Toker DE, Kattah JC, Alvernia JE, et al. (2008). Normal head impulse test differentiates acute cerebellar strokes from vestibular neuritis. *Neurology*, 70, 2378–85.
16. Kidwell CS, Chalela JA, Saver JL, et al. (2004). Comparison of MRI and CT for detection of acute intracerebral hemorrhage. *JAMA*, 292, 1823–30.
17. Chalela JA, Kidwell CS, Nentwich LM, et al. (2007). Magnetic resonance imaging and computed tomography in emergency assessment of patients with suspected acute stroke: a prospective comparison. *Lancet*, 369, 293–8.
18. Seemungal BM. (2007). Neuro-otological emergencies. *Curr Opin Neurol*, 20, 32–9.

Chapter 12

Thalamic Stroke

12.1 Introduction

The thalamus belongs to a region of the brain called the diencephalon (Figure 1). The thalamus is often described as a relay center because of the massive amount of information it transmits. The thalamus has multiple different nuclei that specialize in various functions including regulating sensory, motor, arousal, sleep-related, and memory processes. Thalamic stroke is difficult to evaluate because it can cause any type of stroke deficit including motor weakness, aphasia, neglect, and cognitive or visual abnormalities. One distinctive feature of the thalamus is that its medial nuclei have an important role in maintaining arousal and vigilance. Typically, ischemic stroke does not cause a loss of consciousness. While it would be difficult to remember the arterial supply to each of the thalamic nuclei, the thalamus can be divided into four vascular regions. When affected by stroke, each region has a consistent constellation of symptoms. However, before these four vascular regions of the thalamus can be discussed, a more in-depth review of the posterior circulation is warranted.

FIGURE 1. The Thalamus

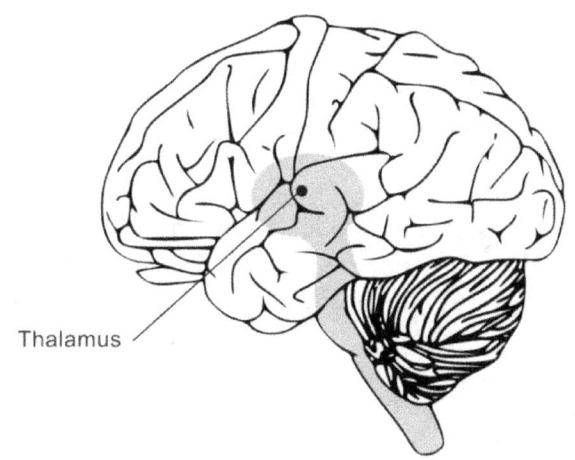

12.2 Vascular Anatomy

The basilar artery divides into two, paired posterior cerebral arteries (PCAs) that extend laterally and posteriorly to curve around the brainstem (Figure 2). The PCA (like the internal carotid artery, middle cerebral, and vertebral artery) is divided into four segments (Figure 2). The first segment (P1) is from the origin of the PCA to the origin of the PCoA. Recall that the PCA can also originate from the anterior circulation (arising from the supraclinoid segment of the ICA). When this occurs, this is termed a *fetal* origin of the posterior cerebral artery (fPCA) and the P1 segment is either congenitally absent or hypoplastic (Figure 3). The second segment (P2) is from the takeoff of the PCoA to the posterior margin of the midbrain. The P3 segment extends from the posterior margin of the midbrain through the quadrigeminal cistern and terminates at the bifurcation of the parieto-occipital and calcarine arteries. The P4 segment includes the parieto-occipital and calcarine arteries and their terminal or cortical branches. These terminal or cortical branches of the PCA supply the inferomedial region of the temporal lobe, the medial aspects of the occipital lobe, and even portions of the brainstem. Due to the variety of structures they supply and the heterogeneity of their functions, **PCA stroke, more than any other intracranial artery occlusion, presents with the greatest variety of clinical deficits.**

FIGURE 2. The 4 Segments of the Posterior Cerebral Artery

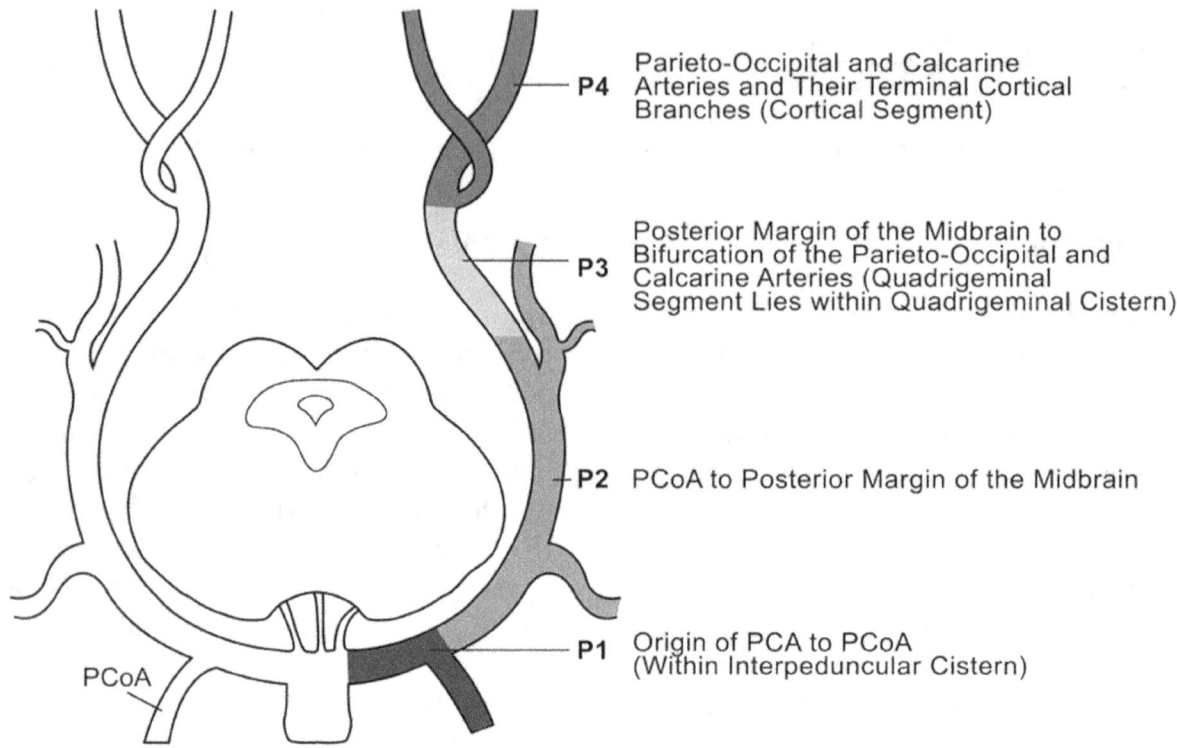

FIGURE 3. Fetal Origin of the Posterior Cerebral Artery (fPCA)

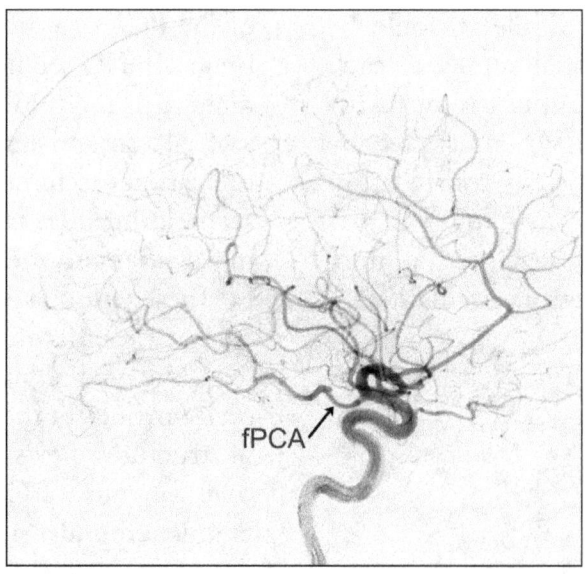

Recall that the posterior communicating artery (PCoA) connects the PCA to the supraclinoid segment of the internal carotid artery (ICA) (Figure 4). Perforating vessels originating from the PCoA, the P1 and P2 segments supply the immensely packed collection of nuclei and fibers located within the thalamus. The thalamus itself is located directly above the arteries that supply it (Figure 5).

FIGURE 4. The Posterior Communicating Artery (PCoA)

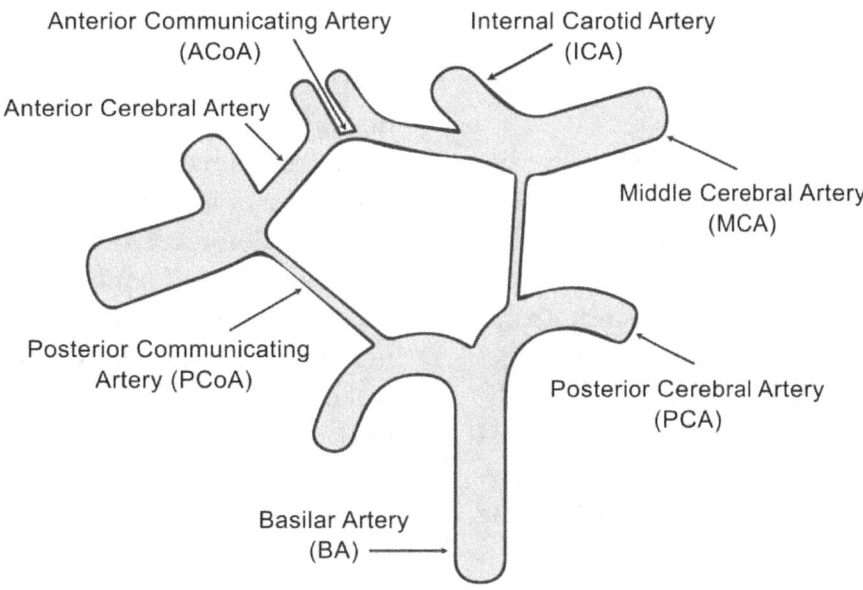

FIGURE 5. The Thalamus in Relationship to Its Vascular Supply

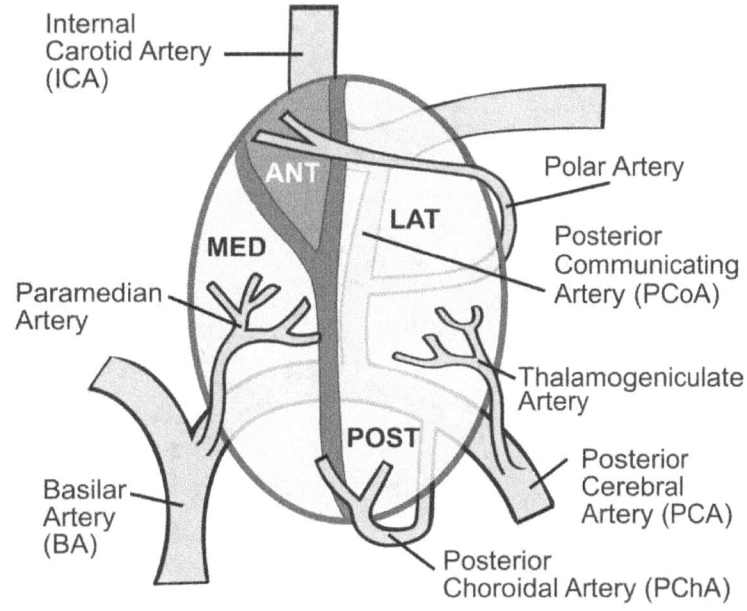

12.3 The 4 Vascular Regions of the Thalamus

The thalamus can be separated into four regions and each of these regions derives its arterial supply from branches of the PCA. These four vascular regions and their corresponding artery supply include the: (1) anterior region supplied by the polar artery (also called the *anterior thalamoperforating artery*), (2) medial region supplied by the paramedian artery, (3) lateral region supplied by the thalamogeniculate artery, and (4) posterior region supplied by the posterior choroidal artery (Figure 5). While thalamic stroke can cause a myriad of stroke symptoms, certain deficits have been consistently reported to correspond to the following regions of the thalamus: language and memory (anterior region), motor and sensory (lateral region), arousal, vigilance and memory (medial region), and optic or visual (posterior region)

(Figure 6).[1] An easy way to remember these symptoms is with the mnemonic 'LMAO' (Table 1). Consider thalamic stroke when symptoms cannot be located in a single cortical distribution or the patient has loss of consciousness.

There are three last noteworthy points to discuss concerning the thalamus. First, the central artery of Percheron variant is a single vessel that arises from either the right or left P1 segment. This artery can supply the medial aspect (paramedian) of the thalamus or the rostral aspect of the midbrain bilaterally (Figure 7). Usually, paired paramedian arteries arising from the posterior cerebral arteries supply the thalami. However, variable configurations exist that include the artery of Percheron which can result in bilateral medial thalamic infarcts or rostral midbrain infarction (Figure 8).[2] This single, lateralized artery can cause a bilateral thalamic and mesencephalic infarct (Figure 7 and 8). Clinically, patients can be obtunded, comatose, or agitated, with associated hemiplegia or hemisensory loss. Secondly, this entire discussion focused on ischemic stroke involving the thalamus. Hemorrhagic and venous stroke can also involve the thalamus. The venous structure most often associated with a thalamic venous stroke is the straight sinus (Figure 9). Finally, do not forget that lacunar infarcts can also involve the thalamus (Table 2).

FIGURE 6. The Four Vascular Regions of the Thalamus and Associated Deficits

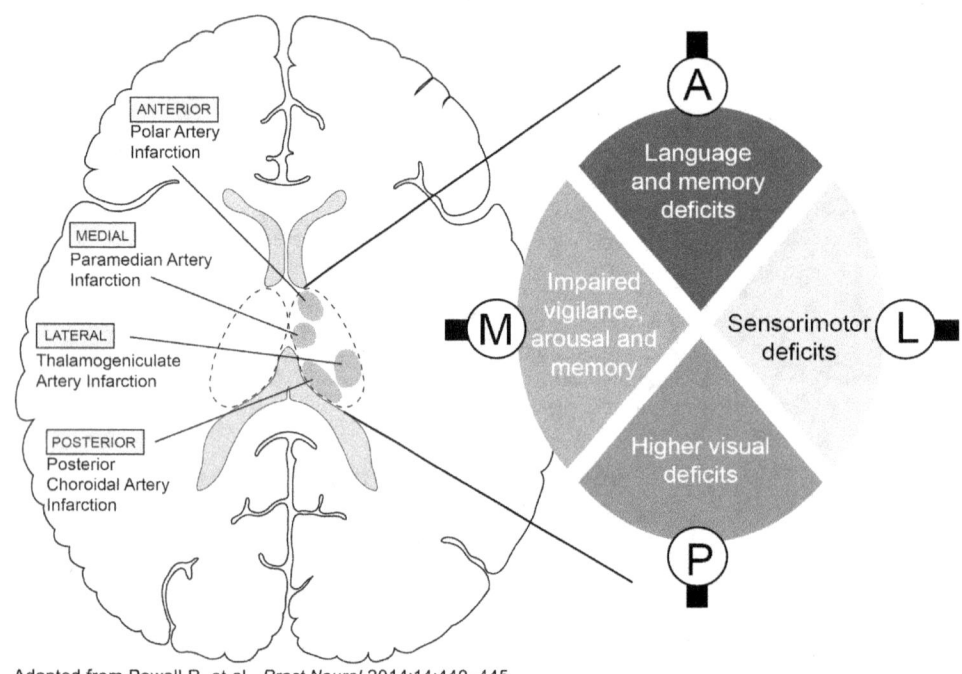

Adapted from Powell R, et al. *Pract Neurol* 2014;14:440–445

TABLE 1. Thalamic Stroke Symptoms: **LMAO**

	Deficit	Region	Artery	Origin
L	Language, (Dominant) and Memory	Anterior	Polar Artery (Absent in 40%)	PCoA
M	Motor and Sensory	Lateral	Thalamogeniculate Artery	P2
A	Arousal, Vigilance and Memory	Medial	Paramedian Artery	P1
O	Optic or Visual	Posterior	Posterior Choroidal Artery	P2

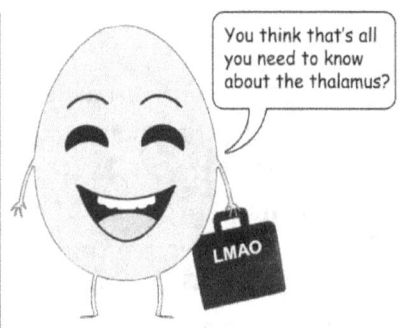

FIGURE 7. The Artery of Percheron

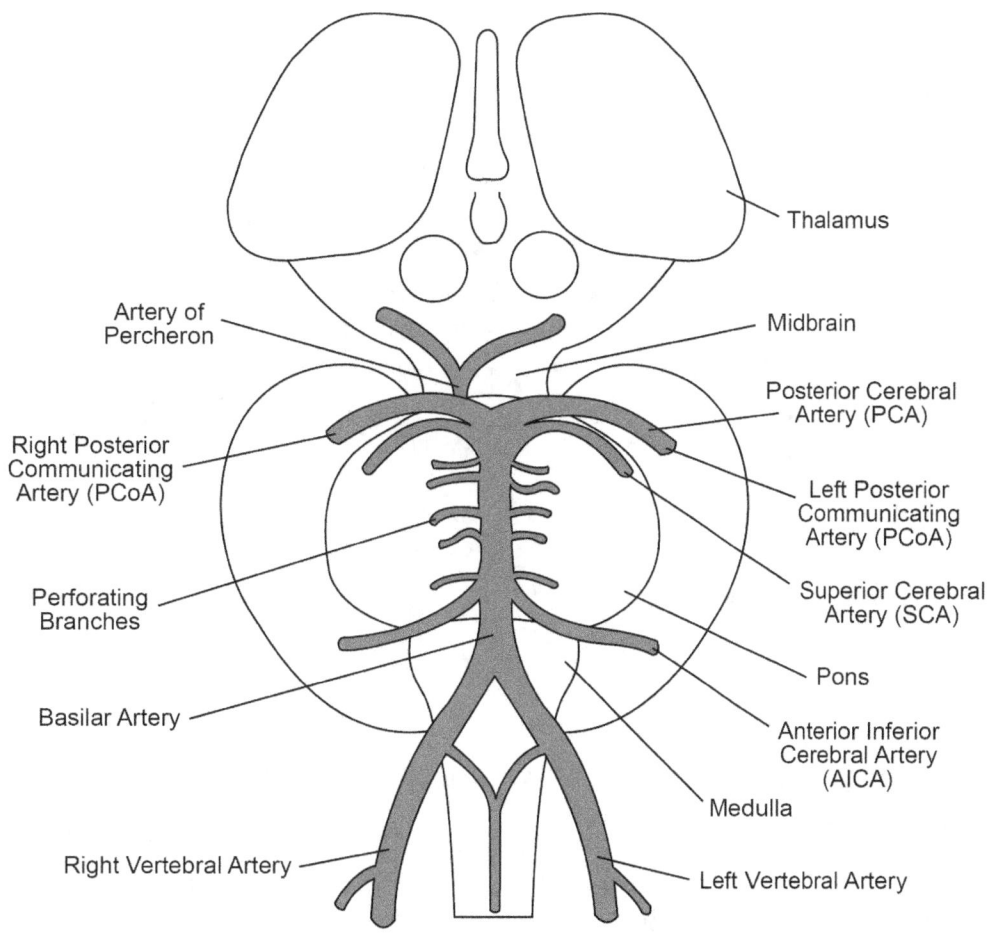

FIGURE 8. Axial DWI MRI Demonstrates Bilateral Thalamic and Midbrain Artery of Percheron Infarcts

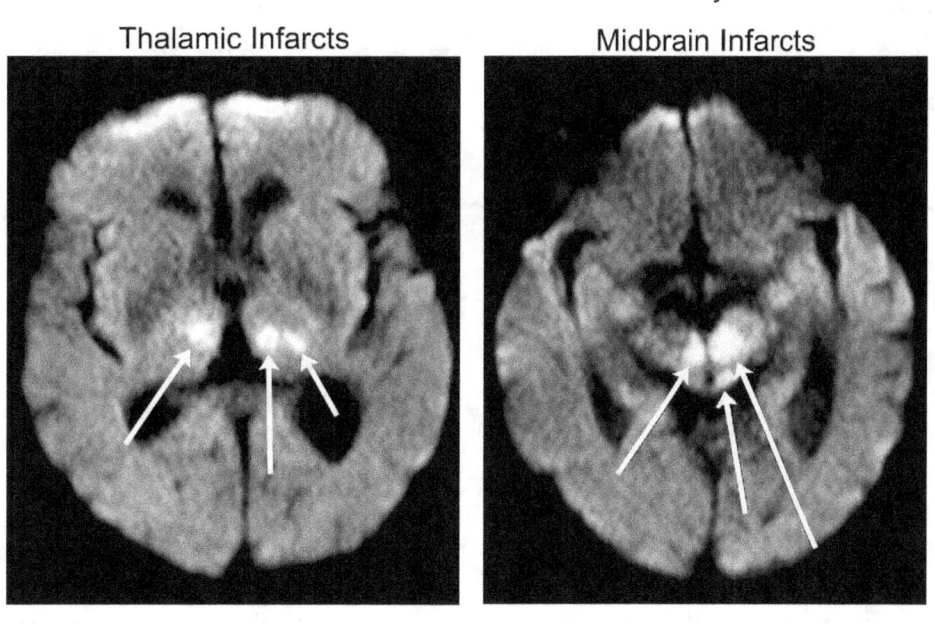

FIGURE 9. Intracranial Venous Drainage

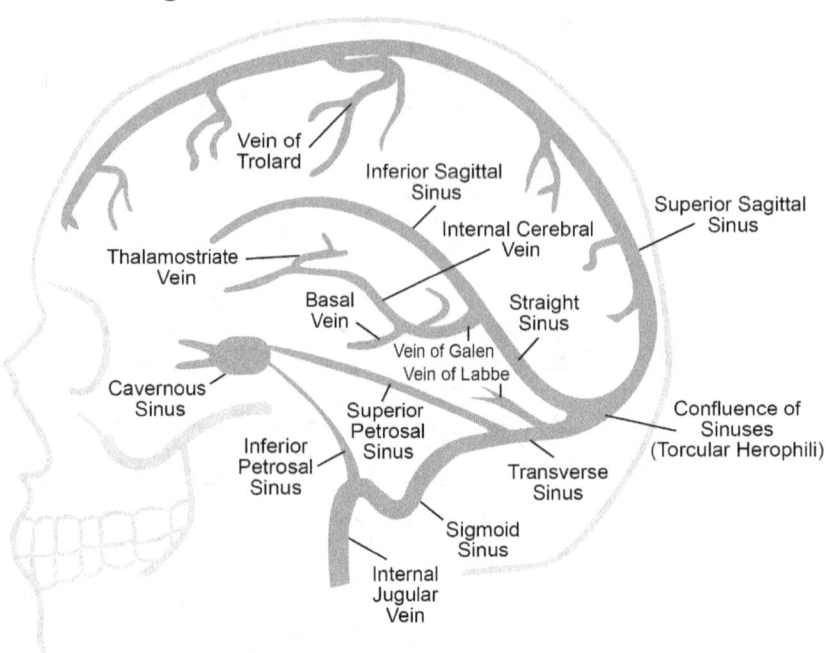

TABLE 2. Lacunar Syndromes and Deficits

Syndrome	Arterial Territory	Brain Location	Symptoms
Pure Motor Hemiparesis	Lenticulostriate/ Pontine Perforator	Internal Capsule, Pons	Contralateral Weakness
Ataxic Hemiparesis	Pontine Perforators	Ventral Pons	Hemiparesis with Prominent Ataxia
Pure Sensory	Thalamogeniculate Artery	VPL Nucleus, Thalamus	Contralateral Sensory Loss
Dysarthria/ Clumsy Hand	Lenticulostriate/ Pontine Perforator	Internal Capsule, Pons	Dysarthria and Hand Clumsiness
Mixed Motor/ Sensory	Lenticulostriate/ Thalamic Perforator	Internal Capsule, Thalamus	Hemiparesis and Contralateral Sensory Impairment

12.4 Summary

The thalamus has multiple different nuclei specializing in different functions that include regulating sensory, motor, arousal, sleep-related, and memory activities. Thalamic stroke is difficult to evaluate because it can present with any type of stroke deficit including motor weakness, aphasia, neglect, or cognitive and visual abnormalities. Dividing the thalamus into four vascular regions makes thalamic stroke more manageable. Do not forget to consider a thalamic stroke when presenting symptoms cannot be located in a single cortical distribution and particularly in patients with impaired arousal or vigilance.

Abbreviations list

fPCA, fetal origin of the posterior cerebral artery; ICA, internal carotid artery; PCAs, posterior cerebral arteries; PCoA, posterior communicating artery.

References

1. Powell R, Hughes T. (2014). A chamber of secrets. The neurology of the thalamus: lessons from acute stroke. Pract Neurol, Dec, 14(6), 440-5.

2. Reilly M, Connolly S, Stack J, et al. (1992). Bilateral paramedian thalamic infarction: a distinct but poorly recognized stroke syndrome. QJM, 82, 63–70.

Chapter 13

Brainstem Stroke

13.1 Introduction

One reason the posterior circulation gives healthcare providers so much angst is because of the numerous, different, and complex structures it contains. The brainstem is no exception to this dilemma. From top to bottom, the brainstem consists of the midbrain (also called the mesencephalon), the pons, and the medulla (Figure 1). The blood supply to the brainstem and each of its components is provided laterally by *long circumferential branches* arising from the SCA, AICA, and PICA depending on the level of the brainstem, and medially by *paramedian* branches of the same arteries (Figure 2).

FIGURE 1. The Brainstem

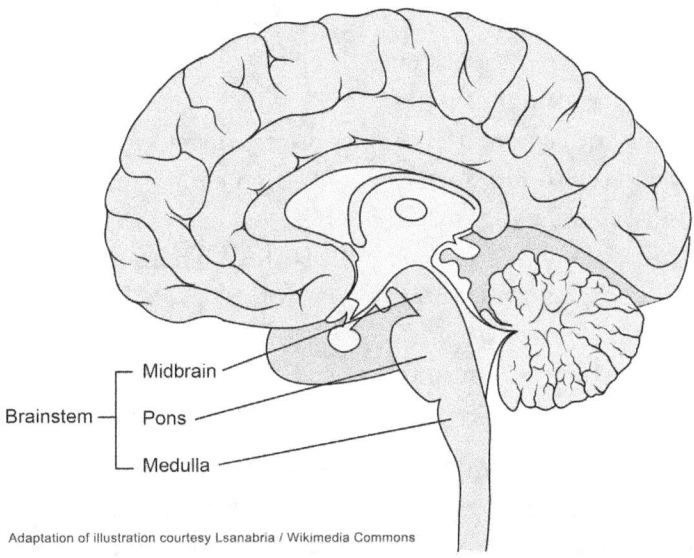

FIGURE 2. Vascular Supply to the Brainstem

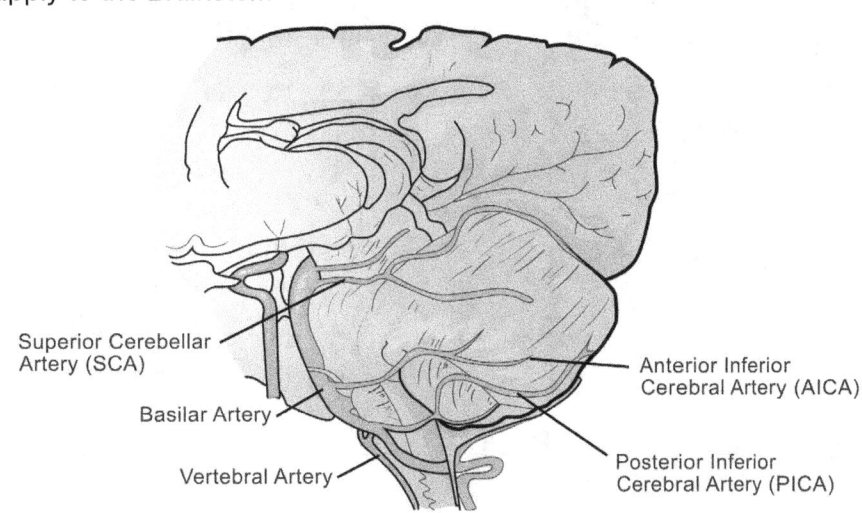

A paramedian branch occlusion results in a medial brainstem stroke whereas a long circumferential branch occlusion results in a lateral brainstem stroke. Different regions of the brainstem contain specific structures causing specific symptoms when affected by stroke. These symptoms are characterized by specific brainstem syndromes. Specific arterial involvement (SCA, AICA, or PICA) is dependent on the level or region of the brainstem. Most brainstem syndromes are either medially or laterally oriented infarcts that affect the midbrain, pons, or medulla. However, one scary exception to this observation is a basilar artery occlusion, which will be discussed separately in Chapter 15.

13.2 The 4 Rules of the Brainstem

Essentially, a brainstem stroke is determined by its level and laterality. The trick is to remember what neural structures (cranial nerves and neural pathways) are located at each level and whether they are medially or laterally oriented. To aid in this process, Peter Gates wrote an amazing paper titled, *"The rule of 4 of the brainstem: a simplified method for understanding brainstem anatomy and brainstem vascular syndromes for the non-neurologist."*[1] In this paper published in 2005, Gates described a simple method using four basic rules to establish lesion localization which allows the examiner to determine the level of the brainstem affected and whether the stroke is medial or lateral.[1] As stated earlier, blood supply to the brainstem is from either medial or lateral branches which arise from the SCA, ACA, or PICA, depending on the level of the brainstem. Typically, a **paramedian branch** occlusion results in a **medial** brainstem syndrome, whereas an occlusion of a **long circumferential branch** results in a **lateral** brainstem syndrome (Table 1).

TABLE 1. Medial Versus Lateral Brainstem Syndrome Arterial Supply

Arterial Branch	Syndrome
Paramedian	Medial Brainstem Syndrome
Long Circumferential	Lateral Brainstem Syndrome

Gates developed **4 rules** concerning the brainstem which can be summarized below.

Rule 1. There are 4 MIDLINE structures beginning with 'M' (Table 2).

TABLE 2. The 4 Midline Structures Beginning with 'M' and Associated Deficits

MIDLINE STRUCTURE	DEFICITS
Motor Pathway (Corticospinal Tract)	**Contralateral** Hemibody (Arm and Leg) Weakness
Medial Lemniscus	**Contralateral** Hemibody Numbness (Loss of Vibration and Proprioception)
Medial Longitudinal Fasciculus	**Ipsilateral** Internuclear Ophthalmoplegia
Motor Nucleus and Nerve	**Ipsilateral** Cranial Neuropathy (3, 4, 6 or 12)

NOTE: Cranial neuropathies are ipsilateral

TABLE 3. Brainstem Midline Structure Deficits: **MOAN**

M	Motor Weakness, Contralateral (Corticospinal Tract)
O	Ophthalmoplegia, Intranuclear, Ipsilateral (Medial Longitudinal Fasciculus)
A	Arm and Leg Numbness, Contralateral (Medial Lemniscus)
N	Neuropathy, Cranial, Ipsilateral (Motor Nucleus and Nerve)

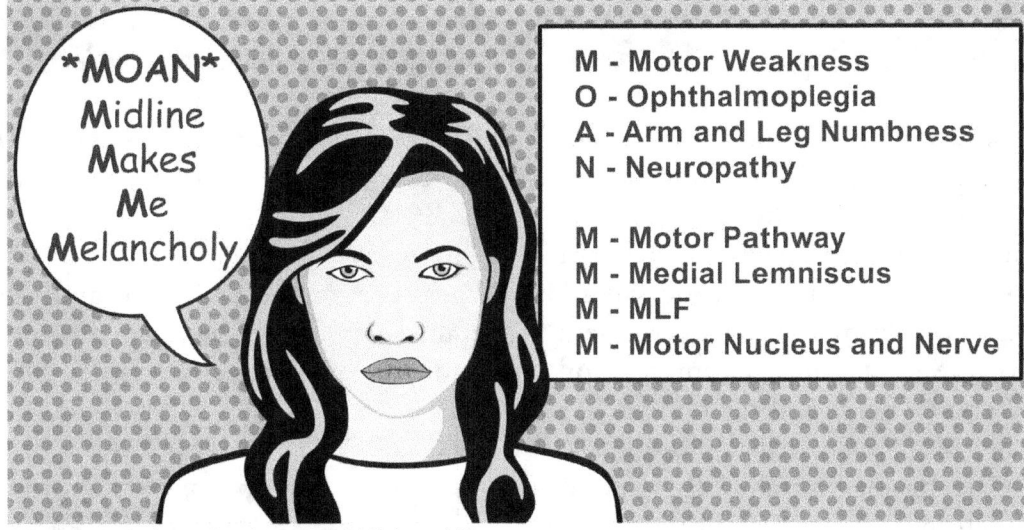

The mouth (required to MOAN) is midline

A simple way to remember the brainstem midline structure deficits is with the mnemonic 'MOAN' (Table 3).

Rule 2. There are 4 SIDE (lateral) structures beginning with 'S' (Table 4).

TABLE 4. **4 SIDE** (Lateral) Structures Beginning with '**S**' and Associated Deficits

LATERAL STRUCTURE	DEFICITS
Spinocerebellar Pathway	**Ipsilateral** Hemibody Ataxia
Spinothalamic Pathway	**Contralateral** Hemibody Numbness
Sensory Nucleus of CN V	**Ipsilateral** Facial Numbness (CN V Distribution)
Sympathetic Pathway	**Ipsilateral** Horner's Syndrome

A simple way to remember the deficits caused by brainstem lateral structures is with the mnemonic 'HAND' (Table 5).

TABLE 5. Brainstem Lateral Structure Deficits: **HAND**

H	Horner's Syndrome, Ipsilateral (Sympathetic Pathway)
A	Ataxia, Hemibody Ipsilateral (Spinocerebellar)
N	Numbness, Hemibody Contralateral (Spinothalamic)
D	Distribution of CN V, Ipsilateral Facial Numbness

The hand is lateral

A simple mnemonic to remember the deficits associated with Horner's syndrome is 'MISHAP' (Table 6).

TABLE 6. Horner's Syndrome: **MISHAP**

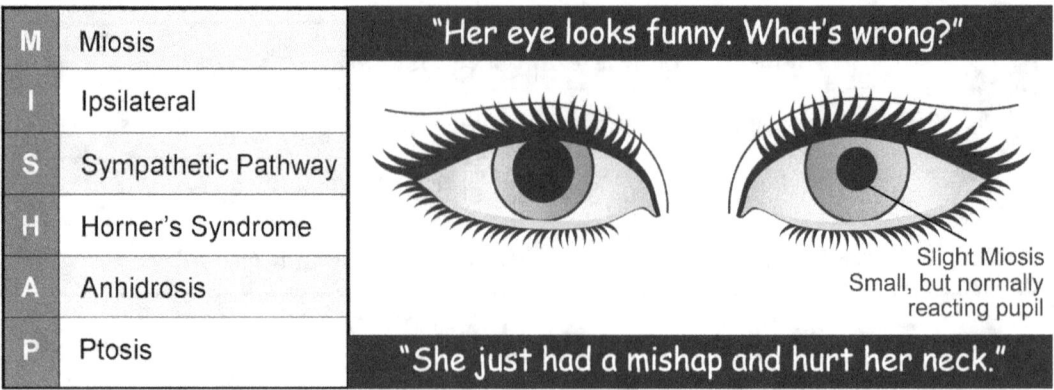

M	Miosis
I	Ipsilateral
S	Sympathetic Pathway
H	Horner's Syndrome
A	Anhidrosis
P	Ptosis

These pathways, located either medially or laterally (rules 1 and 2), run up and down the brainstem in a cranial-caudal direction. The cranial nerves that will be discussed next run front-to-back or side-to-side in the brainstem. Thus, identifying the cranial nerve involvement will determine a specific level of the brainstem. The intersection of the affected cranial nerve and neural pathway will provide the site of the brainstem lesion. As Gates stated in his original article: "These pathways pass through the entire length of the brainstem and can be linked to 'meridians of longitude' whereas the various cranial nerves can be regarded as 'parallels of latitude.' If you establish where the meridians of longitude and parallels of latitude intersect, then you have established the site of the lesion."[1] Gates's next rule describes the levels of the brainstem where the cranial nuclei are located.

Rule 3. There are 4 cranial nerves in the medulla, 4 in the pons, and 4 above the pons (M4/P4/P>4).

Each level of the brainstem and their associated cranial nerves, deficits, and mnemonics are presented below (Tables 7, 8, 9, 10, 11, 12 and 13).

TABLE 7. 4 CNs in the MEDULLA: IX, X, XI and XII

CRANIAL NERVE	DEFICITS
CN IX (Glossopharyngeal)	Ipsilateral Loss of Pharyngeal Sensation
CN X (Vagus)	Ipsilateral Palatal Weakness
CN XI (Spinal Accessory)	Ipsilateral Trapezius and Sternocleidomastoid Weakness
CN XII (Hypoglossal)	Ispilateral Tongue Weakness

A simple way to remember the cranial nuclei at the level of the medulla is with the mnemonic 'V-HAG' (Table 8).

TABLE 8. Cranial Nuclei at the Level of the Medulla: **V-HAG**

V	Vagus
H	Hypoglossal
A	Accessory
G	Glossopharyngeal

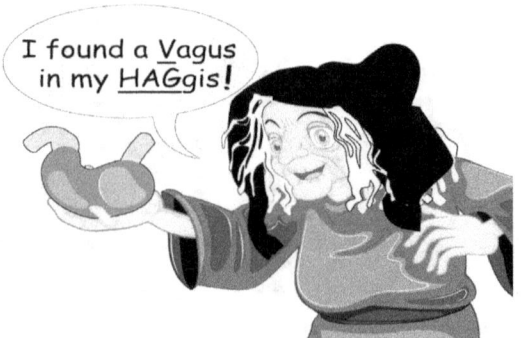

TABLE 9. 4 CNs in the PONS: V, VI, VII and VIII

CRANIAL NERVE	DEFICITS
CN V (Trigeminal)	Ipsilateral Facial Numbness (Anterior 2/3 of Scalp, Spares Jaw)
CN VI (Abducens)	Ipsilateral Weakness Lateral Movement (Abduction) of the Eye
CN VII (Facial)	Ipsilateral Facial Weakness
CN VIII (Auditory)	Ispilateral Deafness

A simple way to remember the cranial nuclei at the level of the pons is with the mnemonic 'V-FAT' (Table 10).

TABLE 10. Cranial Nuclei at the Level of the Pons: **V-FAT**

V	Vestibulocochlear (CN VIII)
F	Facial (CN VII)
A	Abducens (CN VI)
T	Trigeminal (CN V)

TABLE 11. 4 CNs Above the PONS: I, II, II, IV (ONLY 2 IN MIDBRAIN)

CRANIAL NERVE	DEFICITS
CN I (Olfactory)	Above the Midbrain
CN II (Optic)	Above the Midbrain
CN III (Oculomotor)	Ipsilateral Eye Turned Out and Slightly Down
CN IV (Trochlear)	Ispilateral Eye Unable to Look Down Toward the Nose (Superior Oblique)

A simple way to remember the two cranial nuclei contained within the midbrain and above is with the mnemonic 'TOO' (Table 12).

TABLE 12. Cranial Nuclei Within the Midbrain and Above: **TOO**

T	Trochlear (CN IV)
O	Oculomotor (CN III)
O	Optic and Olfactory - Above the Midbrain

To recall the 10 cranial nerves located in the brainstem, just remember 'TOO VERY FAT, VERY HAG.' (Table 13).

TABLE 13. Brainstem Cranial Nerves: **TOOVFATVHAG**

T	Trochlear (CN IV)
O	Oculomotor (CN III)
O	Optic and Olfactory - Above the Midbrain
V	Vestibulocochlear (CN VIII)
F	Facial (CN VII)
A	Abducens (CN VI)
T	Trigeminal (CN V)
V	Vagus (CN X)
H	Hypoglossal (CN XII)
A	Accessory (CN XI)
G	Glossopharyngeal (CN IX)

The last and 4th rule indicates which cranial nerves are medially located.

Rule 4. 4 MOTOR NUCLEI are MEDIALLY MAPPED and MATHEMATICALLY DIVISIBLE BY 12-3, 4, 6 & 12. By default, the remainder are lateral. (Figure 3).

FIGURE 3. Rule 4. 4 MOTOR NUCLEI are MEDIALLY MAPPED and MATHEMATICALLY DIVISIBLE BY 12-3, 4, 6 & 12.

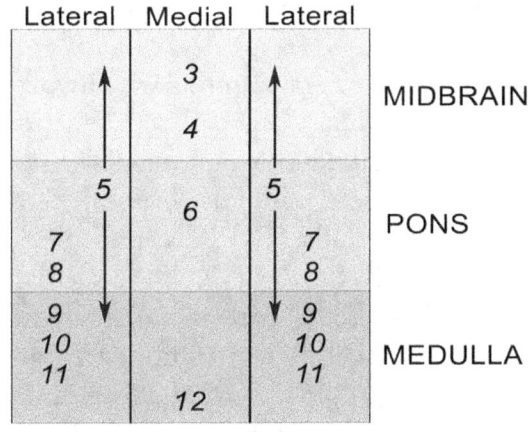

The function of all the cranial nerves is summarized in Table 14.

13.3 Applying the 4 Rules of the Brainstem

To summarize, the medial and lateral pathways running up and down the brainstem will intersect with medial or lateral-oriented cranial nerves situated perpendicular to them. This intersection will determine the level and laterality of the brainstem lesion causing a specific syndrome. Recall that most brainstem lesions (based upon vascular supply) are located either medially or laterally. A medial brainstem syndrome will consist of the four 'M' (medial) structures (**M**otor pathway, **M**edial lemniscus, **M**edial longitudinal fasciculus, and **M**otor nucleus and nerve). Also remember that the **4 MOTOR NUCLEI** that are **MIDLINE** are **3, 4, 6 & 12** (**MMMM**-4 **M**OTOR NUCLEI, **M**EDIALLY **M**APPED and **M**ATHEMATICALLY DIVISIBLE BY 12: 3, 4, 6, & 12).

TABLE 14. The Cranial Nerves

#	Name	Nerve Type	Function
I	Olfactory	Sensory	Smell
II	Optic	Sensory	Vision
III	Oculomotor	Motor	Most Eye Movement
IV	Trochlear	Motor	Moves Eye
V	Trigeminal	Both	Face Sensation, Mastication
VI	Abducens	Motor	Abducts the Eye
VII	Facial	Both	Facial Expression, Taste
VIII	Vestibulochoclear	Sensory	Hearing, Balance
IX	Glossopharyngeal	Both	Taste, Gag Reflex
X	Vagus	Both	Gag Reflex, Parasympathetic Innervation
XI	Accessory	Motor	Shoulder Shrug
XII	Hypoglossal	Motor	Swallowing, Speech

A medial brainstem syndrome will involve the motor (corticospinal tract) pathway and result in contralateral weakness. Motor cranial nerve involvement will determine the level of the brainstem lesion—medulla (CN XII), pons (CN VI), or midbrain (CN III and IV). If the medial lemniscus is affected, the patient will present with contralateral arm and leg numbness. Typically, the medial longitudinal fasciculus is not affected when hemiparesis is present due to its posterior location in the brainstem. However, lacunar infarcts of the MLF can result in ipsilateral internuclear ophthalmoplegia (inability to adduct eye or move towards the nose, and nystagmus on looking laterally to the opposite side of the lesion with the contralateral eye). The MLF is discussed in greater detail in Chapter 14 (Stroke and Vision). For the purposes of this chapter, just be aware that an infarct involving the MLF results in ipsilateral intranuclear ophthalmoplegia.

A lateral brainstem syndrome will consist of the four 'S' (side or lateral) structures (**S**pinocerebellar pathway, **S**pinothalamic pathway, **S**ensory nucleus of CN V, and **S**ympathetic pathway) and cranial nerve involvement depending on which level of the brainstem is affected. For example, CNs IX, X, and XI are laterally located at the level of the medulla and therefore are involved in lateral brainstem lesions at the level of the medulla. (Recall that CN XII is a **M**edially **M**apped, **M**otor CN, **M**athematically divisible by 12). CNs V, VII, and VIII are located at the level of the pons—Therefore, a lateral brainstem syndrome at the level of the pons will consist of the four 'S' (side or lateral) structures and CNs V, VII, or VIII. (Recall that CN VI is a **M**edially **M**apped, **M**otor CN, **M**athematically divisible by 12). Recall also that the CNs III and IV are the only CNs located in the midbrain. Both CNs are **M**edially **M**apped, **M**otor CN, **M**athematically divisible by 12. Since there are no laterally located cranial nuclei at the level of the midbrain, our discussion is only relevant to medially located cranial nerves within the midbrain (CNs III and IV). However, the midbrain deviates from the 4 brainstem rules that have been discussed. This point will be addressed shortly.

Now that the 4 rules of the brainstem have been reviewed, it's time to apply them. Again, the three components of the brainstem top to bottom are the midbrain, pons, and medulla (Figure 1). Each of these levels have specific vascular syndromes based on medial or lateral involvement. Each brainstem vascular syndrome has specific clinical signs which can be deduced by applying the 4 rules of the brainstem mentioned earlier and these are summarized in Figure 4. This image succinctly encapsulates all 4 brainstem rules and will be used for the remainder of the chapter to apply them.

FIGURE 4. Pictorial Representation of the 4 Brainstem Rules

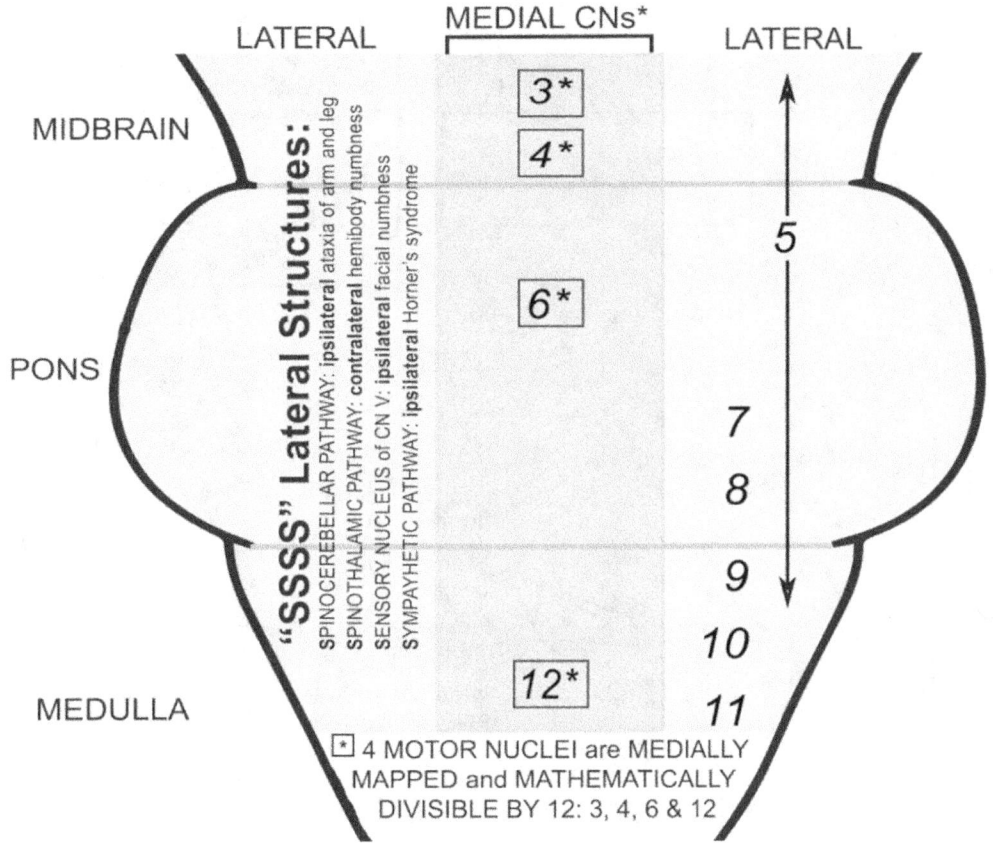

13.4 Medulla Oblongata

13.4.1 Lateral Medullary Syndrome

Lateral medullary syndrome, also referred to as Wallenberg syndrome, is typically due to infarction of the posterior inferior cerebellar artery (PICA) (Figure 5). The vascular distribution of PICA is the lateral aspect of the medulla. Since it is a lateral brainstem syndrome, only the lateral pathways and cranial nerves are affected. Figure 4 shows these to be the four lateral structures from Rule #2 which states there are 4 SIDE (lateral) structures beginning with 'S.' Remember, this is only half the battle. In addition to these tracts, one must recall Rule #3 which states that cranial nerves IX through XII are located in the medulla. Furthermore, Rule #4 states that cranial nerve XII is located medially, so it cannot be associated with this vascular syndrome which affects the lateral aspect of the medulla.

Thus, only cranial nerves IX, X, and XI can be involved. Lateral medullary syndrome typically involves cranial nerves IX and X and usually spares cranial nerve XI. Therefore, cranial nerve deficits that are specific to lateral medullary syndrome include loss of function of cranial nerves IX and X (glossopharyngeal and vagus) which results in hoarseness and dysphagia. The saying "Never pick a (PICA) horse (hoarseness) that cannot eat (dysphagia)" is a simple way to remember these involved cranial nerves and artery (PICA).[2] Lateral medullary (Wallenberg) syndrome consists of lateral brainstem structure deficits combined with cranial nerve IX and X involvement (Figure 5).

FIGURE 5. Lateral Medullary (Wallenberg) Syndrome

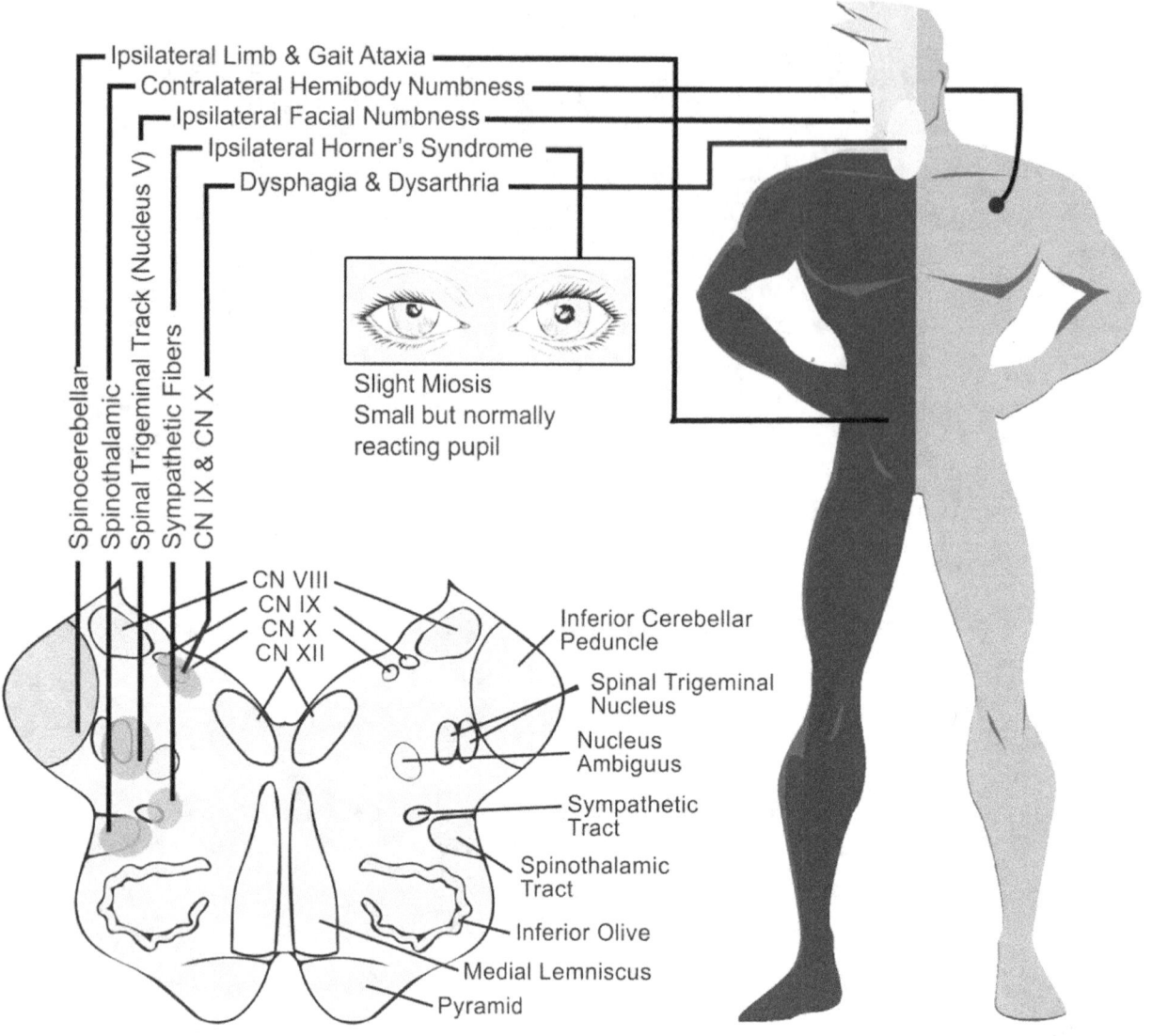

13.4.2 Medial Medullary Syndrome

Medial medullary syndrome, also known as Dejerine syndrome, is most commonly caused by infarction of the anterior spinal artery which arises from the vertebral artery (Figure 6).[3] Because the medial medulla is affected, one must apply the first rule of the brainstem which states "There are 4 MIDLINE structures beginning with 'M' (Figure 4). These four structures are again the **m**otor pathways (corticospinal tract) which result in contralateral hemibody weakness, the **m**edial lemniscus which results in contralateral hemibody numbness, the **m**edial longitudinal fasciculus which results in ipsilateral internuclear ophthalmoplegia, and the **m**otor nucleus and nerve which result in ipsilateral cranial neuropathy. Recall that the third rule states: "The medulla has **4** cranial nerves; the pons has **4** and **4** are above the pons" (Figure 4). Applying this rule, the medulla has 4 cranial nerves. However, Rule #4 states, "4 MOTOR NUCLEI are MEDIALLY MAPPED and MATHEMATICALLY DIVISIBLE BY 12: III, IV, VI and XII." Cranial nerve XII is the only cranial nerve that is located (mapped) within the medial medulla. Thus, a medial medullary infarct results in loss of cranial nerve XII (hypoglossal nerve) function which results in ipsilateral tongue deviation—that is, the tongue deviates towards the side of the involved cranial nerve.

FIGURE 6. Medial Medullary Syndrome

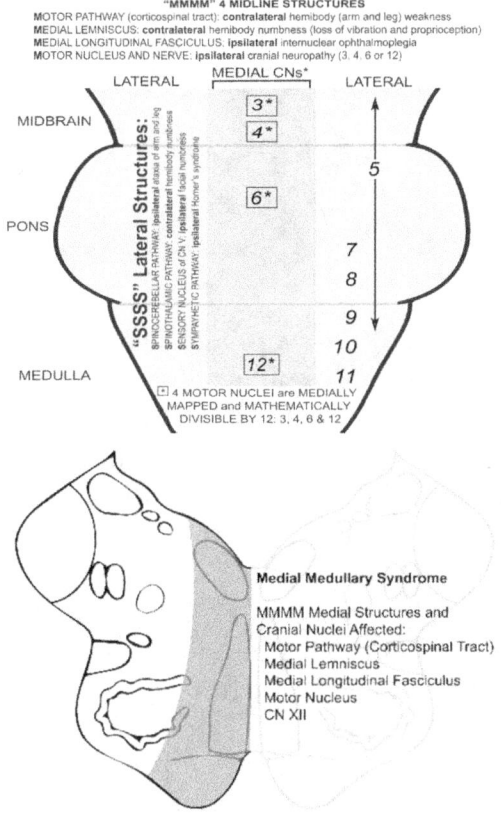

TABLE 16. Deficits Caused by Lateral Brainstem Structures: **HAND**

H	Horner's Syndrome, Ipsilateral (Sympathetic Pathway)
A	Ataxia, Hemibody Ipsilateral (Spinocerebellar)
N	Numbness, Hemibody Contralateral (Spinothalamic)
D	Distribution of CN V, Ipsilateral Facial Numbness

The hand is lateral

13.5 Vascular Syndromes of the Pons

13.5.1 Lateral Pontine Syndrome

Lateral pontine syndrome is usually due to an infarction of the anterior inferior cerebellar artery (AICA).[3] Since the lateral pons is affected, the second rule of the brainstem which states "There are 4 SIDE (lateral) structures beginning with 'S' is applied here (Figure 4). The deficits caused by involvement of these four lateral structures can be remembered by the mnemonic: 'HAND' (Table 16).

To summarize, patients with lateral pontine syndrome present with similar pathway deficits as patients with lateral medullary syndrome. What separates the two syndromes is the level of cranial nerve involvement. Remember, Rule #3 states that cranial nerves V through VIII are located in the pons (Figure 4). Rule #4 states that cranial nerve VI is located medially and thus excludes this nerve from lateral pontine syndrome (Figure 4). Therefore, only cranial nerves V, VII, and VIII can be associated with lateral pontine syndrome. This syndrome typically affects cranial nerve VII (facial nerve) causing facial paralysis (Figure 7). A simple mnemonic to remember the features of lateral pontine syndrome is '7-HAND.' (Table 17).

To sum up, patients with medial medullary syndrome present with contralateral hemibody weakness (corticospinal tract), contralateral hemibody numbness (medial lemniscus), intranuclear ophthalmoplegia of the ipsilateral eye (medial longitudinal fasciculus), and ipsilateral deviation of the tongue (CN XII) (Table 15). These symptoms are again based on the medial location of their associated pathways and cranial nerves within the medulla. Once this medial location is determined, one must correlate the cranial nerve deficit with the level of the brainstem involved—i.e. CN IX-XII (medulla), CN V-VIII (pons), and CN III and IV (midbrain) (Figure 4).

TABLE 15. Deficits Associated with Medial Medullary Syndrome: **MINT**

M	Motor Weakness - Contralateral Hemibody (Corticospinal Tract)
I	Intranuclear Ophthalmoplegia, Ipsilateral (Medial Longitudinal Fasciculus)
N	Numbness - Contralateral Hemibody (Medial Lemniscus)
T	Tongue Deviation - Ipsilateral (CN XII)

TABLE 17. Lateral Pontine Syndrome: **7-HAND**

7	CN VII - Ipsilateral Facial Paralysis
H	Horner's Syndrome, Ipsilateral (Sympathetic Pathway)
A	Ataxia, Hemibody Ipsilateral (Spinocerebellar)
N	Numbness, Hemibody Contralateral (Spinothalamic)
D	Distribution of CN V, Ipsilateral Facial Numbness

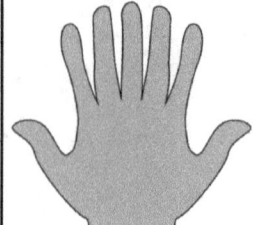

FIGURE 7. Lateral Pontine Syndrome

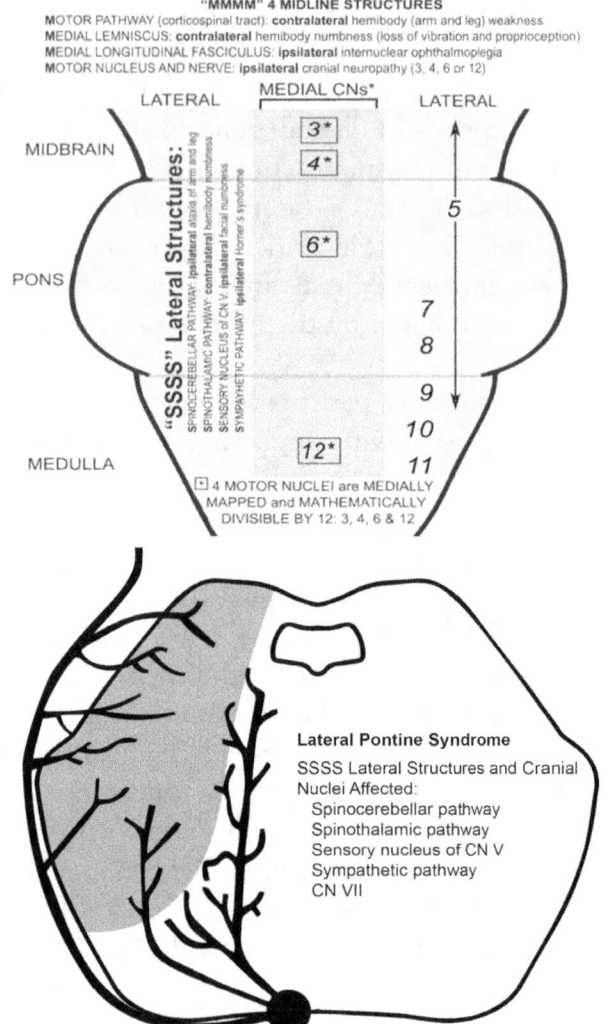

Lateral Pontine Syndrome
SSSS Lateral Structures and Cranial Nuclei Affected:
  Spinocerebellar pathway
  Spinothalamic pathway
  Sensory nucleus of CN V
  Sympathetic pathway
  CN VII

13.5.2 Medial Pontine Syndrome

Medial pontine syndrome is usually caused by infarction of the paramedian branches of the basilar artery.[3] Since the medial pons is affected, the first rule of the brainstem stating that "There are 4 MIDLINE structures beginning with "M" applies to this vascular syndrome (Figure 4). These four structures are again the **m**otor pathways (corticospinal tract) which result in contralateral weakness of the arm and leg, the **m**edial lemniscus which results in contralateral hemibody numbness, the **m**edial longitudinal fasciculus which results in ipsilateral internuclear ophthalmoplegia, and the **m**otor nucleus and nerve which result in an ipsilateral cranial neuropathy. The mnemonic used to remember the deficits associated with the midbrain structures of the brainstem is 'MOAN' (Table 18).

TABLE 18. Brainstem Midline Structures: **MOAN**

M	Motor Weakness, Contralateral (Corticospinal Tract)
O	Ophthalmoplegia, Intranuclear, Ipsilateral (Medial Longitudinal Fasciculus)
A	Arm and Leg Numbness, Contralateral (Medial Lemniscus)
N	Neuropathy, Cranial, Ipsilateral (Motor Nucleus and Nerve)

Recall that the third rules states: "The medulla has **4** cranial nerves; the pons has **4** and **4** are above the pons (Figure 4)." Applying this rule, the pons has 4 cranial nerves. However, Rule #4 states that "4 MOTOR NUCLEI are MEDIALLY MAPPED and MATHEMATICALLY DIVISIBLE BY 12: III, IV, VI and XII." Cranial nerve VI is the only cranial nerve that is located (mapped) within the medial pons. Thus, a medial pontine infarct results in loss of cranial nerve VI (abducens nerve) function that leads to ipsilateral paralysis of the lateral rectus muscle—that is, the ipsilateral eye will be unable to track laterally (Figure 8). Thus, patients with medial pontine syndrome present with weakness of the contralateral arm and leg (corticospinal tract), numbness of the contralateral arm and leg (medial meniscus), intranuclear ophthalmoplegia of the ipsilateral eye (medial longitudinal fasciculus), and ipsilateral paralysis of the lateral rectus muscle (CN VI) (Figure 9). A simple mnemonic to remember the features of medial pontine syndrome is 'MOANA' (Table 19).

FIGURE 8. Left Abducent (CN VI) Nerve Palsy

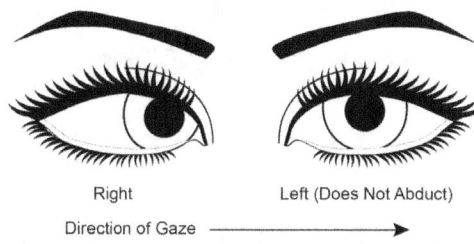

FIGURE 9. Medial Pontine Syndrome

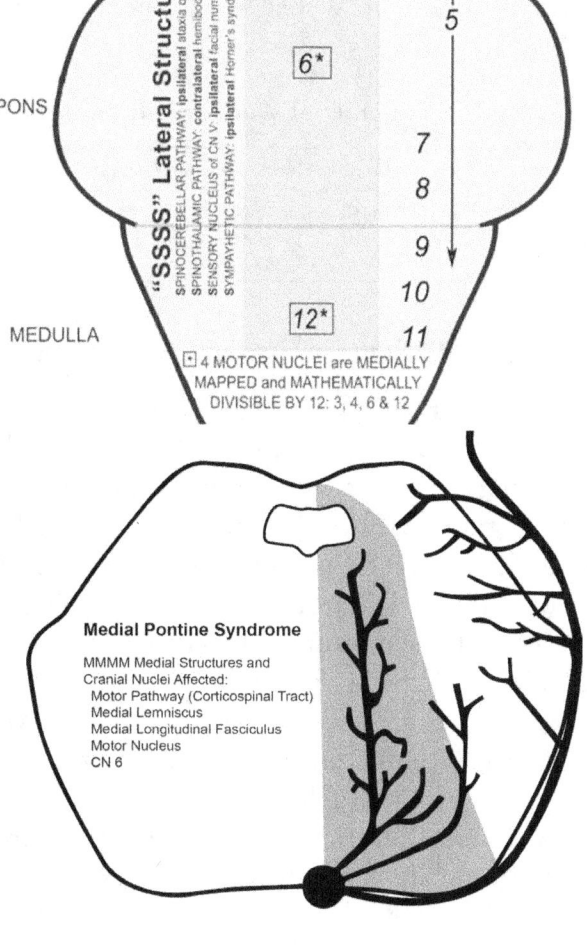

TABLE 19. Medial Pontine Syndrome: **MOANA**

M	Motor Weakness, Contralateral (Corticospinal Tract)
O	Ophthalmoplegia, Intranuclear, Ipsilateral (Medial Longitudinal Fasciculus)
A	Arm and Leg Numbness, Contralateral (Medial Lemniscus)
N	Neuropathy, Cranial, Ipsilateral (Motor Nucleus and Nerve)
A	Abducens (CN VI) Ipsilateral Paralysis of the Lateral Rectus Muscle

13.5.3 Ventral Pontine Syndrome

Locked-in syndrome (LIS) or ventral pontine syndrome is a devastating clinical condition which is typically the result of a ventral pontine infarct due to an acute basilar occlusion (Figure 10). It can also be caused by any other process that can affect the ventral pons such as hemorrhage, dissection, tumor, central pontine myelolysis, and multiple sclerosis.[4] Because this condition affects the midline pathways bilaterally, both the corticospinal tract and medial lemniscus are involved. Cranial nerves V through VIII dysfunction can be variable.

LIS is characterized by quadriplegia and the inability to speak (anarthria), with the preservation of consciousness and eye movements (blinking). Communication in patients with locked-in syndrome is accomplished by either moving or blinking their eyes.[3] A patient acutely presenting with LIS should be immediately evaluated with noncontrast brain CT and CTA which may demonstrate a hyperdense basilar artery sign (Figure 11). Just like a hyperdense MCA sign, this should be considered a neurointerventional emergency unless proven otherwise.

FIGURE 10. Locked-In Syndrome (Ventral Pontine Syndrome)

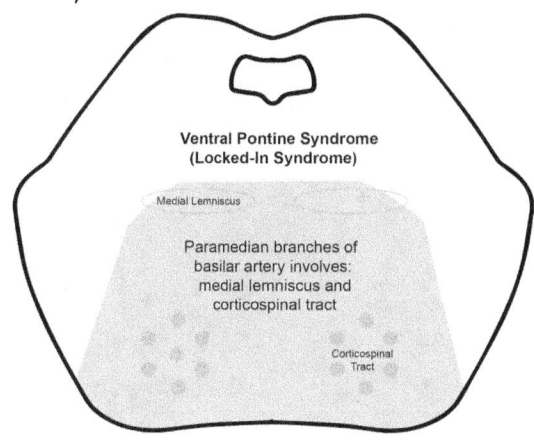

FIGURE 11. Hyperdense Basilar Artery Sign

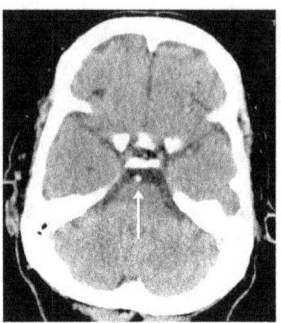

13.6 Vascular Syndromes of the Midbrain

Vascular syndromes of the midbrain do not conform to Gates's rules of the brainstem. This is because the vascular supply to the midbrain is more diverse and therefore less predictable than either the pons or medulla (Figure 12). Medial, lateral, and dorsal midbrain syndromes will be reviewed and a summary will be provided to include other midbrain syndromes. Due to the complex and variable presentation of these syndromes, neuroimaging is highly recommended.

13.6.1 Medial Midbrain (Weber) Syndrome

Medial midbrain syndrome, also known as Weber syndrome, results from infarction of the penetrating branches of the posterior cerebral artery (Figure 13).[3] Occlusion of these branches typically involves the oculomotor nerve, the corticobulbar tract, and the cortical spinal tract (Figure 13). Thus, the symptoms associated with medial midbrain or Weber syndrome include the ipsilateral eye being "down and out," a dilated, unresponsive pupil, and contralateral weakness of the face, arm, and leg (Table 20).

FIGURE 12. Diverse Vascular Supply to the Midbrain

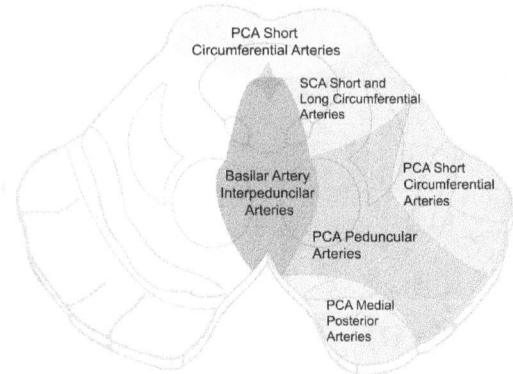

FIGURE 13. Midbrain Vascular Syndromes

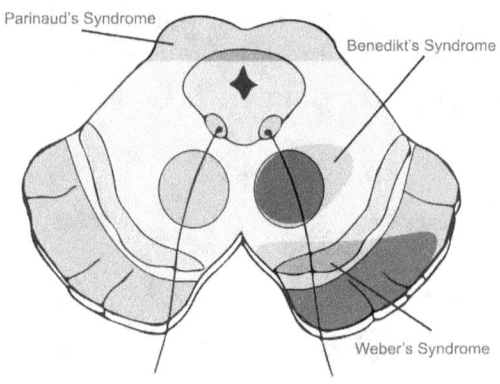

TABLE 20. Medial Midbrain (Weber) Syndrome

Structure	Deficit
Oculomotor Nerve (CN III)	Ipsilateral Eye "Down and Out" with Dilation, Unresponsive Pupil
Corticobulbar Tract	Contralateral Weakness of the Face
Corticospinal Tract	Contralateral Weakness of the Arm and Leg

A simple mnemonic to remember the features of medial midbrain or Weber syndrome is 'WEB' (Table 21).

TABLE 21. Medial Midbrain or Weber Syndrome: **WEB**

W	Weakness, Face and Hemibody (Corticobulbar and Corticospinal Tracts)
E	Eye "Down and Out," Unresponsive Pupil, Ipsilateral (DUI)
B	Both Face and Hemibody Weakness, Contralateral

13.6.2 Lateral Midbrain (Benedikt) Syndrome

Lateral midbrain syndrome, also known as Benedikt syndrome, results from infarction of the penetrating branches of the posterior cerebral artery (Figure 13).[3] Occlusion of these branches typically involves the oculomotor nerve, the red nucleus, and the dentarubrothalamic tract (Figure 13). Thus, the symptoms associated with lateral midbrain or Benedikt syndrome include the ipsilateral eye being "down and out" with dilation, unresponsive pupil, ataxia of the contralateral body, and tremor (Tables 22, 23 and 24). This syndrome also affects the dentarubrothalamic tract resulting in hemiatheosis and hemichorea. Athetosis is a deficit manifested by slow, involuntary, convoluted, writhing movements of the fingers, hands, toes, and feet and to a lesser extent, the arms, legs, neck, and tongue. Chorea is characterized by nonrhythmic, jerky, rapid, non-suppressible involuntary movement that involves the distal muscles and face.

A simple mnemonic to remember the features of lateral midbrain or Benedikt syndrome is 'HATE' (Table 23).

TABLE 22. Lateral Midbrain (Benedikt) Syndrome

Structure	Deficit
Oculomotor Nerve (CN III)	Ipsilateral Eye "Down and Out" with Dilation, Unresponsive Pupil
Red Nucleus	Contralateral Body Ataxia
Dentarubrothalamic Tract	Tremor, Hemichorea or Hemiathetosis

TABLE 23. Lateral Midbrain Syndrome: **HATE**

H	Hemichorea or Hemiathetosis (Dentatorubrothalamic Tract)	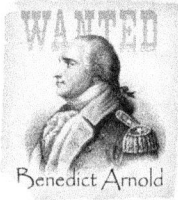 Benedict Arnold
A	Ataxia, Contralateral Body (Red Nucleus)	
T	Tremor (Dentatorubrothalamic Tract)	
E	Eye "Down and Out", Unresponsive Pupil, Ipsilateral (CNIII)	

I Hate Benedict Arnold

TABLE 24. Cranial Nerve III Deficits: **DUI**

D	Down and Out
U	Unresponsive Pupil
I	Ipsilateral

13.6.3 Dorsal Midbrain (Parinaud's) Syndrome

Dorsal midbrain syndrome (also known as Parinaud's syndrome) and vertical gaze palsy most commonly result from a pinealoma which compresses the superior colliculus affecting the rostral interstitial nucleus of the medial longitudinal fasciculus (Figure 13).[3] This results in paralysis of upward gaze (involvement of the rostral interstitial nucleus of the medial longitudinal fasciculus) and retraction of the eyelids. Multiple sclerosis and occlusion of the posterior thalamo-subthalamic paramedian artery is also known to cause this syndrome.[5] The midbrain syndromes discussed above and a few others are summarized in Table 25.

13.7 Summary

The brainstem is perhaps the most conceptually difficult region of the posterior circulation to comprehend. However, the 4 rules of the brainstem provide a straightforward method for understanding vascular syndromes at the level of the medulla and pons. Unfortunately, the vasculature diversity of the midbrain prevents the application of these rules for this level of the brainstem. Nonetheless, application of the 4 rules of the brainstem and understanding the mnemonics for the midbrain should yield an understanding of brainstem anatomy that is more than sufficient for stroke management. Always remember the stroke plan and include neuroimaging in your assessment of the brainstem (Table 26).

Abbreviations list

AICA, anterior inferior cerebellar artery; LIS, locked-in syndrome or ventral pontine syndrome; MLF, medial longitudinal fasciculus; PICA, posterior inferior cerebellar artery.

Stroke Made Simple

TABLE 25. Midbrain Vascular Syndromes

Syndrome	Structure	Cranial Nerve	Tracts	Deficits
Weber	Base	III	Corticospinal	Oculomotor palsy with crossed hemiplegia
Claude	Tegmentum	III	Red nucleus and brachium conjunctivum	Oculomotor palsy with contralateral cerebellar ataxia and tremor
Benedikt	Tegmentum	III	Red nucleus, corticospinal and brachium conjunctivum	Oculomotor palsy with contralateral cerebellar ataxia, tremor and corticospinal signs
Nothnagel	Tectum	Unilateral or Bilateral III	Superior cerebellar peduncle	Ocular palsies; paralysis of gaze and cerebellar ataxia
Parinaud	Dorsal		Supranuclear mechanism for upward gaze and other structures in periaqueductal gray matter	Paralysis of upward gaze and accommodation, fixed pupils

TABLE 26. The Stroke Plan: **S-PLAN**

S	Source (embolic or thrombotic)
P	Pathophysiology (etiology)
L	Location (of brain affected)
A	Artery (arterial territory involved)
N	Neuroimaging

Source	Pathophysiology	Location	Artery	Neuroimaging
• Embolic • Thrombotic	**C**: Cardioembolic (20%) **A**: Atherosclerotic large vessel disease (30%) **U**: Undetermined etiology - ESUS (30%) **S**: Small vessel disease or lacunar infarct (15%) **E**: Everything else or other (5%)	• Frontal • Parietal • Temporal • Occipital • Cerebellar • Thalamic • Brainstem	• ICA • MCA • ACA • Vertebral • Basilar • PICA • ACA • SCA	• CT • CTA • CTP • MRI • MRA • Angio

References

1. The rule of 4 of the brainstem: a simplified method for understanding brainstem anatomy and brainstem vascular syndromes for the non-neurologist. (2005). *Intern Med J*, Apr,35(4), 263-6.
2. Le T, Bhushan V, Sochart M. (2016). First Aid for the USMLE Step 1. New York, NY: McGraw Hill, 46.
3. Longo DL, Fauci AS, Kasper DL, Hauser SL, Jameson JL, Loscalzo J. eds. (2012). Harrison's Principles of Internal Medicine. 18ed. New York, NY: McGraw Hill, 3288–93.
4. Smith E, Delargy M. (2005). Locked-in syndrome. *Br Med J*, 330, 406–9.
5. Serino J, Martins J, Páris L, Duarte A, Ribeiro I. (2015). Parinaud's syndrome due to a unilateral vascular ischemic lesion. *Int Ophthalmol*, Apr, 35(2), 275–9.

Chapter 14

Stroke and Vision

14.1 Introduction

This chapter will discuss the relationship between stroke and vision. The visual pathway and cortical structures associated with vision will be reviewed. Specifically, symptoms involving different arterial territories within the visual pathway and occipital cortex will be discussed. This chapter will also review cranial nerve innervation and extraocular muscle function. Lastly, pupil abnormalities will also be presented.

14.2 The Visual Pathway

Visual input is transmitted to the optic nerve by retinal neurons within the eye. Each optic nerve contains fibers that represent each eye's visual field. These fibers consist of both nasal (medial) fibers and temporal (lateral) fibers (Figure 1). The nasal (medial) fibers transmit information from the lateral aspect of visual field and cross in the optic chiasm (Figure 1). Thus, the optic tract behind the optic chiasm consists of fibers from one half of the visual field (Figure 1). For example, the right optic tract consists of temporal (lateral) fibers from the right eye and nasal (medial) fibers from the left eye. Therefore, each optic tract transmits one half of the visual field (Figure 1). For this reason, pre-chiasmal lesions affect vision in the ipsilateral eye (Figure 2). However, retrochiasmal lesions result in deficits in the contralateral half of the visual field of both eyes (Figure 2). To illustrate, an infarct involving the right optic tract will result in a contralateral or left homonymous hemianopia (Figure 2).

The neurons from the optic tracts terminate and synapse in the lateral geniculate nuclei (Figure 2). Here, the optic radiations transmit information to the primary visual or calcarine cortex (Brodmann Area 17) which is located in the posterior aspect of the occipital lobe (Figures 2 and 3).

FIGURE 1. The Optic Chiasm

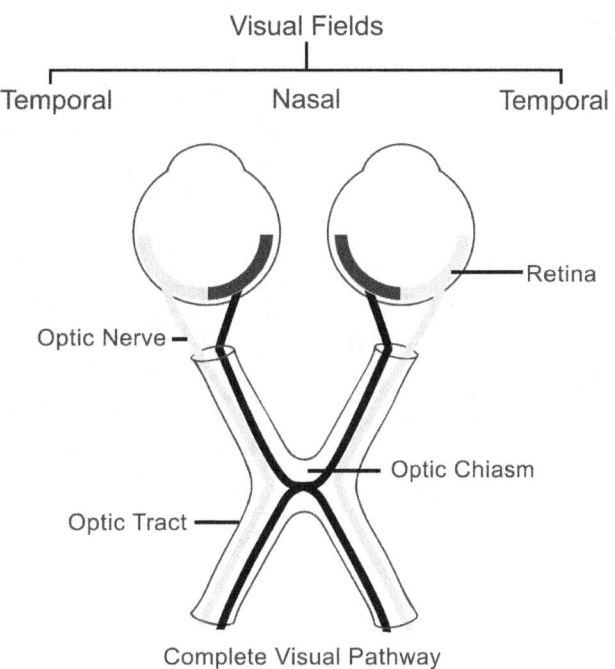

FIGURE 2. The Visual Pathway and Localized Deficits

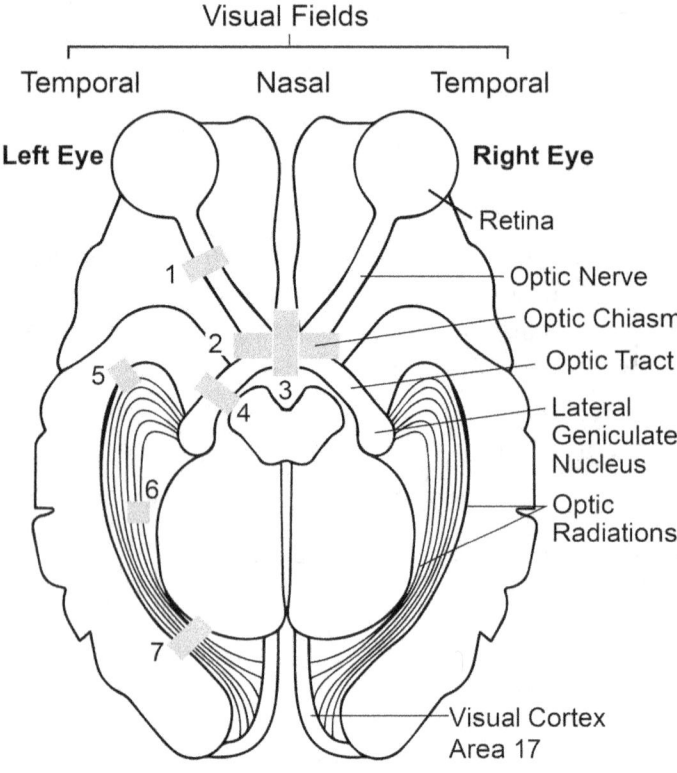

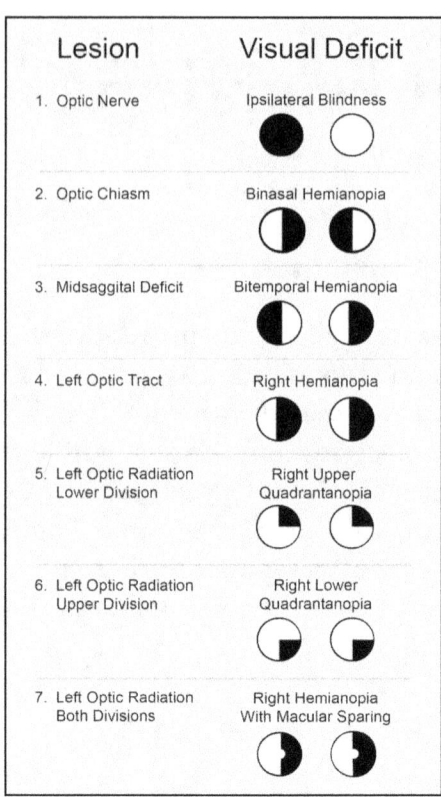

FIGURE 3. The Primary Visual Cortex

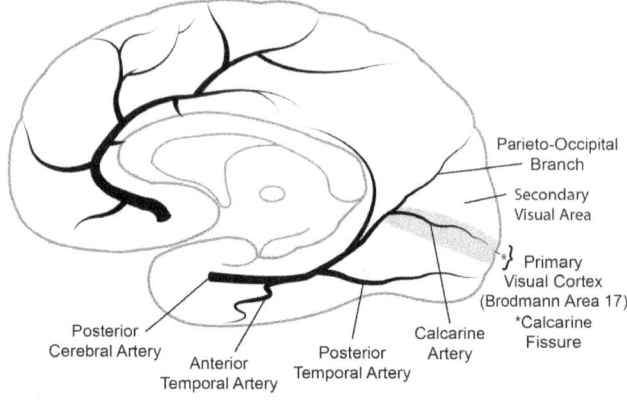

Adjacent to the primary visual cortex are visual association areas (Brodmann areas 18 and 19). Prior to reaching the primary visual cortex, the arterial supply to the visual pathway is diverse. The vascular supply to the visual pathway is derived from the internal carotid artery (ophthalmic and anterior choroidal arteries), the middle cerebral, and posterior cerebral arteries (Figure 4). Thus, stroke involving any of these arterial territories can produce visual field deficits specific to the arterial territory compromised (Figure 4).

The optic nerve receives its arterial supply from the ophthalmic artery (Figure 4). The optic radiations are predominantly supplied by branches of the middle cerebral artery (MCA) (Figure 4). Thus, MCA infarcts can result in vision loss of the contralateral visual field (Figure 2 and 5). The primary visual cortex is located above and below the calcarine fissure within the occipital lobe and supplied by cortical branches from the posterior cerebral artery (PCA) (Figure 5). Like a MCA stroke, a posterior cerebral artery occlusion also results in vision loss of the contralateral visual field. However, distinct from an MCA occlusion, macular vision is typically spared in a PCA occlusion (Figure 2).

FIGURE 4. The Arterial Territories of the Visual Pathway

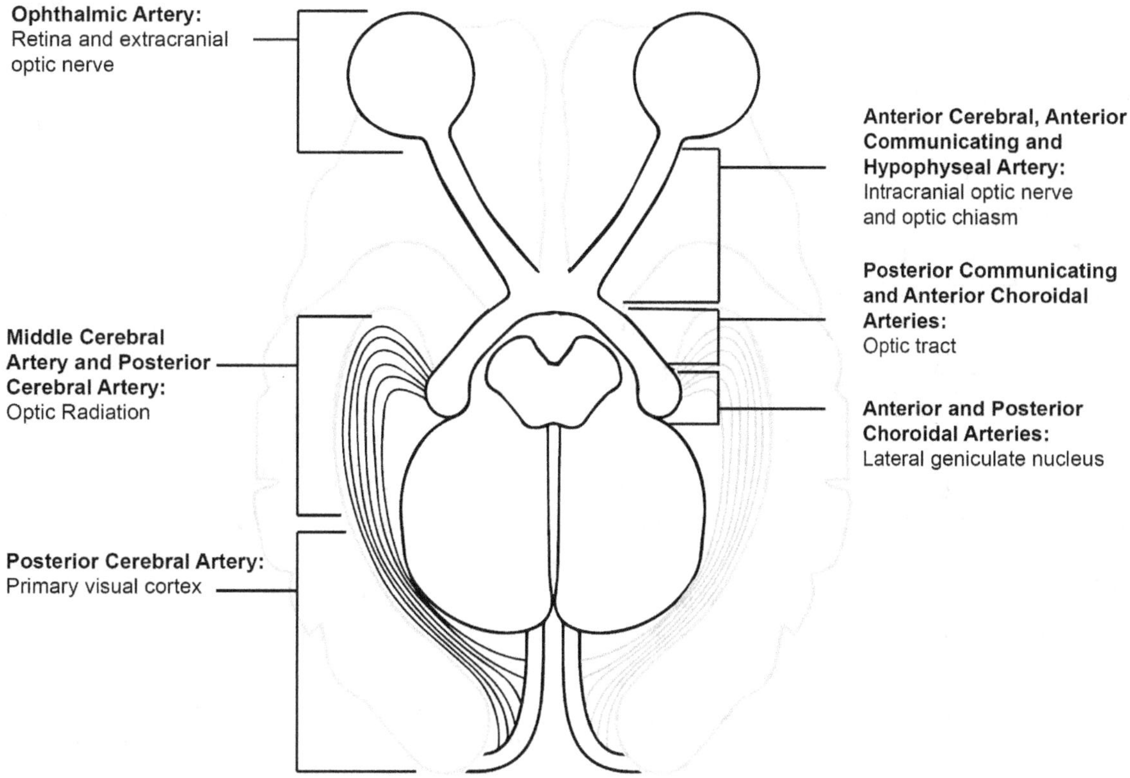

Ophthalmic Artery: Retina and extracranial optic nerve

Middle Cerebral Artery and Posterior Cerebral Artery: Optic Radiation

Posterior Cerebral Artery: Primary visual cortex

Anterior Cerebral, Anterior Communicating and Hypophyseal Artery: Intracranial optic nerve and optic chiasm

Posterior Communicating and Anterior Choroidal Arteries: Optic tract

Anterior and Posterior Choroidal Arteries: Lateral geniculate nucleus

FIGURE 5. Cortical Branches of the Posterior Cerebral Artery

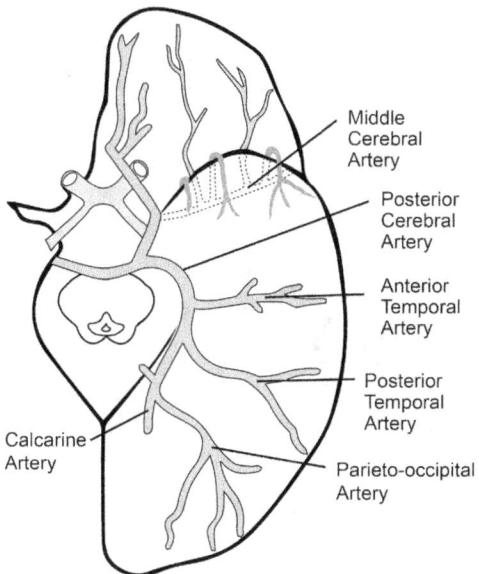

14.3 Posterior Circulation Cortical Stroke

The next segment of this chapter will discuss the distal, cortical branches of the posterior cerebral artery (PCA) and the territories they supply (Figure 5). Cortical PCA stroke most commonly presents as a visual abnormality. A unilateral cortical PCA stroke usually presents as a contralateral visual field deficit, a homonymous hemianopia with macular sparing (Figure 2). Again, this differs from a homonymous hemianopia resulting from injury to the optic tract which is commonly caused by a middle cerebral artery (MCA) infarct. The homonymous hemianopsia associated with a unilateral cortical PCA stroke usually has macular sparing, whereas a MCA stroke involving the optic tract typically presents with homonymous hemianopsia without macular sparing (Figure 2).

Bilateral cortical PCA occlusions affecting the primary visual (calcarine) cortex can produce bilateral homonymous hemianopia. Variations in cortical blindness are based on the extent of the stroke and the degree of collateral circulation. A basilar artery or tip of the basilar artery occlusion can cause bilateral occipital lobe infarction resulting in cortical blindness (bilateral homonymous hemianopia). One commonly encountered presentation is *Anton's syndrome* where patients believe they retain the ability to see. When asked to describe objects, they often provide great detail, oblivious to the fact that they are completely wrong. Another encountered deficit is *visual agnosia*, a disorder in which patients are unable to recognize objects visually but can distinguish them by a nonvisual sensory system such as touch or sound (e.g. the feel or clicking of a pen).

Visuospatial processing abnormalities can also occur. *Balint syndrome* is a triad of visual simultanagnosia (inability to integrate components of a visual scene into a cohesive format), optic ataxia (loss of hand-eye coordination), and apraxia of gaze (defect of controlled, voluntary, and purposeful eye movement). Balint syndrome can be caused by bilateral parieto-occipital infarctions most commonly in watershed distributions of the PCA and MCA territories. *Prosopagnosia*, another deficit caused by a PCA cortical infarct, is the inability to recognize faces. Cortical deficits can also include illusory phenomenon including palinopsia, micropsia and macropsia. *Palinopsi*a is the persistence of a visual image in a partially blind hemifield for seconds or even days. *Micropsia* is the appearance of images smaller than they actually are and *macropsia* is the opposite.

14.4 The Extraocular Muscles and Their Cranial Nerve Innervation

The preceding chapter (Brainstem Stroke) provided a cursory review of the cranial nerves within the midbrain and pons that are responsible for eye movements. However, a more in-depth discussion is warranted because understanding ocular muscle cranial nerve innervation can be quite complex. The fictitious chemical formula 'LR6SO4' provides an easy way to remember these cranial nerves (Figures 6 and 7)—that is, the lateral rectus muscle (LR) is innervated by CN VI and the superior oblique muscle (SO) is innervated by CN IV. The remaining extraocular muscles (superior rectus, inferior oblique, inferior rectus, and medial rectus) are innervated by CN III. To recall the extraocular muscles innervated by CN III, remember the mnemonic 'SIMI' (Table 1).

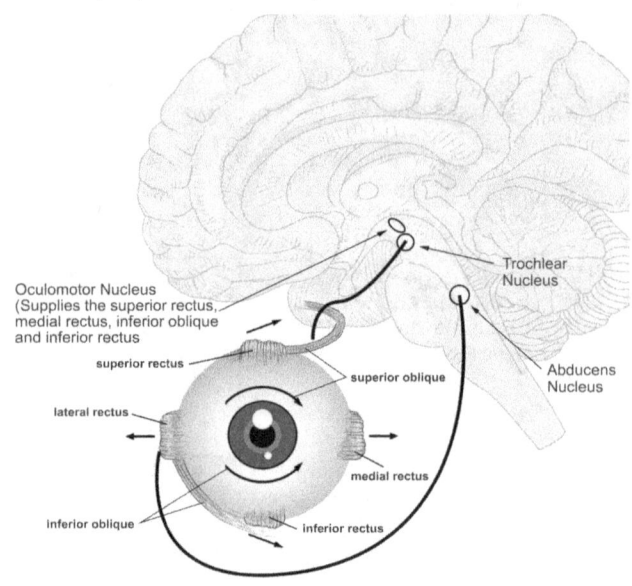

FIGURE 6. LR6SO4: The Lateral Rectus Muscle (LR) Innervated by CN VI and the Superior Oblique Muscle (SO) Innervated by CN IV

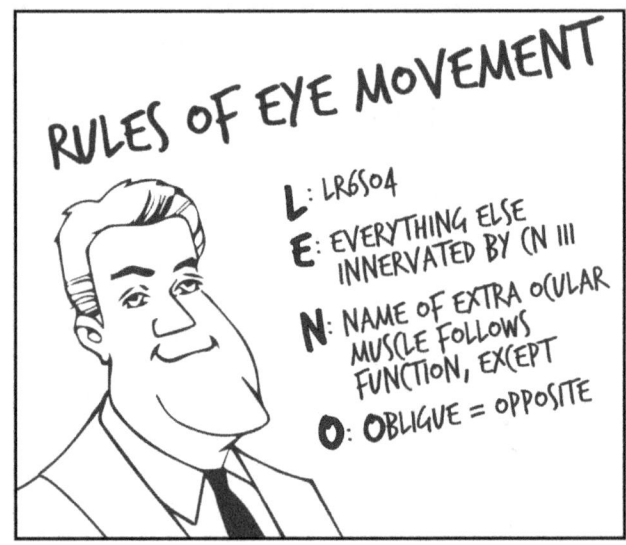

FIGURE 7. Rules of Eye Movement: **LENO**

TABLE 1. Extraocular Muscles Innervated by Cranial Nerve III: **SIMI**

S	Superior Rectus
I	Inferior Rectus
M	Medial Rectus
I	Inferior Oblique

In addition to understanding their cranial nerve innervation, understanding the functions of the extraocular muscles can also be challenging. Eye movement is coordinated by the action of six extraocular muscles which are attached to each globe. There are two groups of extraocular muscles - the **rectus muscles** and the **oblique muscles**. The rectus muscles are relatively straightforward to understand because they are named after the movement they control (Figure 8). The lateral rectus muscle moves the eyes laterally while the superior rectus muscle moves the eye superiorly (up and out). The inferior rectus muscle moves the eye inferiorly (down and out) and the medial rectus muscle moves the eye medially (Figure 8). Understanding the oblique muscles, however, is a bit more complex. That is because their actions appear to contradict what their names suggest. The superior oblique muscle moves the eye down and medially (intorsion) while the inferior oblique muscle moves the eye up and medially (Figure 8). Remember the oblique muscles start with the letter **'O'** and move the eye in the **O**pposite direction that their name suggests (Oblique = Opposite) (Figure 7 and 8).

FIGURE 8. The Extraocular Muscles

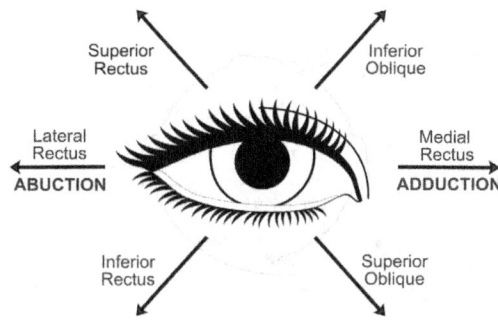

14.5 The Medial Longitudinal Fasciculus (MLF)

The MLF is a fiber tract that allows synchronous eye movement. The MLF connects the abducens nucleus (CN VI) within the pons to the oculomotor nucleus (CN III) which is located in the midbrain. Certain muscles in both eyes are coordinated through the actions of the MLF but only through indirect brainstem pathways. The right CN VI nucleus is connected to the left CN III nucleus by the left MLF. The left MLF connects the right CN VI nucleus to the left CN III, coordinating synchronous eye movement towards the right (right-sided gaze). In a similar fashion, the right MLF connects the left CN VI nucleus to the right CN III nucleus and directs synchronous eye movements towards the left (left-sided gaze) (Figure 9).

Lateral conjugate gaze requires the coordination of abduction (lateral rectus muscle, CN VI—look laterally towards the ipsilateral ear) in one eye and adduction (medial rectus muscle, CN III—look medially towards the nose) in the other eye. Sometimes, the definitions of abduction and adduction can be hard to remember. However, remembering the mnemonic 'ABE' (**AB**duction is eye movement towards the **E**ar) will help. These coordinated movements are controlled by the paramedian pontine reticular formation (PPRF) which is also termed the *pontine gaze center*. The PPRF receives cortical input from the contralateral frontal lobe's frontal eye field. For example, the left frontal eye field transmits cortical input to the right PPRF and the right frontal eye field transmits cortical input to the left PPRF. Thus, stroke involving the frontal cortex will inhibit contralateral horizontal gaze, resulting in a gaze preference toward the side of the infarct. However, frontal lobe seizures may cause gaze preference away from the side of the lesion. The pathway that includes the PPRF, MLF, and cranial nerves VI and III is the following:

1. To look to the right (right gaze), the left frontal eye field (FEF) sends signals to the right PPRF.
2. The right PPRF innervates the right abducens (CN VI) nucleus, which controls the right lateral rectus muscle and causes the right eye to ABduct (look towards the right).
3. The medial longitudinal fasciculus (MLF) connects the CN VI nucleus to the contralateral CNIII nucleus. The left oculomotor (CNIII) nucleus innervates the left medial rectus muscle and causes the left eye to adduct (look towards the midline).

FIGURE 9. The Medial Longitudinal Fasciculus (MLF)

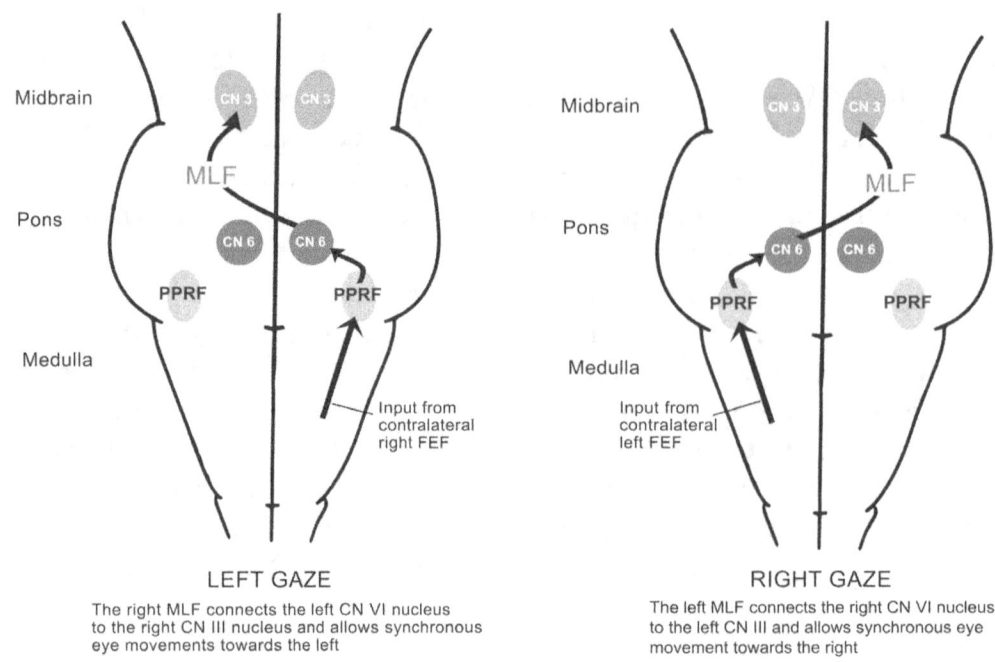

LEFT GAZE
The right MLF connects the left CN VI nucleus to the right CN III nucleus and allows synchronous eye movements towards the left

RIGHT GAZE
The left MLF connects the right CN VI nucleus to the left CN III and allows synchronous eye movement towards the right

FEF - frontal eye field; MLF - medial longitudinal fasciculus; PPRF - paramedian pontine reticular formation

FIGURE 10. Internuclear Ophthalmoplegia (INO)

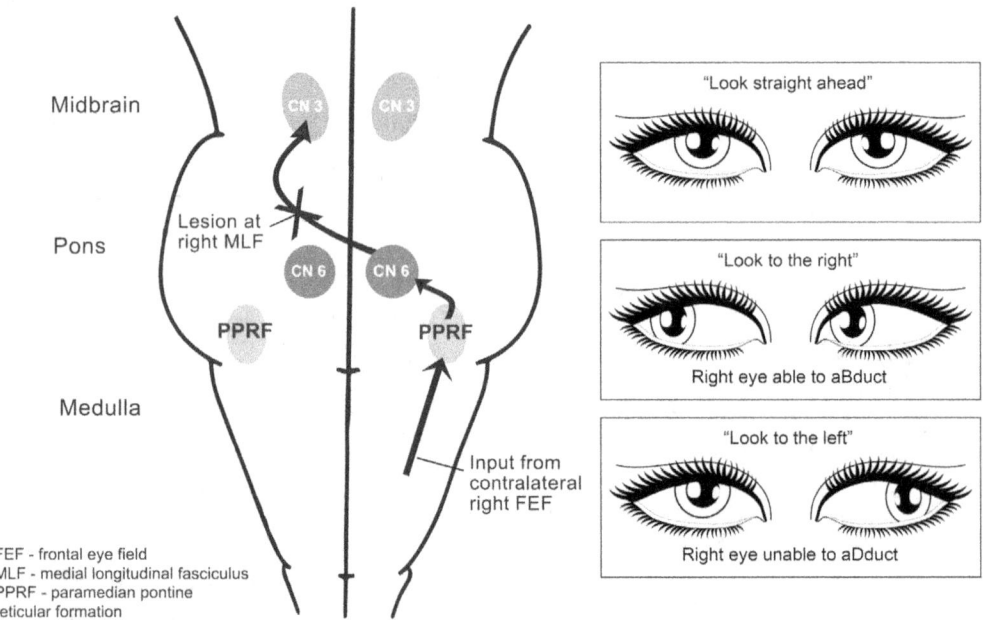

FEF - frontal eye field
MLF - medial longitudinal fasciculus
PPRF - paramedian pontine reticular formation

Internuclear ophthalmoplegia (INO) is a lateral conjugate gaze deficit (both eyes looking laterally) caused by a medial longitudinal fasciculus (MLF) lesion. This results in the inability to adduct the corresponding eye during conjugate lateral gaze but preserves convergence (eye crossing, which involves a different pathway). A right intranuclear ophthalmoplegia (INO) results from damage to the right medial longitudinal fasciculus (MLF). Thus, the right eye can ABduct (lateral rectus muscle, CN VI-look laterally towards the ear) to look towards the right but cannot ADduct (medial rectus muscle, CN III, look medially towards the nose) to look to the left (Figure 10).

14.6 Pupil Abnormalities and Stroke

Pupil abnormalities present commonly with brainstem vascular syndromes. Pupillary dilation is mediated by the sympathetic division of the autonomic nervous system. This is balanced by the parasympathetic division of the autonomic nervous system which controls pupillary constriction. Specifically, the Edinger-Westphal nucleus of cranial nerve III has preganglionic fibers which synapse at the ciliary ganglion in the posterior orbit. Here, the postganglionic fibers innervate the sphincter muscle of the iris resulting in constriction. Mass effect from brain injury or stroke compresses the third cranial nerve. In this manner, parasympathetic supply to the pupil can be compromised, resulting in unopposed sympathetic innervation and dilation. (Figure 11). For this reason, unilateral or bilateral fixed pupils are suggestive of unilateral compression of the oculomotor nerve (CN III) (uncal herniation) or a bilateral midbrain (tectal) process. Pinpoint pupils that are minimally reactive to light are strongly suggestive of a pontine lesion. Other conditions and affected regions of the brain can also vary pupillary size (Figure 12).

FIGURE 11. Pupillary Constriction and Autonomic Nervous System

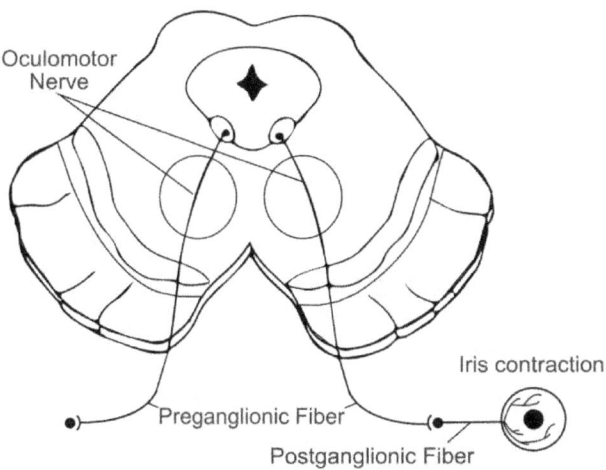

14.7 Summary

This chapter reviewed the relationship between vision and stroke. First, the visual pathway was discussed. It is essential to be familiar with and recognize deficits caused by stroke within any part of the visual pathway. In addition, the extraocular muscles of the eye and their cranial nerve innervation were also reviewed. Finally, different pupillary abnormalities were also presented. Both the extraocular muscles of the eye and pupillary abnormalities can be easily assessed on physical examination. Understanding abnormalities and their presentation can yield important insights into cranial nerve and brainstem pathology, respectively.

Abbreviations list

FEF, frontal eye field; INO, intranuclear ophthalmoplegia; LR, lateral rectus muscle; MCA, middle cerebral artery; MLF, medial longitudinal fasciculus; PCA, posterior cerebral artery; PPRF, paramedian pontine reticular formation; SO, superior oblique muscle.

FIGURE 12. Pupil Abnormalities and Associated Regions of the Brain

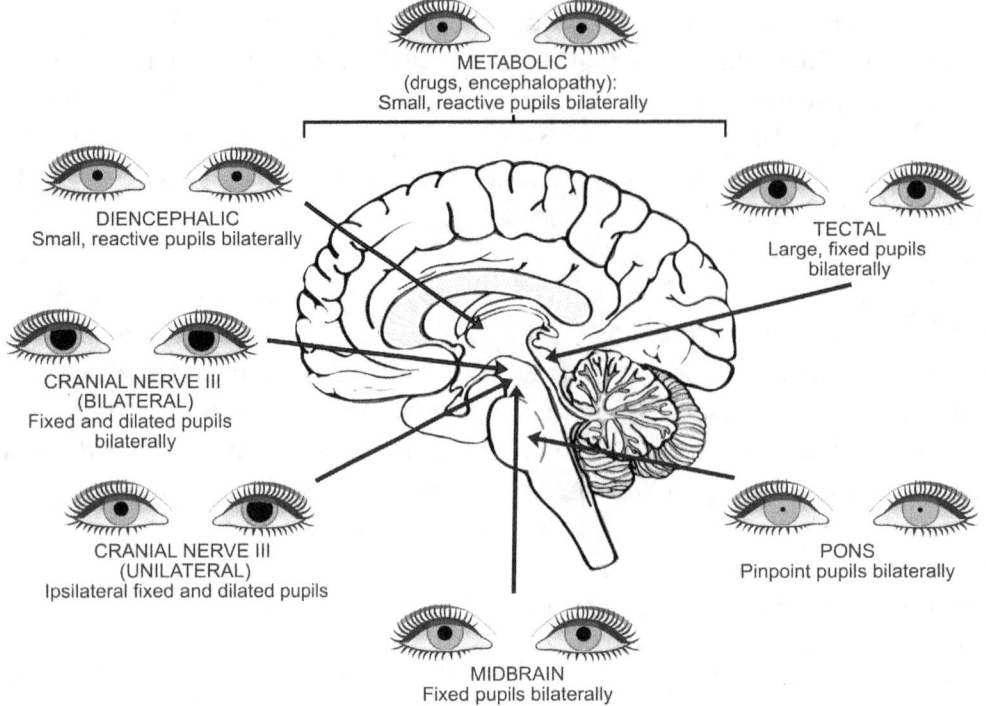

Chapter 15

Basilar Artery Occlusion

The basilar artery is the largest and most important artery of the posterior circulation. The major regions of the brain supplied by the posterior circulation include the thalamus, the occipital lobe, parietal lobe, the cerebellum, and the brainstem. Acute basilar artery occlusion (BAO) can involve these structures to different degrees. Acute BAO represents 1%-3% of all strokes but is associated with a devastating prognosis and carries the highest mortality rate (80 to 90%) among intracranial large vessel occlusion (LVO).[1-3] The primary objective in the treatment of AIS is the restoration of cerebral blood flow and the treatment of BAO is certainly no exception.

Unlike most LVOs, BAO is predominantly a result of atherosclerotic (thrombotic) disease.[4] This pathophysiology can confound the diagnosis and treatment of BAO due to its heterogeneous and ill-defined symptoms.[5] Basilar artery thrombosis may present in three typical fashions:

1. A sudden onset of severe motor and bulbar symptoms with impaired consciousness.
2. A gradual or progressive course of a combination of symptoms such as motor deficits, dysarthria and speech impairment, vertigo, nausea and vomiting, headache, visual disturbances, and altered consciousness that may progress into disabling motor and bulbar symptoms, impaired consciousness, or the combination of both.
3. A waxing or waning course of prodromal symptoms that may include loss of vision, diplopia, vertigo, hemiparesis, paresthesia, imbalance, and dysarthria days or months before a BAO.

BAO is another form of LVO AIS that warrants advanced neuroimaging. Like every other form of LVO AIS, poor functional outcome is directly related to the time required for recanalization.

Top of the basilar syndrome is a variant of BAO which results from a thromboembolic occlusion of the top of the basilar artery (Figure 1).

FIGURE 1. Top of the Basilar Syndrome

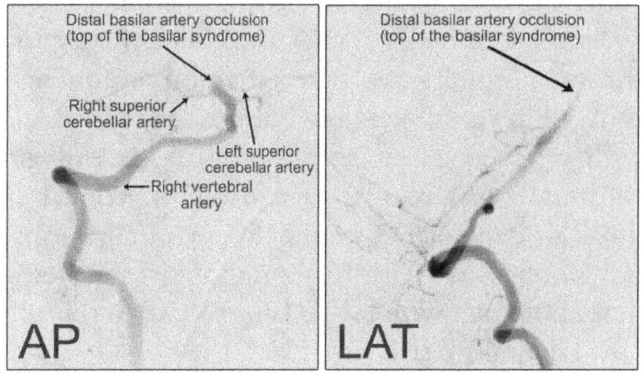

Clinically, this is characterized by visual and oculomotor deficits, behavioral abnormalities, and somnolence typically with the absence of motor dysfunction. An easy mnemonic to help recall these symptoms is 'SOB' (Table 1). This can be associated with a hyperdense basilar artery sign on nonenhanced brain CT (Figure 2). Top of the basilar syndrome can result in bilateral thalamic ischemia due to the occlusion of perforator vessels arising from the posterior cerebral artery (PCA).

TABLE 1. Top of the Basilar Syndrome Symptoms: **SOB**

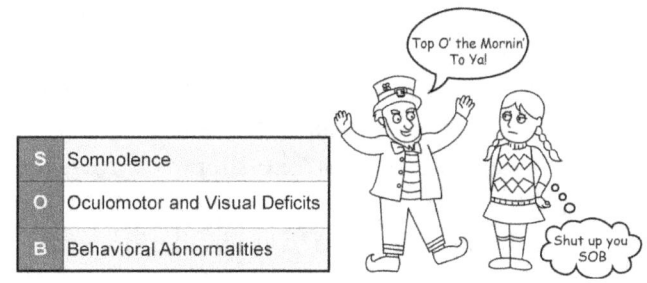

S	Somnolence
O	Oculomotor and Visual Deficits
B	Behavioral Abnormalities

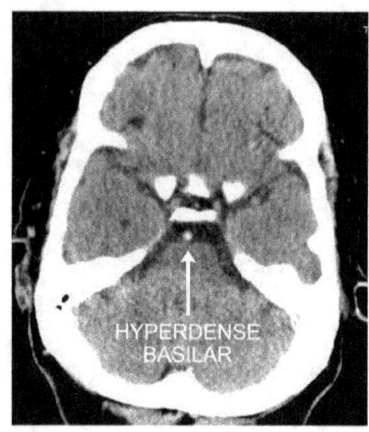

FIGURE 2. Hyperdense Basilar Artery Sign

Early recanalization improves functional outcome in BAO patients.[6] Recanalization can be performed using IV or IA thrombolytic agents, thrombo-aspiration, or mechanical thrombectomy. However, previous treatments for BAO with intravenous or intra-arterial pharmacologic thrombolysis were unsatisfactory, with the rates of death or dependency being 78% with IV thrombolysis and 76% with IA thrombolysis.[7] The recanalization rates with IV TPA for LVO are typically low, ranging from 17 to 38%.[8-11]

While the degree of recanalization does not correlate to functional outcome, higher rates of functional independence and reduced mortality were observed in patients with recanalization compared to patients without recanalization.[8] Furthermore, patients with early recanalization typically had better outcomes than those with late recanalization.[8] These principles will underscore our mantra for LVO AIS: **Find them fast and fix them fast**. We need to identify LVO AIS patients quickly because treatment with IV TPA alone has low recanalization rates and poor functional outcomes. Once LVO AIS patients are identified, they need to be recanalized quickly as early recanalization demonstrates better functional outcomes.

Newer stroke devices called stent retrievers have heralded a "Stroke Renaissance" in AIS management and endovascular stroke therapy. However, the trials that demonstrated the efficacy of these devices only pertained to anterior circulation stroke.

While no formal BAO mechanical thrombectomy trials have been performed to demonstrate safety, technical success, and clinical efficacy, both single center studies and case series have demonstrated favorable clinical results.[6, 12-13] A large and recent meta-analysis demonstrated a high recanalization rate of 80% and good functional outcome rates of 42.8% for acute BAO treated with stent retriever mechanical thrombectomy.[14] Another large meta-analysis of 45 studies involving 2,056 patients with basilar artery occlusion (BAO) demonstrated recanalization rates of 75% with new generation thrombectomy devices and showed the number needed to treat (NNT) of three to decrease death or functional dependency.[15]

Basilar artery occlusion is a very lethal neurologic condition with a mortality rate of 80%-90% if not treated. While multiple endovascular trials have recently (2015) demonstrated the efficacy of endovascular treatment for anterior circulation stroke, none have been performed to evaluate basilar artery occlusion. This leads to many unanswered questions due to the lack of prospective studies. Certainly, randomized control trials are warranted, but until that time, the data that exists today demonstrate EVT must always be considered in the treatment of acute BAO. While different presentations of acute BAO were described earlier, the sudden onset of severe motor and bulbar symptoms with loss of consciousness is frequently encountered in the emergency department. Carefully review the brain CT of these patients and look for a hyperdense basilar artery sign. Unless contraindicated, these patients should receive EVT immediately. The 2018 AHA/ASA guidelines state, "Although the benefits are uncertain, the use of mechanical thrombectomy with stent retrievers may be reasonable for carefully selected patients with AIS in whom treatment can be initiated (groin puncture) within 6 hours of symptoms onset and who have causative occlusion of the anterior cerebral arteries, *vertebral* arteries, *basilar* artery, or posterior cerebral arteries."[16]

Abbreviations list

AIS, acute ischemic stroke; BAO, basilar artery occlusion; EVT, endovascular therapy; LVO, large vessel occlusion; NNT, number needed to treat; PCA, posterior cerebral artery.

References

1. Lindsberg PJ, Soinne L, Tatlisumak T, et al. (2004). Long-term outcome after intravenous thrombolysis of basilar artery occlusion. *JAMA*, Oct 20, 292(15), 1862-6.
2. Schonewille WJ, Wijman CA, Michel P, et al. (2009). Treatment and outcomes of acute basilar artery occlusion in the basilar artery international cooperation study (BASICS): a prospective registry study. *Lancet Neurol*, 8, 724–30.
3. Hacke W, Zeumer H, Ferbert A, et al. (1988). Intra-arterial thrombolytic therapy improves outcome in patients with acute vertebrobasilar occlusive disease. *Stroke*, 19, 1216–22.
4. Voetsch B, DeWitt LD, Pessin MS, Caplan LR. (2004). Basilar artery occlusive disease in the New England Medical Center Posterior Circulation Registry. *Arch Neurol*, 61, 496–504.
5. Vergouwen MD, Algra A, Pfefferkorn T, et al. (2012). Time is brain(stem) in basilar artery occlusion. *Stroke*, 43, 3003–06.
6. Espinosa de Rueda M, Parrilla G, Zamarro J, et al. (2013). Treatment of acute vertebrobasilar occlusion using thrombectomy with stent retrievers: initial experience with 18 patients. *AJNR Am J Neuroradiol*, 34, 1044–48.
7. Lindsberg PJ, Mattle HP. (2006). Therapy of basilar artery occlusion: a systematic analysis comparing intra-arterial and intravenous thrombolysis. *Stroke*, 37, 922–28.
8. Bhatia R, Hill MD, Shobha N, et al. (2010). Low rates of acute recanalization with intravenous recombinant tissue plasminogen activator in ischemic stroke: real-world experience and a call for action. *Stroke*, 41, 2254–58.
9. Alexandrov AV, Molina CA, Grotta JC, et al. (2004). Ultrasound-enhanced systemic thrombolysis for acute ischemic stroke. *N Engl J Med*, 351, 2170–78.
10. del Zoppo GJ, Poeck K, Pessin MS, et al. (1992). Recombinant tissue plasminogen activator in acute thrombotic and embolic stroke. *Ann Neurol*, 32, 78–86.
11. Ribo M, Alvarez-Sabin J, Montaner J, et al. (2006). Temporal profile of recanalization after intravenous tissue plasminogen activator: selecting patients for rescue reperfusion techniques. *Stroke*, 37, 1000–100.
12. Mordasini P, Brekenfeld C, Byrne JV, et al. (2013). Technical feasibility and application of mechanical thrombectomy with the Solitaire FR revascularization device in acute basilar artery occlusion. *AJNR Am J Neuroradiol*, 34, 159–63.
13. Mourand I, Machi P, Milhaud D, et al. (2013). Mechanical thrombectomy with the Solitaire device in acute basilar artery occlusion. *J Neurointervent Surg*, May 4, [Epub ahead of print].
14. Phan K, Phan S, Huo YR, et al. (2016). Outcomes of endovascular treatment of basilar artery occlusion in the stent retriever era: a systematic review and meta-analysis. *Journal of NeuroInterventional Surgery*, 8, 1107-15.
15. Kumar G, Shahripour RB, Alexandrov AV. (2014). Recanalization of acute basilar artery occlusion improves outcomes: A meta-analysis. *Journal of neurointerventional surgery*.
16. Powers WJ, Rabinstein AA, Ackerson T, Adeoye OM, Bambakidis NC, Becker K, Biller J, Brown M, Demaerschalk BM, Hoh B, et al. (2018). Guidelines for the Early Management of Patients With Acute Ischemic Stroke: A Guideline for Healthcare Professionals From the American Heart Association/American Stroke Association. *Stroke*, Jan 24.

Chapter 16

Anterior Circulation Stroke

16.1 Introduction

Both cerebrovascular anatomy and acute ischemic stroke (AIS) have already been discussed. However, as stated earlier, understanding cerebrovascular anatomy by itself is insufficient to manage stroke. In addition, knowledge of what regions of the brain are supplied by this vasculature and their functions is essential. Remember, this is all part of the stroke plan (Table 1). This chapter serves as a brief description of the anterior circulation, the regions of the brain it supplies, and their functions.

16.2 Cortical Anatomy

As mentioned earlier, the cerebral cortex has different anatomic designations which, in turn, have both specific and integrated functions (Figure 1, Table 2). These regions of the cortex have already been discussed in Chapter 3 (The Brain) but bear repeating due to their particular relevance to stroke. The frontal eye fields (FEF) are located in the frontal cortex (Brodmann Area 8) and are responsible for initiating and tracking eye movements. The primary motor cortex is contained within the frontal lobe and separated anteriorly from the parietal lobe by the central sulcus. It contains the cell bodies of the pyramidal tract which control voluntary movement. The gyrus immediately posterior to the central sulcus which is the most anterior gyrus of the parietal lobe is called the *postcentral gyrus* (Brodmann Areas 3, 1 and 2). This is also referred to as the primary sensory cortex and is the main somatic sensory reception center of the brain.

TABLE 1. The Stroke Plan: S-PLAN

S	Source (embolic or thrombotic)
P	Pathophysiology (etiology)
L	Location (of brain affected)
A	Artery (arterial territory involved)
N	Neuroimaging

Source	Pathophysiology	Location	Artery	Neuroimaging
• Embolic • Thrombotic	**C**: Cardioembolic (20%) **A**: Atherosclerotic large vessel disease (30%) **U**: Undetermined etiology - ESUS (30%) **S**: Small vessel disease or lacunar infarct (15%) **E**: Everything else or other (5%)	• Frontal • Parietal • Temporal • Occipital • Cerebellar • Thalamic • Brainstem	• ICA • MCA • ACA • Vertebral • Basilar • PICA • ACA • SCA	• CT • CTA • CTP • MRI • MRA • Angio

Broca's area is located within the frontal cortex of the dominant lobe (usually left hemisphere) of the brain and is responsible for the production of speech. The Sylvian fissure separates the frontal lobe superiorly from the temporal lobe inferiorly. The most superiorly located gyrus of the temporal lobe (immediately beneath the Sylvian fissure) is called *the superior temporal gyrus*. Portions of this gyrus plus Brodmann areas 41 and 42 comprise Wernicke's area which is responsible for understanding speech (Figure 1). Wernicke's area is also located in the cortex of the dominant temporal lobe (usually left hemisphere) of the brain. The primary visual cortex is located within the occipital lobe and is responsible for vision.

FIGURE 1. Cortical Regions and Associated Deficits

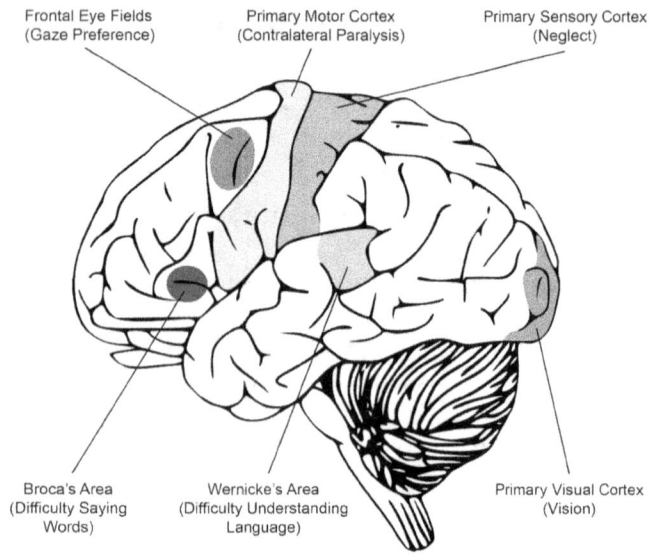

TABLE 2. Cortical Regions and Associated Functions

Cortical Structure	Location	Function
Frontal Eye Fields (FEF)	Frontal Lobe	Eye Movement
Primary Motor Cortex	Frontal Lobe	Voluntary Movement
Broca's Area	Frontal Lobe	Production of Speech
Primary Sensory Cortex	Parietal Lobe	Sensation
Wernicke's Area	Temporal Lobe	Language Comprehension
Primary Visual Cortex	Occipital Lobe	Vision

16.3 Internal Carotid Artery Stroke (ICA)

As discussed in Chapter 4 (*Cerebrovascular Anatomy*), blood supply to the brain is divided into an anterior circulation and a posterior circulation. The anterior circulation consists of three basic components: (1) the internal carotid artery (ICA), (2) the middle cerebral artery (MCA), and (3) the anterior cerebral artery (ACA) (Figure 2). Recall that the internal carotid artery has four segments but only the supraclinoid segment is located within the brain (intradural). As discussed earlier, the supraclinoid segment has three major vessels: (1) the ophthalmic artery (OA), (2) the posterior communicating artery (PCoA), and (3) the anterior choroidal artery (AChA). An easy way to remember the three vessels that arise from the supraclinoid segment is the mnemonic 'OPA' (Table 3). The supraclinoid segment bifurcates into the MCA laterally and the ACA medially (Figure 4). Understanding anterior circulation stroke is dependent upon understanding these three components. The mnemonic 'SAM' is an easy way remember them (Table 4).

FIGURE 2. The Supraclinoid Segment, Middle and Anterior Cerebral Arteries

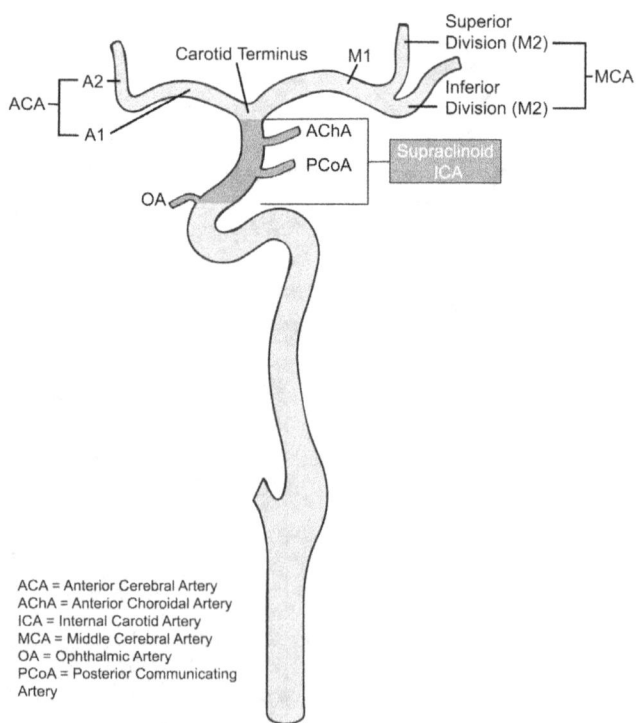

ACA = Anterior Cerebral Artery
AChA = Anterior Choroidal Artery
ICA = Internal Carotid Artery
MCA = Middle Cerebral Artery
OA = Ophthalmic Artery
PCoA = Posterior Communicating Artery

TABLE 3. Supraclinoid ICA Segment Vessels: **OPA**

O	Ophthalmic Artery (OA)
P	Posterior Communicating Artery (PCoA)
A	Anterior Choroidal Artery (AChA)

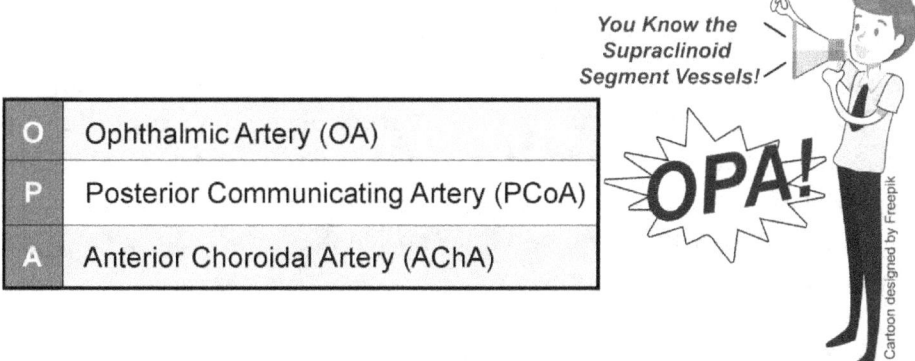

TABLE 4. The Three Vascular Components of the Anterior Circulation: **SAM**

S	Supraclinoid segment of internal carotid artery
A	Anterior cerebral artery (ACA)
M	Middle cerebral artery (MCA)

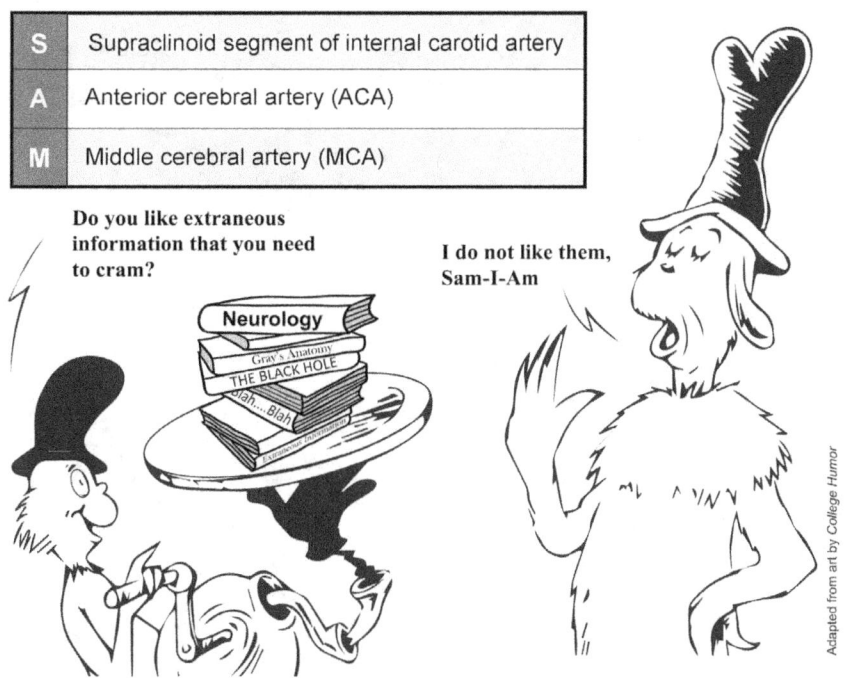

The ICA is the most proximal component of the anterior circulation. The internal carotid arteries supply the cerebral hemispheres and the eyes. Because of its proximal location, pathologic stroke processes occurring in the ICA can theoretically affect all the remaining components in the anterior circulation (all the branches of the supraclinoid segment, MCA, ACA, and watershed infarcts). The mechanisms by which the ICA can contribute to anterior circulation stroke are varied, but five clinical scenarios are particularly common and include amaurosis fugax, occlusion of the AChA, watershed infarcts, and infarcts involving the MCA and ACA, either alone or in combination. This is because embolic material can affect any region of the anterior circulation, making its presentation variable.

Recall that the OA is the most proximal vessel to arise from the supraclinoid segment of the ICA. Thus, the ICA perfuses both the optic nerve and retina via the OA and its branches. *Amaurosis fugax* is a temporary loss of vision in one or both eyes due to a lack of blood flow to the retina and presents in 25% of symptomatic ICA disease. **Amaurosis** (meaning *darkening*) **fugax** (meaning *fleeting*) is temporary loss of vision due to lack of blood flow or emboli affecting the retina. This is because emboli from the ICA travel to the ophthalmic artery and into the central retinal artery, causing focal, repetitive retinal ischemia (Figure 3). A history of amaurosis fugax is strongly suggestive of ICA disease proximal to the origin of the ophthalmic artery and prompts further investigation to exclude atherosclerotic stenosis of the ipsilateral carotid origin.

The next vessel that arises from the supraclinoid segment is the PCoA. Keep in mind that this is an important anastomotic channel which connects the anterior and posterior circulation (Figure 4).

The PCoA has many perforating branches (perforators) that supply the posterior part of the optic chiasm and optic tract, the posterior part of the hypothalamus, the mammillary body, and a portion of the thalamus. PCoA-related perforator infarcts are considered a form of posterior circulation stroke and this was previously discussed in earlier chapters.

FIGURE 3. The Ophthalmic Artery and Central Retinal Artery

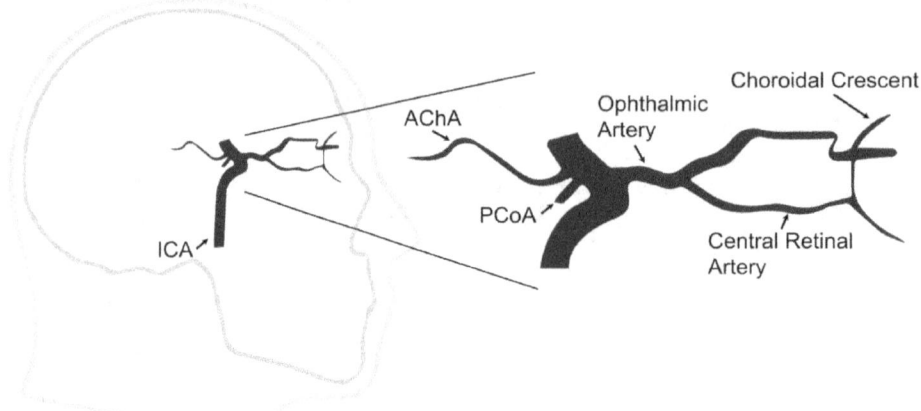

ICA - Internal Carotid Artery, AChA - Anterior Choroidal Artery, PCoA - Posterior Communicating Artery

FIGURE 4. The Posterior Communicating Artery (PCoA)

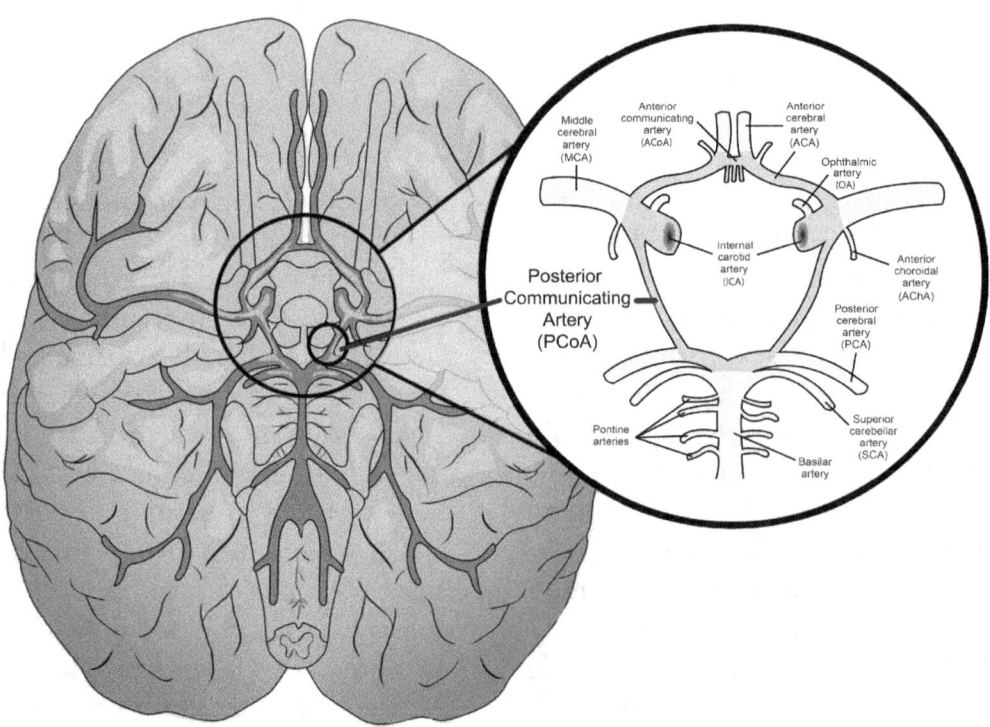

One important and common anatomic variant is a fetal origin of the posterior cerebral artery (fPCA) (Figure 5). Here, the PCoA is enlarged (larger than the P1 segment of the ipsilateral posterior cerebral artery) and supplies most blood flow to the ipsilateral PCA (PCA). In this situation, anterior circulation stroke affecting the ipsilateral carotid artery can involve the fPCA which represents the PCA distribution. In this manner, anterior circulation stroke can affect posterior fossa structures such as the visual cortex. The PCoA also forms a portion of the Circle of Willis (COW) (Figure 4). PCoA artery aneurysms represent 25% of all brain aneurysms and are the second most common form of intracranial aneurysms.[1]

FIGURE 5. Fetal Origin of the Posterior Cerebral Artery (fPCA)

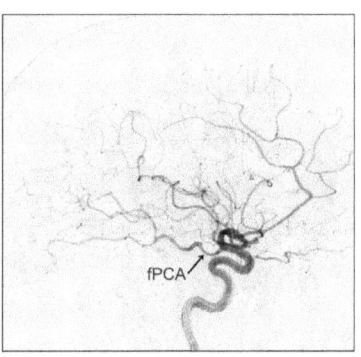

The PCoA is also a frequent site of another entity called an *infundibulum* (Figure 6). Typically, an infundibulum is conically-shaped, less than 3 mm in height, with a normal vessel emanating from its apex.[2] It is important to distinguish the difference between an aneurysm and an infundibulum because infundibula rarely require follow-up evaluation. There are, however, some reports that infundibula can transform into aneurysms, yet this is infrequent.[3]

FIGURE 6. Posterior Communicating Artery Infundibulum

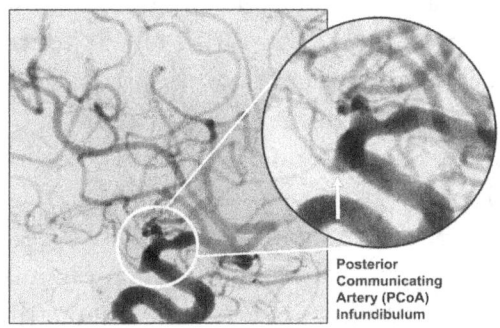

The last branch of the supraclinoid segment of the ICA is the anterior choroidal artery (AChA). The AChA provides specific vascular supply to the choroid plexus, the optic chiasm and tract, the globus pallidus, the internal capsule, the thalamus, the tail of the caudate, hippocampus, amygdala, the substantia nigra, red nucleus, and crus cerebri. An easy way to remember these structures is to recall the mnemonic 'SCORING CHART' (Table 5).

Involvement of the posterior limb of the internal capsule can cause *contralateral hemiplegia*, while involvement of the thalamus can bring about *contralateral hypo-aesthesia*. Additionally, involvement of the optic chiasm and tract can give rise to *homonymous hemianopsia*. An easy way to remember these symptoms is the phrase 'triple H pot' (Table 6). Neglect can result from right-sided involvement. The most common clinical syndrome of an AChA occlusion is contralateral hemiparesis and a contralateral visual field defect. Homonymous hemianopia can sometimes manifest with wedge-shaped visual field defects called *sectoranopia*, which is indicative of an AChA occlusion compromising vascular supply to the lateral geniculate ganglion. For such a small vessel, the AChA has a tremendous vascular distribution (Table 5).

In fact, because its involvement can cause contralateral hemiplegia, sensory loss or homonymous hemianopsia AChA patients can be confused for large vessel occlusion (LVO) AIS stroke patients. For this matter, lacunar infarcts involving lenticulostriate arteries and thalamic or pontine perforators can also cause this dilemma. Stroke caused by the AChA, lenticulostriate arteries, and thalamic or pontine perforators can mimic LVO. AChA infarcts typically have a long-term prognosis worse than lacunar infarcts but better than LVOs.[4] Always consider these vessels in patients presenting with LVO symptoms with no imaging evidence of LVO. An easy way to remember them is with the mnemonic 'PLAT' (Table 7).

TABLE 5. AChA Distribution: **SCORING CHART**

S	Substantia Nigra
C	Choroid Plexus
O	Optic Chiasm
R	Red Nucleus
I	Internal Capsule
N	Neglect - right sided involvement
G	Globus Pallidus
C	Crus Cerebri
H	Hippocampus
A	Amygdala
R	Rear (tail) of Caudate
T	Thalamus

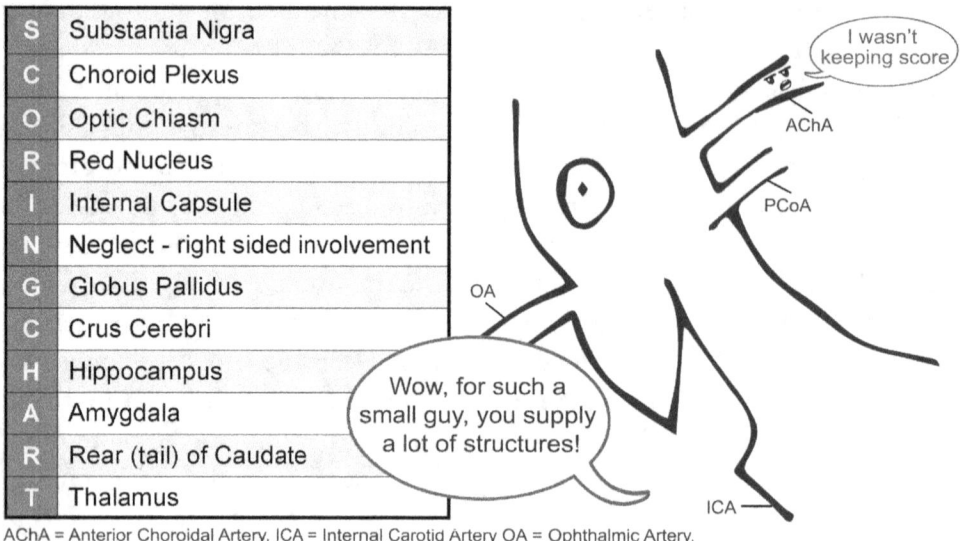

AChA = Anterior Choroidal Artery, ICA = Internal Carotid Artery, OA = Ophthalmic Artery, PCoA = Posterior Communicating Artery

TABLE 6. AChA Symptoms: **TRIPLE H POT**

H	Hemiplegia, Contralateral
H	Homonymous Hemianopia
H	Hypo-aesthesia, Contralateral
P	Posterior Limb Internal Capsule
O	Optic Chiasm and Tract
T	Thalamus

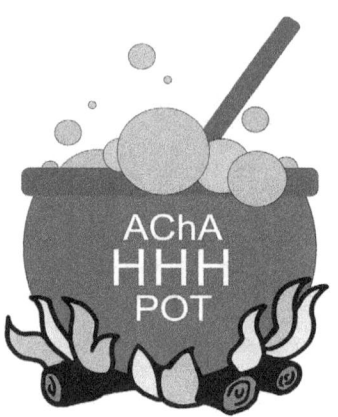

TABLE 7. Small Vessels That Can Mimic Large Vessel Occlusion (LVO): **PLAT**

P	Pontine Perforators
L	Lenticulostriates
A	Anterior Choroidal Artery (AChA)
T	Thalamic Perforator

Atherosclerotic disease affecting the ICA can cause a myriad of symptoms with involvement of branches of the supraclinoid ICA and various distributions of the MCA and ACA arteries. ICA atherosclerotic disease can lead to both embolic disease and hypoperfusion from progressive stenosis with significant reduction in intracranial perfusion. These mechanisms can cause partial or complete occlusion of the internal carotid artery itself, the ACA or the MCA (Figure 7). However, symptoms can be variable with complete ICA occlusion ranging from no symptoms (if good collaterals exist) to severe stroke involving the ACA and MCA distributions (Figure 8).

A carotid T occlusion arises from a clot that involves the distal internal carotid artery, the anterior cerebral artery medially, and the middle cerebral artery laterally. This forms a 'T' pattern (Figure 9). The consequences of these infarcts can be devastating and can involve the distal ICA, ACA, and MCA distributions. Frequently, a carotid T occlusion can produce a similar clinical picture as an MCA occlusion: contralateral hemiplegia, sensory deficits, and aphasia (if dominant hemisphere is involved). In most cases, the ACA distribution is spared from contralateral collaterals but if the ACA is involved, these clinical deficits will also be present. The consequences of carotid T occlusions can be even more devastating if there is an fPCA.

In this case, a carotid T occlusion can involve all the structures mentioned earlier in addition to structures supplied by the PCA.

FIGURE 7. Atherosclerotic and Embolic Disease of ICA

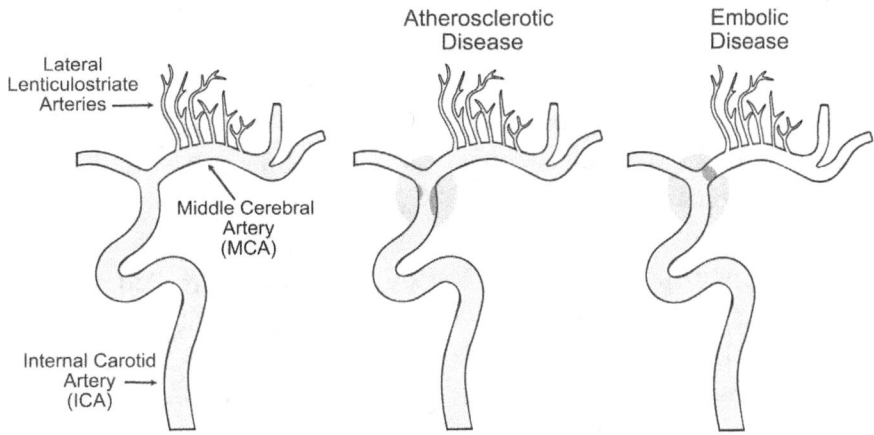

FIGURE 8. Variable Presentations of ICA Stroke

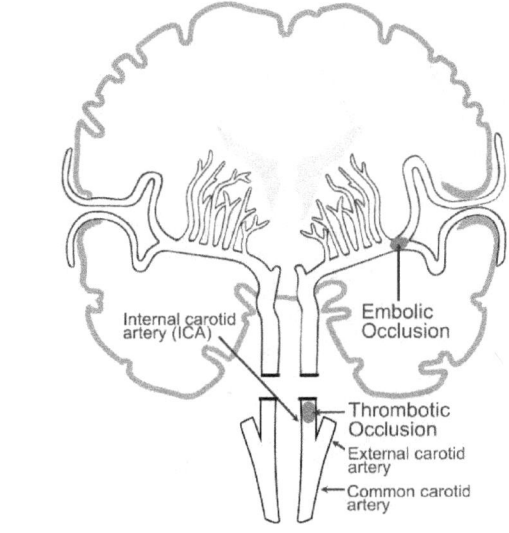

FIGURE 9. Carotid T Occlusion

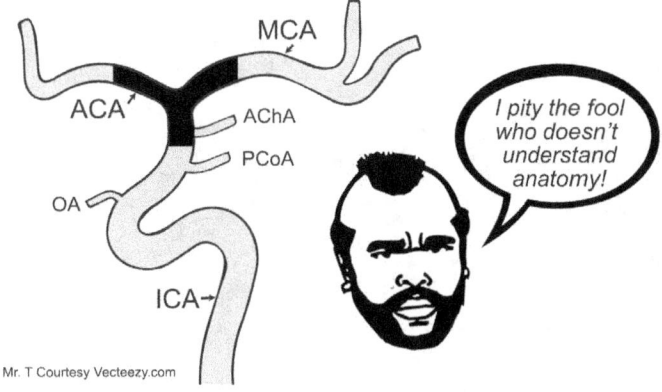

16.4 Middle Cerebral Artery (MCA) Stroke

The MCA supplies the largest portion of the cerebral hemisphere (approximately 80%) and is the most common vascular distribution affected by stroke. The MCA supplies most of the cerebral cortex, almost the entire basal ganglia, and the posterior and anterior limbs of the internal capsule. MCA stroke has clinical symptoms that are dependent on the location of the arterial occlusion, the extent of collateral circulation, the region of the brain that is affected, and the amount of tissue damage (Table 8). MCA strokes are further subdivided as either proximal, large vessel (M1 and M2) or distal, small vessel (M3 and M4) occlusions (Figure 10). Recall that the MCA distribution has an M1 segment which divides into a superior and inferior division. Both divisions have M2, M3, and M4 segments. Understanding the segmental anatomy has two very important and practical consequences. First, proximal MCA occlusions involving the M1 and M2 segments have higher National Institutes of Health Stroke Scale (NIHSS) scores and tend not to be responsive to IV TPA alone. These larger vessels are more accessible to EVT. In addition, proximal LVOs involve vessels distal to them, causing multiple regions of cortical involvement and thereby multiple, diffuse cortical symptoms (Table 8). These symptoms are dependent on the cortical regions involved and thus the arterial territory occluded. In fact, as will be discussed later, identifying multiple cortical symptoms is an ideal method to screen for LVOs. Second, distal MCA occlusions involving the M3 and M4 segments typically have lower NIHSS scores that are currently not amenable to EVT and tend to be more responsive to IV TPA (Figure 10).

TABLE 8. Cortical Regions and Associated Functions

Cortical Structure	Location	Function
Frontal Eye Fields (FEF)	Frontal Lobe	Eye Movement
Primary Motor Cortex	Frontal Lobe	Voluntary Movement
Broca's Area	Frontal Lobe	Production of Speech
Primary Sensory Cortex	Parietal Lobe	Sensation
Wernicke's Area	Temporal Lobe	Language Comprehension
Primary Visual Cortex	Occipital Lobe	Vision

FIGURE 10. The Middle Cerebral Artery (MCA) Segmental Anatomy

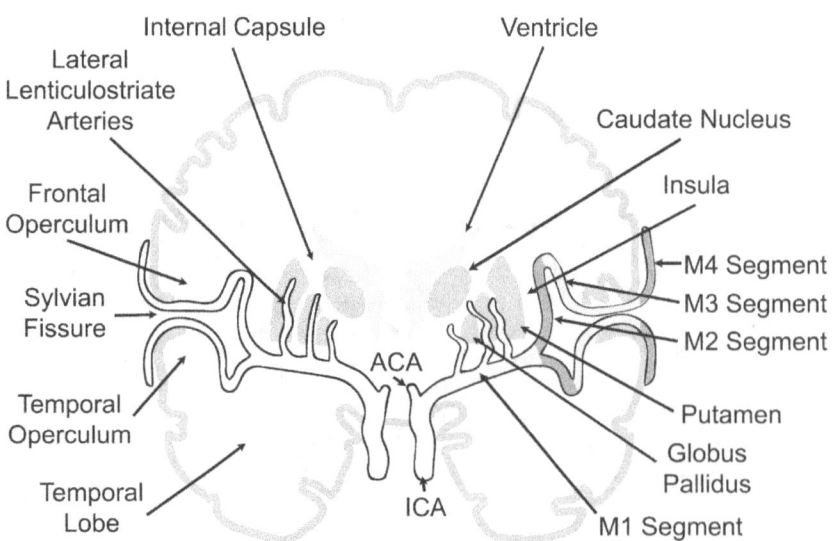

Homunculus is Latin for "little man." The motor and sensory homunculi are the two largest cortical homunculi and act as a map or representation of all the anatomic divisions of the body. The motor homunculus is a proportionate representation of the different parts of the body responsible for motor function and overlays the primary motor cortex (Figure 11). For example, the lower limb extremity motor strip is identified medially and supplied by the anterior cerebral artery (ACA) distribution whereas the upper extremity motor strip is located laterally and supplied by the middle cerebral artery (MCA) distribution (Figure 11). The sensory homunculus is a representation of the region of the brain responsible for sensation and overlays the primary sensory cortex.

Since LVO AIS involves a greater representation of the motor and sensory homunculi, these occlusions present with a more uniform and dense hemiparesis and sensory deficits (Figure 11). Distal MCA infarcts, on the other hand, usually have patchy motor and sensory deficits because of the small distribution on the motor and sensory homunculi, respectively. Small, distal vessel occlusions typically involve single regions of the cortex. There are multiple cortical vessels that branch off the superior and inferior divisions of the MCA which have corresponding syndromes associated with their arterial territory (Figure 12). Rather than reviewing each syndrome specifically associated with each one of these cortical branches, deficits associated with occlusions of the M1 segment as well as superior and inferior divisions of the MCA will be discussed. Again, the arms and face are represented by the lateral motor cortex (Figure 13).

FIGURE 11. The Motor and Sensory Homunculus

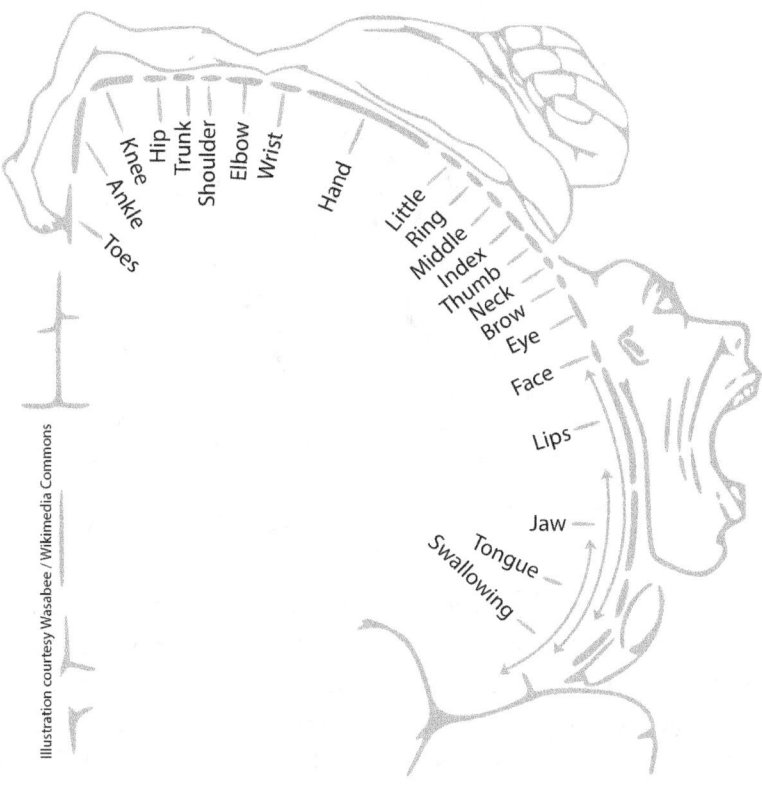

Illustration courtesy Wasabee / Wikimedia Commons

FIGURE 12. The Cortical Branches of the Middle Cerebral Artery

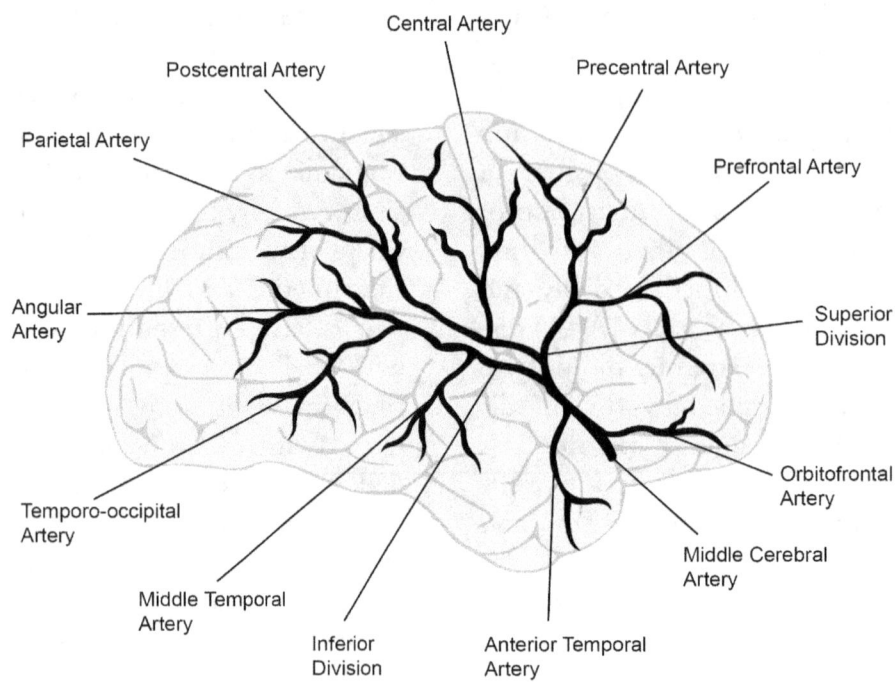

FIGURE 13. Topical Distribution of Motor Cortex

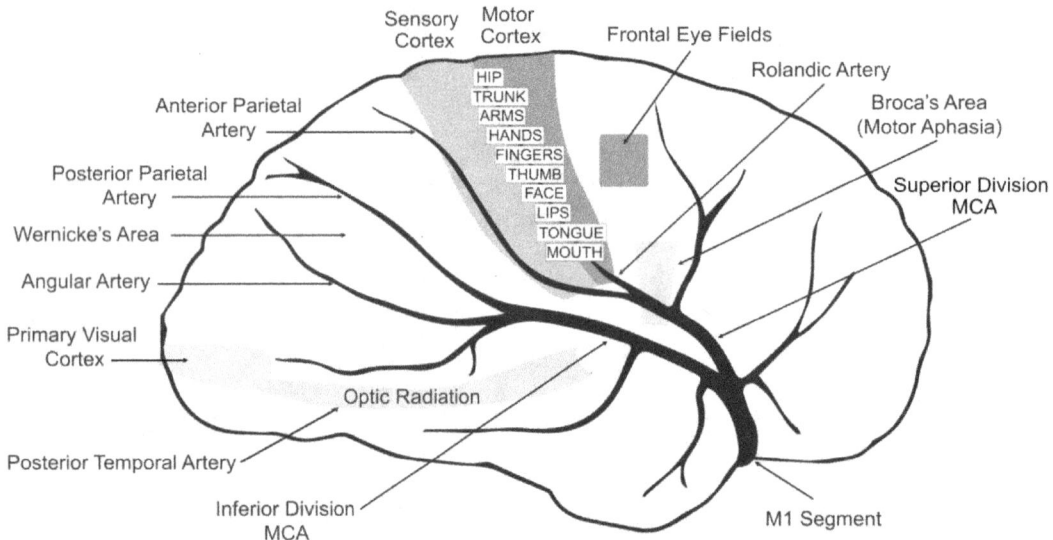

The most proximal segment of the MCA is the M1 segment (Figure 14). Arising from this segment are the lateral lenticulostriate arteries, which are end arteries that have no collateral supply. These small vessels are commonly involved in lacunar strokes symptoms that were discussed in Chapter 5 (Ischemic Stroke). Recall that chapter explained that the pathophysiology of lacunar strokes was predominantly thrombotic vascular small vessel disease. Lacunar syndromes involving lateral lenticulostriate arteries originating from the M1 segment of the MCA may affect the internal capsule (genu and posterior limb), the lentiform nucleus, putamen, internal capsule, centrum semiovale, and corona radiata (Figure 15). An easy way to remember these structures affected by lacunar infarcts (mostly involving the lateral lenticulostriate arteries in the M1 segment of the MCA) is the mnemonic 'SPLIT LIP' (Table 9).

FIGURE 14. The Middle Cerebral Artery (MCA)

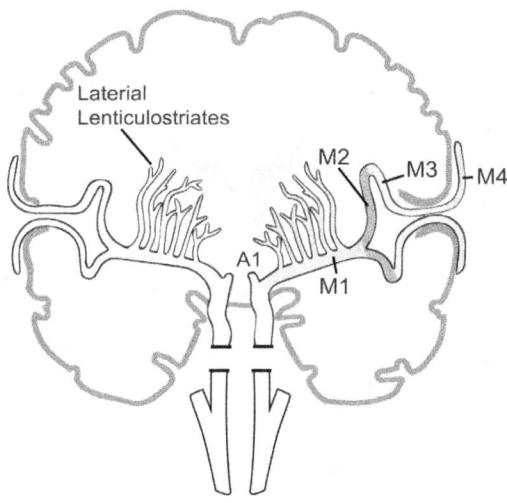

FIGURE 15. Anatomic Structures Commonly Involved in Lacunar Infarcts

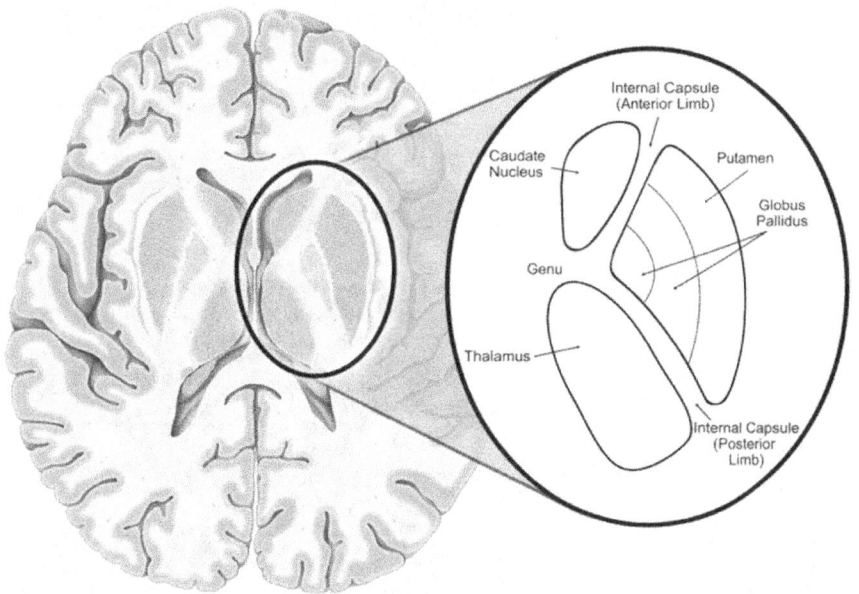

TABLE 9. Structures Involved in Lacunar Infarcts: **SPLIT LIP**

S	Semiovale, Centrum and Corona Radiata
P	Putamen
L	Lentiform Nucleus
I	Internal Capsule - Genu
T	Thalamus
L	Lenticulostriates - Most Common
I	Internal Capsule - Posterior Limb
P	Pontine Perforators

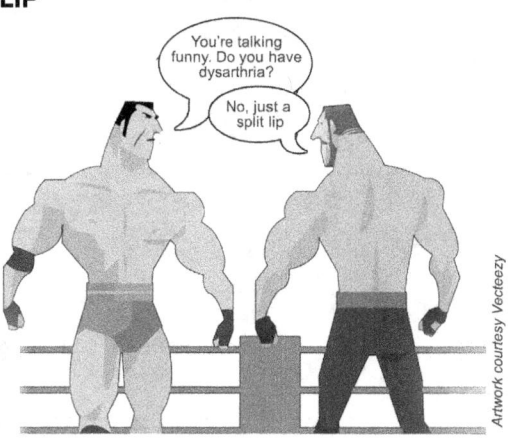

In addition to lateral lenticulostriate arteries involvement, a complete M1 occlusion also involves superior and inferior divisions of the MCA and the cortical structures supplied by them. Because this infarct involves the lateral lenticulostriate arteries and the motor fibers in the internal capsule, it results in paralysis of the face, hand, arm, and leg as well as contralateral sensory loss within the same distribution (Box 1). This stroke also causes gaze preference and head deviation toward the side of the stroke and homonymous hemianopia (Figure 16). A dominant hemisphere (typically left hemisphere) M1 occlusion will cause global aphasia. A non-dominant (typically right hemisphere) M1 occlusion will also cause left spatial neglect, cortical sensory loss, anosognosia (a person's ability to understand and perceive their illness), and amorphosynthesis (patient is unaware of somatic sensations from one side of the body; there is a loss of proprioception and spatial relationships). An easy way to remember these deficits is with the mnemonic 'SHAGS' (Table 10).

BOX 1. Motor Weakness Terminology

Term	Paralysis
Hemiplegia	Paralysis of an ipsilateral upper and lower limb
Monoplegia	Paralysis of either upper or lower limb
Paraplegia	Paralysis of both lower limbs
Quadriplegia	Paralysis of all four limbs

FIGURE 16. Middle Cerebral Artery (MCA) Segmental Syndromes

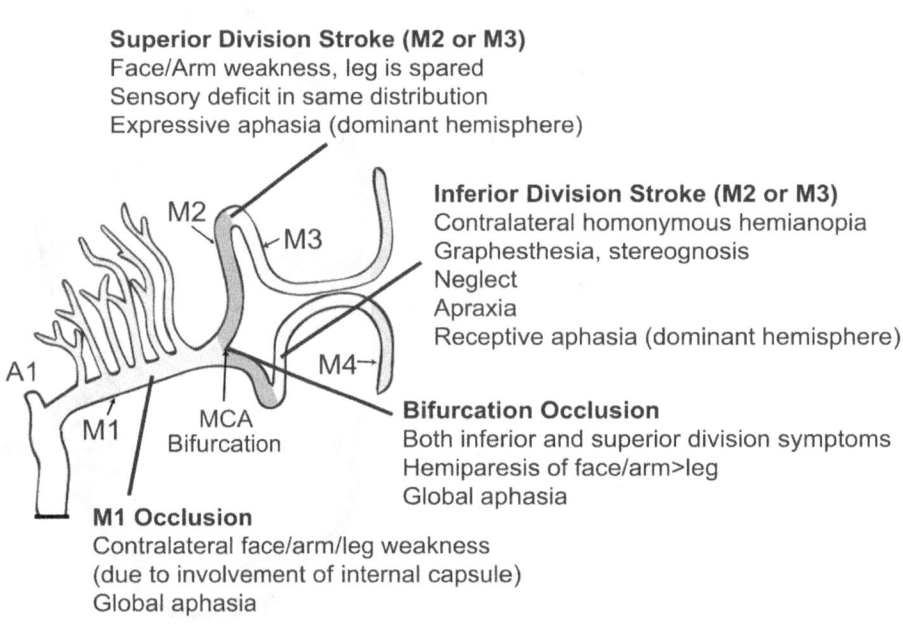

TABLE 10. M1 Occlusion Symptoms: **SHAGS**

S	Sensory loss, contralateral
H	Hemiplegia, contralateral
A	Aphasia, global (dominant)
G	Gaze preference towards infarct
S	Spatial Neglect

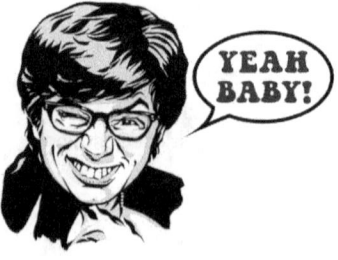

Cortical sensory loss can be evaluated by testing position sense and assessing for *stereognosis* (inability to perceive the form of an object by touch) and *graphesthesia* (the ability to recognize writing on the skin purely by touch). The inability to identify a number written on the patient's hand is termed *agraphesthesia*. The inability to identify an object in a patient's hand is termed *astereognosis*. M1 occlusion MCA infarcts can also have the unfortunate consequence of malignant MCA syndrome (rapid neurological deterioration due to mass effect from cerebral edema following large MCA territory stroke). These patients have a guarded prognosis with mortality rates as high as 80%. This is precisely why AIS patients with LVOs must be identified and treated promptly.

Stroke involving the superior division of the MCA involves the frontal convexity and the anterior parietal lobe. Like an M1 occlusion, a superior division MCA occlusion presents with contralateral hemiparesis, hemisensory loss, forced gaze and head deviation toward the infarct, and variable degrees of aphasia and neglect (Figure 18). Typically, patients present with Broca's (expressive) aphasia characterized by impairment of language expression, although comprehension generally remains intact. In distinction to an M1 occlusion, motor deficits are caused by cortical structures with sparing of the internal capsule resulting in contralateral face and arm weakness greater than the leg. Again, a superior division MCA infarct causes a dense sensorimotor deficit of the contralateral face and arm, but to a lesser extent of the leg (Figure 17). This differs from an M1 occlusion by sparing the contralateral leg and foot. Recall that the face and arm are represented more laterally on the motor strip and the leg is represented more medially (Figure 11). Sensory deficits can be profound but are usually less severe than motor deficits and present as stereoanesthesia (inability to recognize objects by touch), agraphesthesia (inability to recognize letters or numbers drawn by the examiner on skin), impaired position sense, tactile localization, and two-point discrimination deficits.

Patients still have gaze preference because the MCA also supplies the middle frontal gyrus which contains the frontal eye fields (FEF) and is responsible for initiating and tracking eye movements. (Figure 1 and Table 2). Left-sided (dominant) superior division MCA infarcts present with global aphasia (Figure 17). In the non-acute phase, symptoms will improve to Broca's or expressive aphasia and speech apraxia. This is because in the acute setting, aphasias are often global and not anatomically defined in their presentation. If the superior division of the non-dominant hemisphere (usually right hemisphere) of the MCA is affected, patients present with left spatial neglect. Typically, visual field deficits (homonymous hemianopia) are not associated with MCA superior division occlusions. Thus, symptoms do not include homonymous hemianopsia. Single cortical branch occlusion of the superior division of the MCA is the most common vascular distribution of AIS.

FIGURE 17. Superior Division Stroke

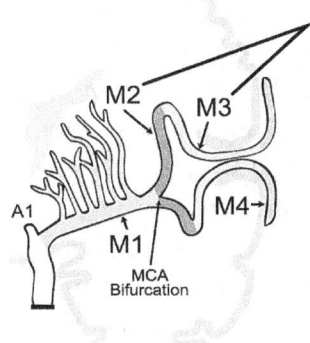

Inferior division MCA stroke is less common than superior division and involves the lateral temporal and inferior parietal lobes, typically sparing the motor or sensory cortex (Figure 18). Therefore, inferior division MCA stroke patients do not have hemiparesis, sensory deficits, or gaze preference. The lack of motor and sensory symptoms can make inferior division MCA strokes difficult to diagnose. Contralateral, homonymous hemianopia may result from vascular compromise to the optic radiations. However, language and behavioral deficits are the most reliable findings. If the inferior division of the left MCA (dominant hemisphere) is affected, patients present with Wernicke's or receptive aphasia. If the inferior division of the right (non-dominant hemisphere) MCA is affected, patients can have behavioral abnormalities such as confusion and delirium, as well as mild left visuospatial neglect or inattention (Figure 18). Involvement of the non-dominant hemisphere can result in acute confusional states. A receptive aphasia with a visual field cut localizes the stroke to the inferior division of the MCA and strengthens this diagnosis.

16.5 Anterior Cerebral Artery (ACA) Stroke

Stroke involving the anterior cerebral artery (ACA) is less common than MCA infarcts due to preferential flow from the ICA into the MCA. The cortical branches of the ACA supply three quarters of the medial surface of the frontal lobe and its deeper penetrating branches supply the anterior limb of the internal capsule, the caudate nucleus, and the anterior portion of the globus pallidus. Just like stroke affecting the MCA, the major determinants of ACA stroke symptoms are the proximity of the occlusion, collateral circulation, the region of the brain affected, and the degree of tissue damage. Due to the medial representation of the leg on both the motor and sensory homunculus, ACA infarcts typically result in contralateral leg weakness with sparing of the arm and face (Figure 11). Note, however, that leg weakness is not unique to ACA stroke and can also present with MCA stroke that involves the internal capsule. Left-sided ACA infarcts can cause contralateral leg weakness with sparing of the arm and face, transient akinetic mutism (abulia), and cortical motor aphasia. Abulia is the inability to act decisively or the absence of willpower. Right-sided ACA infarcts can cause acute confusion, motor hemineglect, transient akinetic mutism (abulia), and contralateral hemiparesis. Bilateral ACA infarcts can result in prolonged akinetic mutism, urinary incontinence, and paraplegia. Recall that bilateral ACA infarcts can result when one ACA trunk supplies both hemispheres (azygos ACA variant). In this situation when the medial portions of both cerebral hemispheres are supplied by a single vessel, paraplegia, incontinence, abulia (abnormal lack of ability to act or to make decisions), and frontal lobe personality changes result.

16.6 Summary

The purpose of this chapter was to incorporate prior discussions concerning neuroanatomy and cerebrovascular anatomy with anterior circulation ischemic stroke. The arterial anatomy of the anterior circulation is summarized in Figure 19. Deficits produced by this territory are summarized in Table 11. The intent of this book is to have these chapters progressively build upon each other to reinforce key concepts in the diagnosis and treatment of stroke. In a similar manner, the next chapter will attempt to do the same with the discussion of transient ischemic attack (TIA).

Abbreviations list

ACA, anterior cerebral artery; AChA, anterior choroidal artery; AIS, acute ischemic stroke; COW, Circle of Willis; EVT, endovascular therapy; FEF, frontal eye field; fPCA, fetal origin of the posterior cerebral artery; ICA, internal carotid artery; LVO, large vessel occlusion; MCA, middle cerebral artery; NIHSS, National Institutes of Health Stroke Scale; OA, ophthalmic artery; PCA, posterior cerebral artery; PCoA, posterior communicating artery; TIA, transient ischemic attack.

FIGURE 18. Inferior Division Stroke

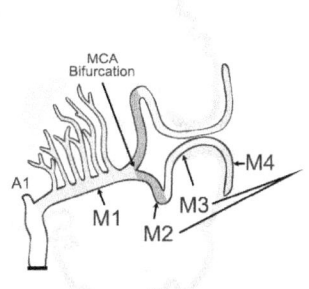

Inferior Division MCA Stroke:
Left side = Wernicke's aphasia
Right side = Behavioral Changes

Inferior Division Stroke (M2 or M3)
Contralateral homonymous hemianopia
Receptive aphasia (dominant hemisphere)
Behavioral changes (nondominant hemisphere)

FIGURE 19. Arterial Territory of the Anterior Circulation

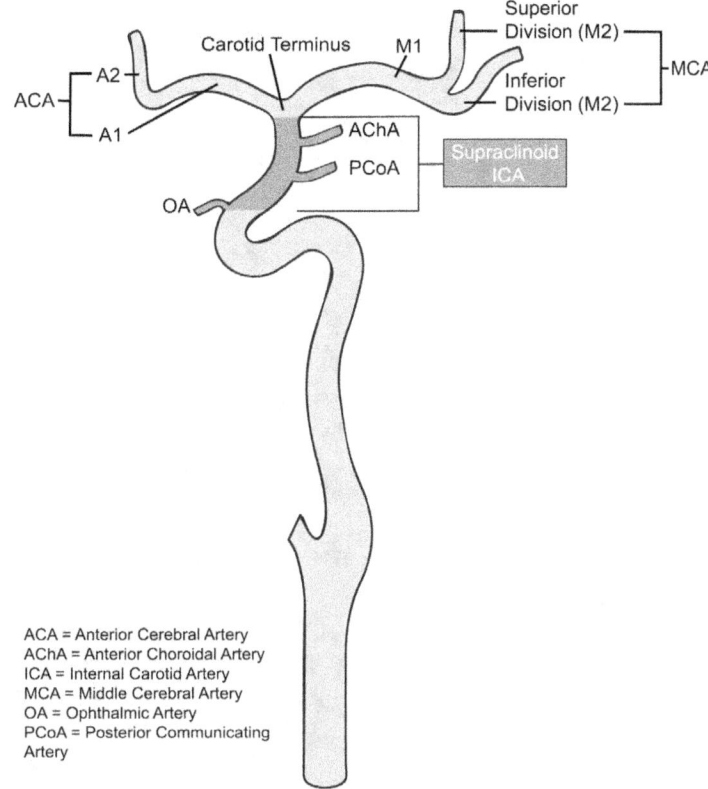

ACA = Anterior Cerebral Artery
AChA = Anterior Choroidal Artery
ICA = Internal Carotid Artery
MCA = Middle Cerebral Artery
OA = Ophthalmic Artery
PCoA = Posterior Communicating Artery

TABLE 11. Anterior Circulation Localization and Deficits

Artery	Lobe	Sign
Right ACA	Frontal, parietal	Left leg weakness
Right MCA: Superior division	Frontal, parietal	Left arm/face weakness/ sensation loss, hemineglect, right gaze preference
Right MCA: Inferior division	Temporal, parietal	Profound hemineglect, left homonymous hemianopia
Left ACA	Frontal, parietal	Right leg weakness
Left MCA: Superior division	Frontal, parietal	Right face/arm weakness/ sensation loss, Broca's aphasia
Left MCA: Inferior division	Temporal, parietal	Wernicke's aphasia, right homonymous hemianopia

References

1. Ojemann RG, Crowell RM. (1988). Surgical Management of Cerebrovascular Disease. 2nd ed. Baltimore: Williams and Wilkins, Internal carotid artery aneurysms, 179–98.
2. Archer CR, Silbert S. (1978). Infundibula may be clinically significant. Neuroradiology, 15, 247-51.
3. Marshman LA, Ward PJ, Walter PH, Dossetor RS. (1998). The progression of an infundibulum to aneurysm formation and rupture: case report and literature review. Neurosurgery, Dec, 43(6), 1445–49.
4. Ois A, Cuadrado-Godia E, Solano A, et al. (2009). Acute ischemic stroke in anterior choroidal artery territory. J Neurol Sci, 281, 80.

Transient Ischemic Attack (TIA)

17.1 Introduction

Every year, approximately 200,000 to 500,000 transient ischemic attacks (TIAs) are diagnosed in the United States.[1] Despite these high figures, even more people with TIA-like symptoms never seek medical attention.[2] TIAs can be associated with a high risk of recurrent stroke in approximately 10%-20% of patients (most occurring within 48 hours).[3-6] The risk of recurrent stroke makes TIAs a medical emergency which requires immediate diagnosis and treatment. The goals of TIA management are to determine which patients are at high risk of recurrent stroke and prevent it. The purpose of this chapter is to explain why an outdated definition of TIAs based on arbitrary time points is not very helpful. Additionally, it will review the importance of a more helpful, image-based TIA definition.

17.2 TIA Definition

A transient ischemic attack (TIA) results from the same pathophysiologic mechanism(s) as an acute ischemic stroke (AIS) (Figure 1). Both can result from an occluded blood vessel that supplies oxygen to the brain. In 1990, The National Institute of Neurological Disorders and Stroke Report defined TIAs as "brief episodes of focal loss of brain function of *less than 24-hour duration*, thought to be due to ischemia that can usually be localized to that portion of the brain supplied by one vascular system."[7] This *older*, time-based definition and other traditional definitions like it assume that rapid resolution of TIA symptoms indicates a transient (non-permanent) ischemic insult. That is, these traditional definitions of TIAs correlate rapidly resolving symptoms with a non-permanent ischemic insult of brain tissue, i.e. symptoms lasting less than 24 hours.[8] For this reason, TIAs have been dangerously mislabeled as "mini strokes." This is a misleading and critically flawed label for several reasons.

First, the 24-hour time point definition is arbitrary and unrelated to any underlying pathophysiologic mechanism. Furthermore, a significant number of patients who are incorrectly diagnosed with TIAs have ischemic stroke. An arbitrary 24-hour time point does not have the ability to discriminate TIA from AIS.

FIGURE 1. Common Pathophysiology of Ischemic Disease

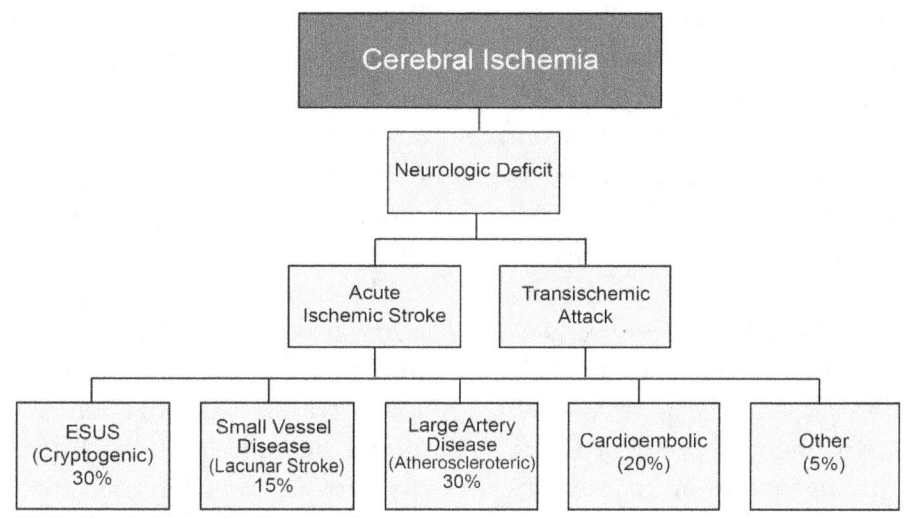

ESUS - Embolic Stroke of Undetermined Source

In fact, MRI-documented tissue infarction has been identified in a significant number of patients incorrectly diagnosed with rapidly resolving (< one hour) "TIAs." Additionally, recurrent stroke rate is higher in patients with rapid recovery than those with slower recovery. TIA symptom resolution time has no correlation to brain tissue infarction and, therefore, cannot be used to assess the severity of either TIA or AIS.

17.3 TIA and Neuroimaging

Advances in neuroimaging have dramatically changed our understanding of TIAs. These advances have led to a *newer* tissue-based definition of TIAs that is endorsed by the American Heart Association, the American Stroke Council, and the American Academy of Neurology.[9] TIAs are now described as a transient episode of neurologic dysfunction caused by focal brain, spinal cord, or retinal ischemia, *without evidence of acute infarction*. This newer definition of TIAs tremendously assists in distinguishing a TIA from an AIS because MRI can be utilized to recognize tiny DWI-positive lesions as AIS, *regardless of whether symptoms are transient and regardless of the duration*. MRI DWI can discern AIS and enables better detection of smaller lesions that are representative of AIS and not TIA.

How does this new definition affect our current work-up of stroke? Most stroke centers evaluate AIS with CT imaging, but in this regard, CT has limited sensitivity and is less preferred. However, MRI imaging is rarely the first line of imaging in TIA patients.[10] Hospital systems must endorse rapid access to MRI to enhance the diagnostic evaluation of TIA. It is important to understand that even tiny signal abnormalities identified by MRI DWI represent stroke and not TIAs.[11]

What exactly is MRI DWI data demonstrating? First, patients with neurologic deficits that resolved in less than 24 hours but also have DWI positive lesions on MRI have AIS, and are at the highest risk of in-hospital recurrent stroke. In many ways, a TIA involving the brain is what unstable angina is to the heart. In both conditions, unstable, fluctuating tissue perfusion threatens brain and cardiac tissue viability, respectively. At this point, threatened brain tissue can either improve (no stroke) or progress into a core infarct (AIS). MRI DWI can differentiate TIAs (no imaging findings) from actual AIS (DWI positive imaging).

17.4 TIA and Antiplatelet Therapy

MRI DWI positive lesions are considered ischemic stroke regardless of symptom duration and are at a higher risk for recurrent stroke. In the absence of cardioembolic events, this patient population should receive antithrombotic therapy for secondary stroke prevention. But which antiplatelet regimen should be implemented? The **Clopidogrel in High-risk patients with Acute Non-disabling Cerebrovascular Events (CHANCE) Trial** randomized 5,170 patients with either minor stroke or high risk TIAs within 24 hours of symptom onset, comparing the combination of aspirin and clopidogrel versus aspirin alone.[12] Specifically, clopidogrel (300 mg loading dose followed by 75 mg daily for 90 days) plus aspirin (75 mg once daily for the initial 21 days) versus aspirin monotherapy (75 mg daily for 90 days) demonstrated patients receiving dual antiplatelet therapy had a lower risk of recurrent stroke (primary endpoint) within 90 days compared to aspirin monotherapy (8.2% versus 11.7%), with no increase in intracranial hemorrhage or other major bleeding events (Figure 2).

The CHANCE Trial demonstrates a paradigm shift towards early antiplatelet therapy in AIS management. While other studies have investigated the role of antiplatelet therapy for secondary stroke prevention, the CHANCE Trial specifically focused on the early, high-risk period after the initial stroke. Again, it is within this time point (within 48 hours) when the risk of recurrent stroke is at its greatest. To this end, while the trial required randomization within 24 hours after initial stroke, almost half of the patients were enrolled within 12 hours and treated shortly thereafter. The CHANCE Trial demonstrated secondary stroke prevention was best achieved with early combination antiplatelet therapy, which reduced this risk by 32% when compared with aspirin alone. This equates to a number needed to treat (NNT) of 29 patients to prevent one recurrent stroke. Note that antiplatelet treatment cannot be initiated within 24 hours of IV TPA administration, and no patients enrolled in the CHANCE Trial received IV TPA.

FIGURE 2. Dual Antiplatelet Therapy and Recurrent Stroke Risk Reduction

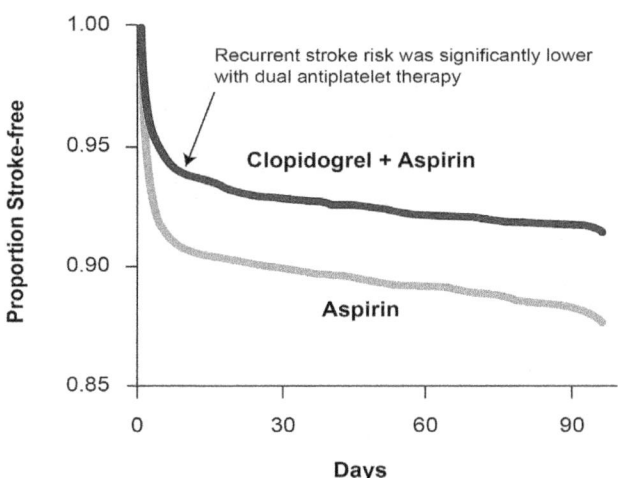

However, several additional points must be considered and these can be recalled by the mnemonic 'CAT' (Table 1). First, prior to initiating antithrombotic therapy, cardioembolic mechanisms must be excluded. If cardioembolic mechanisms exist, anticoagulation should be considered. In the absence of cardioembolic mechanisms, dual antiplatelet therapy should not be initiated within 24 hours of IV TPA administration. Despite the results from the CHANCE Trial, a recent meta-analysis comparing long-term clopidogrel monotherapy to dual antiplatelet therapy (aspirin plus clopidogrel) demonstrated comparable risk reductions for recurrent stroke, but a higher risk of intracranial hemorrhage was associated with dual antiplatelet therapy.[13]

TABLE 1. Antiplatelet Therapy for Recurrent Stroke Prevention: **CAT**

C	Cardioembolic Etiology Must be Excluded
A	Aspirin and Clopidogrel Therapy Initiated Early
T	TPA Precludes Treatment for 24 Hours After its Administration

These varied results can be due to differences between US and Chinese patients with the latter having a larger proportion of untreated, modifiable risk factors (such as diabetes and hypertension) and a higher incidence of large vessel atherosclerotic disease. The authors of the CHANCE Trial themselves state, "Our findings may not apply to other populations of patients with ischemic events." To address this issue, the NIH-sponsored Platelet-Oriented Inhibition in New TIA and Minor Ischemic Stroke (POINT Trial) is enrolling patients to investigate dual antiplatelet therapy in the United States. While the POINT Trial will have a similar design, the loading dose of clopidogrel will be 600 mg instead of 300 mg as used in the CHANCE Trial.

It is reasonable for practitioners unable to enroll patients in the POINT Trial to treat either minor AIS or high-risk TIA patients with a short period of dual antiplatelet therapy followed by clopidogrel alone. Since 75 mg is the low-dose form of aspirin in the United States, the dual antiplatelet protocol consists of a loading dose of 300 mg of clopidogrel (or 600 mg if enrolled in the POINT Trial) and 75 mg daily thereafter, plus aspirin for the first 21 days in the absence of cardioembolic etiology (Box 1). These recommendations have been adopted by the new 2018 AHA/ASA stroke guidelines which state: "In patients presenting with minor stroke, treatment for 21 days with dual antiplatelet therapy (aspirin and clopidogrel) begun within 24 hours can be beneficial for early secondary stroke prevention for a period of up to 90 days from symptom onset."[14]

BOX 1. Ischemic Dual Antiplatelet Protocol

Drug	Loading Dose	Maintenance Dose
Clopidrogel*	300mg	75mg Daily After Loading Dose
Aspirin*	81mg	81mg Daily After Loading Dose

* Must exclude cardioembolic etiology and cannot be administered within 24 hrs of IV TPA bolus

17.5 TIA Diagnosis and Treatment

MRI DWI is required to effectively diagnose AIS and exclude TIA after obtaining a non-contrast brain CT. Patients whose deficits resolve in less than 24 hours but have DWI-positive lesions on MRI have AIS and are at the highest risk of in-hospital recurrent stroke. However, one can tremendously reduce the incidence of subsequent stroke to 0.4% by simply applying the newer tissue-based definition (TIA with no DWI-confirmed infarction). MRI imaging can distinguish TIAs (no imaging findings) from ischemic stroke (positive DWI lesions) regardless of symptom duration. MRI DWI-positive lesions are considered ischemic stroke regardless of symptom duration and these patients are at a higher risk for recurrent stroke. This allows the distinction between high-risk ischemic stroke (DWI-positive imaging) and low-risk TIA (no imaging findings) groups, with high-risk patients benefiting from specialized stroke centers and low-risk patients not requiring hospitalization (Figure 3). Note that the ischemic stroke (DWI-positive) pathway leads to admission and does not recommend dual antiplatelet therapy because one cannot assume the diagnosis of a minor stroke. The treatment of minor stroke is discussed in Chapter 28.

The 2018 AHA/ASA guidelines state: "In some patients with AIS, the use of MRI might be considered to provide additional information for initial diagnosis or to plan subsequent treatment, although the fact on outcome is uncertain."[14] The protocol certainly satisfies these criteria because MRI determines whether or not the patient has a TIA or AIS, and whether or not they are at an increased risk for recurrent stroke (DWI-positive MRI). The 2018 AHA/ASA evidence committee considered what additional information diagnostic imaging provided and whether or not this additional information led to a change in treatment. The TIA protocol above includes MRI and satisfies these conditions because it does lead to a change in treatment, whether the patient is DWI MRI-negative (TIA) or DWI MRI-positive (AIS). Therefore, the aforementioned protocol (which includes MRI) changes treatment and leads to better clinical outcome.

FIGURE 3. Transient Ischemic Attack (TIA) Diagnostic and Treatment Protocol

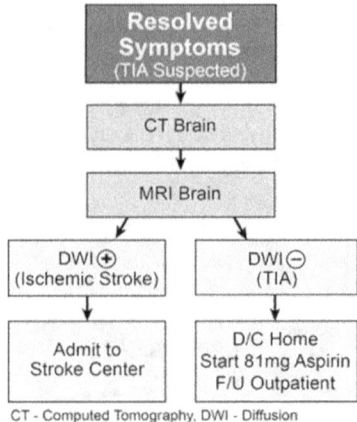

CT - Computed Tomography, DWI - Diffusion Weighted Imaging, D/C - Discharge, F/U - Follow-up MRI - Magnetic Resonance Imaging, TIA - Transient Ischemic Attack

17.6 Summary

The original temporal (<24 hours) definition of TIA was arbitrary in nature and lacked specific pathophysiologic meaning. Severe limitations in this definition led to an image-guided, tissue-based definition of TIA. These advances in neuroimaging enable the early identification of brain tissue ischemic injury. This chapter emphasized the advantages of the newer tissue-based definition of TIAs (imaging-based) and the disadvantages of the arbitrary, time-based concept of TIAs. Advances in neuroimaging have substantially improved our ability to understand and manage TIAs. TIAs, as defined by newer, tissue-based criteria, are associated with a much lower risk of subsequent stroke (0.4%). However, neuroimaging signs (DWI-positive MRI) of AIS can have recurrent stroke risk that can be 20 times higher than the risk of TIA associated with normal imaging. To recall these concepts, remember the mnemonic 'TIA' (Table 2).

TABLE 2. Transient Ischemic Attack: **TIA**

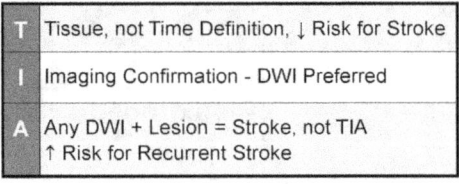

Abbreviations list

AIS, acute ischemic stroke; DWI, diffusion weighted imaging; MRI, magnetic resonance imaging; NNT, number needed to treat; TIA, transient ischemic attack.

References

1. Heart disease and stroke statistics--2010 update: a report from the American Heart Association.
2. Johnston SC, Fayad PB, Gorelick PB, Hanley DF, Shwayder P, van Husen D, Weiskopf T. (2003). Prevalence and knowledge of transient ischemic attack among US adults. *Neurology*, May 13, 60(9), 1429-34.
3. Kleindorfer D, Panagos P, Pancioli A, et al. (2005). Incidence and short-term prognosis of transient ischemic attack in a population-based study. *Stroke*, 36, 720-23.
4. Coull AJ, Lovett JK, Rothwell PM. (2004). Population based study of early risk of stroke after transient ischaemic attack or minor stroke: implications for public education and organisation of services. *BMJ*, 328, 326.
5. Johnston SC, Gress DR, Browner WS, Sidney S. (2000). Short-term prognosis after emergency department diagnosis of TIA. *JAMA*, 284, 2901-06.
6. Lovett JK, Coull AJ, Rothwell PM. (2004). Early risk of recurrence by subtype of ischemic stroke in population-based incidence studies. *Neurology*, 62, 569-73.
7. National Institute of Neurological Disorders and Stroke. (1990). Special report from the National Institute of Neurological Disorders and Stroke: classification of cerebrovascular diseases, III. *Stroke*, 21, 637–76.
8. Special report from the National Institute of Neurological Disorders and Stroke. (1990). Classification of cerebrovascular diseases III. *Stroke*, Apr, 21(4), 637-76.
9. Easton JD, Saver JL, Albers GW, Alberts MJ, Chaturvedi S, Feldmann E, Hatsukam Tsi, Higashida RT, Claiborne Johnston S, Kidwell CS, Lutsep HL, Miller E, and Sacco RL. (2009). Definition and Evaluation of Transient Ischemic Attack. *Stroke*, 40, 2276-93.
10. Edlow JA, Kim S, Pelletier AJ, Camargo CA Jr. (2006). National study on emergency department visits for transient ischemic attack, 1992-2001. *Acad Emerg Med*, Jun, 13(6), 666-72.
11. Ay H, Koroshetz WJ, Benner T, et al. (2005). Transient ischemic attack with infarction: a unique syndrome? *Ann Neurol*, 57, 679–86.
12. Wang Y, Wang Y, Zhao X, Liu L, Wang D, Wang C, et al. (2013). Clopidogrel with aspirin in acute minor stroke or transient ischemic attack. *N Engl J Med*, 369, 11–19.
13. Lee M, Saver JL, Hong KS, Rao NM, Wu YL, Ovbiagele B. (2013). Risk-benefit profile of long-term dual- versus single- antiplatelet therapy among patients with ischemic stroke: a systematic review and meta-analysis. *Ann Intern Med*, 159, 463–70.
14. Powers WJ, Rabinstein AA, Ackerson T, Adeoye OM, Bambakidis NC, Becker K, Biller J, Brown M, Demaerschalk BM, Hoh B, et al. (2018) 2018 Guidelines for the Early Management of Patients With Acute Ischemic Stroke: A Guideline for Healthcare Professionals From the American Heart Association/American Stroke Association. *Stroke*, Jan 24, Epub 2018.

Chapter 18

Platelets, Stents, and Stroke

18.1 Introduction

Platelets, stents, and stroke may seem to be unrelated topics but they are all relevant to microembolic disease. This disease process is reduced by carotid stenting which demonstrates superiority to medical management. This disease process also has a higher rate of occurrence with intracranial stenting, yielding the current aggressive medical management protocol for the treatment of intracranial stenosis. Furthermore, microembolic disease is also implicated in secondary stroke for which antiplatelet therapy is advocated.

18.2 Carotid Endarterectomy (CEA)

Extracranial carotid stenosis has been implicated in the pathophysiology of ischemic stroke for almost 70 years and is responsible for nearly 20% of all ischemic stroke.[1] Since that time, carotid endarterectomy (CEA) has shown superiority to *earlier* medical therapy (aspirin) for stroke prevention.[2] The *North American Symptomatic Carotid Endarterectomy Trial (NASCET)* examined CEA versus medical therapy in patients with *symptomatic* carotid stenosis and found a two-year ipsilateral stroke risk of 26% in the medical arm versus 9% in the surgical arm for patients with severe (> 70%) symptomatic stenosis.[3] Note that during the NASCET Trial, medical therapy consisted of only aspirin. This point will be addressed later in this chapter. Other studies also confirmed the benefits of surgery compared to earlier (aspirin only) medical therapy. For example, the *European Carotid Surgery (ECS) Trial* demonstrated CEA reduced the risk of disabling stroke and mortality in patients with carotid stenosis > 70%.

18.3 Asymptomatic Carotid Stenosis

For patients with *asymptomatic* carotid stenosis, one must determine if revascularization is required, and if so, which type of revascularization should be performed. In this regard, two large randomized trials comparing carotid endarterectomy to medical therapy for stroke prevention support the use of CEA in asymptomatic carotid stenosis patients. First, the *Asymptomatic Carotid Atherosclerosis Study (ACAS)* demonstrated that patients with > 60% angiographic carotid stenosis had only a 5.1% five-year surgical risk of ipsilateral stroke, perioperative stroke, or death versus 11% with medical therapy. Second, the *Asymptomatic Carotid Surgery Trial (ACST)* demonstrated that patients with asymptomatic significant carotid stenosis (≥60%) had a 6.4% five-year surgical risk of perioperative stroke, myocardial infarction (MI), death, or non-operative stroke compared to 11.8% with medical therapy. A 10-year follow-up study also demonstrated stroke risk at 10.8% in the surgical (CEA) arm versus 16.9% in the medical arm.

18.4 Carotid Stenting

In the last 20 years, studies have demonstrated safety, feasibility, and equivalency of carotid artery stenting (CAS) compared to CEA. CAS is accepted as a valid alternative to CEA for appropriate patients.[4] The *Carotid Revascularization Endarterectomy versus Stenting Trial (CREST)* was a randomized trial consisting of both symptomatic and asymptomatic carotid stenosis patients which compared CAS to CEA. *Asymptomatic* patients required either a > 60% angiographic stenosis or > 70% ultrasonographic stenosis. Primary outcomes included periprocedural stroke, death, or MI and ipsilateral stroke within the four-year follow-up. Carotid stenting and angioplasty had a 7.2% risk and CEA had a 6.8% risk, which were not significantly different. Perioperative strokes were more common with CAS whereas MI was more prevalent following CEA. Younger patients (<70 y.o.) had better outcomes with CAS and older patients (>70 y.o.) had better outcomes with CEA. While CREST demonstrated no significant difference between CAS and CEA for the treatment of *asymptomatic* carotid stenosis, it was insufficiently powered to determine equivalency of the two procedures in *symptomatic* carotid stenosis patients. After 10 years of follow-up, CREST showed no difference in the rate of stroke, death, MI, or post-procedural ipsilateral stroke between CAS and CEA for asymptomatic patients of average surgical risk.[5]

The CREST results were supported by the *ACT-1 (Asymptomatic Carotid Trial)*, another trial which showed no difference between CAS and CEA for death, stroke, or MI within 30 days of the procedure or ipsilateral stroke within one year in patients < 80 y.o. with *asymptomatic* carotid stenosis >70%.[6] The cumulative five-year rate of stroke-free survival was 93.1% for CAS patients and 94.7% for CEA patients. This study evaluated patients who were at a *standard* risk for surgical complications. The *SAPPHIRE (Stenting and Angioplasty with Protection in Patients at High-Risk for Endarterectomy) Trial* compared CAS versus CEA in patients at *high* surgical risk based on anatomical characteristics or coexisting conditions. This study demonstrated no difference in one-year stroke, death, and MI in *symptomatic* patients but found CAS had a better one-year outcome in *asymptomatic* patients compared to CEA.[7] *Thus, CAS is preferred over CEA in the treatment of high surgical risk, asymptomatic patients*. The current American Heart and Stroke Association guidelines recommend CAS in average surgical risk *symptomatic* patients who have an anticipated risk of periprocedural stroke or mortality of < 6%. CAS was preferred for anatomically unfavorable cases (high cervical lesion, restenosis, or radiation therapy). CAS may also be considered in asymptomatic patients with a ≥70% stenosis "if the risk of perioperative stroke, MI and death is low."[8] However, reimbursement for CAS is limited to patients who have > 70% stenosis and considered to be at high surgical risk or are enrolled in an FDA-sanctioned clinical trial.[9]

Periprocedural thromboembolic events are the major risks associated with CAS and other neurologic stent-related procedures. For example, CREST identified age determinant differences between CAS and CEA. CAS had a small benefit for patients younger than 70. Conversely in patients over 70 years, a small benefit was found in favor of surgery. This is theorized to be caused by increased thromboembolic events associated with age-related vascular disease. Thromboembolic theory is also supported by antiplatelet therapy. For example, a recently published study determined clopidogrel resistance was a significant risk factor for CAS-related post-procedural cerebral ischemic events.[10] For these reasons, dual antiplatelet therapy in combination with heparin is recommended to reduce CAS-related periprocedural and post-procedural thromboembolic events.

Despite these recommendations, clinicians should always consider each patient individually. While some patients are better candidates for CEA (i.e., those with difficult vasculature, heavily calcified stenoses, soft plaque or high plaque burden) and some are better candidates for CAS (i.e., high surgical risk patients, stable plaque, not heavily calcified stenoses), most patients can be treated with either procedure. CAS is increasing in frequency but always consider the following: Are there anatomic or technical features that would prolong procedure time and favor CEA over CAS? Are there anatomical constraints that would impede the delivery of a distal embolic protection device? Other considerations such as vascular access and chronic renal failure should also be kept in mind.

18.5 Vertebrobasilar Atherosclerotic Disease

The management of vertebrobasilar atherosclerotic disease has no specific indications for invasive treatment as data from randomized controlled trials is virtually nonexistent. A non-randomized single center perspective study from the Borgess Medical Center investigated 114 patients who underwent ostial stenting for symptomatic vertebral stenosis of > 50%.[11] This study found a 2% stroke recurrence rate at one year and a 25% restenosis rate of > 50%. A systematic review on stenting of the extracranial vertebral artery published the same year found a 1.1% 30-day periprocedural stroke rate, as well as a 2-year in-stent stenosis rate of 11% for drug-eluting stents and 30% for bare-metal stents.[12] The *Stenting of SYmptomatic atherosclerotic Lesions in the Vertebral or Intracranial Arteries (SSYLVIA) Trial* demonstrated a 30-day perioperative stroke rate of 6.6% for intracranial stenting.[13] It also reported a 35% restenosis rate at six months, with almost one third of patients being symptomatic.

18.6 The SAMMPRIS Trial

Intracranial angioplasty with stenting plus aggressive medical management (AMM) was compared to AMM by itself in the *Stenting vs. Aggressive Medical Management for Preventing Recurrent Stroke in Intracranial Stenosis (SAMMPRIS) Trial* (Box 1).[14] AMM included dual antiplatelet therapy (aspirin plus clopidogrel) for 90 days, statins for a target LDL ≤ 70 mg/dL, and blood pressure management. Patients randomized to percutaneous angioplasty and stenting had a 14.7% rate of stroke and death at 30 days compared to the AMM arm which was 5.8%. For this reason, the trial was prematurely ended due to the higher risk of the percutaneous angioplasty and stenting group.

I still encounter this question from referring physicians: "I know the SAMMPRIS Trial says not to stent but can you still stent that intracranial stenosis?" And to them I respond, "Don't be an Ass Hat." Actually, based on data from the SAMMPRIS Trial, the FDA has revised the use of the Wingspan® stent in August 2012. Currently, it has limited application to patients aged between 22 and 80 who have experienced two or more strokes despite aggressive medical management. Additionally, the most recent stroke must have occurred more than 7 days prior to the procedure. Patients must also have a 70-99% intracranial stenosis related to the recurrent stroke(s) and a modified Rankin score of 3 or less prior to Wingspan® treatment. A simple mnemonic to remember these criteria is 'ASS HAT' (Table 1).

BOX 1. SAMMPRIS and Aggressive Medical Management (AMM)

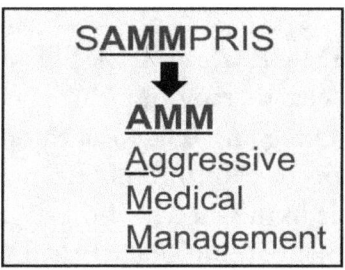

Interestingly, the SAMMPRIS Trial demonstrated no differences in stroke distal to the arterial territory treated beyond the initial 30 days and up to a median of 32.4 months between the two groups.[15] Only 13% of patients in the SAMMPRIS Trial had vertebrobasilar stenosis and most thromboembolic complications occurred due to basilar artery paramedian branch occlusions.[16] Thus, the findings of this trial predominantly apply to angioplasty and stenting of the intracranial anterior circulation. The SAMMPRIS Trial demonstrated that periprocedural thromboembolic events are the major risk associated with intracranial stenting.

TABLE 1. Wingspan® Criteria: **ASS HAT**

A	Age 22 - 80
S	Strokes - Two or More Despite Aggressive Medical Management
S	Seven - Most Recent Stroke Within Seven Days Prior to Treatment
H	Have 70% - 99% Intracranial Stenosis Related to Recurrent Strokes
A	Aggressive Medical Management Failure
T	Treatment - mRS ≤ 3 Prior to Treatment

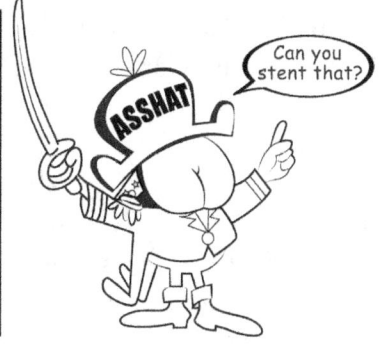

This observation was further enforced by the *Vitesse Intracranial Stent Study for Ischemic Stroke Therapy (VISSIT) Trial*.[17] The VISSIT Trial randomized 112 patients with symptomatic intracranial stenosis to receive balloon angioplasty and stenting and compared the outcomes with AMM. Like the SAMMPRIS Trial, this trial was also negative for the stenting group. Specifically, the primary endpoints including stroke, death, or intracranial hemorrhage within 30 days were observed in 24% of the intracranial stented group versus 9% of patients who received AMM. Further, the rate of either stroke or TIA at one year was 36% for the intracranial stented group versus 15% in the AMM group.

Both SAMMPRIS and VISSIT incorporated dual antiplatelet therapy (aspirin 81-325 mg and clopidogrel 75 mg for 90 days) as part of the AMM arm. This specific antithrombotic regimen likely had a key role in the success of the aggressive medical management arm in both trials. In addition to antiplatelet therapy, aggressive medical management in both trials consisted of aggressive blood pressure control targeted at <140/90 mmHg (or 130/80 if diabetic), lipid management of LDL <70 mg/dL, diabetes management, smoking cessation, weight loss, and exercise. The American Heart Association/ American Stroke Association guidelines endorse the use of high intensity statins (if tolerated) for secondary stroke prevention in patients with intracranial atherosclerotic disease. This regimen includes atorvastatin 40-80 mg or rosuvastatin 20-40 mg. Both the SAMMPRIS and VISSIT Trials demonstrated that AMM currently is the most effective option for the treatment of patients with intracranial atherosclerotic disease. In these patients, unless there is significant risk of bleeding, the short-term use of dual antiplatelet agents is reasonable.

Despite the findings of the SAMMPRIS and VISSIT Trials, the Wingspan stEnt system post mArket surVEillance (WEAVE) Trial which has yet to be published, followed the on-label, FDA-approved WINGSPAN® stent indications listed above (ASS HAT mnemonic) and demonstrated an extremely low 72-hour periprocedural stroke and death rate of 2.6%. After an interim safety analysis, this trial was halted early on October 25, 2017 and its results were presented at the International Stroke Conference 2018.[18] This trial was designed so that experienced interventionalists performed these procedures. The interventionalists that participated in this trial had a mean procedural experience of 37 Wingspan® stent cases prior to enrollment. These results suggest proper patient selection in combination with an experienced interventionalist are necessary for good outcomes and may represent a paradigm shift in our understanding of intracranial atherosclerotic disease.

The WEAVE Trial results substantially differ from those of the SAMMPRIS and VISSIT Trials. The results of the SAMMPRIS Trial again led the FDA to approve label changes in August 2012 which limited the use of Wingspan® stent procedures to patients with 70 to 99% intracranial stenosis, recurrent stroke despite optimal medical management, and no new stroke symptoms within seven days prior to treatment. One reason for the different outcomes between the WEAVE and SAMPPRIS Trials was interventionalist experience, with the average number of procedures performed by operators in the SAMMPRIS Trial being 10 compared to 37 in the WEAVE Trial. The favorable data of the WEAVE Trial may swing the pendulum back to intracranial stenting but the current criteria required to perform on-label intracranial stenting is still extremely limited. As will be presented in Chapter 25 (Endovascular Treatment), mechanical thrombectomy was initially also considered ineffective. At the very least, these trial results suggest re-evaluation of intracranial stenting as a treatment option for symptomatic intracranial atherosclerotic disease.

18.7 The Implications of Aggressive Medical Management

The efficacy of AMM in both the SAMMPRIS and VISSIT Trials raises fundamental concerns. First, going back to CAS and CEA, there is one critical flaw in the comparison studies of surgical carotid revascularization and medical therapy that led the approval of CEA. That is, medical therapy in these initial studies consisted only of aspirin. As seen in the SAMMPRIS and VISSIT Trials, AMM consisted of a cocktail of antiplatelet, antihypertensive, statin, and behavioral modification therapies, and not just aspirin exclusively. However, before the SAMMPRIS Trial, the *Warfarin-Aspirin Symptomatic Intracranial Disease (WASID) Trial* compared warfarin to aspirin in symptomatic patients with intracranial stenoses.[19] Prior to the WASID Trial, research suggested that warfarin may have a possible benefit over aspirin for secondary stroke prevention in patients with intracranial stenosis.

The WASID Trial demonstrated warfarin was associated with higher rates of adverse events yet provided no additional benefit over aspirin. As a result, it recommended the use of aspirin for patients with intracranial stenosis.

The stroke and death outcomes for the aspirin group were 10.7% at 30 days and 25.7% at one year, respectively. Compare this to the SAMMPRIS results which compared angioplasty and stenting with AMM and AMM alone, again in patients with intracranial stenotic disease (Table 2). Similarly, the *Cervical Artery Dissection In Stroke Study (CADISS)* demonstrated no difference in the risk of stroke recurrence in patients with either carotid or vertebral artery dissections when treated with either oral anticoagulation or antiplatelet therapy.[20]

Interestingly, patients from the AMM arm of the SAMMPRIS Trial (who also had intracranial stenoses) had half the rate of negative outcomes when compared to those in the WASID Trial (Table 2). The SAMMPRIS Trial demonstrated that AMM was superior to angioplasty and stenting in patients with intracranial arterial stenosis using the Wingspan® stent system. However, the SAMMPRIS data led to another powerful but often overlooked observation—**the risk of stroke with AMM was much lower than anticipated.** If this risk is almost half the risk seen with aspirin alone (WASID Trial), how would the stroke and death rate of CEA or CAS compare to modern AMM (antiplatelet, antihypertensive, and statin therapy) versus the medical therapy to which CEA was originally assessed (aspirin alone)? Carotid revascularization (CEA or CAS) must be compared to modern AMM and not just aspirin alone, which is precisely the purpose of the **CREST 2 Trial**. In this trial, two separate patient groups will have either CAS or CEA and each of these categories will be compared to AMM (Figure 1). Primary endpoints will include stroke and death within the first 30 days and ipsilateral stroke thereafter up to four years.

FIGURE 1. Crest-2 Parallel Study

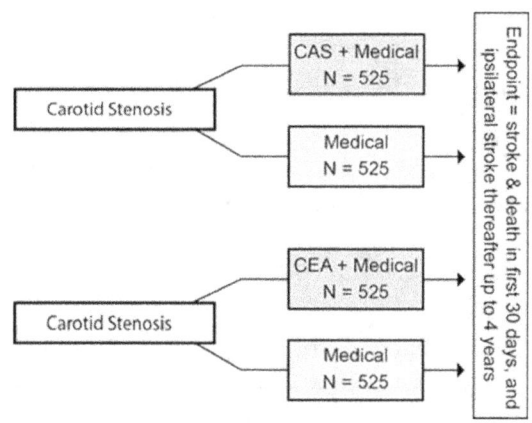

TABLE 2. Intracranial Medical Therapy Trials in Intracranial Atherosclerotic Disease (WASID vs SAMMPRIS)

FEATURES	WASID TRIAL	SAMMPRIS TRIAL
Year	1999 - 2003	2008 - 2012
Patients	Symptomatic High Grade Intracranial Atherosclerotic Stenosis	Symptomatic High Grade Intracranial Atherosclerotic Stenosis
Study Design	ASA vs. Warfarin	Stenting vs. AMM
30 Day DS	10.7%	5.8% in AMM

ASA - Aspirin; AMM - Aggressive Medical Management; DS - Death or Stroke

18.8 Dual Antiplatelet Therapy

The development of medical therapies with proven efficacy has resulted in a significant reduction of stroke and recurrent stroke within the last five decades, with antiplatelet therapy leading the pack. The most often used antiplatelet agents in clinical practice are **aspirin**, which inhibits cyclooxygenase, and **clopidogrel**, which irreversibly blocks the P2Y12 subtype of the adenosine diphosphate receptor. P2Y12 values, platelet inhibition, and receptor agonists are outlined below (Tables 3 and 4). The combined use of clopidogrel and aspirin gives dual antiplatelet therapy the potential to simultaneously block multiple platelet activation pathways and thus, reduce ischemic vascular events to a greater degree than antiplatelet monotherapy alone. Antiplatelet agents such as aspirin and clopidogrel have played an enormous role in secondary stroke prevention by reducing the risk of stroke, myocardial infarction, and death by 22%.[21] However, the use of dual antiplatelet therapy for non-cardioembolic ischemic stroke reduction continues to be investigated.

The *Clopidogrel in High-risk patients with Acute Non-disabling Cerebrovascular Events (CHANCE) Trial* compared a daily dose of 75 mg clopidogrel (loading dose 300 mg) and 75 mg aspirin for the first 21 days and then clopidogrel alone for days 22 to 90 versus 75 mg of aspirin alone with placebo for 90 days in 5,170 patients.[22]

TABLE 3. P2Y12 Values and Platelet Inhibition

P2Y12 Resistance Units	Percent Platelet Inhibition
259	10%
237	20%
214	30%
187	40%
159	50%
131	60%

Patients receiving dual antiplatelet therapy had a lower risk of recurrent stroke (primary endpoint) within 90 days compared to aspirin monotherapy (8.2% versus 11.7%), with no increase in intracranial hemorrhage or other major bleeding events. While the results of the CHANCE Trial are intriguing, certain points are worth considering.[22]

First, the rate of stroke in China is approximately five times higher than that in America.[22] Next, a recent meta-analysis comparing long-term clopidogrel monotherapy to dual antiplatelet therapy (aspirin plus clopidogrel) demonstrated comparable risk reductions for recurrent stroke but a higher risk of intracranial hemorrhage associated with dual antiplatelet therapy.[23] Other studies including the *MATCH (Management of Atherothrombosis with Clopidogrel in High-risk patients)* and *FASTER (Fast Assessment of Stroke and*

TABLE 4. Antiplatelet Drug Comparison Chart

	Clopidogrel (Plavix®)	Prasugrel (Effient®)	Ticagrelor (Brilinta®)	Cangrelor (Kengreal®)
Prodrug	Yes	Yes	No	No
Route	Oral	Oral	Oral	Intravenous
Binding	Irreversible	Irreversible	Reversible	Reversible
Peak Effect	6 hours (after load)	4 hours (after load)	2 hours (after load)	Immediate
Duration of Action	After d/c, gradual decline over 5-10 days	After d/c, gradual decline over 5-10 days	After d/c, gradual decline over 2-5 days	Return of platelet function within 1 hour after d/c of infusion
Dosage	Loading dose: 600 mg Maintenance dose: 75 mg/day	Loading dose: 60 mg Maintenance dose: 10 mg/day	Loading dose: 180 mg Maintenance dose: 90 mg bid	
Dual ASA Therapy	75-100 mg/day	81 mg/day, up to 325 mg/day	81 mg/day, up to 100 mg/day	N/A

TIA to prevent Early Recurrence) Trials failed to show a benefit with dual antiplatelet therapy and an increased risk of bleeding.[24,25] The *CHARISMA (Clopidogrel for High Atherothrombotic Risk and Ischemic, Stabilization, Management, and Avoidance) Trial* also failed to show benefit with dual antiplatelet treatment.[26]

All things considered, dual antiplatelet therapy over clopidogrel monotherapy should not be recommended as long-term therapy. Dual antiplatelet therapy initiated early after an ischemic stroke or TIA and during the high-risk period for a recurrent stroke may be superior to antiplatelet monotherapy, with no significant increase in intracranial hemorrhage. However, the long-term use of dual antiplatelet therapy for recurrent stroke prevention has an increased risk of intracranial hemorrhage. Thus, the benefit of dual antiplatelet therapy to prevent stroke recurrence may outweigh the bleeding risk for short-term use but should not be encouraged for long-term use. Currently, The *POINT (Platelet-Oriented Inhibition in New TIA and minor ischemic stroke) Trial* is investigating the use of 75 mg of clopidogrel plus 50 - 325 mg of ASA daily with ASA alone for 90 days in patients presenting within 12 hours of stroke symptoms.[27] This trial is being performed within North America and its data should help elucidate the role of dual antiplatelet therapy for secondary stroke prevention. Regardless, the results of the CHANCE Trial have led to a new recommendation in the 2018 AHA/ASA guidelines which states, "In patients presenting with minor stroke, treatment for 21 days with dual antiplatelet therapy (aspirin and clopidogrel) begun within 24 hours can be beneficial for early secondary stroke prevention for a period of up to 90 days from symptom onset."[28] Reduction in microembolic disease is the proposed mechanism that led to the **reduction in recurrent stroke** in the **CHANCE Trial** and the efficacy of dual antiplatelet therapy in both the **SAMMPRIS** and **VISSIT Trials**.

If aspirin is used in conjunction with clopidogrel, it should be administered within 24 hours of stroke or TIA and continued for up to 90 days.[21] One very important exception is to hold antiplatelet therapy for 24 hours after IV TPA administration. Long-term dual antiplatelet therapy with aspirin and clopidogrel (i.e., more than 90 days) is not recommended due to the increased risk of hemorrhage unless other indications exist (i.e., cardiac stent). Other antiplatelet agents such as ticagelor and prasugrel failed to show benefit for secondary stroke prevention when compared to aspirin.[29] Further, prasugrel is contraindicated in patients with a history of either stroke or TIA as was demonstrated to have an increased risk in patients in the *TRITON-TIMI 38 (Trial to Assess Improvement in Therapeutic Outcomes by Optimizing Platelet Inhibition with Prasugrel–Thrombolysis in Myocardial Infarction) Trial*.[30]

18.9 Antithrombotic Concerns

The use of aspirin and Plavix can cause several clinical concerns. Aspirin can cause direct mucosal injury to the gastrointestinal (GI) tract whereas Plavix may promote bleeding in pre-existing gastric lesions.[31] In many of the dual antiplatelet trials mentioned above, most hemorrhagic complications were G.I. bleeds.[24] This issue will be addressed in the POINT Trial which will have a similar design to the CHANCE Trial but with a loading dose of 600 mg clopidogrel instead of 300 mg. In addition to hemorrhagic risk, previous concerns existed based on an observational study suggesting omeprazole inhibited the conversion of clopidogrel to its active form resulting in a reduced efficacy.[32] However, a randomized controlled trial demonstrated no clinically significant interaction.[33] Regardless, the availability of several other proton pump inhibitors should discourage the use of either omeprazole or esomeprazole in patients currently taking clopidogrel.

18.10 Carotid Revascularization

The 2018 AHA/ASA guidelines have specific recommendations for patients with nondisabling ipsilateral stroke and symptomatic carotid stenosis. These recommendations apply to vascular imaging and carotid revascularization. In terms of vascular imaging, the 2018 AHA/ASA guidelines state: "For patients with non-disabling (mRS score 0-2) AIS in the internal carotid artery territory who are candidates for CEA or stenting, noninvasive imaging of the cervical vessels should be performed routinely within 24 hours of admission."[28]

A meta-analysis performed by De Rango et al demonstrates high rates of complications for carotid revascularization procedures (CEA and CAS) performed <48 hours, and no difference in procedural risk when performed between 0-7 days and 0-15 days.[34] Additional research supports carotid revascularization for nondisabling stroke (mRS score 0-2) between 48 hours and seven days after initial stroke.[35] This led to the 2018 AHA/ASA guidelines recommendation which states: "When revascularization is indicated for secondary prevention in patients with minor, nondisabling stroke (mRS score 0-2), it is reasonable to perform the procedure between 48 hours and 7 days of the index event rather than delay treatment if there are no contraindications to early revascularization."[28]

Essentially, observational data has demonstrated a high risk of recurrent stroke in patients with symptomatic carotid stenosis within the first several days and weeks. Thus, the efficacy of carotid revascularization (CEA or CAS) would be best during this high-risk period. However, researchers have also demonstrated that the risk of complications from these revascularization procedures is highest within the first 48 hours. Thus the 2018 AHA/ASA guidelines recommend noninvasive imaging within 24 hours of admission and revascularization treatment (CEA or CAS) from 48 hours to seven days (Table 5).

18.11 Conclusion

The objectives of this chapter were to review the current literature regarding carotid stenting, intracranial stenting, and the use of dual antiplatelet therapy for non-cardioembolic, secondary ischemic stroke prevention. Both CEA and CAS are effective procedures for extracranial vascular reperfusion. CAS is a good alternative to CEA for most patients requiring revascularization. However, CAS should be performed in a complementary fashion based on individual patient characteristics and local center experience. In terms of symptomatic intracranial stenosis, aggressive medical management is preferred to intracranial angioplasty and stenting. However, specific criteria do exist that permit intracranial stenting.

Antiplatelet treatment has been found beneficial for secondary stroke prevention, carotid stenting, intracranial stenting, and extracranial dissection. Again, this is likely attributed to its ability to reduce microemboli from symptomatic intracranial stenosis and other sources that can lead to stroke. Nonetheless, long-term dual antiplatelet therapy (i.e., > 90 days) is associated with increased morbidity (hemorrhage) and mortality and is not recommended unless other indications exist (i.e., cardiac stent). Further investigation regarding dual antiplatelet treatment and aggressive medical management may rapidly alter current protocols for the treatment of carotid stenosis, intracranial stenosis, and secondary stroke prevention.

TABLE 5. Summary of 2018 AHA/ASA Carotid Revascularization Recommendations

Summary of 2018 AHA/ASA Carotid Revascularization Recommendations	
Stroke Severity	Non-disabling stroke (mRS score 0-2)
Imaging	Cervical vessel noninvasive imaging <24 hours
Revascularization	48 hours - 7 days from the index event

mRS - Modified Rankin Scale

Abbreviations list

AMM, aggressive medical management; CAS, carotid artery stenting; CEA, carotid endarterectomy; GI, gastrointestinal.

References

1. Fisher M. (1951). Occlusion of the internal carotid artery. *AMA Arch Neurol Psychiatry*, 65, 346–77.
2. Mayberg MR, Wilson SE, Yatsu F, Weiss DG, Messina L, Hershey LA, et al. (1991). Carotid endarterectomy and prevention of cerebral ischemia in symptomatic carotid stenosis. Veterans affairs cooperative studies program 309 trialist group. *J Am Med Assoc*, 266, 3289–94.
3. North American Symptomatic Carotid Endarterectomy Trial Collaborators. (1991). Beneficial effect of carotid endarterectomy in symptomatic patients with high-grade stenosis. *N Engl J Med*, 325, 445–53.
4. Brott TG, Hobson RW II, Howard G, et al. (2010). Stenting versus endarterectomy for treatment of carotid-artery stenosis. *N Engl J Med*, 363(1), 11-23.
5. Brott TG, Howard G, Roubin GS, et al. (2016). Long-term results of stenting versus endarterectomy for carotid-artery stenosis. *N Engl J Med*, 374, 1021-31.
6. Rosenfield K, Matsumura JS, Chaturvedi S, et al. (2016). Randomized trial of stent versus surgery for asymptomatic carotid stenosis. *N Engl J Med*, 374, 1011-20.
7. Yadav JS, Wholey MH, Kuntz RE, Fayad P, Katzen BT, Mishkel GJ, et al. (2004). Protected carotid-artery stenting versus endarterectomy in high-risk patients. *N Engl J Med*, 351, 1493–501.
8. Brott TG, Halperin JL, Abbara S, et al. (2011). ASA/ACCF/AHA/AANN/AANS/ACR/ASNR/CNS/SAIP/SCAI/SIR/ SNIS/SVM/SVS guideline on the management of patients with extracranial carotid and vertebral artery disease: executive summary: a report of the American College of Cardiology Foundation/American Heart Association Task Force on Practice Guidelines, and the American Stroke Association, American Association of Neuroscience Nurses, American Association of Neurological Surgeons, American College of Radiology, American Society of Neuro-radiology, Congress of Neurological Surgeons, Society of Atherosclerosis Imaging and Prevention, Society for Cardiovascular Angiography and Interventions, Society of Interventional Radiology, Society of NeuroInterventional Surgery, Society for Vascular Medicine, and Society for Vascular Surgery. *J Am Coll Cardiol*, 57, 1002-44.
9. White CJ. (2014). Carotid artery stenting. *J Am Coll Cardiol*, 64, 722–31.
10. Song TJ, Suh SH, Min PK, et al. (2013). The influence of anti-platelet resistance on the development of cerebral ischemic lesion after carotid artery stenting. *Yonsei Med J*, 54(2), 288-94.
11. Al-Ali F, Barrow T, Duan L, Jefferson A, Louis S, Luke K, et al. (2011). Vertebral artery ostium atherosclerotic plaque as a potential source of posterior circulation ischemic stroke result from Borgess Medical Center vertebral artery ostium stenting registry. *Stroke*, 42(9), 2544–910.
12. Stayman AN, Nogueira RG, Gupta R. (2011). A systematic review of stenting and angioplasty of symptomatic extracranial vertebral artery stenosis. *Stroke*, 42(8), 2212–610.
13. Lutsep HL, Barnwell S, Mawad M, Chiu D, Hartmann M, Hacke W, et al. (2004). Stenting of symptomatic atherosclerotic lesions in the vertebral or intracranial arteries (SSYLVIA) study results. *Stroke*, 35(6), 1388–9210.
14. Chimowitz MI, Lynn MJ, Derdeyn CP, Turan TN, Fiorella D, Lane BF, et al. (2011). SAMMPRIS trial investigators. Stenting versus aggressive medical therapy for intracranial arterial stenosis. *N Engl J Med*, 365(11), 993–1003.
15. Derdeyn CP, Chimowitz MI, Lynn MJ, Fiorella D, Turan TN, Janis LS, et al. (2014). Aggressive medical treatment with or without stenting in high-risk patients with intracranial artery stenosis (SAMMPRIS): the final results of a randomised trial. *Lancet*, 383(9914), 333–411.
16. Derdeyn CP, Fiorella D, Lynn MJ, Rumboldt Z, Cloft HJ, Gibson D, et al. (2013). Mechanisms of Stroke after intracranial angioplasty and stenting in the SAMMPRIS trial. *Neurosurgery*, 72(5), 777–951.
17. Zaidat OO, Fitzimmons BF, Woodward BK, et al. for the VISSIT trial investigators. (2015). Effect of a balloon-expandable intracranial stent vs medical therapy on risk of stroke in patients with symptomatic intracranial stenosis: the VISSIT randomized clinical trial. *JAMA*, 313, 1240-48.

18. Alexander MJ, Chaloupka, JC, Zauner A, Baxter B, Callison R, Yu W. (2017). Abstract 6: Interim Report of the Weave Trial: First 102 Consecutive on Label Patients. *Stroke*, 48, A6. Pub. First: 21 February 2017.
19. Kasner SE, Lynn MJ, Chimowitz MI, Frankel MR, Howlett-Smith H, Hertzberg VS, et al. (2006). Warfarin vs aspirin for symptomatic intracranial stenosis: subgroup analyses from wasid. *Neurology*, 67, 1275–78.
20. CADISS trial investigators. (2015). Antiplatelet treatment compared with anticoagulation treatment for cervical artery dissection (CADISS): a randomised trial. *Lancet Neurol*, 14, 361-67.
21. Kernan WN, Ovbiagele B, Black HR, Bravata DM, Chimowitz MI, Ezekowitz MD, et al. (2014). Guidelines for the prevention of stroke in patients with stroke and transient ischemic attack: a guideline for healthcare professionals from the American Heart Association/American Stroke Association. *Stoke* 45(7), 2160–236. Erratum in: *Stroke* (2015), 46(2), e54.
22. Wang Y, Wang Y, Zhao X, Liu L, Wang D, Wang C, et al. (2013). Clopidogrel with aspirin in acute minor stroke or transient ischemic attack. *N Engl J Med*, 369, 11–19.
23. Lee M, Saver JL, Hong KS, Rao NM, Wu YL, Ovbiagele B. (2013). Risk-benefit profile of long-term dual- versus single-antiplatelet therapy among patients with ischemic stroke: a systematic review and meta-analysis. *Ann Intern Med.*, 159, 463–70.
24. Diener HC, Bogousslavsky J, Brass LM, Cimminiello C, Csiba L, Kaste M, et al. (2004). Aspirin and clopidogrel compared with clopidogrel alone after recent ischaemic stroke or transient ischaemic attack in high-risk patients (MATCH): randomised, double-blind, placebo-controlled trial. *Lancet*, 364(9431), 331–7.
25. Kennedy J, Hill MD, Ryckborst KJ, Eliasziw M, Demchuk AM, Buchan AM. (2007). Fast assessment of stroke and transient ischaemic attack to prevent early recurrence (FASTER): a randomised controlled pilot trial. *Lancet Neurol*, 6(11), 961–69.
26. Bhatt DL, Fox KA, Hacke W, Berger PB, Black HR, Boden WE, et al. (2006). Clopidogrel and aspirin versus aspirin alone for the prevention of atherothrombotic events. *N Engl J Med*, 354(16), 1706–17.
27. ClinicalTrials.gov [website] (2016). Platelet-Oriented Inhibition in New TIA and minor ischemic stroke (POINT) trial. Bethesda, MD: US National Institutes of Health.
28. Powers WJ, Rabinstein AA, Ackerson T, Adeoye OM, Bambakidis NC, Becker K, Biller J, Brown M, Demaerschalk BM, Hoh B, et al. (2018) Guidelines for the Early Management of Patients With Acute Ischemic Stroke: A Guideline for Healthcare Professionals From the American Heart Association/American Stroke Association.. *Stroke,* Jan 24, Epub 2018 Jan 24.
29. AstraZeneca [website]. (2016). AstraZeneca reports top-line results from the Brilinta SOCRATES trial in stroke. Cambridge, UK: AstraZeneca. Available from:
30. www.astrazeneca.com/media-centre/press-releases/2016/astrazeneca-reports-top-line-results-from-the-brilinta-socrates-trial-in-stroke-23032016.html.
31. Wiviott SD, Braunwald E, McCabe CH, Montalescot G, Ruzyllo W, Gottlieb S, et al. (2007). Prasugrel versus clopidogrel in patients with acute coronary syndromes. *N Engl J Med*, 357(20), 2001–15.
32. Agewall S, Cattaneo M, Collet JP, Andreotti F, Lip GY, Verheugt FW, et al. (2013). Expert position paper on the use of proton pump inhibitors in patients with cardiovascular disease and antithrombotic therapy. *Eur Heart J*, 34(23), 1708–13.
33. Juurlink DN, Gomes T, Ko D, Szmitko PE, Austin PC, Tu JV, et al. (2009). A population-based study of the drug interaction between proton pump inhibitors and clopidogrel. *CMAJ*, 180(7), 713–18.
34. Bhatt DL, Cryer BL, Contant CF, Cohen M, Lanas A, Schnitzer TJ, et al. (2010). Clopidogrel with or without omeprazole in coronary artery disease. *N Engl J Med*, 363(20), 1909–17.
35. De Rango P, Brown MM, Chaturvedi S, Howard VJ, Jovin T, Mazya MV, Paciaroni M, Manzone A, Farchioni L, Caso V. (2015) Summary of evidence on early carotid intervention for recently symptomatic stenosis based on meta-analysis of current risks. Stroke, 46, 3423–36.
36. Ferguson GG, Eliasziw M, Barr HW, Clagett GP, Barnes RW, Wallace MC, Taylor DW, Haynes RB, Finan JW, Hachinski VC, Barnett HJ. (1999). The North American Symptomatic Carotid Endarterectomy Trial: surgical results in 1415 patients. Stroke, 30, 1751–58.

Chapter 19

Stroke Mimics

19.1 Introduction

The term *stroke mimic* is used for manifestations of disease processes that can mimic stroke and thus confound its diagnosis. The ability to discern acute ischemic stroke (AIS) from other conditions that can mimic its presentation is essential. Yet, stroke mimics continue to be often misdiagnosed as AIS and, in some reports, this can happen up to 31% of the time.[1] The purpose of this chapter is to review common stroke mimics and their distinguishing features that differentiate them from AIS. This distinction is important because while mimics may produce symptoms similar to stroke, they generally have very different therapeutic implications.

The most common stroke mimics include seizures, hypoglycemia, intracranial lesions, migraine headaches, vestibular dysfunction, encephalopathy, sepsis, and multiple sclerosis. These can be remembered by the stroke mimic mnemonic 'MIMICKERS™' (Table 1). Again, the recognition of stroke mimics is important because they have different therapeutic implications than AIS. Stroke mimics can also be summarized in terms of stroke misdiagnosis frequency (Table 2). Stroke mimics often lack cardiovascular risk factors such as hypertension, hyperlipidemia, and atrial fibrillation.[2] However, stroke mimics have characteristic features that aid in distinguishing them from AIS.

TABLE 1. Stroke Mimickers: **MIMICKERS**™

M	Metabolic-Hypoglycemia or Hyperglycemia
I	Ictal-Seizures
M	Multiple Sclerosis
I	Intracranial Lesions (traumatic, infectious, hemorrhagic and neoplastic)
C	Classic and Specific Migraine Subtypes
K	Keep Balance? (Vestibular Dysfunction)
E	Encephalopathy
R	Regular Diastolic Pressure
S	Sepsis

19.2 Seizure Mimic

Seizure is a common stroke mimic and can account for up to one third of stroke mimics.[3-6] A patient with witnessed seizure activity, a known history of epilepsy, or one who demonstrates typical symptoms such as generalized convulsions, involuntary movements, confusion, tongue biting, and incontinence is less likely to be confused with an acute stroke patient. However, post-seizure paresis (Todd's paralysis) can easily be confused with an acute stroke presentation.[7] This is because in addition to focal motor deficits, postictal paresis has also been reported in dominant hemisphere seizures.[8] Todd's paralysis is usually localized to one side of the body and occurs in approximately 13% of all seizures.[9] Occasionally, seizure may cause diffusion abnormalities on MRI but can be distinguished from stroke by a nonvascular distribution in the absence of vascular occlusion.[10] Incidentally, seizure at the onset of stroke symptoms was originally but is no longer considered a contraindication to IV TPA.[11] Seizures can substantially increase intracranial pressure and worsen functional outcome. For this reason, benzodiazepines including IV lorazepam or diazepam are recommended as first-line agents.

TABLE 2. Stroke Mimics and Frequency of Stroke Misdiagnosis

Mimic	Misdiagnosed as Stroke (%)
Brain tumor	7-15
Labyrinthitis	5-6
Metabolic disorder	3-13
Migraine	11-47
Psychiatric disorder	1-40
Seizures	11-40
Sepsis	14-17
Syncope	5-22
Transient global amnesia	3-10
Other	11-37

Adapted from *J Fam Pract.* 2010 January; 59(1):26-30

19.3 Metabolic Disorders Mimic

Metabolic disorders can also present as stroke mimics, with diabetic hypoglycemia being the "classic" stroke mimic within this category. Thus, early evaluation of blood glucose is a critical step in the assessment of a patient suspected of having an acute ischemic stroke. Hypoglycemia may mimic stroke with focal neurologic deficits such as hemiplegia and aphasia.[12] Hypoglycemia secondary to alcoholism can present similarly. Fortunately, the wide use of bedside rapid laboratory testing for glucose makes this condition easily detectable and treatable. Typically, most symptoms related to hypoglycemia such as diaphoresis resolve immediately with administration of intravenous glucose; however, delays in resolution have also been reported.[13] Patients with significant hypoglycemia are bolused with 50% IV dextrose or receive insulin for blood sugar > 300 mg/dL. Other metabolic disorders that may present with focal stroke-like symptoms include hyperglycemic nonketotic hyperosmolar states, severe hyponatremia, and hepatic encephalopathy.

19.4 Vertigo Mimic

Each year, over four million Americans visit the emergency department for dizziness or vertigo. Vertigo is a medical condition wherein a person feels as if they or the objects in their surroundings are spinning or moving in the absence of any movement. This can be caused by pathology within the ear, the brain, or the nerve pathways that connect them. The emergency department evaluation of vertigo is complex. While most of these patients who present with isolated vertigo have benign disorders, up to 3% can have cerebellar infarcts.[14] Worse, 35% of patients having a cerebellar stroke are not diagnosed.[15] Thus, vertigo can be benign or caused by a cerebellar stroke. Please refer to Chapter 11 (Cerebellar Stroke) for a detailed discussion on the evaluation of vertigo and cerebellar infarct.

19.5 Migraine Mimic

Migraine and migraine auras are other stroke mimics. Migraine disproportionally affects females three times more often than males and has a peak incidence around age 40. Most migraines do not present with an aura. However, 20-30% of migraines known as *classic migraines* are associated with an aura that can include visual, sensory, motor, or speech disturbances. This is a further diagnostic challenge when a migraine occurs with minimal or no headache. In such cases, it is known as an *acephalgic migraine*.[16] One important diagnostic clue is that migraine auras often occur sequentially, with one resolving as the other begins, rather than simultaneously as in stroke.

Specific migraine presentations are worth noting. Ophthalmoplegic migraine can involve cranial nerves III, IV, or VI with associated oculomotor dysfunction and pupil involvement. A retinal migraine can present with blindness. Complex and hemiplegic migraines can present as hemiparesis or hemiplegia. Basilar type migraines have auras that can affect the vascular territory of the brainstem and can present with multiple symptoms such as visual loss, dysarthria, tinnitus, vertigo, bilateral paresthesia, and paresis. Vertiginous migraines may also frequently present with isolated vertigo. Finally, the vascular distribution of an aura can progress into an actual infarct, termed *migrainous infarction*.[13] Migraines are not just stroke mimics but can also progress into a stroke. In fact, migrainous stroke can account for 15% of strokes in patients less than 45 years of age.[17]

19.6 Intracranial Mimics

Intracranial infectious, neoplastic, hemorrhagic, or traumatic lesions that produce mass effect on the brain can also cause stroke-like symptoms. These symptoms are believed to occur secondary to mass effect resulting in partial impairment of cerebral blood flow.[18] Typically, intracranial lesions such as tumors tend to have more gradual, progressive symptoms. However acute deterioration of a tumor such as hemorrhage or infarction can rapidly raise intracranial pressure and present with acute symptomatology. Other intracranial hemorrhages such as subdural hematomas, epidural hematomas, and subarachnoid hemorrhages can also be clinically confused with stroke. Every stroke workup involves a noncontrast brain CT which will likely demonstrate most intracranial processes related to mass effect. Focal lesions within the brain can also occur from microbial seeding of the CNS from an infectious agent and may result in focal stroke-like symptoms. Generally, sepsis from any infectious agent can result in less specific stroke-like symptoms such as weakness, altered speech, and delirium.

19.7 Encephalopathy Mimic

Another stroke mimic is *encephalopathy*, which is a general term describing a disease process that damages the brain. For example, *posterior reversible encephalopathy syndrome (PRES)* is one such encephalopathy related to high blood pressure. Elevated blood pressure causes a hyperperfusion state which elevates capillary hydrostatic pressure and results in vascular autoregulation dysfunction. Subsequently, there is blood-brain barrier breakdown and extravasation of fluids which result in edema. This type of encephalopathy has mimicked focal stroke deficits.[19] However, it is important to distinguish this encephalopathy from stroke because the symptoms associated with PRES usually resolve with blood pressure control. Sustained high blood pressure levels, on the other hand, will only cause PRES to progress. Confusing PRES with AIS invokes the opposite end of the treatment spectrum. Typically, blood pressures are desired to run high with AIS, which is the opposite treatment for PRES. This mimic is particularly tricky as it can present with elevated blood pressure just like AIS. However, excluding this exception, diastolic blood pressure of > 90 mm Hg can distinguish between a stroke and a stroke mimic.[20]

19.8 Multiple Sclerosis Mimic

Multiple sclerosis can present with two types of paroxysmal symptoms that can mimic ischemic stroke. Fortunately, these are highly characteristic of multiple sclerosis. Paroxysmal dysarthria is characterized by recurrent stereotyped episodes of slurred speech. Recent reports have attributed this symptom to demyelinating midbrain lesions.[21] Tonic spasms (dystonia) that typically affect a single upper limb have also been attributable to multiple sclerosis.[22] These symptoms typically occur in younger people devoid of cardiovascular risk factors. These stroke mimics should be considered in patients with an established history of multiple sclerosis.

19.9 Stroke Mimic Rule

What if a stroke mimic cannot be distinguished from AIS? For example, what if one cannot discriminate a stroke mimic from an actual stroke? How does one determine delayed resolution of stroke-like symptoms in patients with either hypoglycemia or postictal states from seizures representing delayed resolution or actual AIS? If the stroke practitioner "rides it out" and waits for the symptoms to dissipate, they may miss the narrow therapeutic window available for IV TPA administration. Thus, waiting for symptom improvement to confirm the diagnosis of a stroke mimic such as a seizure or migraine would exclude the ability to administer IV TPA. Weighing the risks against the benefits, studies have demonstrated that patients presenting with stroke mimics who nonetheless received IV TPA rarely had hemorrhagic complications, with symptomatic intracranial hemorrhage rates of approximately 1%.[5, 23-24]

This makes sense when one considers that hemorrhagic rates from IV TPA administration are directly related to stroke severity represented by higher NIHSS and lower ASPECT scores. That is, patients with severe stroke (high NIHSS and low ASPECT scores) tend to have higher hemorrhagic complications with IV TPA than patients with less severe stroke (lower NIHSS and higher ASPECT scores). This brings us to the stroke mimic rule: **If the diagnosis of a stroke mimic cannot be confirmed before or within the IV TPA treatment time window (4.5 hours), assume the patient has an AIS and administer IV TPA.** Again, multiple studies where stroke mimic patients received IV TPA have demonstrated a low risk of symptomatic intracranial hemorrhage. The 2018 AHA/ASA guidelines state that the risk of symptomatic intracranial hemorrhage in the stroke population is quite low; thus, starting IV alteplase is probably recommended in preference over delaying treatment to pursue additional diagnostic studies.[25] The benefit of giving IV TPA to a potential AIS patient far exceeds the risk of erroneously treating a stroke mimic with IV TPA.

19.10 Conclusion

This chapter is a summary of stroke mimics. Recall, however, the importance of always using the stroke plan when addressing stroke (S-PLAN) (Table 3). The proper understanding of these elements of stroke will enable its accurate diagnosis. While stroke mimics may produce stroke-like symptoms, they typically have very different therapeutic implications. The mnemonic 'MIMICKERS™' should be considered in the workup of every suspected AIS patient (Table 1). Stroke mimics generally lack cardiovascular risk factors such as hypertension, hyperlipidemia, and atrial fibrillation. If one has difficulty discerning a stroke mimic from AIS, remember the *stroke mimic rule*: **If the diagnosis of a stroke mimic cannot be confirmed before or within the IV TPA treatment time window (4.5 hours), assume the patient has an AIS and administer IV TPA.** Fortunately, the iatrogenic use of IV TPA given to stroke mimics has been demonstrated to be safe.[5, 23-24] The 2018 AHA/ASA guidelines state that "the risk of symptomatic intracranial hemorrhage in the stroke population is quite low; thus, starting IV alteplase is probably recommended in preference over delaying treatment to pursue additional diagnostic studies."[25] The stroke mimic (no stroke diagnostic/treatment) protocol is summarized below (Figure 1).

FIGURE 1. Stroke Mimic/No Stroke Diagnostic and Treatment Protocol

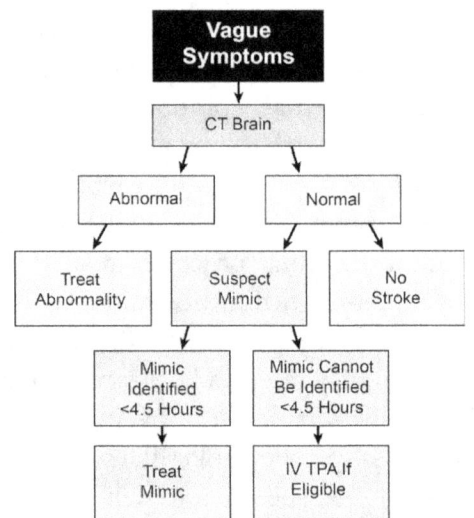

TABLE 3. Acute Ischemic Stroke Plan: **S-PLAN**

S	Source (embolic or thrombotic)
P	Pathophysiology (etiology)
L	Location (of brain affected)
A	Artery (arterial territory involved)
N	Neuroimaging

<u>S</u>ource	<u>P</u>atho-physiology	<u>L</u>ocation	<u>A</u>rtery	<u>N</u>euro-imaging
• Embolic • Thrombotic	**C**: Cardioembolic (20%) **A**: Atherosclerotic large vessel disease (30%) **U**: Undetermined etiology - ESUS (30%) **S**: Small vessel disease or lacunar infarct (15%) **E**: Everything else or other (5%)	• Frontal • Parietal • Temporal • Occipital • Cerebellar • Thalamic • Brainstem	• ICA • MCA • ACA • Vertebral • Basilar • PICA • ACA • SCA	• CT • CTA • CTP • MRI • MRA • Angio

Abbreviations list

AIS, acute ischemic stroke; CNS, central nervous system; MRI, magnetic resonance imaging; PRES, posterior reversible encephalopathy syndrome.

References

1. Kothari R, Barsan W, Brott T, et al. (1995). Frequency and accuracy of prehospital diagnosis of acute stroke. *Stroke, A Journal of Cerebral Circulation,* 26, 937–41.
2. Merino JG, Luby M, Benson RT, et al. (2013). Predictors of acute stroke mimics in 8187 patients referred to a stroke service. *J Stroke Cerebrovasc Dis,* 22, 397-403.
3. Forster A, Griebe M, Wolf ME, et al. (2012). How to identify stroke mimics in patients eligible for intravenous thrombolysis? *J Neurol,* 259, 1247-53.
4. Tsivgoulis G, Alexandrov AV, Chang J, et al. (2011). Safety and outcomes of intravenous thrombolysis in stroke mimics. *Stroke,* 42, 1771-74.
5. Brunser AM, Illanes S, Lavados PM, Munoz P, Carcamo D, Hoppe A, et al. (2013). Exclusion criteria for intravenous thrombolysis in stroke mimics: An observational study. *J Stroke Cerebrovasc Di,* 22, 1140–45.
6. Zinkstok SM, Engelter ST, Gensicke H, Lyrer PA, Ringleb PA, Artto V, et al. (2013). Safety of thrombolysis in stroke mimics: Results from a multicenter cohort study. *Stroke,* 44, 1080–84.
7. Magauran BG, Nitka M. (2012). Stroke mimics. *Emerg Med Clin North Am,* 30, 795-804.
8. Nadarajan V, Perry RJ, Johnson J, et al. (2014). Transient ischaemic attacks: Mimics and chameleons. *Pract Neurol,* 14, 23–31.
9. Gallmetzer P, Leutmezer F, Serles W, et al. (2004). Postictal paresis in focal epilepsies: incidence, duration, and causes. *Neurology,* 12, 2160-64.
10. Di Bonaventura C, Bonini F, Fattouch J, Mari F, Petrucci S, Carni M, et al. (2009). Diffusion-weighted magnetic resonance imaging in patients with partial status epilepticus. *Epilepsia,* 50, Suppl 1, 45–52.

11. Jauch EC, Saver JL, Adams HP, et al. (2013). Guidelines for the early management of patients with acute ischemic stroke: a guideline for healthcare professionals from the American Heart Association/American Stroke Association. *Stroke*, 44(3), 870-947.
12. Montgomery BM, Pinner CA, Newberry SC. (1964). Transient hypoglycemic hemiplegia. *Arch Int Med*, 114, 680-84.
13. Wallis WE, Donaldson I, Scott RS, Wilson J. (1985). Hypoglycemia masquerading as cerebrovascular disease (hypoglycemic hemiplegia). *Ann Neurol*, 18, 510-12.
14. Kerber KA, Brown DL, Lisabeth LD, et al. (2006). Stroke among patients with dizziness, vertigo, and imbalance in the emergency department: a population-based study. *Stroke*, 37, 2484–87.
15. Savitz SI, Caplan LR, Edlow JA. (2007). Pitfalls in the diagnosis of cerebellar infarction. *Acad Emerg Med*, 14, 63-8.
16. Headache Classification Committee of the International Headache Society. (2013). The International Classification of Headache Disorders, 3rd ed. *Cephalalgia*, 33, 629-808.
17. Arboix A, Massons J, Garcia-Eroles L, Oliveres M, Balcells M, Targa C. (2003). Migrainous cerebral infarction in the sagrat cor hospital of barcelona stroke registry. *Cephalalgia*, 23, 389–94.
18. Ueno Y, Tanaka A, Nakayama Y. (1998). Transient neurological deficits simulating transient ischemic attacks in a patient with meningioma--case report. *Neurol Med Chir (Tokyo)*, 38, 661–65.
19. Terranova S, Kumar JD, Libman RB. (2012). Posterior Reversible Encephalopathy Syndrome Mimicking a Left Middle Cerebral Artery Stroke. *The Open Neuroimaging Journal*, 6, 10-12.
20. Libman RB, Wirkowski E, Alvir J, Rao TH. (1995). Conditions that mimic stroke in the emergency department. Implications for acute stroke trials. *Arch Neurol*, 52, 1119–22.
21. Isolated paroxysmal dysarthria caused by a single demyelinating midbrain lesion, BMJ Case Rep. (2013): bcr2013200777.
22. Berger JR, Sheremata WA, Melamed E. (1984). Paroxysmal dystonia as the initial manifestation of multiple sclerosis. *Arch Neurol*, 41(7), 747-50.
23. Chernyshev OY, Martin-Schild S, Albright KC, et al. (2010). Safety of tPA in stroke mimics and neuroimaging-negative cerebral ischemia. *Neurology*, 74, 1340–45.
24. Tsivgoulis G, Zand R, Katsanos AH, Goyal N, Uchino K, Chang J, Dardiotis E, Putaala J, Alexandrov AW, Malkoff MD, and Alexandrov AV. (2015). Safety of Intravenous Thrombolysis in Stroke Mimics. *Stroke*, 46, 1281-87.
25. Powers WJ, Rabinstein AA, Ackerson T, Adeoye OM, Bambakidis NC, Becker K, Biller J, Brown M, Demaerschalk BM, Hoh B, et al. (2018). Guidelines for the Early Management of Patients With Acute Ischemic Stroke: A Guideline for Healthcare Professionals From the American Heart Association/American Stroke Association. *Stroke*, Jan 24, Epub 2018 Jan 24.

Chapter 20

NIHSS

20.1 Introduction

The objective of this chapter is to discuss the purpose of the National Institutes of Health Stroke Scale (NIHSS), describe how to perform it, and make it simpler to understand. Recall that the distinguishing clinical feature of an acute ischemic stroke (AIS) is the sudden onset of a neurologic deficit caused by arterial occlusion. The source of this occlusion and its pathophysiology are important for both stroke diagnosis and treatment. Stroke symptoms reflect perfusion-compromised regions within the brain. These symptoms allow the examiner to localize the region(s) of the brain affected and their arterial territory. The affected regions of the brain and arterial territory can also be determined by neuroimaging. Don't forget to utilize the stroke plan (Table 1).

The National Institutes of Health Stroke Scale (NIHSS) is a clinical assessment tool consisting of 11 elements that objectively measure the level of impairment caused by stroke (Table 2). While the NIHSS can quantitate stroke severity, it is neither a diagnostic scale nor does it possess a localization or etiological component. The NIHSS was originally developed as a research tool to determine the neurologic baseline for clinical trials but subsequently has been implemented to objectively quantify neurologic impairment. Additionally, it has reliable reproducibility and can predict infarct size and functional outcome. The new 2018 AHA/ASA Guidelines state, "The use of a stroke severity rating scale, *preferably* the NIHSS, is recommended."[1] While it is predominantly used for AIS assessment, the NIHSS can also be utilized for other neurologic evaluations.

TABLE 1. Acute Ischemic Stroke Plan: **S-PLAN**

S	Source (embolic or thrombotic)
P	Pathophysiology (etiology)
L	Location (of brain affected)
A	Artery (arterial territory involved)
N	Neuroimaging

Source	Pathophysiology	Location	Artery	Neuroimaging
• Embolic • Thrombotic	C: Cardioembolic (20%) A: Atherosclerotic large vessel disease (30%) U: Undetermined etiology - ESUS (30%) S: Small vessel disease or lacunar infarct (15%) E: Everything else or other (5%)	• Frontal • Parietal • Temporal • Occipital • Cerebellar • Thalamic • Brainstem	• ICA • MCA • ACA • Vertebral • Basilar • PICA • ACA • SCA	• CT • CTA • CTP • MRI • MRA • Angio

TABLE 2. National Institutes of Health Stroke Scale (NIHSS)

Item	Score
1a. Level of consciousness	0 = alert, readily responsive to questions 1 = not alert but arousal with minor stimulus 2 = not alert, requires repetitive or painful stimulation (if obtunded) for response 3 = unresponsive, flaccid, response only with reflex motor or autonomic effects
1b. Level of consciousness Questions (month and age)	0 = answers both correctly 1 = answers one correctly 2 = answers neither correctly
1c. Level of consciousness Commands	0 = performs both tasks correctly 1 = performs one task correctly 2 = performs neither task correctly
2. Gaze	0 = normal 1 = partial gaze palsy 2 = total gaze palsy
3. Visual fields	0 = no visual loss 1 = partial hemianopsia 2 = complete hemianopsia 3 = bilateral hemianopsia
4. Facial palsy	0 = normal 1 = minor paralysis 2 = partial paralysis 3 = complete paralysis

5. Motor arm
  a. Left
  b. Right
	0 = no drift
	1 = drifts before 10 sec
	2 = falls before 10 sec
	3 = no effort against gravity
	4 = no movement

6. Motor leg
  a. Left
  b. Right
	0 = no drift
	1 = drifts before 5 sec
	2 = falls before 5 sec
	3 = no effort against gravity
	4 = no movement

7. Ataxia	0 = absent 1 = 1 limb 2 = 2 limbs
8. Sensory	0 = normal 1 = mild loss 2 = severe loss
9. Language	0 = normal 1 = mild aphasia 2 = severe aphasia 3 = mute or global aphasia
10. Dysarthria	0 = normal 1 = mild 2 = severe
11. Extinction/inattention	0 = no neglect 1 = partial neglect 2 = complete neglect

20.2 NIHSS Examination

The NIHSS has 11 categories. The first section assesses the patient's level of consciousness (LOC) and consists of three separate subcomponents. The first component (Item 1a) should begin by introducing yourself to the patient and asking questions like "How are you feeling?" and "Do you have any pain?" (Table 2). Patients without impairment should respond readily and verbally if no speech deficits are present. However, this section of the NIHSS is evaluating the level of consciousness and not speech. For this reason, do not confuse alertness with the inability to talk. If the patient is normal, awake and alert, they would receive a score of '0'. If the patient appears confused and requires the question repeated, additional stimulation such as touch to invoke a response may be necessary. In this case, they will receive a score of '1' or '2' depending on the degree of stimulation. Patients who are completely non-responsive (comatose) or only display reflexive posturing to noxious stimuli (sternal rub) receive a score of '3'.

The second component of the NIHSS LOC assessment (Item 1b) is the ability to answer questions. The patient is asked their age and the month. It is very important to understand that the first response is the most reliable and most reproducible response. Patients should not be coached ("almost" or "you're so close") and no partial credit is given. Additionally, written responses are valid in patients that cannot speak. Patients who can correctly answer both questions appropriately are scored '0'. Patients who are suffering aphasia or cannot speak (intubation) and cannot respond in writing are given a score of '1'. Unresponsive aphasic or comatose patients are given a score of '2'.

The third component of the LOC assessment (Item 1c) evaluates the ability to follow or execute commands. The examiner asks the patient to open their eyes and then close them. The patient is then asked to make a tight fist and then relax their hand. In this section, credit is given if an attempt is made to demonstrate understanding. For example, the patient attempts to make a fist but is too weak to do so. During this component of the NIHSS, the patient must be focused on the examiner's instruction. Whenever possible, demonstrate the action required to be performed by the patient. For example, state "I want you to make a fist and then open your hand" and then demonstrate this action to the patient. If the patient performs both tasks correctly they receive a score of '0'. One task performed correctly receives a score of '1' and if neither task is performed correctly, they receive a score of '2'. These four components within this section can be recalled with the mnemonic 'LAME' (Table 3). Please refer to Table 2 or 3 for scoring of this and the remaining sections.

The next two sections (Items 2 and 3) of the NIHSS test gaze and visual fields. Refer to Table 2 or 3 for scoring. This does not serve as a complete eye neurologic examination. While the NIHSS can quantify severity of symptoms, it is not a replacement for a complete neurologic examination. Neurologic examination provides localization of symptoms which the NIHSS does not in its limited capacity. The NIHSS has utility because it is quick, easy to perform, standardized, reproducible, and a useful means of communication to other healthcare professionals.

Prior to evaluating vision, it is important to determine if the patient normally wears glasses. Often, glasses are removed by first responders. If this is the case, please make sure the patient's glasses are returned prior to any visual examination. This is equally important when using NIHSS images during language assessment (Item 9).

Item 2 of the NIHSS is entitled "Best Gaze." This is determined by asking the patient to follow your finger with their eyes to assess horizontal eye movement. The objective of this exam is to evaluate horizontal eye movement. Thus, if the patient is aphasic or confused, the examiner may move around the room to see if the patient tracks them. Coaching is also permissible to elicit horizontal movement of the eyes. If the patient is unconscious, sometimes the examiner may require to hold the eyelids open. Certain strokes may cause forced gaze deviation to the side of the stroke. If present, an oculocephalic maneuver can be performed to determine if one or both eyes have reflexive movement. This is carried out by holding the patient's head and turning it side to side while assessing eye movement. Normally, the eyes should deviate away from the side the head is turned and then return to midline. If no such corrective movement is demonstrated, the patient receives a score of '2'. If the patient has voluntary or partial gaze (eyes are able to cross the midline), they will receive a score of '1'. Those with an isolated cranial neuropathy (CN, III, IV or VI) will also receive a score of '1.' If the patient has involuntary or forced gaze (eyes are unable to cross the midline), they will receive a score of '2'.

Item 3 assesses the visual fields. The patient is instructed to look at the examiner's eyes or nose and then each visual quadrant is individually tested. Finger counting is preferred over motion due to its greater sensitivity for the detection of visual deficits. Visual field testing is accomplished by covering one eye and checking all four visual fields of each eye separately. It is essential to assess all four quadrants of each eye. Patients with unilateral blindness should only have their functional eye scored.

Patients who are unable to communicate can still be tested with visual "threats". One method involves holding the hand approximately 12 inches away from the eye and moving the hand quickly towards it to test all four visual quadrants. Observe the patient for defensive responses (closing the eye). Vision that is absent or impaired on one side of visual field (both the upper and lower quadrants) is termed *hemianopia*. When hemianopia occurs on the same side of both eyes, this is termed homonymous hemianopia. If only one quadrant of the visual field is affected, this is termed quadrantanopia. If the same quadrant defect occurs in both eyes, this is termed homonymous quadrantanopia. Visual deficits are usually contralateral. That is, a left hemispheric stroke produces right visual field deficits and a right hemispheric stroke produces left visual field deficits.

TABLE 3. NIHSS: **LEG PLEASED**™

	National Institutes of Health Stroke Scale (NIHSS)		
		Item	Score
L	Level of Consciousness* *LAME	L: Level of consciousness	0 = alert (alert and responsive) 1 = not alert (arousable to minor stimulation) 2 = obtunded (arousable only to painful stimulation) 3 = unresponsive (reflex responses or unarousable)
		A: Age? M: Month?	0 = answers both correctly 1 = answers one correctly 2 = answers neither correctly
		E: Executes Commands	0 = performs both tasks correctly 1 = performs one task correctly 2 = performs neither task correctly
E	Eyes - Visual Fields	Visual fields	0 = no visual loss 1 = partial hemianopsia 2 = complete hemianopsia 3 = bilateral hemianopsia
G	Gaze	Gaze	0 = normal 1 = partial gaze palsy 2 = total gaze palsy
P	Palsy of Face	Facial palsy	0 = normal 1 = minor paralysis 2 = partial paralysis 3 = complete paralysis
L	Language	Language	0 = normal 1 = mild aphasia 2 = severe aphasia 3 = mute or global aphasia
E	Each Limb	Motor assessment each arm and each leg	0 = no drift 1 = drifts before 5 sec 2 = falls before 5 sec 3 = no effort against gravity 4 = no movement
A	Ataxia	Ataxia	0 = absent 1 = 1 limb 2 = 2 limbs
S	Sensation	Sensory	0 = normal 1 = mild loss 2 = severe loss
E	Extinction / Inattention	Extinction/inattention	0 = no neglect 1 = partial neglect 2 = complete neglect
D	Dysarthria	Dysarthria	0 = normal 1 = mild 2 = severe

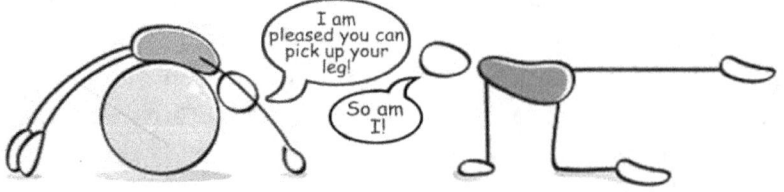

Visual fields are scored on a scale of 0 to 3. Intact vision in all four quadrants receives a normal score of '0'. Partial hemianopia or quadrantanopia receives a score of '1'. Complete hemianopia receives a score of '2'. Bilateral hemianopia (blindness of one side of the visual field in both eyes) or total blindness receives a score of '3'. Neglect (see section 11) is also tested using the technique of double simultaneous stimulation. Visual stimuli are initially presented to each side separately, and then to both sides simultaneously. If vision is extinguished on one side when bilateral, simultaneous visual stimulation is presented, the patient receives a score of '1'.

Facial palsy (Item 4) is tested next. Refer to Table 2 or 3 for scoring. This is accomplished by asking the patient to smile and assessing for an asymmetric smile. The patient is also asked to raise their eyebrows or close their eyes. If the patient is either aphasic or confused, noxious stimuli can be used to elicit a grimace which can be scored for symmetry. A normal symmetric smile or grimace receives a score of '0'. Minor paralysis or asymmetry of the lower face (asymmetric smile or grimace) receives a score of '1'. Partial paralysis (total or near total paralysis) of the lower face receives a score of '2'. Complete paralysis of the upper and lower face receives a score of '3'.

The next items of the NIHSS (Items 5 and 6) examine the motor strength of both arms and legs. Refer to Table 2 or 3 for scoring. This assessment should be performed with each limb independently and should start with the non-paretic arm. During this evaluation, count out loud and use your fingers to encourage patients, especially those who are aphasic. Have the patient extend their arms (palms down) 90° if seated or 45° if supine. Each leg must also be extended at a 30° angle. If either arm (before 10 seconds) or either leg (before 5 seconds) demonstrates drift, the patient is scored positive for drift (score of '1'). It's very important to separate a "drift" from a "dip." A "dip" in the arm or leg is a very small change in arm or leg positioning with an instantaneous correction. This receives no points. However, a "drift" occurs when the patient's arm or leg is lowered to a significant degree. Limb drift that does not hit the bed or other support is scored a '1'. If the arm or leg drifts down to the bed but has effort against gravity, the patient will receive a score of '2'. The patient will receive a score of '3' if the arm or leg drops to the bed but maintains the ability to move side to side with no effort against. A patient unable to move their limb side to side or against gravity (no movement) will receive a score of '4'. Amputated limbs are not scored.

Next, the patient is assessed for limb ataxia (Item 7) which may be indicative of a unilateral cerebellar infarct. Refer to Table 2 or 3 for scoring. Ataxia can be secondary to weakness. It is important to distinguish muscle control and coordination (ataxia) from general weakness. Thus, in order for ataxia to be scored on the NIHSS, it must be out of proportion to weakness. Each limb should be assessed separately by performing finger-nose-finger and heel-shin tests bilaterally. Again, ataxia is scored positive only if present or out of proportion to weakness. Also, ataxia is only scored if present. For example, a patient who cannot understand or is paralyzed would receive no points for ataxia. A patient without ataxia would receive a score of '0'. Ataxia present in one limb would receive a score of '1' and if present in two limbs would receive a score of '2'.

Next, sensation or withdrawal from noxious stimuli (in a nonresponsive patient, i.e. aphasic) is tested in the face, trunk, arms, and legs (Item 8). Refer to Table 2 or 3 for scoring. Sensation is assessed using a sterile safety needle or other sharp object. Testing should always be performed on the skin as clothing can blunt sensation. Testing of the hands and feet should be avoided as pre-existing neuropathy may impair evaluation. Only sensory loss from acute stroke should be scored. Testing is typically performed on each side of the face, the proximal regions of the limbs, and above the wrists and ankles. Scoring for sensation is straightforward with '0' being normal, '2' representing total sensory loss, and '1' being anything between these two values. If the patient is unable to respond verbally, evaluate their face while testing for sensation and look for signs of discomfort.

Sensation is only scored if sensory loss is clearly demonstrated.

By this point, the examiner has likely determined the patient's language capacity yet this section (Item 9) should still be performed for confirmation. Refer to Table 2 or 3 for scoring. In addition, several visual aids are available for this portion of the NIHSS. If necessary, make sure the patient has their glasses before proceeding. Patients can be asked to perform several tasks when assessing language. Typically, naming, repetition, and comprehension are assessed during these tasks. If the patient has no visual deficits, ask them to describe the contents of the famous "cookie jar/dishwashing" picture (Figure 1). This is done by presenting the picture to the patient and asking, "Can you tell me what you see in this picture?" This response allows the examiner to evaluate fluency, naming and inattention to one side of space. As they respond, listen carefully to the patient's articulation and be cognizant of any slurring or difficulty expressing ideas. There are many responses that can be elicited but the primary elements of this picture are (1) the boy is sneaking cookies from the cookie jar while the girl reaches for a cookie, (2) the mother is washing dishes, (3) the boy's stool is unstable or falling, and (4) the sink is overflowing. If the patient speaks slowly but can adequately describe the picture, they receive a normal score. However, the examiner should not coach the patient to notice additional findings within the picture.

FIGURE 1. Image Used with the NIH Stroke Scale

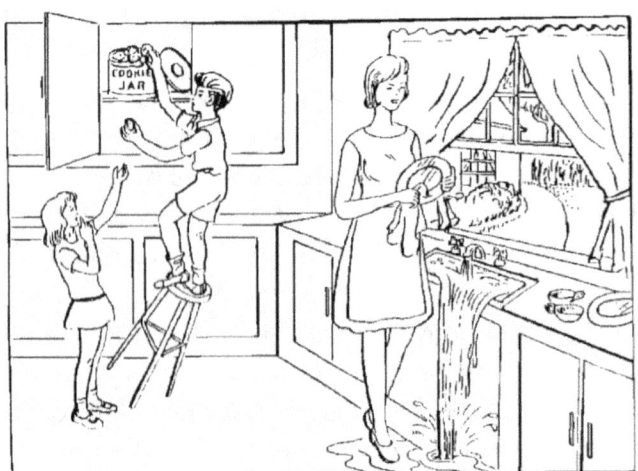

FIGURE 2. Image Used with the NIH Stroke Scale

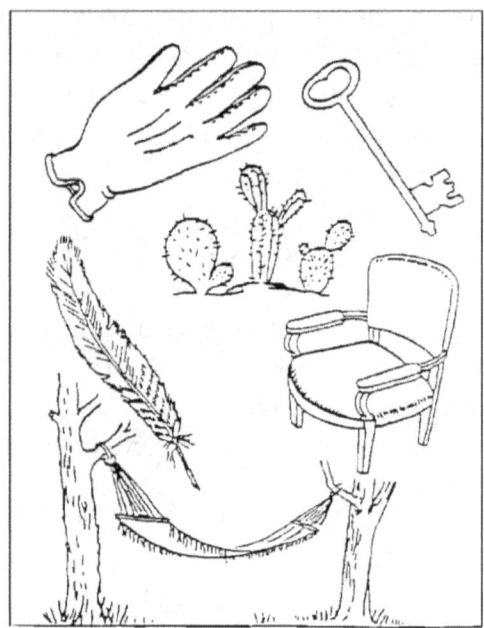

Another method used to evaluate language is identifying objects on cards (Figure 2). This task involves showing the patient drawings of relatively common items and asking them to name specific items. Remember the primary purpose of this task is to assess the patient's ability to use language and speak clearly. Thus, if the patient identifies the "glove" as a "hand", they should be scored without a language deficit. Language can also be evaluated by requesting the patient to read a list of sentences. (Figure 3).

FIGURE 3. Image Used with the NIH Stroke Scale

You know how.

Down to earth.

I got home from work.

Near the table in the dining room.

They heard him speak on the radio last night.

Obviously, these visual aids are of no use if the patient has a severe visual deficit or blindness. In this case, language can be assessed by asking the patient to feel items such as a pen, watch or phone. Language can be further tested by asking the patient what the function of a pen, watch or phone is. Similarly, cultural issues may play a part in language assessment. For example, cacti are not common in all parts of the world. Thus, people who don't live in deserts may have trouble identifying them on naming cards and may perceive them as something else. So long as their answer is reasonable it should be considered correct.

Despite what method of language evaluation is used, this item's scale ranges from 0 to 3. A score of '0' indicates no aphasia with normal fluency and comprehension. A score of '1' indicates mild to moderate aphasia with loss of fluency or comprehension. In this situation, the examiner is able to understand what the patient is trying to convey. A score of '2' represents severe aphasia with extremely limited communication. Here, the examiner is unable to understand what the patient is trying to convey. A score of '3' is indicative of an unresponsive, mute and globally aphasic patient.

Other methods to assess language should also be considered. For example, if the patient has a severe visual deficit or blindness, language can be assessed by asking the patient to feel items such as a pen, watch or phone. Additionally, requesting the patient to write out answers can help discern whether or not they are aphasic as writing should parallel spoken deficits.

Dysarthria (Item 10) or slurred speech is evaluated next by both listening to the patient and having them read from cards (Figure 4). Refer to Table 2 or 3 for scoring. Again, the examiner may feel confident they understand the patient's language deficits at this point of the NIHSS. However, this item should still be examined. During this evaluation, the examiner asks the patient to read a list of words and listens very closely for evidence of slurring while observing the patient's mouth and lips. Here, the examiner should evaluate different motor processes of the mouth required for the production of certain words. For example, the

FIGURE 4. Image Used with the NIH Stroke Scale

```
MAMA
TIP – TOP
FIFTY – FIFTY
THANKS
HUCKLEBERRY
BASEBALL PLAYER
```

word "mama" requires bringing the lips together twice to make this repetitive sound. The word "huckleberry" is a multisyllable word requiring repositioning of the mouth and tongue to produce each syllable and can be used to better elicit dysarthria. Similarly, "baseball player" is a multisyllable term that also requires repositioning of the mouth and tongue for its pronunciation.

Speech that is clearly enunciated and normal in sound receives a score of '0'. Mild to moderate slurring of words that is still understandable receives a score of '1'. Speech that is severely slurred and not understandable in any meaningful way or if the patient is mute or comatose receives a score of '2'. Patients who are intubated or cannot be evaluated (trauma) are scored as UN for untested.

The last section of the NIHSS (Item 11) entitled "Extinction and Inattention" evaluates neglect. Refer to Table 2 or 3 for scoring. Neglect is a symptom in which patients fail to attend to one aspect of their environment or even their own body and tends to occur with severe right MCA territory infarcts. These patients have impaired attention and only attend to items on one side of space (usually the right).

Neglect is assessed by the NIHSS with both visual and tactile stimulation. As discussed above (visual fields, Item 3), assessment of the visual fields is also performed by providing double simultaneous stimulation. Extinction or the inability of the patient to discern stimuli on one side of the body when double simultaneous stimulation is provided results in a score of '1'. Tactile neglect is tested by *double simultaneous stimulation* of the body. Extinction which is typically on the left (usually associated with severe right MCA territory infarcts) with double simultaneous stimulation results in a score of '1'. Note however, the patient must have intact sensation on the left in order discern neglect from a sensation deficit.

Essentially, extinction and inattention (Item 11) determines if double simultaneous stimulation impairs attention on one side of the body whether affecting the visual fields or tactile sensation. Although sensation has already been assessed, additional evaluation should be performed by having the patient close their eyes and then lightly touch the right side, then left, and then both sides of the face together. Assess both the upper and lower extremities in a similar manner. If the patient responds normally to double simultaneous stimulation with both visual and somatosensory stimuli, the patient does not suffer from neglect. If the patient demonstrates neglect on one side of the body with somatosensory stimulation but has no neglect with visual stimuli, this is indicative of mild neglect. The patient receives a score of '1' for this item. Neglect on one side of the body to both visual and somatosensory stimulation indicates severe neglect and the patient will receive a score of '2.' Patients suffering severe neglect may not recognize their own body part (such as the hand) and will also receive a score of '2.' Anosognosia, a form of severe neglect, impairs a person's ability to understand and perceive their own illness. This is also referred to as "lack of insight" and patients unaware of their deficits insist there is nothing wrong with them.

The NIHSS consists of 11 items. Each item is scored and totaled to determine the patient's NIHSS score.[2] An easy way to remember the NIHSS is to recall the mnemonic '**LEG PLEASED**™' (Table 3). This may sound lame, but **LAME** is also the mnemonic to recall the components of the level of consciousness section of the NIHSS (Table 3). Realize that many experts within this field stress that it is extremely important to perform the NIHSS beginning with item 1 and moving through the assessment to item number 11. However, the purpose of this mnemonic is to simply remember the components of the NIHSS.

Abbreviated NIHSS tables and phone applications are also very helpful (Table 4). The different categories of the NIHSS may overlap. It can be difficult to discern neglect versus a visual field cut, or ataxia from motor weakness. For these reasons, training and certification of the practitioner conducting the NIHSS are encouraged.[3] Such training is readily available (NIHSS.com or NIHStrokeScale.org).

TABLE 4. Abbreviated National Institutes of Health Stroke Scale (NIHSS)

Score	Item
	Abbreviated NIH Stroke Scale
	1. Level of consciousness
0 - 3	A. Alertness
0 - 2	B. Orientation
0 - 2	C. Follows command
0 - 2	2. Best gaze
0 - 2	3. Visual fields
0 - 2	4. Facial palsy
	5. Motor function (arm)
0 - 4	A. Right
0 - 4	B. Left
	6. Motor function (leg)
0 - 4	A. Right
0 - 4	B. Left
0 - 2	7. Limb ataxia
0 - 2	8. Sensory
0 - 3	9. Language (aphasia)
0 - 2	10. Dysarthria (articulation)
0 - 2	11. Neglect

20.3 NIHSS Utility

The NIHSS serves several important functions. First, it allows a baseline stroke severity to be determined in an AIS patient. A normal exam has a score of zero, with the maximal score of 42 signifying a severe stroke. A score of 1-4 is indicative of a mild stroke, 5-15 is considered a moderate stroke, 15-20 is a moderate to severe stroke, and 21-42 indicates severe stroke (Table 5). Realize that these NIHSS score ranges are not exact. For example, one definition of mild stroke (as will be discussed later) is an NIHSS score ≤ 5. Instead, these categories provide a gestalt of stroke severity but the NIHSS score by itself should never be a determinant to either administer or not administer IV TPA.

TABLE 5. National Institutes of Health Stroke Scale (NIHSS) and Stroke Severity

Stroke Severity	Score
No Stroke Symptoms	0
Minor Stroke	1-4
Moderate Stroke	5-15
Moderate to Severe Stroke	16-20
Severe Stroke	21-42

The NIHSS Stroke Scale is a tool used by healthcare providers to objectively quantify and succinctly communicate the impairment caused by a stroke.

While the use of the NIHSS score by itself to manage IV TPA administration is discouraged, the NIHSS score in conjunction with other factors can be utilized to manage stroke. For example, the risk of intracerebral hemorrhage rises with increasing stroke severity as evaluated by the NIHSS. The risk of intracerebral hemorrhage following the administration of IV TPA varies from 2% (NIHSS < 6) to 17% (NIHSS >20). Furthermore, an NIHSS of ≥ 9 in the 0 to 3-hour window or an NIHSS > 7 in the 3 to 6-hour window is a predictor of large vessel occlusion (LVO) (Table 6).[4] However, as will be discussed in greater detail in subsequent chapters, suspected LVO requires image confirmation. This is because LVO AIS patients may have a low NIHSS score.[5] The NIHSS also serves as a useful predictor of three-month outcomes. In addition, examining a stroke patient using the NIHSS allows the examiner to track changes in stroke severity and provides a standardized means for clear communication of stroke severity between caregivers.

TABLE 6. NIHHS Predictors of Large Vessel Occlusion (LVO)

NIHSS	Hours Since Onset
≥ 9	0-3
> 7	3-6

20.4 NIHSS Limitations

The NIHSS is not without limitations. For example, the NIHSS disproportionately evaluates language function over sensory function. For this reason, left MCA infarcts average 4 points higher than right MCA infarcts when evaluated by the NIHSS. The NIHSS also disproportionately evaluates the posterior circulation, with minimal evaluation of brainstem and cerebellar function. This means the NIHSS underestimates the severity of non-dominant hemisphere and posterior circulation stroke. Thus, these strokes may have a worse outcome than what a low-scoring NIHSS may suggest. Despite these limitations, the NIHSS is utilized in virtually every stroke center.

One of the largest concerns regarding the NIHSS is that patients with a low NIHSS may still have an LVO.[5] In fact, a recent study demonstrated LVO AIS patients can have a low NIHSS score.[6] This study further stresses the importance of emergent imaging (CTA and/or CTP) in addition to clinical examination in the evaluation of AIS patients. Simply put, the NIHSS cannot reliably exclude an LVO or distinguish threatened but still recoverable brain tissue (ischemic penumbra) from a completed stroke (core infarct).

20.5 Conclusion

The NIHSS is an excellent clinical tool for the evaluation of AIS. To recall the NIHSS, remember the mnemonic '**LEG PLEASED**™' (Table 3). Many authorities consider the NIHSS the most efficient manner to assess patients with AIS.[7] The NIHSS can quantify the degree of ischemic stroke, facilitate communication, and aid in acute stroke intervention. While the NIHSS is routinely utilized for the evaluation of AIS, it is not without its limitations. Despite these constraints, the NIHSS is still an excellent tool to quantify stroke and is employed by virtually every stroke center for this purpose.

Abbreviations list

AIS, acute ischemic stroke; CTA, computed tomography angiography; CTP, CT perfusion; LOC, level of consciousness; LVO, large vessel occlusion; MCA, middle cerebral artery; NIHSS, National Institutes of Health Stroke Scale.

References

1. Powers WJ, Rabinstein AA, Ackerson T, Adeoye OM, Bambakidis NC, Becker K, Biller J, Brown M, Demaerschalk BM, Hoh B, et al. (2018). Guidelines for the Early Management of Patients With Acute Ischemic Stroke: A Guideline for Healthcare Professionals From the American Heart Association/American Stroke Association. *Stroke,* Jan 24, Epub 2018 Jan 24.
2. NIH Stroke Scale Training, Part 2. Basic Instruction. Department of Health and Human Services, National Institute of Neurological Disorders and Stroke. The National Institute of Neurological Disorders and Stroke (NINDS) Version 2.0.
3. Summers D, Leonard A, Wentworth D, Saver JL, Simpson J, Spilker JA, et al. (2009). American Heart Association Council on Cardiovascular Nursing and the Stroke Council. Comprehensive overview of nursing and interdisciplinary care of the acute ischemic stroke patient: a scientific statement from the American Heart Association. *Stroke,* 40, 2911–44.
4. Heldner MR, Zubler C, Mattle HP, et al. (2013). National Institutes of Health stroke scale score and vessel occlusion in 2152 patients with acute ischemic stroke. *Stroke,* 44(4), 1153–57.
5. Fink JN, Selim MH, Kumar S, Silver B, Linfante I, Caplan LR. (2002). Is the association of national institutes of health stroke scale scores and acute magnetic resonance imaging stroke volume equal for patients with right- and left-hemisphere ischemic stroke? *Stroke,* 33, 954-58.
6. Kim JT, Park MS, Chang J, Lee JS, Choi KH, Cho KH. (2013). Proximal arterial occlusion in acute ischemic stroke with low NIHSS scores should not be considered as mild stroke. *PLoS One,* 8(8), e70996.
7. Spilker J, Kongable G, Barch C, Braimah J, Brattina P, Daley S, et al. (1997). Using the NIH Stroke Scale to assess stroke patients. The NINDS rt-PA Stroke Study Group. *J Neurosci Nurs,* 29, 384-92.

Chapter 21

Stroke Imaging

21.1 Introduction

Throughout this book, neuroimaging related to acute ischemic stroke (AIS) has been discussed. Neuroimaging is a necessary component in the diagnosis and treatment of AIS.[1] This is because only neuroimaging can distinguish between normal brain tissue, threatened ischemic penumbra, and irreparably damaged core infarct. Salvageable brain tissue or ischemic penumbra cannot be determined by a clinical exam. The ability to identify and distinguish ischemic penumbra from core infarct is one of the major goals of modern acute stroke intervention. The effective treatment of AIS requires both a greater understanding of existing neuroimaging and the implementation of more advanced neuroimaging techniques.

Image confirmation is required for the diagnosis and treatment of AIS. While the decision whether to give IV TPA may be guided by clinical exam, it is regulated by CT findings. Clinical exam alone cannot differentiate ischemic from hemorrhagic infarct. Similarly, large vessel occlusion (LVO), core infarct size, or ischemic penumbra cannot be determined by a clinical exam. By verifying clot location and collateral status, CTA can determine AIS diagnosis and guide its management. Additionally, CT perfusion (CTP) or CTA (dual or multiphase) can distinguish between potentially salvageable brain tissue at risk (ischemic penumbra) and irreparably damaged core infarct.

Imaging is a balance between anatomic knowledge and interpretive skills. Only when the normal appearance of anatomic structures is understood can interpretive skills determine the presence of an abnormality. To be able to interpret a stroke on brain CT, one must understand normal neuroanatomy. Is there an MCA stroke? Is there an MCA occlusion? Is there a basilar artery occlusion? We can only answer these questions by knowing the normal anatomy of these structures. Interpretive conclusions based on anatomic knowledge is essential for stroke diagnosis and treatment.

The only FDA-approved treatment options for AIS are **IV TPA** and **endovascular treatment (EVT)**. The aim of both treatment options is to reestablish blood flow to areas of the brain that are underperfused (threatened) but still contain salvageable brain tissue (ischemic penumbra). While a noncontrast brain CT can confirm IV TPA eligibility, more information is generally required to evaluate EVT candidacy. This chapter will consist of two segments to follow in a logical progression. The first portion will discuss IV TPA and the necessary imaging (noncontrast brain CT) surrounding its use. The second part will discuss the relationship between neuroimaging and EVT. Neuroimaging of brain tissue and not arbitrary time points determine EVT candidacy. This chapter will also discuss terms such as *core infarct, ischemic penumbra, collateral circulation, CT perfusion (CTP), multiphase CTA* and *dual-phase CTA*. Please familiarize yourself with these terms and concepts and urge your colleagues to do the same. Efficient stroke care requires effective communication which necessitates the competent understanding of relevant terminology.

In 1996, the FDA approved IV TPA for AIS that presented within three hours of symptom onset. ECASS III subsequently demonstrated the benefit of IV TPA for up to 4.5 hours from symptom onset. Details pertaining to the use of IV TPA including inclusion and exclusion criteria will be discussed in Chapter 23 (IV TPA). Prior to the administration of IV TPA, a noncontrast brain CT scan must demonstrate neither hemorrhage nor infarct (hypodensity) greater than one third the MCA territory. This is because the incidence of hemorrhagic complications significantly increases when infarct size is greater than one-third the MCA territory. In fact, brain CT is the only imaging study that is usually performed before the administration of IV TPA. This stems from the NINDS trial performed over 20 years ago which only used brain CT as a neuroimaging protocol to determine IV TPA administration.[2] Since that time, however, a paradigm shift which can greatly improve functional outcome in AIS patients has occurred in stroke imaging. Isn't it time to adopt newer imaging protocols proven to improve AIS outcome?

21.2 Brain CT and Early Ischemic Changes

Even if imaging protocols were expanded to include more than noncontrast brain CT, it is still the initial step and remains a mandatory study. In addition to its utilization for stroke, brain CT is also utilized to exclude stroke mimics such as neoplasm. Since a brain CT is the first-line imaging modality for the evaluation of AIS, we as healthcare providers must do an outstanding job interpreting it. Realize that a brain CT can look completely normal if no imaging findings related to stroke have occurred. However, imaging findings related to stroke often occur but are not properly identified. In fact, about one-third of brain CTs that were initially read as having no early ischemic changes (EICs) in the NINDS trial were subsequently reanalyzed and determined to have EICs. Fortunately, newer and more reliable methods have been devised to interpret brain CTs since this trial.

Proper interpretation of brain CTs relies on the ability to identify imaging characteristics associated with stroke. However, before this process can be discussed, confusing issues related to these imaging findings must be addressed and clarified. First, the use of the term "EICs" is common parlance in stroke-related imaging vocabulary. However, the definition of EICs can vary in the literature. Different definitions result in different image interpretations which can result in different methods of treatment. Second, EICs can be difficult to interpret, yielding differences in interpretation among different radiologists.[3,4]

The Alberta Stroke Program Early CT Score (ASPECTS) was one of the first methods used to address EICs.[5] The ASPECTS authors defined EICs as "focal swelling or parenchymal hypoattenuation." Parenchymal hypoattenuation was further defined as "abnormally decreased attenuation brain structures relative to attenuation of other parts of the same structures or of the contralateral hemisphere." They also defined focal brain swelling or mass effect as "any focal narrowing of the CSF space due to compression by adjacent structures, such as effacement of cortical sulci or ventricular compression." In short, the ASPECTS study placed both brain tissue swelling and hypodensity into one category—EICs.

However, since the publication of ASPECTS, the stroke-related literature has demonstrated that while both parenchymal hypoattenuation or focal swelling and mass effect have been described as EICs, they each have different connotations. It is now recognized that focal swelling or mass effect represents a separate process that is distinct from parenchymal hypoattenuation. Cortical swelling by itself is representative of threatened brain tissue or salvageable ischemic penumbra (Figure 1).[6,7] Hypodense tissue, and not tissue swelling, is representative of irreversibly damaged brain tissue or core infarct (Figure 2).[8,9] Again, isodense swelling represents threatened brain tissue (ischemic penumbra) while parenchymal hypodensity represents irreparably damaged core infarct (Box 1).[10]

BOX 1. Imaging Characteristic of Penumbra Versus Core

Puffy = Penumbra
HypoDense Brain = Dead Core

Recent recommendations and guidelines by the American Heart Association and American Stroke Association (AHA/ASA) have also discussed these imaging criteria. The 2018 AHA/ASA guidelines and 2015 AHA/ASA scientific rationale paper have classified focal brain swelling and parenchymal (brain tissue) hypodensity as two separate processes. Isodense brain swelling, mass effect, or loss of gray-white matter junction represent threatened brain tissue or ischemic penumbra. Parenchymal hypodensity, on the other hand, is now considered representative of irreparably damaged brain tissue or core infarct. The presence of parenchymal hypodensity greater than one third the MCA territory discourages the use of intravenous thrombolysis. There is confounding evidence regarding the use of IV TPA and early ischemic changes related to stroke. Extensive *brain tissue hypodensity* correlates with poor outcome and higher bleeding risk in thrombolytic trials and prospective studies.[8,11]

However, other studies suggest no definitive evidence that IV TPA is ineffective or harmful when there are extensive *early ischemic changes*.[12] These baffling results from different researchers emanate from the failure to distinguish isodense brain tissue swelling (representative of ischemic penumbra) from hypodense brain tissue (representative of core infarct).[13] Unfortunately, the stroke literature continues to categorize both isodense and hypodense brain tissue as EICs. Thus, instead of using the term *EICs* to describe acute ischemic changes on brain CT, one should **only use the terms *isodense* or *hypodense* brain tissue**.

FIGURE 1. Parenchymal Swelling Representing Ischemic Penumbra

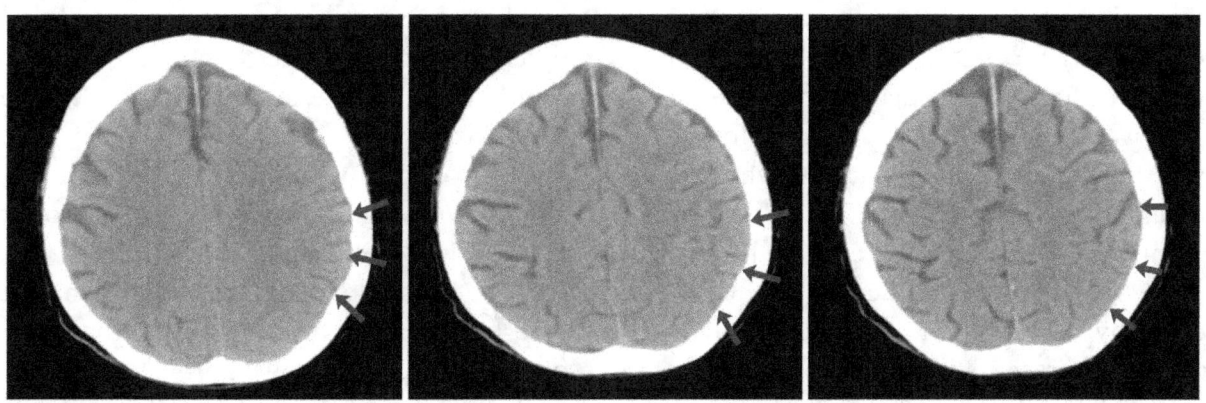

Notice the gyri of the left hemisphere (arrows) are swollen when compared to the right. However, this brain tissue is isodense consistent with ischemic penumbra and not hypodense which would indicate core infarct.

FIGURE 2. Noncontrast Brain CT: Hypodensity > One Third the Right MCA Territory

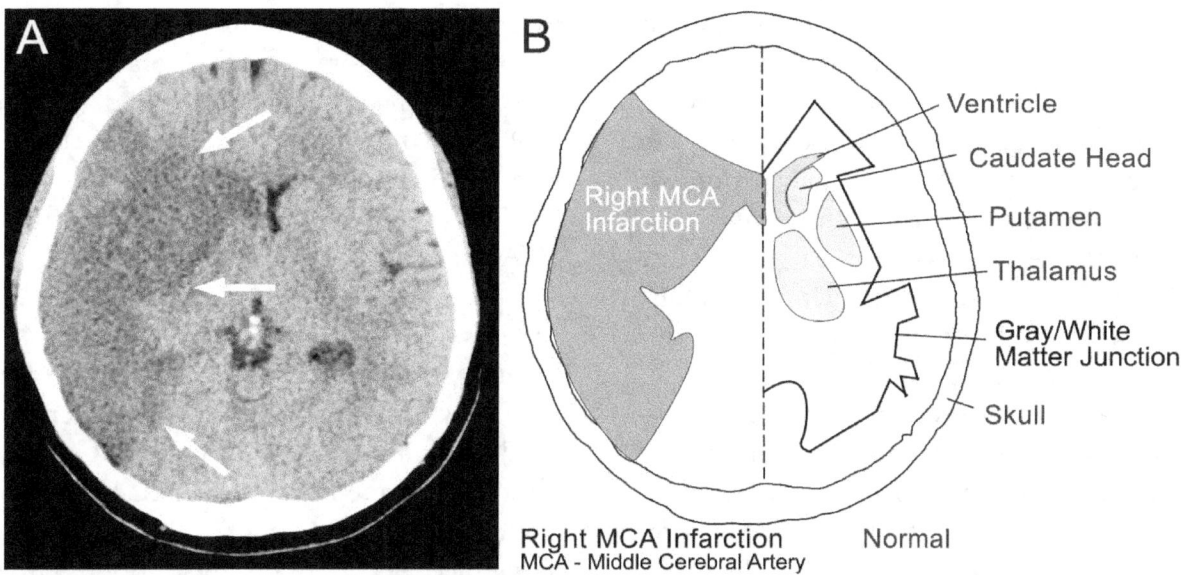

(A) Noncontrast brain CT demonstrating hypodense brain tissue (arrows) consistent with right MCA core infarct. (B) Diagram of right MCA infarct and involved structures.

Both the earlier 2013 and new 2018 AHA/ASA guidelines recommend IV TPA even with the presence of EICs (brain swelling) on CT but also cautioned that hypodensity on CT can increase the risk of intracranial hemorrhage.[14] This makes sense because isodense brain tissue (brain tissue swelling, mass effect, or loss of gray-white matter junction) is suggestive of ischemic penumbra. Recall that parenchymal hypodensity represents core infarct. Recommendations from the recent 2018 AHA/ASA guidelines state, "There remains insufficient evidence to identify a threshold of acute CT hypoattenuation severity or extent that affects treatment response to IV alteplase. The extent severity of acute hypoattenuation or early ischemic changes should not be used as a criterion to withhold therapy for such patients who otherwise qualify." Nevertheless, immediately after this statement, the very next sentence states, "However, administering IV alteplase to patients whose CT brain imaging exhibits extensive regions of clear hypoattenuation is **not recommended**. These patients have a poor prognosis despite IV alteplase and severe hypoattenuation defined as **obvious hypodensity represents irreversible injury**."

So what does all this really mean? It seems as if the 2018 AHA/ASA guideline recommendations may be lumping hypodense brain tissue and early ischemic changes together when they state, "The extent severity of acute hypo-attenuation or early ischemic changes should not be used as a criterion to withhold therapy for such patients who otherwise qualify." I somewhat agree with this statement because swollen, isodense brain tissue represents salvageable ischemic penumbra whereas hypodense brain tissue represents irreparably damaged core infarct. If early ischemic changes refer to isodense and swollen brain tissue (which represent salvageable ischemic penumbra), then their presence should not be used as criteria to withhold thrombolytic therapy. However, hypodense brain tissue represents irreparably damaged core infarct, and for this reason, I agree with the guidelines when they state, "However administering IV alteplase to patients whose CT brain imaging exhibits extensive regions of clear hypoattenuation is **not recommended**. These patients have a poor prognosis despite IV alteplase and severe hypoattenuation defined as obvious hypodensity represents irreversible injury." Thus, IV TPA administration is **not recommended** when extensive regions of clear hypoattenuation are present on noncontrast brain CT. This point will be readdressed when IV TPA restrictions are discussed in Chapter 23 (IV TPA). Again, hypodense brain tissue that represents more than one-third of the MCA territory is an increased risk for symptomatic intracranial hemorrhage and represents irreversible injury (core infarct). This confusion can be eliminated by not categorizing both isodense and hypodense brain tissue as EICs. Furthermore, instead of using the term EICs to describe acute ischemic changes on brain CT, one should **only use the terms *isodense* or *hypodense* brain tissue**.

The parenchymal hypodensity *more than one-third of the MCA territory rule* was introduced by ECASS I.[15] There is an increased risk for symptomatic intracranial hemorrhage when parenchymal hypodensity involves more than one-third of the MCA territory (Figure 3).[16] A subsequent analysis of this study determined imaging findings were an important predictor of IV TPA success.[17] Both isodense and hypodense brain tissue continue to be described as EICs in stroke literature. Please be certain to differentiate isodense brain tissue (ischemic penumbra) from parenchymal hypodensities (core infarct). A brain CT is not the only neuroimaging study that can determine if IV TPA is warranted. In fact, many neuroimaging techniques have far surpassed this popular diagnostic tool. For example, information from brain CTA studies can increase the diagnostic certainty and likelihood of treatment with IV TPA in AIS patients.[18]

It is essential to identify parenchymal hypodensity and determine if it is greater than one third the middle cerebral artery (MCA) territory. If more than one-third of the MCA territory is infarcted (hypodense tissue) or if there is an intracerebral bleed, IV TPA administration is either "not recommended" or "contraindicated." However, reliably determining if the extent of parenchymal hypodensity (core infarct) is greater than one third the MCA territory is often complicated. Even experienced stroke physicians and radiologists have difficulty with this.[17] A better method to reliably recognize and quantitate parenchymal hypodensity is required.

21.3 ASPECTS

One reliable method to help improve brain CT interpretation is the *Alberta Stroke Program Early CT Score (ASPECTS)*. ASPECTS is a 10-point quantitative topographic CT scan score developed to increase reader reliability and thus reduce interobserver variability (Figure 3). ASPECT scoring accomplishes this by evaluating two levels of the brain predominantly supplied by the MCA. The first is the level of the basal ganglia and the second is the supraganglionic level. The level of the basal ganglia is referred to as the *ganglionic level* and includes assessing the caudate head, internal capsule, the lentiform nucleus, insular cortex, and cortical regions supplied by the middle cerebral artery at this level. The *supraganglionic level* evaluates three cortical regions supplied by the middle cerebral artery at that level.

At the ganglionic level, seven structures are assessed: the caudate head, the internal capsule, the lentiform nucleus, the insular cortex and M1, M2, and M3 (Figure 3). M1, M2, and M3 represent different cortical regions supplied by the middle cerebral artery at the level of the basal ganglia. The most anteriorly located cortical region is denoted M1. Just lateral to the insular cortex is M2 and posterior to M2 is M3 (Figure 3). Do not confuse these cortical regions with the segmental anatomy of the MCA which includes the M1, M2, M3, and M4 segments (Figure 4). At the supraganglionic level, there are only three structures: M4, M5, and M6 (Figure 3). Again, just like at the ganglionic level, M4, M5, and M6 represent cortical regions supplied by the middle cerebral artery. M4 represents the most anterior cortical region, M5 is located in the middle, and M6 represents the most posterior cortical region.

FIGURE 3. ASPECTS: Ganglionic and Supraganglionic Levels

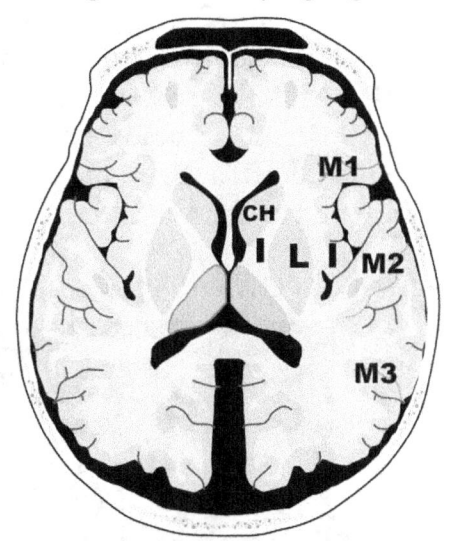
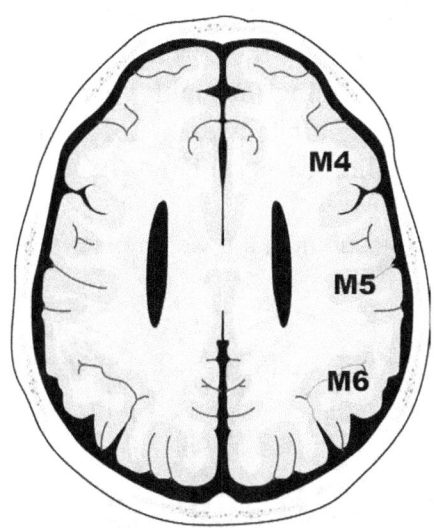

GANGLIONIC LEVEL
- CH: Caudate Head
- I: Internal Capsule
- L: Lentiform Nucleus
- I: Insular Cortex
- M1: Inferior Anterior MCA Territory
- M2: Inferior Middle MCA Territory
- M3: Inferior Posterior MCA Territory

SUPRAGANGLIONIC LEVEL
- M4: Superior Anterior MCA Territory
- M5: Superior Middle MCA Territory
- M6: Superior Posterior MCA Territory

FIGURE 4. The Four Segments of the Middle Cerebral Artery

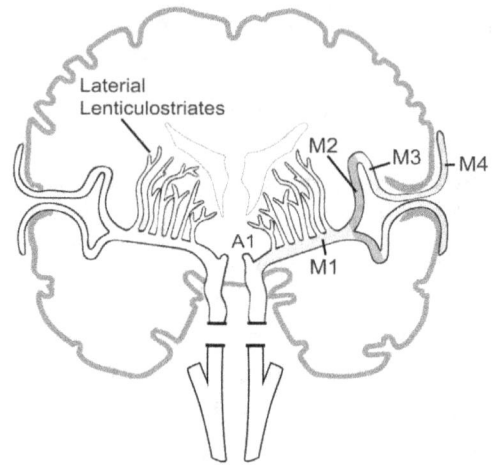

How does one distinguish the ganglionic level from the supraganglionic level? To identify the ganglionic level, look for the frontal horns of the lateral ventricle which look like a pair of rabbit ears (Figure 5). Just lateral to them is the caudate head and lateral to the caudate head is the anterior limb of the internal capsule. Lateral to this is the lentiform nucleus and lateral to the lentiform nucleus is the insular cortex. Lateral to the insular cortex is the M2 region of the cortex. Anterior to the M2 region of the cortex is the M1 region and posterior to the M2 region of the cortex is the M3 region. So, by simply finding the "rabbit ears" on a brain CT, you can identify all seven ASPECTS structures at the ganglionic level (Figure 6).

FIGURE 5. ASPECTS: Determining the Ganglionic Level

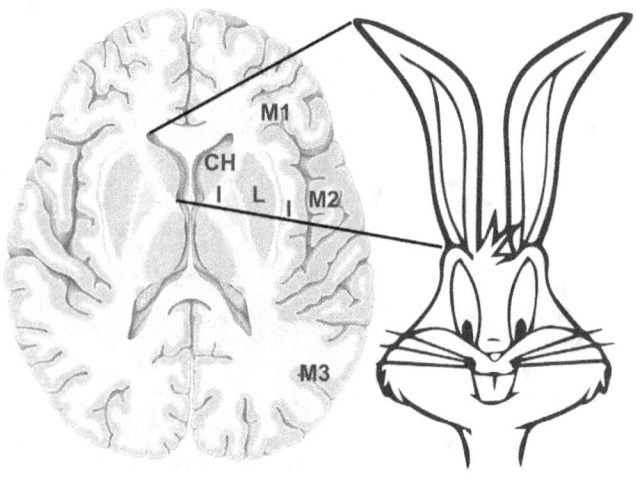

CH - Caudate Head; I - Internal Capsule; L - Lentiform Nucleus; I - Insular Cortex; M1 - Anterior MCA Cortex, M2 - MCA Cortex Lateral to the Insular Cortex; M3 - Posterior MCA Cortex

FIGURE 6. ASPECTS: The Ganglionic Level

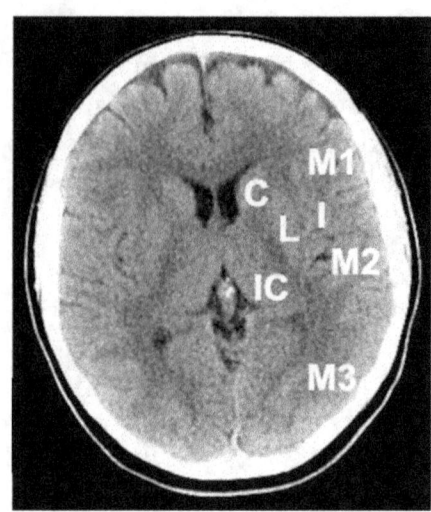

The identification of the supraganglionic level is even easier—just look for the bodies of both lateral ventricles (Figure 7). By looking at the cortex lateral to the body of the lateral ventricle and traveling anterior to posterior, M4, M5, and M6 are identified. Given that it is not difficult to identify all 10 structures utilizing ASPECTS plus the fact that most of the 2015 EVT trials used ASPECTS, why don't more physicians use ASPECTS? One reason is that many people find it difficult to recall all 10 ASPECTS structures. An easy way to remember these structures is with the mnemonic 'CHILI-6™' (Table 1). In this mnemonic, 'CH' stands for caudate head, 'I' for internal capsule, 'L' for lentiform nucleus, the second 'I' for insular cortex, and '6' for M1-M6.

FIGURE 7. ASPECTS: The Supraganglionic Level

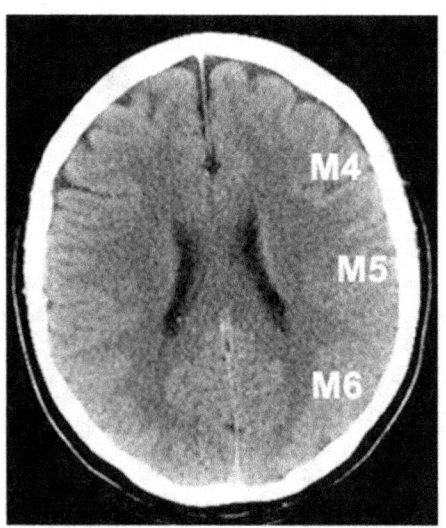

TABLE 1. ASPECTS Mnemonic: **CHILI-6**™

CH	Caudate Head
I	Internal Capsule
L	Lentiform Nucleus
I	Insular Cortex
6	M1 - M6 (GL and SGL)

GL - Ganglionic Level; SGL - Supraganglionic Level

ASPECTS is important for several reasons. First, it increases the ability to detect stroke on noncontrast brain CT. Second, it reduces interobserver variability. These factors allow ASPECTS to assist in the management of stroke. For example, an ASPECTS value ≤7 increases the risk of symptomatic intracerebral hemorrhage by 14 times versus an ASPECTS value > 7.[11] Also, per the most recent American Heart Association/American Stroke Association (AHA/ASA) guidelines for EVT (as will be discussed in greater detail in Chapter 25, Endovascular Treatment), patients with an ASPECTS of ≥ 6 (in conjunction with other criteria) are eligible for EVT. Conversely, those with ASPECTS ≤ 5 are not.

Two important points regarding these criteria must be considered. First, these are not exclusionary criteria and exceptions can always be made. Second, these criteria are relevant to EVT and not IV TPA AIS treatment. However, an argument could be made that an ASPECT score of 5 corresponds to approximately a one-third the middle cerebral artery distribution infarct. So what is ASPECTS really telling us? Every hypodense ASPECT structure is irreparably damaged by stroke and their totality determines core infarct size. Higher ASPECTS values indicate smaller core infarct and better patient prognosis whereas lower ASPECTS values are indicative of larger core infarct and a worse prognosis (Table 2).

The size of irreparably damaged brain tissue (core infarct) is important for two major reasons. First, larger core infarcts have a higher risk of hemorrhage, especially when given IV TPA. For this reason, the administration of IV TPA is not recommended in patients with hypodense parenchyma greater than one third the MCA distribution. Incidentally, an ASPECTS value of 4-6 is equivalent to the involvement of one-third of the MCA territory.[19] Second, as will be discussed later, the most important determinant for potential EVT is core infarct size. Smaller core infarcts with ASPECTS ranging from 6-10 are ideal candidates for EVT (ASPECTS values are indirectly related to core size: ↑ASPECTS=↓ CORE). However larger core infarcts with ASPECTS from 0-5 are typically poor EVT candidates (ASPECTS values are indirectly related to core size: ↓ASPECTS = ↑ CORE) (Table 2). The better way to remember this is that ASPECTS is directly related to EVT candidacy, with higher ASPECT scores favoring EVT and lower scores discouraging it. Most of the published EVT trials performed in 2015 utilized ASPECTS to determine EVT candidacy (Table 3).

TABLE 2. ASPECTS is Indirectly Related to Core Size

↑ CORE = ↓ ASPECTS Value = ↓ EVT Candidacy
↓ CORE = ↑ ASPECTS Value = ↑ EVT Candidacy

TABLE 3. ASPECTS and 2015 EVT Randomized Controlled Trials (RCT)

RCT	Lowest ASPECTS
MR CLEAN	N/A
ESCAPE	6
EXTEND-IA	N/A
SWIFT PRIME	6
REVASCAT	7 (CT)

RCT - Randomized Controlled Trial

21.4 Hyperdense Arterial Signs

Acute thrombus in an intracranial vessel may appear as an area of increased density on a noncontrast brain CT. There are three important vascular signs related to AIS that can be visualized on noncontrast brain CT. These are the **hyperdense MCA sign**, the **MCA dot sign**, and the **hyperdense basilar artery sign**. Recall the segmental anatomy of the middle cerebral artery (Figure 4).

The first segment of the MCA or horizontal segment is called the "M1" segment. When occluded, this can become hyperdense on noncontrast brain CT (Figure 8). Because this structure is parallel to an axial brain CT image, a *hyperdense MCA sign* has linear morphology. The next segment is called the "M2" segment, which is perpendicular to an axial sectioned brain CT. For this reason, the *MCA dot sign* is round like a dot in its morphology (Figure 9). Recall also that the basilar artery runs perpendicular to an axial oriented brain CT. Because of this, a *hyperdense basilar artery sign* will also be round in configuration (Figure 10). These vessels must be denser (hyperdense) than other cerebral vessels to be considered occluded. Since these signs (the hyperdense MCA sign, the MCA dot sign, and the hyperdense basilar artery sign) involve relatively large vessels (M1, M2 segments, and basilar artery, respectively), these are endovascular candidates unless proven otherwise. This is because IV TPA, by itself, is relatively ineffective in treating proximal LVOs.

FIGURE 8. Hyperdense MCA Sign

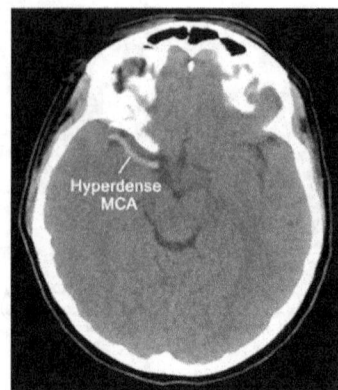

FIGURE 9. MCA Dot Sign

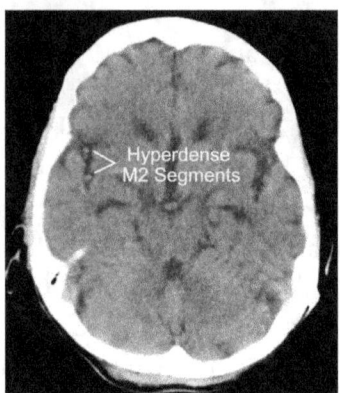

FIGURE 10. Hyperdense Basilar Artery Sign

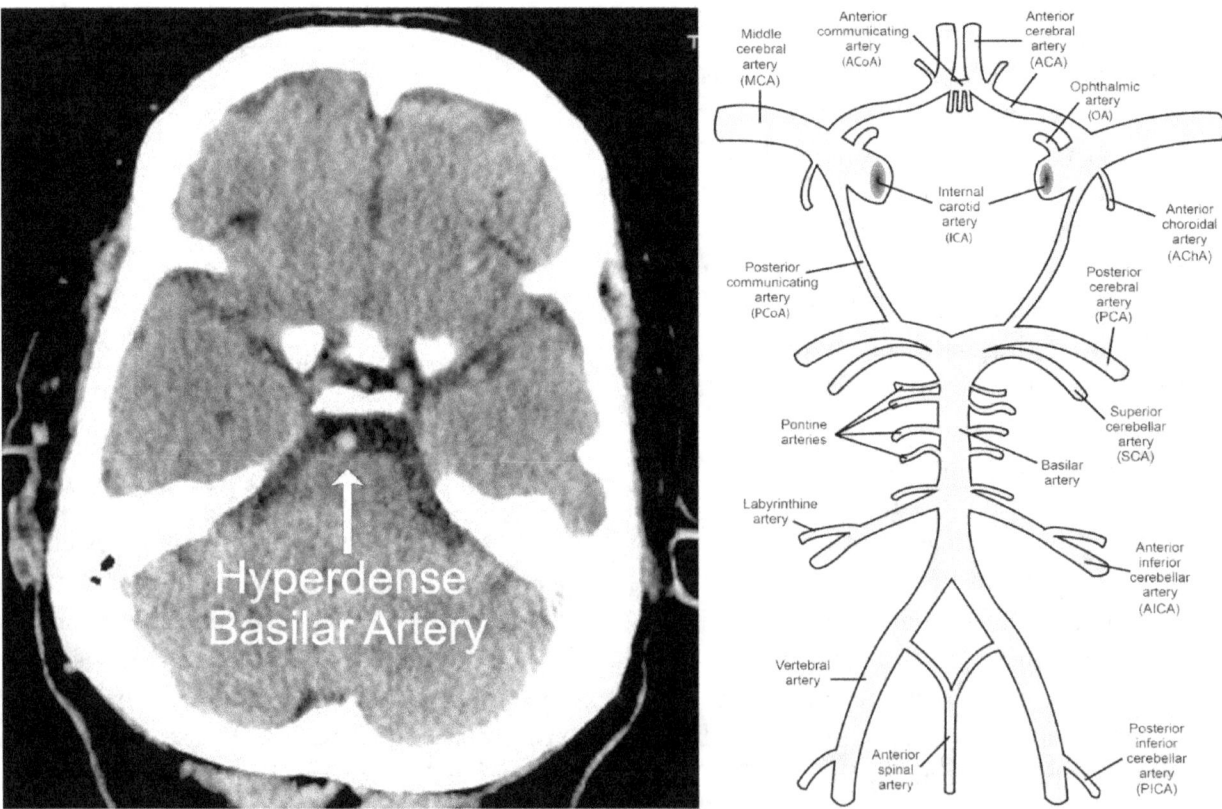

21.5 Neuroimaging and Endovascular Treatment (EVT) Candidacy

Eleven percent of ischemic stroke is caused by LVO which can involve the internal carotid artery, the proximal MCA, the proximal ACA, or the vertebral or basilar arteries. An easy way to remember the large vessels of the brain is with the mnemonic 'BAMBI' (Table 4). It is important to identify LVO because it accounts for nearly all AIS deaths, 90% of AIS cost, and 80% of functional disability. The treatment algorithm for LVO is relatively straightforward. LVO patients are EVT candidates provided they do not have an intracerebral hemorrhage or a significant core infarct and still have salvageable ischemic penumbra (Figure 11).

The most important criterion in the determination of EVT candidacy is **core infarct size** (irreversibly damaged brain tissue) (Figure 12). This is the single most important prognostic indicator of long-term outcome in patients with AIS. Patients with a core infarct (irreversibly damaged brain tissue) of greater than 70 cc in the anterior circulation or one that involves the midbrain bilaterally in the posterior circulation will likely have a poor prognosis regardless of therapeutic intervention. Therefore, it is essential to identify core infarct (irreparably damaged brain tissue) rapidly and reliably.

The best indicator of irreversibly damaged brain tissue or core infarct is diffusion MRI. However, CT imaging requires shorter scanning times and is usually more accessible in the emergency setting compared to MRI. In addition, most EVT trials utilized and proved the efficiency of CT evaluation for stroke diagnosis and treatment. Also, because of the overwhelming speed requirement for AIS treatment, it is unlikely that most hospitals can perform MRI in a timely fashion. For these reasons, this discussion will be limited to the use of CT imaging for both the determination of core infarct (irreparably damaged brain tissue) and ischemic penumbra (threatened but still salvageable brain tissue).

TABLE 4. Large Vessels of the Brain: **BAMBI**

B	Basilar Artery
A	Anterior Cerebral Artery
M	Middle Cerebral Artery
B	Both Vertebral Arteries
I	Internal Carotid Artery

FIGURE 11. Endovascular Treatment (EVT) Acute Ischemic Stroke (AIS) Algorithm

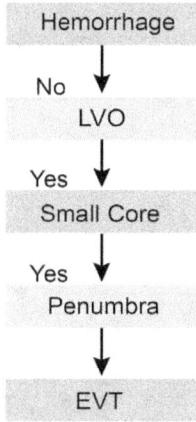

FIGURE 12. Core Infarct

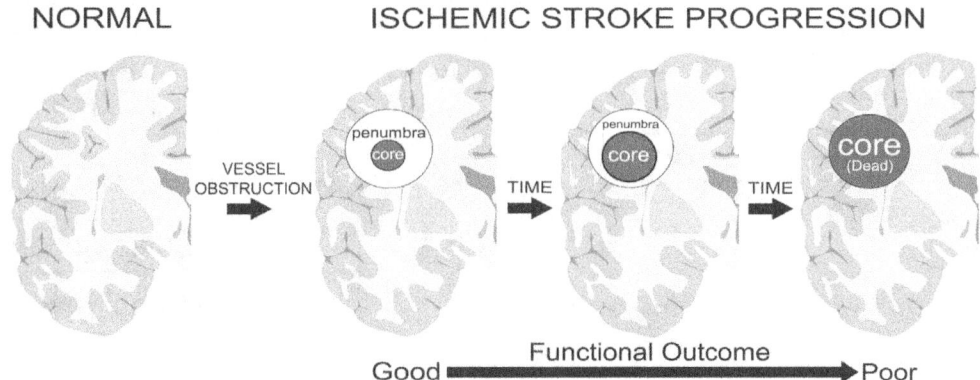

CT-based markers for core infarct include low cerebral blood volume on CTP, poor collaterals on multiphase or dual phase CTA, or hypodense parenchyma on a noncontrast brain CT. Once the size of a core infarct has been established, the next step is to determine if there is salvageable brain tissue. That is, are there regions of the brain that are underperfused but still viable? These hypoperfused regions are threatened by an arterial occlusion and will be irreparably damaged if the occluded vessel is not recanalized (Figure 12). So how is the presence of ischemic penumbra or core infarct determined? Recall that endovascular reperfusion treatment has three principal questions that must be answered (Figure 13). First, is there an LVO? If there is an LVO, how large is the core infarct (the region of irreversibly injured brain tissue)? Finally, if there's a small core infarct, are there regions of the brain that are currently being threatened but not yet irreparably damaged by underperfusion (ischemic penumbra)? In short, an LVO, small core infarct, and significant ischemic penumbra are required for EVT candidacy.

FIGURE 13. Three Determinants Related to EVT Candidacy

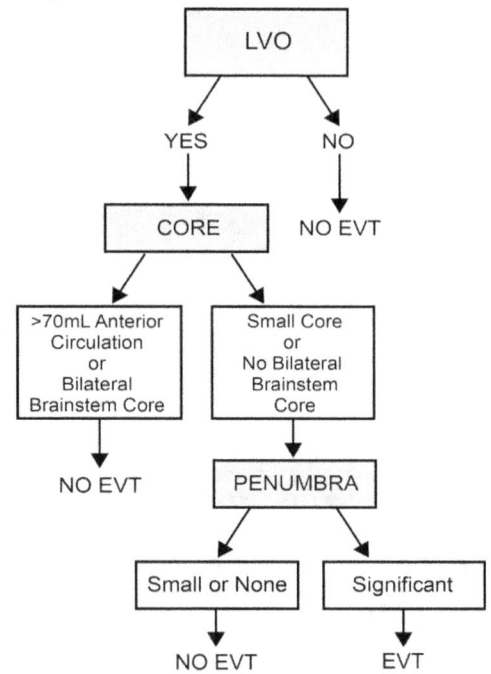

All AIS therapy targets the treatment of an ischemic penumbra by restoring blood flow to an occluded arterial territory. Once brain tissue is threatened by an occluded artery, collaterals prevent threatened brain tissue (ischemic penumbra) from being irreparably damaged for a certain period. This is accomplished by temporarily rerouting blood flow to threatened, under perfused regions of the brain. However, the collateral circulation can only do this for a certain time period which varies for everyone. That is why arbitrary time points used in the management of AIS must be abandoned and replaced with precise neuroimaging that can assess an individual's specific physiology. Healthier individuals tend to have better collaterals and, therefore, can maintain an ischemic penumbra for a longer period. We can all agree that the collateral circulation of a 92-year-old patient is not the same as a 30-year-old patient. The same arbitrary time points should not be used in the management of these two vastly different patients. That is why the use of arbitrary time points for AIS management must be reconsidered. EVT candidacy and all AIS management is dependent on physiology and not on an arbitrary time window.

21.6 CT Angiography (CTA) and CT Perfusion (CTP)

To determine if there is a large vessel occlusion, substantial core, and penumbra, many stroke centers utilize *CT angiography (CTA)* and *CT perfusion (CTP)*. As stated earlier, the focus of this text is CT-based imaging because it is usually associated with lower cost, greater availability, and increased speed. CT angiography or CTA examines the anatomy of the blood vessels in the brain. It allows visualization of these vessels and determines if there is an LVO. Think of it this way: CT '**A**' assesses '**A**'natomy (Box 2). Specifically, CTA assesses the arterial circulation and determines the presence and location of an LVO (Figure 14).

BOX 2. CT Angiography and Perfusion

CT**A** determines **A**natomy
CT**P** determines **P**hysiology

FIGURE 14. CT Angiography (CTA) Demonstrating Left M1 Segment Occlusion

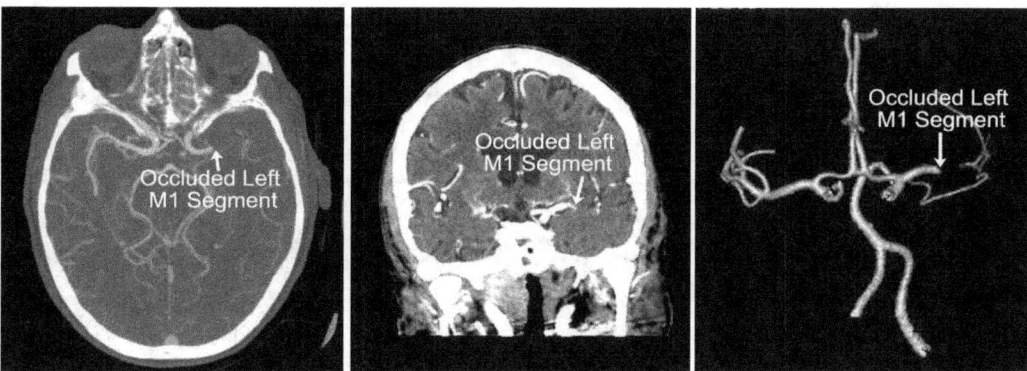

CT perfusion (CTP) identifies areas of the brain that have been irreparably damaged (core infarct) from areas of the brain that are potentially salvageable (ischemic penumbra). That is, CTP images brain physiology and determines whether brain tissue is threatened but still alive (ischemic penumbra) or already irreparably damaged (core infarct). Think of it this way: CT '**P**' assesses '**P**'hysiology. As mentioned earlier, although MRI is more sensitive to early ischemic changes, its clinical application is limited in many institutions. For this reason, this discussion will be limited to CT based imaging.

The fundamental role of CTP is to distinguish a core infarct (irreparably damaged brain tissue) from an ischemic penumbra (threatened but not irrevocably damaged brain tissue). There are three parameters that are utilized to make this distinction. These include *mean transit time (MTT), cerebral blood flow (CBF)* and *cerebral blood volume (CBV)*. MTT represents the time difference between the arterial inflow and venous outflow. CBF is the quantity of blood flow per unit of brain mass per minute (normal range in mixed gray and white matter, 50–60 mL/100 g/min). CBV is the volume of blood per unit of brain mass (normal range in mixed gray and white matter, 4–6 mL/100 g). Typically, the mean transit time (MTT) is elevated in both core infarct (irreparably damaged brain) and ischemic penumbra (threatened brain). MTT, CBF, and CBV are utilized to distinguish ischemic penumbra from core infarct.[20, 21]

Typically, an ischemic penumbra preserves autoregulation, prolongs MTT, and maintains or elevates cerebral blood volume (CBV). Autoregulation causes both vasodilatation and collateral recruitment. A core infarct, on the other hand, results in the loss of autoregulation. In this case, MTT is elevated and cerebral blood volume (CBV) is reduced. In both ischemic penumbra and core infarct, cerebral blood flow (CBF) is reduced. To summarize, cerebral blood flow (CBF) is diminished in both core infarct (irreparably damaged brain) and ischemic penumbra (threatened brain) (Table 5). MTT is elevated in both a core infarct and ischemic penumbra because the time it takes to traverse regions of dead or threatened brain increases. In a similar fashion, CBF is always diminished whether it's dead or threatened brain tissue. Because MTT is consistently elevated in both core infarct (dead brain tissue) and ischemic penumbra (threatened brain tissue) and because CBF is consistently diminished in both core infarct (dead brain tissue) and ischemic penumbra (threatened brain tissue), we can draw an incredible conclusion: **CBV is the most important CTP parameter in the diagnosis and treatment of LVO AIS.**

TABLE 5. AIS CT Perfusion (CTP) Parameters: MTT, CBF and CBV

Etiology	CBF	CBV	MTT
Infarct Core	↓	↓	↑
Ischemic Penumbra	↓	↑	↑
Seizure	↑	↑	↓

CBF - Cerebral Blood Flow; CBV - Cerebral Blood Volume; MTT - Mean Transit Time

This is a very important concept that will be explained one more time. CBV is **near-normal or increased** with ischemic penumbra (threatened brain) and **diminished** with core infarct (irreparably damaged brain). This is because autoregulatory vasodilation causes blood vessels to expand and dilate in attempts to deliver more oxygen, causing CBV to be either normal or elevated in threatened but still salvageable brain tissue (ischemic penumbra) (Figure 15). A core infarct or irreparably damaged brain loses autoregulatory vasodilatation function; thus, blood vessels within dead brain tissue can no longer expand or autoregulate, reducing blood volume. Remember that for both core infarct and ischemic penumbra, **CBF is always reduced**. A core infarct has both reduced CBF and CBV (Figures 15 and 16). This is referred to as a "**matched**" defect. That is, both CBF and CBV are reduced. A matched defect corresponds to a core infarct which represents irreparably damaged brain tissue and makes the patient an unlikely candidate for EVT. It is important to make this distinction because it makes no sense to perform EVT if brain tissue is already dead. More importantly, the use of CTP allows practitioners to make more appropriate individualized selections for EVT candidacy compared to arbitrary time points. Again, individuals have different and specific physiology which allows different patients to maintain an ischemic penumbra for varying time periods.

FIGURE 15. CT Perfusion (CTP) Parameters, Ischemic Penumbra and Core Infarct

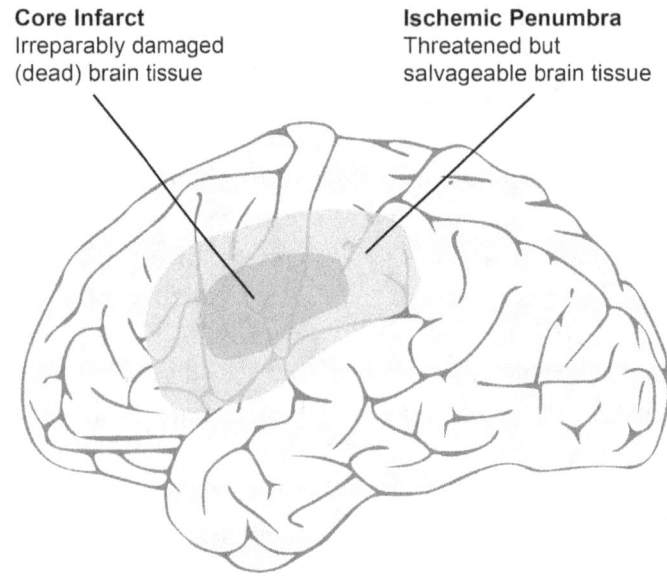

FIGURE 16. Core Infarct (Matched Defect: LOW CBF/LOW CBV)

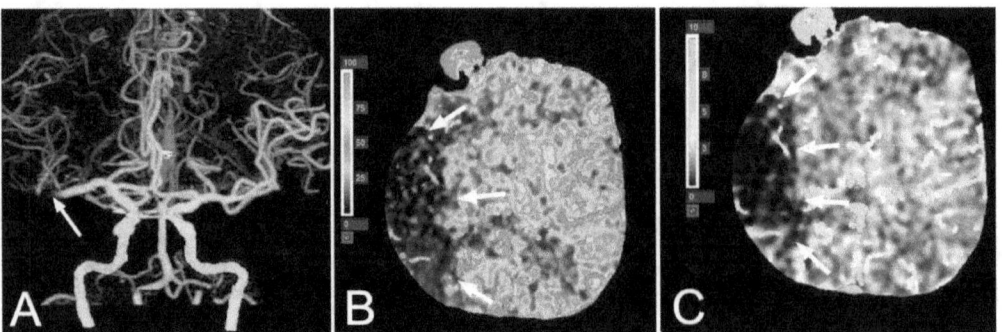

A 68-year-old woman presented with left hemiparesis, dysarthria and neglect. National Institutes of Health Stroke Scale (NIHSS) 19. (A) CT angiography revealed a distal right M1 MCA occlusion. CT perfusion demonstrated (B) reduced right hemispheric cerebral blood flow (CBF) and (C) cerebral blood volume (CBV) indicating core infarct. To view color images, please visit www.strokemadesimple.com/CTP/figures.

An ischemic penumbra (threatened brain) maintains or increases CBV (Figures 15 and 17). This is because the blood vessels within threatened brain tissue are still functional and can still autoregulate. They can still expand in attempts to increase oxygen delivery to the penumbra. Therefore, CBV is either maintained or increased within the threatened brain or the ischemic penumbra. Since an ischemic penumbra has low CBF and either maintains or increases CBV, this is referred to as a "mismatch." A mismatch (elevated CBV and a diminished CBF) represents an ideal candidate for EVT provided there also exists a relatively small or no core infarct (irreparably damaged brain) (Table 6). This is because the penumbra represents threatened but not yet irreparably damaged brain tissue that can survive with collateral circulation. However, this collateral circulation can only maintain the penumbra for a critical time period. This region of threatened but still viable brain tissue (ischemic penumbra) will decay into an irreparably damaged core infarct without timely reperfusion of the occluded artery (Figures 12, 18 and 19).

FIGURE 17. Ischemic Penumbra (Mismatched Defect: LOW CBF/HIGH CBV)

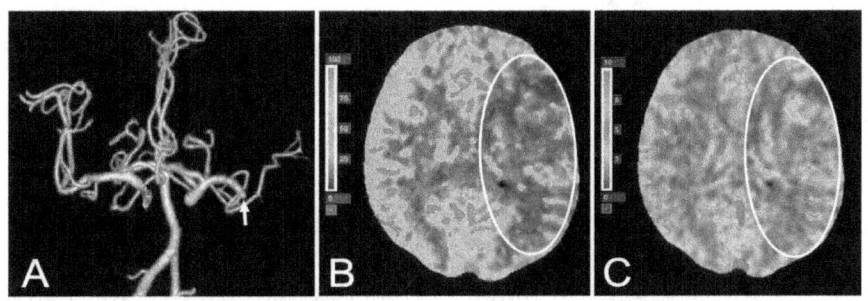

A 96-year-old woman presented with right hemiparesis and global aphasia. National Institutes of Health Stroke Scale (NIHSS) 24. (A) CT angiography revealed a distal left M1 MCA occlusion. CT perfusion demonstrated (B) reduced left hemispheric cerebral blood flow (CBF) and (C) maintained cerebral blood volume (CBV) indicating a mismatch and thus, salvageable ischemic penumbra. To view color images, please visit www.strokemadesimple.com/CTP/figures.

TABLE 6. CTP Matched Versus Mismatched Pattern

| Core | ↓CBF | ↓CBV | Matched Defect |
| Penumbra | ↓CBF | ↑CBV | Mismatched Defect |

FIGURE 18. Ischemic Penumbra Decay

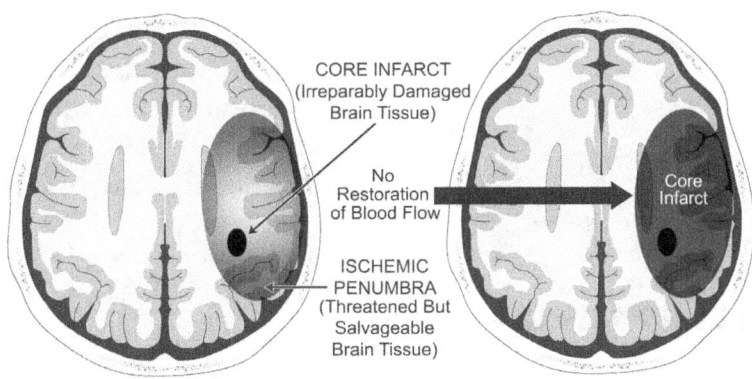

FIGURE 19. Ischemic Penumbra Decay into Core Infarct

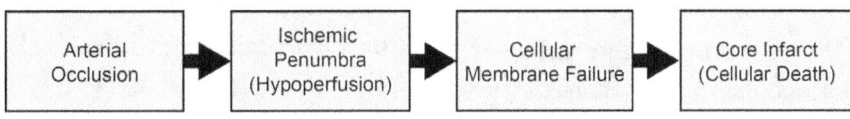

Realize that no clinical exam can distinguish an ischemic penumbra (threatened but still viable brain tissue) from an irreparably damaged core infarct. A patient with an ischemic penumbra presents with stroke-like symptoms because this region of the brain loses its functionality but is not yet irreversibly damaged. Permanent damage does not occur until collateral circulation maintaining these threatened regions of brain tissue is compromised. The goal of EVT and all AIS therapy is to reestablish perfusion to the ischemic penumbra before this region of the brain is irreparably damaged (Figure 20)

The foregoing is a summary of CTA and CTP imaging. If these types of studies provide more information than just a brain CT, why aren't both exams performed on all patients with AIS? For example, what if a patient presents with a stroke due to a completely occluded internal carotid artery or a completely occluded M1 segment? IV TPA is relatively ineffective in treating these larger vessel occlusions by itself. Therefore, identifying these large vessel occlusions with CTA prior to IV TPA use would determine which patients would require EVT in addition to IV TPA administration. It would also increase the efficacy of IV TPA and enhance functional outcome by improving recanalization EVT times.

FIGURE 20. Preservation of Ischemic Penumbra

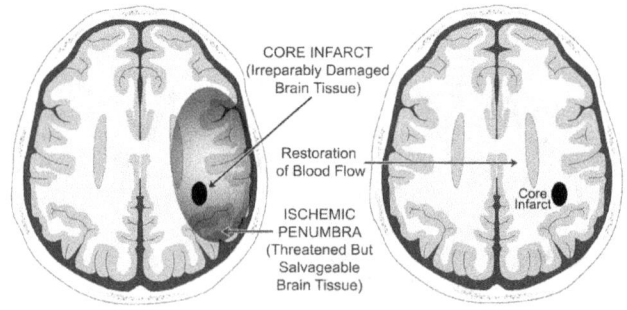

21.7 Multiphase and Dual Phase CTA

Among the primary concerns when performing CTA and CTP in all patients with acute ischemic stroke are increased radiation dose and increased contrast load. Can we somehow determine if there are a large vessel occlusion and an ischemic penumbra without increasing radiation exposure and contrast dose on the patient? One of the 2015 endovascular trials that will be discussed later is the ESCAPE Trial. This was an innovative trial that introduced a new imaging alternative to CTP called **multiphase CTA**. Multiphase CTA performs an arterial bolus CTA (called phase 1) followed by two additional unenhanced CT scans of the brain (called phase 2 and phase 3).

In this manner, this study still retains its properties as a CTA to determine if there is an LVO. Yet, it has the additional benefit of grading the degree of collaterals, which are the vessels that maintain the ischemic penumbra. Multiphase CTA provides additional data to better assess collateral circulation whereas single phase CTA has a single data acquisition during the arterial phase before collateral circulation has time to fill. This leads to an underestimation of collateral circulation and the risk of excluding patients from EVT. The ESCAPE Trial classified the degree of collaterals (which supply the penumbra) as good, intermediate, and poor. If the patient had good or intermediate collaterals, they were determined to be EVT candidates. This trial demonstrated the presence of good or intermediate collaterals as an independent predictor of favorable outcome in AIS EVT. Incidentally, the ESCAPE Trial also validated imaging speed as an independent predictor of functional outcome.

Instead of conducting two separate studies (CTA and CTP), multiphase CTA as a single study can simultaneously assess LVO and collateral status to indicate threatened brain tissue (ischemic penumbra). It does this with a single contrast bolus instead of giving a separate contrast bolus for a CTP and an additional contrast bolus for a CTA. Again, multiphase CTA is a single study that can determine the presence of both LVO and salvageable brain (ischemic penumbra). Additionally, it is a quick and easy-to-use method that requires no further contrast bolus and post-processing. Also, notice how the algorithm for EVT candidacy changes (Figure 21). Now, instead of performing two separate studies (CTA and CTP), a single study (multiphase CTA) can determine EVT candidacy. Note that multiphase CTA is a form of **functional imaging** that identifies collateral circulation, whereas CTP is a form of **physiologic imaging** that discriminates between core infarct and ischemic penumbra. As will be discussed in a separate chapter, stroke treatment is all about the proper assessment of collateral circulation. This is exactly what multiphase CTA allows us to do. It enables the direct visualization and determination of the degree of collateral circulation. Significant collateral circulation indicates the presence of an ischemic penumbra and a small core infarct.

The figure above includes the term "dual-phase" CTA (Figure 21). Dual-phase CTA may make stroke management more efficient than multiphase CTA.[22] Just like multiphase CTA, dual-phase CTA can determine if there is a large vessel occlusion. However, instead of performing two additional phase scans (as done in multiphase CTA), dual-phase CTA finds a sweet spot between both phases and requires only one additional unenhanced scan (Figure 22). That is, dual-phase CTA consists of a single, delayed unenhanced scan that provides an adequate assessment of collaterals in addition to the arterial bolus (required for any CTA). Moreover, dual-phase CTA has been demonstrated to more accurately determine thrombus length when compared to single-phase CTA, which is also an independent predictor of functional outcome in AIS. The bottom line is that multiphase and dual-phase CTA give much more information than single-phase or conventional CTA and may eliminate the need for CTP. Essentially, anything CTA can do, multiphase or dual-phase CTA can do better.[23]

FIGURE 21. CTP vs. Dual Phase CTA

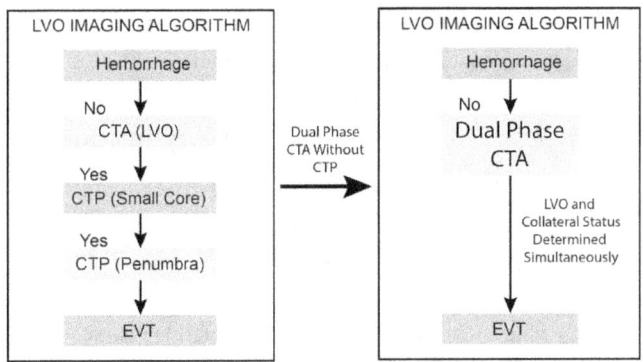

FIGURE 22. Dual Phase CTA

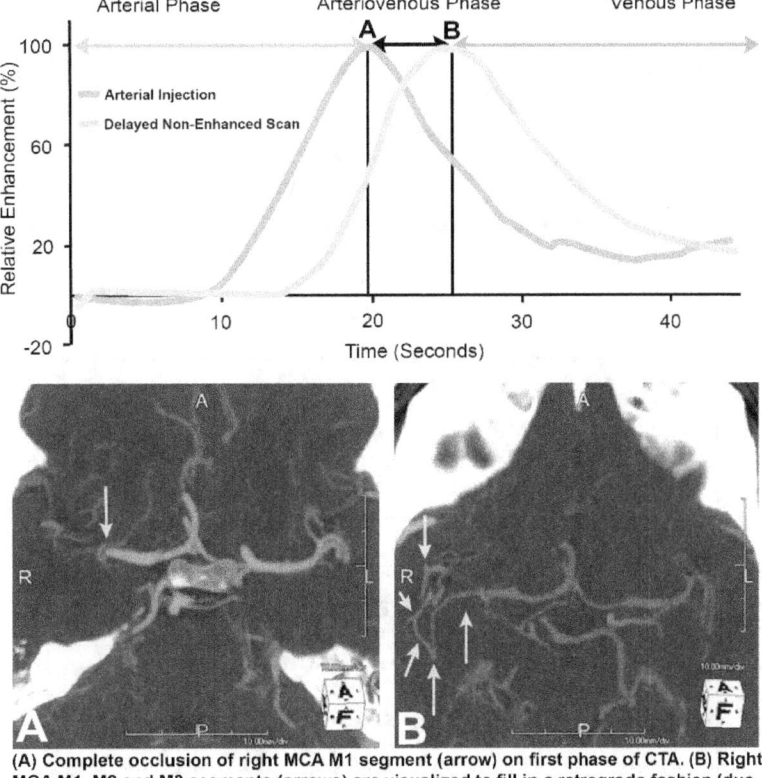

(A) Complete occlusion of right MCA M1 segment (arrow) on first phase of CTA. (B) Right MCA M1, M2 and M3 segments (arrows) are visualized to fill in a retrograde fashion (due to collateral supply from ACA leptomeningeal collaterals) in the second CTA phase.

From a practical standpoint, it is easier to implement dual-phase CTA than multiphase CTA. Also, stroke care centers lacking the ability to perform CT perfusion should strongly consider the use of dual-phase CTA to assess both LVO and collateral circulation status. In addition, stroke care centers that can perform CT perfusion must likewise deliberate the use of dual-phase CTA to assess both LVO and collateral circulation status. It is faster, requires less ionizing radiation, contrast, and post-processing. Dual-phase CTA is also much easier to interpret. When more healthcare providers are able to interpret these studies, more of them can then be directly involved in the diagnosis and treatment of AIS patients. While MRI is the gold standard for acute ischemic stroke pathophysiology, it is often associated with either unacceptable delays or inaccessibility in most institutions. Excluding MRI, there are three major neuroimaging screening options for EVT in stroke centers and other medical or health facilities:

1. CT/CTA
2. CT/Multiphase CTA or Dual-Phase CTA
3. CT/CTP/CTA

21.8 Neuroimaging Categories

Neuroimaging discussed in this chapter can be classified into four separate categories (Table 7). The first category is **exclusion**. A noncontrast brain CT is obtained to either exclude or rule out an intracranial hemorrhage or significant infarct (greater than one third the MCA territory or ASPECTS ≤ 5). Most EVT trials eliminated patients with large ischemic cores using noncontrast brain CT.[24-27] The second category is **anatomic**. Any type of CTA (single, dual, or multiphase) can assess intracranial circulation and determine the presence of an arterial occlusion. For example, a CTA may demonstrate that there is a left M1 segment (MCA) occlusion (Figure 14). In addition, CTA can also determine the length of occlusion. However, both multiphase and dual-phase CTA have been demonstrated to be more accurate in this regard.

The third category is **functional**. In many ways, functional imaging is considered an intermediate category between the anatomic and physiologic categories. Functional imaging is an assessment of collateral circulation using multiphase or dual-phase CTA. It provides a better assessment of clot length, which is an additional independent predictor of functional outcome. Good or intermediate collaterals confirm EVT candidacy in AIS patients. The last category is **physiologic** and includes CTP. Here, three parameters are assessed: MTT, CBF, and CBV. A matched defect (↓CBF/↓CBV) implies irreparably damage brain tissue (core infarct) while a mismatch (↓CBF/↑CBV) implies threatened but salvageable brain tissue (ischemic penumbra). These four categories can be easily remembered with the mnemonic 'RAFT' (Table 8). However, if these categories are too difficult to remember one can always just remember the 3Ps: *parenchyma, pipes,* and *penumbra*.[28]

TABLE 7. Categories of AIS Neuroimaging

Category	Modality	Findings / Significance
Exclusion	CT	Bleed >1/3 MCA APSECTS ≤ 5
Anatomic	CTA	Arterial Anatomy LVO Clot Length, ≥10mm, EVT > IV TPA
Functional	Multiphase or Dual Phase CTA	Intermediate or Good Collaterals (EVT Candidate) Versus Poor Collaterals (Not EVT Candidate)
Physiologic	CTP	Matched Defect (↓CBF/↓CBV) Mismatch (↓CBF/↑CBV)
Exceptions	CT	Swollen Tissue = Penumbra Hypodense Tissue = Core Hyperdense MCA, Basilar Artery and MCA Dot Sign are all Anatomic

TABLE 8. Categories of AIS Neuroimaging: **RAFT**

R	Rule Out - Bleed or >1/3 MCA ASPECTS ≤5
A	Anatomic - Arterial Territory Where is the LVO?
F	Functional - Collateral Status
T	Threatened Brain (Ischemic Penumbra) Versus Completed Infarct (Core Infarct) - Physiologic

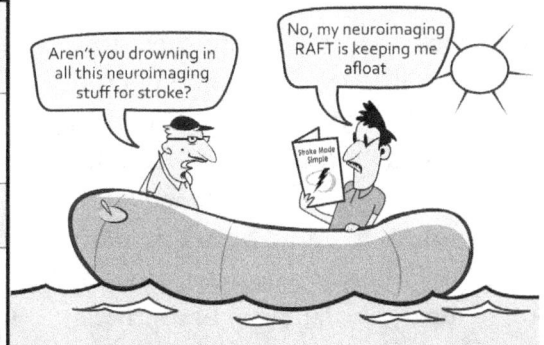

21.9 Conclusion

This chapter reviewed neuroimaging as it pertains to AIS diagnosis and treatment and its role cannot be overemphasized. The evolution of AIS intervention is inseparable from the development of advanced neuroimaging. Neuroimaging is a necessary component that has revolutionized the diagnosis and treatment of AIS. In fact, the success of many stroke centers can be gauged by the neuroimaging protocols set in place for AIS diagnosis and treatment. Some hospitals continue to follow the 20-year-old NINDS standard of a noncontrast brain CT for AIS evaluation even when imaging protocols and AIS treatment have advanced in leaps and bounds, far surpassing noncontrast brain CTs and intravenous thrombolysis. Proof of this lies in the fact that every EVT trial performed in 2015 utilized advanced neuroimaging to determine EVT candidacy (Table 9).

TABLE 9. 2015 EVT Randomized Controlled Trials (RCT) and Relevant Neuroimaging

RCT	Neuroimaging
MR CLEAN	CT/CTA
ESCAPE	CT/CTA/Multiphase
EXTEND-IA	CT/CTA/CTP
SWIFT PRIME	CT/CTA/MRA/MRP/CTP
REVASCAT	CT/CTA/MRA

There is a fundamental relationship between neuroimaging and AIS management. However, two major issues concerning neuroimaging and AIS management continue to occur. First, noncontrast brain CTs are occasionally misread and this directly affects and confuses subsequent AIS management. Fortunately, this problem can be easily remedied by including ASPECTS in every AIS CT interpretation. The success of AIS diagnosis and treatment depends largely on a multidiscipline team approach and proper CT interpretation is a huge factor in this endeavor. A great deal of that success lies in effective communication during time-sensitive AIS management. This communication can be greatly improved by utilizing ASPECTS in all radiographic reports to quantify AIS CT interpretation. **ASPECTS is the imaging equivalent of the NIHSS.** In fact, it is more sensitive in the determination of symptomatic intracranial hemorrhage and outcome than the NIHSS.

Secondly, despite all the evidence regarding the efficiency of imaging (CT/CTA/CTP concomitantly), efficient imaging is not frequently performed. This results in significant treatment delays which translate into worse functional outcomes. Furthermore, without additional imaging, misinterpreted noncontrast brain CTs are the only information emergency department physicians often get. Inaccurate CT interpretation leads to inaccurate stroke care management. For example, it is not uncommon to see a completed stroke interpreted as a "normal head CT." Relying on this information, an ED physician or neurologist may improperly administer IV TPA. Often, hyperdense vessels such as a hyperdense MCA or basilar artery are not identified and the brain CT study is interpreted as a "normal head CT." Unfortunately, these patients who require rapid EVT for LVO never receive proper treatment because no further imaging was performed due to an improper diagnosis resulting from poor image interpretation.

The treatment of all AIS is dependent upon restoration of blood flow to ischemic penumbra (threatened brain tissue). This treatment relies on the proper identification of threatened brain tissue (ischemic penumbra) and irreparably damaged brain tissue (core infarct). The determination of a core infarct (irreparably damaged brain tissue) and ischemic penumbra (threatened but salvageable brain tissue) can be determined anatomically, functionally, and/or physiologically. The presence of a core infarct and ischemic penumbra can be identified by CT, collateral circulation, or by CTP. Neuroimaging allows the precise determination of core infarct or ischemic penumbra compared to arbitrary time points. Neuroimaging determines whether brain tissue is still viable at the moment of imaging rather than assuming viability, for example, at hours. Hypoattenuation or low-density brain tissue on a noncontrast brain CT is indicative of a core infarct. Brain tissue swelling is indicative of an ischemic penumbra. Poor collaterals on multiphase CTA suggest a core infarct. Intermediate or good collaterals point to an ischemic penumbra. A matched defect on CTP (↓CBF and ↓CBV) is indicative of a core infarct. A mismatch on CTP (↓CBF and ↑CBV) indicates an ischemic penumbra (Table 10).

TABLE 10. Neuroimaging Distinguishes Ischemic Penumbra and Core Infarct.

Study	Ischemic Penumbra	Core Infarct
Brain CT	Isodense Tissue Swelling	Hypodensity
Multi- or Dual Phase CTA	Good or Intermediate Collaterals	Poor Collaterals
CTP	Mismatched (↓CBF - ↑CBV)	Matched (↓CBF - ↓CBV)

It is incredibly important to understand neuroimaging in relation to AIS management. Please familiarize yourself with these terms and concepts and urge others you work with to do the same. It will help to review and understand the four different categories of neuroimaging as they pertain to AIS diagnosis and treatment. Effective stroke care requires effective communication, which requires an effective understanding of relevant terminology. Subsequent chapters will discuss AIS treatment advancements and reinforce the importance of neuroimaging in the diagnosis and treatment of AIS.

Abbreviations list

AHA, American Heart Association; AIS, acute ischemic stroke; ASA, American Stroke Association; ASPECTS, Alberta Stroke Program Early CT Score; CBF, cerebral blood flow; CBV, cerebral blood volume; CTA, computed tomography angiography; CTP, CT perfusion; EICs, early ischemic changes; EVT, endovascular treatment; LVO, large vessel occlusion; MCA, middle cerebral artery; MRI, magnetic resonance imaging; MTT, mean transit time; RCT, randomized controlled trial.

References

1. Malhotra K, Liebeskind DS. (2015). Imaging in endovascular stroke trials. *J Neuroimaging,* 25, 51727.
2. Tissue plasminogen activator for acute ischemic stroke. (1995). The National Institute of Neurological Disorders and Stroke rt-PA Stroke Study Group. *N Engl J Med,* 333(24), 1581-87.
3. Grotta JC, Chiu D, Lu M, Patel S, Levine SR, Tilley BC, Brott TG, Haley EC Jr, Lyden PD, Kothari R, Frankel M, Lewandowski CA, Libman R, Kwiatkowski T, Broderick JP, Marler JR, Corrigan J, Huff S, Mitsias P, Talati S, Tanne D. (1999). Agreement and variability in the interpretation of early CT changes in stroke patients qualifying for intravenous rtPA therapy. *Stroke,* 30, 1528–33.
4. Wardlaw JM, Dorman PJ, Lewis SC, Sandercock PA. (1999). Can stroke physicians and neuroradiologists identify signs of early cerebral infarction on CT? *J Neurol Neurosurg Psychiatry,* 67, 651–53.
5. Warwick Pexman JH, Barber PA, Hill MD, Sevick RJ, Demchuk AM, Hudon ME, Hu WY, Buchan AM. (2001). Use of the Alberta Stroke Program Early CT Score (ASPECTS)

for Assessing CT Scans in Patients with Acute Stroke. *Am Jnl Neurorad*, Sep, 22 (8), 1534-42.

6. Muir KW, Baird-Gunning J, Walker L, Baird T, McCormick M, Coutts SB. (2007). Can the ischemic penumbra be identified on noncontrast CT of acute stroke? *Stroke*, 38, 2485–90.

7. Butcher KS, Lee SB, Parsons MW, Allport L, Fink J, Tress B, Donnan G, Davis SM, EPITHET Investigators. 2007). Differential prognosis of isolated cortical swelling and hypoattenuation on CT in acute stroke. *Stroke*, 38, 941–47.

8. Dzialowski I, Hill MD, Coutts SB, Demchuk AM, Kent DM, Wunderlich O, von Kummer R. (2006). Extent of early ischemic changes on computed tomography (CT) before thrombolysis: prognostic value of the Alberta Stroke Program Early CT Score in ECASS II. *Stroke*, 37, 973–78.

9. Puetz V, Dzialowski I, Hill MD, Demchuk AM. (2009). The Alberta Stroke Program Early CT Score in clinical practice: what have we learned? *Int J Stroke*, 4, 354–64.

10. Na DG, Kim EY, Ryoo JW, Lee KH, Roh HG, Kim SS, Song IC, Chang KH. (2005). CT sign of brain swelling without concomitant parenchymal hypoattenuation: comparison with diffusion- and perfusion-weighted MR imaging. *Radiology*, Jun, 235(3), 992-48.

11. Barber PA, Demchuk AM, Zhang J, Buchan AM. (2000). Validity and reliability of a quantitative computed tomography score in predicting outcome of hyperacute stroke before thrombolytic therapy. ASPECTS Study Group. Alberta Stroke Programme Early CT Score. *Lancet*, 355, 1670–74.

12. Demchuk AM, Hill MD, Barber PA, Silver B, Patel SC, Levine SR. (2005). Importance of early ischemic computed tomography changes using ASPECTS in NINDS rtPA Stroke Study. *Stroke*, 36, 2110–15.

13. Hill MD, Rowley HA, Adler F, Eliasziw M, Furlan A, Higashida RT, Wechsler LR, Roberts HC, Dillon WP, Fischbein NJ, Firszt CM, Schulz GA, Buchan AM. (2003). Selection of acute ischemic stroke patients for intra-arterial thrombolysis with pro-urokinase by using ASPECTS. *Stroke*, 34, 1925–31.

14. Jauch EC, Saver JL, Adams HP Jr, Bruno A, Connors JJ, Demaerschalk BM, Khatri P, McMullan PW Jr, Qureshi AI, Rosenfield K, Scott PA, Summers DR, Wang DZ, Wintermark M, Yonas H; on behalf of the American Heart Association Stroke Council; Council on Cardiovascular Nursing; Council on Peripheral Vascular Disease; Council on Clinical Cardiology. (2013). Guidelines for the early management of patients with acute ischemic stroke: a guideline for healthcare professionals from the American Heart Association/American Stroke Association. *Stroke*, 44, 870–947.

15. Hacke W, Kaste M, Fieschi C, Toni D, Lesaffre E, von Kummer R, Boysen G, Bluhmki E, Höxter G, Mahagne MH, Hennerici M. (1995). Intravenous thrombolysis with recombinant tissue plasminogen activator for acute hemispheric stroke: the European Cooperative Acute Stroke Study (ECASS). *JAMA*, 274, 1017–25.

16. Larrue V, von Kummer R, Müller A, Bluhmki E. (2001). Risk factors for severe hemorrhagic transformation in ischemic stroke patients treated with recombinant tissue plasminogen activator: a secondary analysis of the European-Australasian Acute Stroke Study (ECASS II). *Stroke*, 32, 438–41.

17. von Kummer R, Allen KL, Holle R, Bozzao L, Bastianello S, Manelfe C, Bluhmki E, Ringleb P, Meier DH, Hacke W. (1997). Acute stroke: usefulness of early CT findings before thrombolytic therapy. *Radiology*, 205, 327–33.

18. Hopyan J, Ciarallo A, Dowlatshahi D, et al. (2010). Certainty of stroke diagnosis: incremental benefit with CT perfusion over noncontrast CT and CT angiography. *Radiol*, 255(1), 142–53.

19. Demaerschalk BM, Silver B, Wong E, Merino JG, Tamayo A, Hachinski V. (2006). ASPECT scoring to estimate >1/3 middle cerebral artery territory infarction. *Can J Neurol Sci*, May, 33(2), 200-4.

20. Sparacia G, Iaia A, Assadi B, Lagalla R. (2007). Perfusion CT in acute stroke: predictive value of perfusion parameters in assessing tissue viability versus infarction. *Radiol Med (Torino)*, 112, 113–22.

21. Wintermark M, Fischbein NJ, Smith WS, Ko NU, Quist M, Dillon WP. (2005). Accuracy of dynamic perfusion CT with deconvolution in detecting acute hemispheric stroke. *AJNR-Am J Neuroradiol*, 26, 104–12.

22. Shin NY, Kim KE, Park M, Kim YD, Kim DJ, Ahn SJ, et al. (2014) Dual-Phase CT Collateral

Score: A Predictor of Clinical Outcome in Patients with Acute Ischemic Stroke. *PLoS ONE*, 9(9), e107379.
23. Menon B, Demchuk AM. (2011). Computed tomography angiography in the assessment of patients with stroke/TIA. *Neurohospitalist*, 1(4), 187–99.
24. Goyal M, Demchuk AM, Menon BK, et al. (2015). Randomized assessment of rapid endovascular treatment of ischemic stroke. *N Engl J Med*, 372, 1019–30.
25. Saver JL, Goyal M, Bonafe A, et al. (2015). Stent-retriever thrombectomy after intravenous t-PA vs. t-PA alone in stroke. *N Engl J Med*, 372, 2285–95.
26. Campbell BC, Mitchell PJ, Kleinig TJ, et al. (2015). Endovascular therapy for ischemic stroke with perfusion-imaging selection. *N Engl J Med*, 372, 1009–18.
27. Jovin TG, Chamorro A, Cobo E, et al. (2015). Thrombectomy within 8 hours after symptom onset in ischemic stroke. *N Engl J Med*, 372, 2296–306.
28. Rowley HA. (2001). The four Ps of acute stroke imaging: parenchyma, pipes, perfusion, and penumbra. *AJNR-Am J Neuroradiol*, 22, 599–601.

Chapter 22

Contrast-Induced Nephropathy

22.1 Introduction

In every stroke workup, a noncontrast brain CT is required to exclude ischemic stroke mimics such as intracerebral hemorrhage or neoplasm. Furthermore, the completion of a significant ischemic stroke demonstrated by hypodense brain tissue precludes the administration of IV TPA to otherwise eligible patients. Nowadays, neuroimaging has stepped up and revolutionized AIS diagnosis and treatment. Many stroke centers are increasing their use of CTA and CTP imaging protocols as adjunctive studies to further diagnose large vessel occlusion (LVO) and discriminate between threatened brain tissue (ischemic penumbra) and irreparably damaged brain tissue (core infarct). While CTA and CTP imaging protocols permit rapid, noninvasive assessment of the intracranial circulation and brain tissue viability, safety concerns regarding contrast-related renal damage are often raised. The purpose of this chapter is to address these concerns.

22.2 Contrast-Induced Nephropathy (CIN)

Contrast-induced nephropathy (CIN) is defined as a ≥25% increase in baseline creatinine levels within three days following contrast administration.[1,2] Acute stroke patients are frequently incapacitated or cannot communicate. Without a reliable history of renal disease, clinicians are concerned that contrast studies such as CTA or CTP can potentially result in CIN or renal failure. Studies have demonstrated that CTA, CTP, and subsequent cerebral angiography are rarely associated with transient CIN (<3%) and never with renal failure.[3] However, other research has reported a 12 to 26% risk of developing chronic renal disease from contrast-enhanced studies.[4-7]

These divergent results stem from the investigation of two distinct patient populations. Specifically, the higher rates of renal disease reported in non-stroke patients included individuals with pre-existing renal dysfunction and advanced chronic kidney disease, on whom standard pre-hydration protocols were not administered.[4-7] This population is distinct from stroke patient cohorts with little or no history of renal dysfunction in which the overall incidence of CIN remains low (< 3%). While no cases of CIN progressed to renal failure or required dialysis, the most important predictor of CIN was a history of chronic renal disease.[3] For this reason, acute stroke patients who may receive emergent contrast-enhanced CT imaging are recommended to be screened for a history of chronic renal disease or advanced kidney disease whenever possible (realizing AIS patients frequently cannot communicate).

Stroke-specific and random patient population investigations demonstrated differences in CIN development. For example, while diabetes mellitus was associated with the development of CIN in non-stroke patient investigations, it did not contribute to CIN in stroke-specific studies.[2,3,5,8] In a similar manner, stroke-specific investigations did not demonstrate a significant difference in the development of CIN among patients who received low osmolar contrast (Omnipaque®) versus iso-osmolar (Visipaque®), whereas studies have shown such in non-stroke populations.[3,9,10] Research that investigated contrast associated with CTA, CTP, and angiography in acute ischemic stroke patients yielded several other significant observations which are summarized in Box 1.

BOX 1. Summary Data of Contrast-Induced Nephropathy (CIN)

> **Summary Data of Contrast Induced Nephropathy (CIN)**
> 1. Less than 3% of patients developed CIN.
> 2. None of these patients experienced renal failure requiring dialysis.
> 3. A history of renal impairment was the only significant risk factor for the development of CIN.
> 4. CIN was unrelated to diabetes mellitus.
> 5. CIN was not proportional to contrast dose.
> 6. CIN was unrelated to above average contrast dose.
> 7. CIN was unrelated to additional contrast studies even with higher amounts of contrast.
> 8. The use of either iso-osmolar contrast agents (Visipaque®) or non-ionic low osmotic contrast agents (Omnipaque®) were unrelated to the development of CIN.

The diagnosis, management, and treatment of AIS are driven by the mantra 'Time is Brain.'[11] This often translates into immediate CTA and/or CTP imaging even before the results of laboratory values (e.g., creatinine) are available. CTA and CTP greatly assist in management decisions regarding endovascular treatment (EVT) which are driven by knowledge of clot location, collateral status, core size, and presence of an ischemic penumbra. In fact, a similar imaging protocol was developed and stressed in the landmark ESCAPE trial which will be discussed later.[12] Delays in acute stroke management must be avoided because every 15-minute delay between stroke onset and treatment time can result in a significant difference in functional outcome.[13] However, as the ESCAPE Trial has already demonstrated, imaging protocols can be efficiently performed without sacrificing functional outcome.[7] Imaging studies such as CTA are quick, safe, and inexpensive. There is a financial cost to perform studies such as CTA, but these costs are minimal compared to the costs of inappropriately managed and ineffectively treated stroke patients.[14]

One role of a community stroke center is to develop a practical, efficient, and cost-effective protocol to adequately care for acute ischemic stroke (AIS) cases within its territory. The management and treatment of stroke have advanced by leaps and bounds since the NINDS trial performed over 20 years ago.[15] Imaging protocols cannot be constrained by the 20-year-old NINDS standard of a single noncontrast brain CT. Further imaging with either CTA to demonstrate cerebrovascular anatomy and collateral circulation status or CTP to demonstrate brain tissue viability is essential. These additional studies significantly increase diagnostic sensitivity for AIS.[16]

Studies demonstrate that the risk of CIN arising from the administration of contrast media is far less than the risk of hemorrhage from IV TPA administration.[3,15,17,18] Despite the higher risk of hemorrhage associated with IV TPA and the lower risk of CIN associated with contrast-enhanced studies, IV TPA is given reflexively whenever an acute stroke patient is eligible for such treatment. The benefit of receiving this life-sustaining, clot-busting drug is significantly better than the risk of hemorrhage (the benefits outweigh the risks). The risk-versus-benefit profile of performing contrast-enhanced studies such as CTA and CTP without delay and without waiting for a creatinine value must, therefore, be viewed in a similar manner. Clearly, the enormous benefit from minimizing treatment delays serves as justification for the very small risk (< 3%) of CIN. A recently performed meta-analysis of the five major EVT trials performed in 2015 accentuates this point by demonstrating that for every 4-minute delay in emergency department door to EVT reperfusion time, 1 in every 100 treated patients suffers a worse functional outcome. Functional independence at three months was reduced by both increasing emergency department door to reperfusion and neuroimaging to reperfusion times.[19]

Yet for whatever reason, the argument over the risk of CIN or renal failure frequently prevents rapid imaging without a creatinine value. This often results in undesirably prolonged treatment delay while waiting for a creatinine result which in some series took an average of 73 minutes.[18,20] In stark contrast, CT enhanced imaging can be performed quickly without delaying patients from receiving thrombolytic or endovascular therapy.[12,18] The gatekeepers to performing rapid CTA and CTP imaging are mostly radiologists who usually do a phenomenal job. Every stroke center requires the synchronous cooperation of a multidisciplinary team to be successful. Without a doubt, radiology is a key component of this multidisciplinary team. In fact, the majority of AIS management is now image-guided. Radiologists must permit the performance of contrast studies without waiting for creatinine values. Most radiologists already allow this and they are performing a wonderful job in facilitating the diagnosis and treatment of AIS. Unfortunately, a number of radiologists at some stroke centers still continue to require creatinine values (which delay diagnosis and thus treatment) before contrast-enhanced imaging can be performed. In this situation, one must ask: *Quis custodiet ipsos custodes?* Below, I have also included a handy-dandy 'GET OUT RADIOLOGY BS CARD' for your convenience (Figure 1). **Again, most stroke centers do not face this problem and work with incredibly fantastic radiologists.** For the few that do, this practice is unacceptable and must be corrected.

The largest controlled study of acute renal injury following emergency department contrast administration has recently been performed.[21] Investigators divided 17,934 emergency department patients into three groups receiving contrast-enhanced CT, unenhanced CT, or no imaging at all. No increase in the frequency of acute renal injury among these groups was observed. The study also determined patient serum creatinine levels of less than 4.0 mg/dL had no association with the development of contrast-induced nephropathy, chronic renal disease, dialysis, or renal transplantation within six months after receiving IV dye.

FIGURE 1. GET OUT RADIOLOGY BS CARD

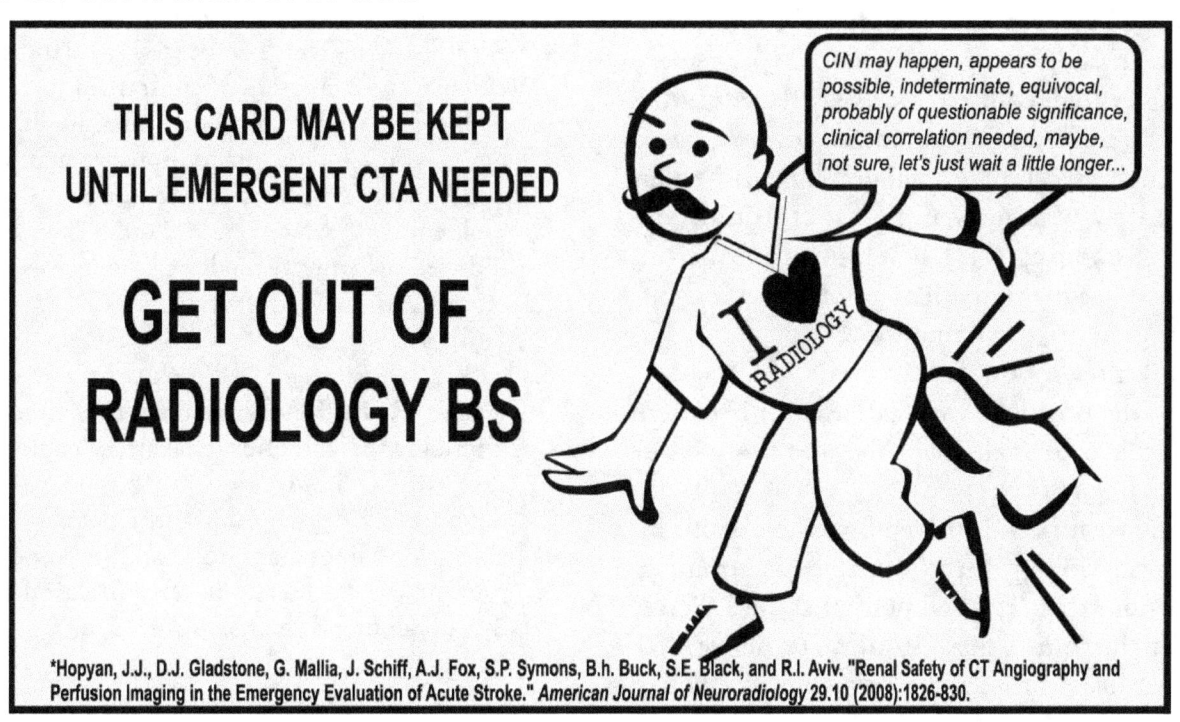

Despite these findings, the authors recommended the continued use of nephroprotective maneuvers to maintain a lower risk of CIN and subsequent renal injury and not to assume that there is no renal risk with contrast-enhanced studies. They also stated, *Our data also suggests that in cases in which contrast–enhanced CT is indicated to avoid delayed or missed diagnosis, the potential morbidity and mortality resulting from a failure to diagnose possibly life-threatening conditions outweigh any potential risk of contrast-induced nephropathy in patients with serum creatinine levels up to 4.0 mg/dL.* In terms of contrast-enhanced CT imaging for AIS evaluation, truer words have never been spoken. Finally, a new recommendation issued by the 2018 AHA/ASA guideline states, "For patients who otherwise meet criteria for EVT, it is reasonable to proceed with CTA if indicated in patients with suspected intracranial LVO before obtaining a serum creatinine concentration in patients without a history of renal impairment."[22]

22.3 Conclusion

In conclusion, studies tailored to address renal toxicity in acute stroke patients demonstrated a very low (<3%) incidence of CIN among stroke patients who underwent emergent CTA and other contrast-based imaging studies. Furthermore, none of these patients experienced permanent renal injury or required dialysis. These studies demonstrate CTA, CTP, and other contrast-based studies such as cerebral angiography can be performed safely without waiting for creatinine values. Long-standing CIN development criticisms and concerns in this patient population are disproportionate to the literature. Performing CTA and CTP after a noncontrast brain CT is a safe and feasible protocol that can expedite patient triage and provide valuable LVO and brain tissue viability information.

Stroke treatment is driven by time. Again, individual physiology (determined by neuroimaging and not arbitrary time points) should dictate treatment but until these studies are performed, we as healthcare professionals must be as efficient and effective as possible. The irrational fear of causing acute kidney injury after the administration of intravenous contrast can impede stroke management and result in significant functional disability. Anything that minimizes delay in AIS management improves functional outcome. Conversely, anything that increases delay in AIS management worsens functional outcome. Don't wait for those creatinine values!

Abbreviations list

AIS, acute ischemic stroke; CIN, contrast-induced nephropathy; CTA, computed tomography angiography; CTP, CT perfusion; EVT, endovascular treatment; LVO, large vessel occlusion.

References

1. Benko A, Fraser-Hill M, Magner P, et al. (2007). Canadian Association of Radiologists: consensus guidelines for the prevention of contrast-induced nephropathy. *Can Assoc Radiol J*, 58, 79–87.
2. Weisbord SD, Palevsky PM. (2005). Radiocontrast-induced acute renal failure. *J Intensive Care Med*, 20, 63–75.
3. Hopyan JJ, Gladstone DJ, Mallia G, et al. (2008). Renal safety of CT angiography and perfusion imaging in the emergency evaluation of acute stroke. *Am J Neuroradiol*, 29(10), 1826–30.
4. Kim SM, Cha RH, Lee JP, et al. (2010). Incidence and outcomes of contrast-induced nephropathy after computed tomography in patients with CKD: a quality improvement report. *Am J Kidney Dis*, 55(6), 1018–25.
5. Goldenberg I, Matetzky S. (2005). Nephropathy induced by contrast media: pathogenesis, risk factors and preventive strategies. *CMAJ*, 172, 1461–71.
6. Sabeti S, Schillinger M, Mlekusch W, et al. (2002). Reduction in renal function after renal arteriography and after renal artery angioplasty. *Eur J Vasc Endovasc Surg*, 24, 156–60.
7. Solomon R, Werner C, Mann D, et al. (1994). Effects of saline, mannitol, and furosemide to prevent acute decreases in renal function induced by radiocontrast agents. *N Engl J Med*, 331, 1416–20.

8. Lautin EM, Freeman NJ, Schoenfeld AH, et al. (1991). Radiocontrast-associated renal dysfunction: incidence and risk factors. *AJR Am J Roentgenol*, 157, 49–58.
9. Aspelin P, Aubry P, Fransson SG, et al. (2003). Nephrotoxic effects in high-risk patients undergoing angiography. *N Engl J Med*, 348, 491–99.
10. Barrett BJ, Carlisle EJ. (1993). Metaanalysis of the relative nephrotoxicity of high- and low-osmolality iodinated contrast media. *Radiology*, 188, 171–78.
11. Saver JL. (2006). Time is brain– quantified. *Stroke*, 37, 263–66.
12. Goyal M, Demchuk AM, Menon BK, et al. (2015). Randomized assessment of rapid endovascular treatment of ischemic stroke. *N Engl J Med*, 372(11), 1019–30.
13. Saver JL, Fonarow GC, Smith EE, et al. (2013). Time to treatment with intravenous tissue plasminogen activator and outcome from acute ischemic stroke. *JAMA*, 309(23), 2480–88.
14. Quinn TJ, Dawson J. (2009). Acute 'strokenomics': efficacy and economic analyses of alteplase for acute ischemic stroke. *Expert Rev Pharmaceoecon Outcomes Res*, 9(6), 513–22.
15. NINDS Study Group. (1995). Tissue plasminogen activator for acute ischemic stroke. *N Engl J Med*, 333(24), 1581–88.
16. Hopyan J, Ciarallo A, Dowlatshahi D, et al. (2010). Certainty of stroke diagnosis: incremental benefit with CT perfusion over non-contrast CT and CT angiography. *Radiol*, 255(1), 142–53.
17. Krol, Andrea L. et al. (2007). Incidence of Radio-contrast Nephropathy in Patients Undergoing Acute Stroke Computed Tomography Angiography. *Stroke,* 38.8, 2364-66.
18. Smith WS, Roberts HC, Chuang NA, Ong KC, Lee TJ, Johnston SC, Dillon WP. (2003). Safety and feasibility of a CT protocol for acute stroke: combined CT, CT angiography, and CT perfusion imaging in 53 consecutive patients. *Am J Neuroradiol,* 24, 688–90.
19. Saver, Jeffrey L., et al. (2016). Time to treatment with endovascular thrombectomy and outcomes from ischemic stroke: A meta-analysis. *Jama,* 316.12 , 1279-88.
20. Josephson SA, Dillon WP, Smith WS. (2005). Incidence of contrast nephropathy from cerebral CT angiography and CT perfusion imaging. *Neurology,* 64, 1805–06.
21. Hinson, JS, et al. (2016). Risk of Acute Kidney Injury After Intravenous Contrast Media Administration. *Ann Emerg Med*, 1-10.
22. Powers WJ, Rabinstein AA, Ackerson T, Adeoye OM, Bambakidis NC, Becker K, Biller J, Brown M, Demaerschalk BM, Hoh B, et al. (2018) Guidelines for the Early Management of Patients With Acute Ischemic Stroke: A Guideline for Healthcare Professionals From the American Heart Association/American Stroke Association. *Stroke,* Epub 24 Jan 2018.

Chapter 23

IV TPA

23.1 Introduction

Intravenous (IV) recombinant tissue plasminogen activator (rtPA) is the only U.S. Food and Drug Administration (FDA)-approved drug for the treatment of acute ischemic stroke. For simplicity, the intravenous administration of recombinant tissue plasminogen activator will be referred to as **IV TPA**. IV TPA converts inactive plasminogen into active plasminogen which is a proteolytic enzyme that can disrupt fibrin cross-links, leading to clot fragmentation and recanalization of occluded arteries in the brain. IV TPA marks a therapeutic milestone in the treatment of stroke as it is the first FDA approved treatment option that could potentially change the devastating consequences of stroke. This chapter will discuss the role, benefits, and limitations of IV TPA in ischemic stroke treatment.

23.2 IV TPA Efficacy

The National Institute of Neurologic Disorders and Stroke (NINDS) trial demonstrated that IV TPA administered within three hours of acute ischemic stroke resulted in significant functional outcome improvement when compared with placebo.[1] The NINDS trial also determined the initial exclusion criteria for the use of IV TPA. Specifically, this trial demonstrated that 50% of patients who received IV TPA recovered to complete functional independence at three months compared to 35% of patients who did not. The NINDS Trial also demonstrated that eight out of every 18 stroke patients (44%) who received IV TPA were functionally independent after three months. Compare this to six out of every 18 stroke patients (33%) who obtained functional independence regardless of treatment (Figure 1).[1]

The NINDS Trial further demonstrated that intracranial hemorrhage occurred in about one out

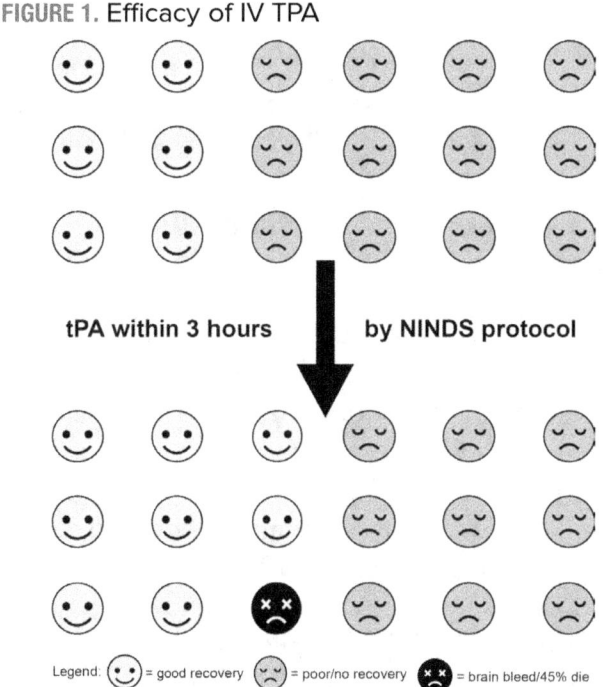

FIGURE 1. Efficacy of IV TPA

of every 18 patients receiving IV TPA (5.8%). In patients who did suffer intracranial hemorrhage, there was a 45% fatality rate (Figure 1). The study also indicated a higher 10-fold risk of symptomatic intracerebral hemorrhage in IV TPA treated patients (6.8%) versus just 0.6% in patients treated with placebo. However, there was no significant difference in mortality. Eight stroke patients needed to be treated (NNT) with IV TPA within three hours for one patient to have significant functional improvement (complete or near complete recovery). If IV TPA was given within two hours, only six patients needed to be treated for one patient to have complete or near complete recovery (Figure 2). If these numbers don't sound impressive, compare them to ST–segment–elevation myocardial infarction (STEMI) patients. In this patient population, 17 patients required treatment to derive treatment benefit to one patient (Figure 2).[2] The NNT is not just a clinically useful indicator of efficacy but is also statistically valid.[3]

FIGURE 2. Need to Treat Number for IV TPA

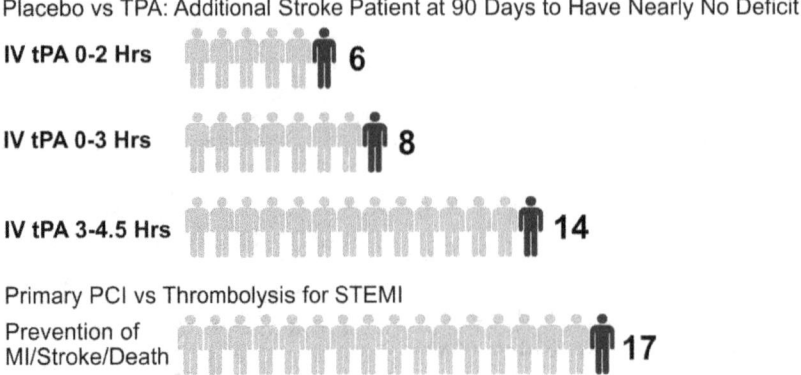

23.3 Initial IV TPA Administration Criteria

Despite its well-documented benefits, very few AIS patients receive IV TPA, with national estimates ranging in the order of 3 to 5%.[4] The most recent IV TPA recommendations provided by the AHA/ASA 2018 guidelines expand past earlier criteria that were predominately based on the NINDS trial published in 1996.[5] Earlier IV TPA administration or restriction criteria were not only based on initial IV TPA pilot studies; they were also derived from other subspecialties and basic science publications.[6-11]

For this reason, previous restriction criteria for IV TPA were considered controversial. Large discrepancies prevail among stroke physicians across the nation as to which exclusion criteria are considered "relative" and which are thought of as "absolute". James Burke famously stated, *"You can only know where you're going if you know where you've been."* This statement applies to all stroke management and treatment. As it pertains to intravenous thrombolysis, it is important to understand the initial inclusion, exclusion, and relative exclusion criteria for IV TPA. Many of these criteria were determined by the NINDS trial which was performed over 20 years ago (1995). Since that time, new recommendations by the American Heart Association and American Stroke Association (AHA/ASA) guidelines in 2018, as well as changes to the prescribing information of alteplase by the FDA in February 2015, have modified these criteria. However, although the initial exclusion and relative exclusion criteria for IV TPA have been revised, they will be reviewed for one very important reason: **Many practitioners continue to base their practice on these criteria.** Understanding how these criteria were once used and how they recently changed will iron out inconsistencies in the appropriate use of IV TPA.

The initial inclusion criteria required to administer IV TPA include patient age over 18 years, a clinical diagnosis of ischemic stroke (measurable deficit), and initiation of treatment within three hours (Table 1). These inclusion criteria can be remembered with the mnemonic 'CAN.' Also, the initial exclusion criteria for IV TPA can be remembered with the mnemonic 'DON'T GIVE TPA' (Table 2). Additionally, the previously considered <u>relative</u> exclusion criteria can be remembered with the mnemonic 'MIGHT DO' (Table 3).

TABLE 1. TPA Inclusion Criteria: CAN

C	Clinical Diagnosis of Ischemic Stroke (Measure Role Neurologic Deficit)
A	Age >18
N	Need to Initiate Treatment Within 3 Hours

TABLE 2. TPA Initial Exclusion Criteria: **DON'T GIVE TPA**

D	Disorders of bleeding (acute bleeding diathesis)
O	Occult SAH or SAH suspicion (even if CT negative for SAH)
N	Not controlled HTN (SBP >185, DBP >110)
T	Tumor, aneurysm or AVM of brain
G	Glucose less than 50 mg/dL (2.7mmol/L)
I	INFARCT (>1/3 MCA) or BLEED on CT
V	VARIABLES for bleeding - ALPHA*
E	Evidence of MAJOR SURGERY or TRAUMA within 3 months
T	Three months - no neurosurgery, head trauma or stroke
P	Previous intracranial hemorrhage history
A	Active internal bleeding w/in 22 days or arterial puncture at non-compressor site within 7 days

*ALPHA

A	aPTT elevated
L	Labs abnormal with use of direct thrombin or direct factor Xa inhibitors (aPTT, INR, platelet count, ECT or TT or factor Xa activity assays)
P	Platelets <100 mm3
H	Heparin w/in 48 hours and aPTT >40
A	Anticoagulant (Warfarin) with INR >1.7 or PT >15

TABLE 3. TPA Initial Relative Exclusion Criteria: **MIGHT DO**

M	Myocardial Infarct Within 3 Months
I	Improving (Rapidly) Stroke Symptoms or Minor Symptoms
G	G.I. or Urinary Tract Hemorrhage Within 21 Days
H	History of Major Surgery or Serious Non-Head Trauma Within 14 Days
T	Tap - Recent Spinal Tap
D	Determined Pregnant
O	Occurrence of Seizure at Onset With Postictal Neurological Impairments

23.4 Current IV TPA Administration Criteria

Since the publication of these recommendations, research has demonstrated inconsistencies in these criteria. Specifically, studies investigating IV TPA use for acute stroke patients have determined it can be safely administered for what was previously considered contraindicated criteria. For example, severe hypertension no longer is an exclusion criterion for IV TPA, provided adequate blood pressure control can be achieved prior to its administration.[12] Currently, a systolic blood pressure of less than 185 mm Hg and a diastolic blood pressure of less than 110 mm Hg are the recommended cutoff values prior to IV TPA treatment. Blood pressure management guidelines for patients during and for the first 24 hours after receiving IV thrombolytic is < 180 mmHg systolic pressure and < 105 mmHg diastolic pressure.[5]

These older exclusion criteria have been reviewed by the American Heart Association/American Stroke Association (AHA/ASA). The latest guidelines now recommend that the provider make more independent, patient-specific clinical judgments when weighing the risks and benefits of IV TPA administration. These recommendations coincide with the most recent changes to the prescribing information of alteplase by the FDA in February 2015. In addition, a newer 2015 AHA/ASA scientific statement and 2018 AHA/ASA guidelines discussing IV TPA indications for acute ischemic stroke have been issued.[5]

The recent changes to the prescribing information of alteplase by the FDA in February 2015 are summarized below (Box 1). However, writers of the AHA/ASA scientific statement for the inclusion and exclusion criteria for IV TPA strongly recommend that clinicians apply the contents of this document in conjunction with previous AHA/ASA guidelines for acute ischemic stroke treatment and management. However, new 2018 AHA/ASA guidelines have now been published and will be discussed shortly.[5] Rather than merely listing these recommendations in a manner that is impossible to remember, IV TPA administration criteria will be designated as follows:

- **permissible criteria** that allow the administration of IV TPA on a case-by-case basis, if reasonable
- **laboratory criteria** that would prevent the administration of IV TPA
- **anticoagulants**
- **not permissible criteria** for the administration of IV TPA
- **temporally related criteria** for the administration of IV TPA

These categories will purposely overlap to make it easier to remember them. The majority of these recommendations persisted in the new 2018 AHA/ASA guidelines. However, any differences will favor the newer 2018 AHA/ASA guidelines. An easy way to recall these different categories is with the mnemonic 'PLANT' (Table 4).

BOX 1. 2015 IV TPA (Activase) Labeling

Activase 2015 Labeling	Previous Activase Labeling
1. Current intracranial hemorrhage	1. History of intracranial hemorrhage
2. Subarachnoid hemorrhage	2. Suspicion of subarachnoid hemorrhage
3. Active internal bleeding	3. Active internal bleeding
4. Recent surgery (intracranial or spinal) or serious head trauma within 3 months	4. Recent surgery (intracranial or spinal) or serious head trauma within 3 months
5. Intracranial lesions associated with increased risk of bleeding (aneurysms, AVMs or neoplasms)	5. Intracranial lesions associated with increased risk of bleeding (aneurysms, AVMs or neoplasms)
6. Current severe uncontrolled hypertension	6. Systolic blood pressure >185 mm Hg or DBP >110 mm Hg
7. Bleeding diathesis	7. Acute bleeding diathesis
	8. Seizure at onset of stroke

TABLE 4. Different Criteria Related to IV TPA Administration: **PLANT**

P	Permissible Criteria
L	Laboratory Criteria
A	Anticoagulants
N	Not Permissible Criteria
T	Temporally Related Criteria

23.4.1 Permissible Criteria

The 2015 AHA/ASA scientific statement and 2018 AHA/ASA guidelines state that IV TPA may be administered on a case-by-case basis, if the following are present:

1. Pregnant and postpartum patients
2. Patients with a clinical history of a potential bleeding diathesis or coagulopathy
3. Warfarin use and INR ≤ 1.7
4. Pericarditis
5. Severe hypertension if it can be safely lowered (< 185/110 mmHg)
6. Intracranial aneurysm (<10 mm)
7. Extra-axial intracranial neoplasm
8. Pre-existing neurologic or psychiatric disability
9. Glucose levels < 50 or > 400 mg/dL that are subsequently normalized
10. Seizure at the time of stroke onset

An easy way to remember these permissible criteria is with the mnemonic 'CAN HAPPEN' (Table 5).

23.4.2 Laboratory Criteria

IV TPA is not recommended if INR >1.7, aPTT >40 seconds, PT >15 seconds, or platelet count <100,000/mm3. An easy way to remember these impermissible laboratory criteria is with the mnemonic 'PAPI' (Table 6). Despite these restrictions, the new 2018 AHA/ASA guidelines state that given the extremely low risk of these laboratory values being abnormal, IV TPA treatment should not be delayed waiting for results if there is no reason to suspect an abnormal test.[5]

TABLE 6. Impermissible IV TPA Laboratory Criteria

P	PT >15
A	aPTT >40
P	Platelets <100,000/mm3
I	INR >1.7

TABLE 5. Permissible Criteria for IV TPA: **CAN HAPPEN**

C	Coumadin Use and INR ≤ 1.7
A	Aneurysm (< 10 mm) or AVM
N	Normalized Hyperglycemia
H	Hypertension That can be Lowered Safely (< 185/110 mmHg)
A	A Potential Bleeding Diathesis or Coagulopathy
P	Pregnant and Postpartum Patients
P	Pericarditis
E	Epilepsy/Seizure at Stroke Onset
N	Neoplasm

23.4.3 Anticoagulants

Vitamin K antagonists, factor Xa inhibitors (including heparin and derivative substances), and direct thrombin inhibitors are three types of anticoagulants commonly encountered with atrial fibrillation patients suffering stroke (Table 7). IV TPA is permissible with warfarin (Coumadin®) use if the INR ≤ 1.7 and not permissible if INR > 1.7. IV TPA is not recommended if therapeutic (but not prophylactic) low molecular weight heparins (LMWHs) have been administered within the previous 24 hours. IV TPA use is likewise currently not recommended with direct thrombin inhibitors such as dabigatran (Pradaxa®), bivalirudin (Angiomax®), and argatroban (Acova®), or factor Xa inhibitors such as apixaban (Eliquis®), edoxaban (Savaysa®) or rivaroxaban (Xarelto®).

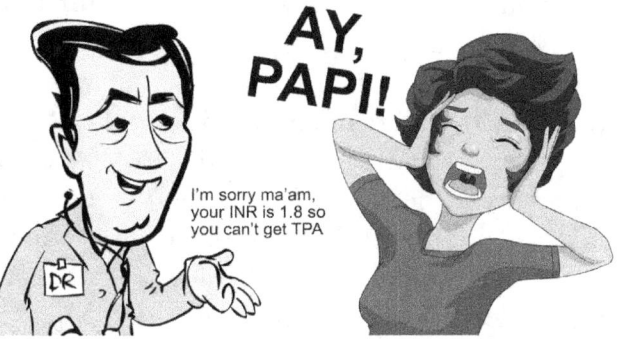

TABLE 7. Anticoagulant and IV TPA Use

ANTICOAGULANT CLASS	ANTICOAGULANT	TPA USE
Vitamin K Antagonists	Warfarin (Coumadin®)	YES - If INR ≤ 1.7 NO - If INR > 1.7
Factor Xa Inhibitors	Low Molecular Weight Heparins (LMWHs)	YES - If LMWH is administered > 24 hours NO - If ≤ 24 Hours
	Apixaban (Eliquis®) Edoxaban (Savaysa®) Rivaroxaban (Xarelto®)	NO*
Direct Thrombin Inhibitors	Dabigatran (Pradaxa®) Bivalirudin (Angiomax®) Argatroban (Acova)	NO*

*unless normal laboratory tests or were taken >48 hours

23.4.4 Temporally Related Criteria

Temporally related criteria regarding IV TPA administration are determined at 7 days, 14 days, 21 days and 3 months. The safety and efficacy of IV TPA administration to AIS patients who have received an arterial puncture of a noncompressible vessel in the preceding seven days is uncertain. IV TPA can be given to AIS patients who have undergone a lumbar puncture within the preceding seven days.[5] The administration of IV TPA can be considered in both major trauma (excluding severe head trauma) and major surgery (excluding intracranial and spinal) within 14 days. In both cases, bleeding from traumatic injury or the surgical site should be weighed against the potential stroke-related disability or anticipated benefits of IV TPA. Gastrointestinal structural malignancies or recent hemorrhage within 21 days of an acute stroke are considered high risk and IV TPA administration is potentially harmful.

IV TPA is contraindicated in patients who have experienced severe head trauma and can be potentially harmful following central nervous system (intracranial or spinal) surgery or an ischemic (or hemorrhagic) stroke within three months. One should notice a trend here. Essentially, IV TPA is contraindicated or potentially harmful to any central nervous system (brain or spinal cord) event such as surgery, ischemia, or trauma within three months. For these patients, this means you have to 'SIT' on IV TPA and not administer it. That's the mnemonic to help recall exclusions in TPA administration within three months of certain CNS processes (Table 8).

TABLE 8. Three Months CNS Events That Exclude IV TPA Administration: **SIT**

S	Surgery, Intracranial or Spinal Within Three Months
I	Ischemic or Hemorrhagic Stroke Within Three Months
T	Trauma, Severe Head Trauma Within Three Months

However, if the patient has a history of a recent MI in the last three months, the decision of whether or not to administer IV TPA is dependent on the AIS patient's ST–segment–elevation myocardial infarction (STEMI) status. The administration of IV TPA is reasonable if the recent MI (< 3 months) was non-STEMI. IV TPA administration is also reasonable if the recent MI (< 3 months) was a STEMI involving the left anterior myocardium or the right or inferior myocardium.[5] The administration of IV TPA is also reasonable in those AIS patients presenting with concurrent AIS and acute MI.[5]

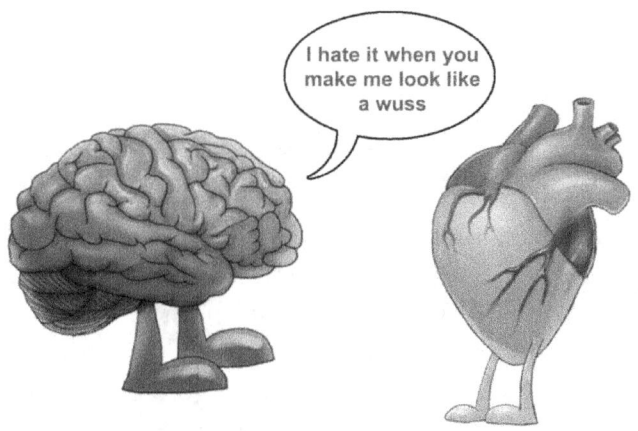

Again, IV TPA administration in patients with a history of intracranial hemorrhage is potentially harmful. Intracranial hemorrhage includes subarachnoid hemorrhage, parenchymal hemorrhage, and intraventricular hemorrhage, hemorrhagic conversion of infarction, epidural hematoma, and subdural hematoma. However, ≤ 10 asymptomatic cerebral microbleeds detected by gradient echo sequences and magnetic resonance imaging (MRI) is not a contraindication to the administration of IV TPA (see Section 23.7).[13] The new 2018 AHA/ASA guidelines also state, "Routine use of magnetic resonance imaging (MRI) to exclude cerebral microbleeds (CMBs) before administration of IV alteplase is not recommended."[5] An easy way to remember the different types of intracranial hemorrhage, all of which prohibit the use of IV TPA, is with the mnemonic 'SPICES' (Table 9).

TABLE 9. Different Types of Intracranial Hemorrhage: **SPICES**

S	Subarachnoid Hemorrhage
P	Parenchymal Hemorrhage
I	Intraventricular Hemorrhage
C	Conversion – Hemorrhagic Conversion of Infarct
E	Epidural Hematoma
S	Subdural Hematoma

23.4.5 IV TPA Restricted Criteria

All of the 2018 AHA/ASA guidelines are based on the strength of the recommendation which is referred to as a *class* and the quality of evidence which is referred to as a *level*. The level of evidence is further broken down into greater distinctions based on the type of data used and the origin of such data (i.e., randomized controlled trials). This information demonstrates how the recommendation was created along with its supporting evidence. There are several IV TPA contraindications, 16 additional recommendations that reach Class IIa level of evidence, and 25 additional recommendations that reach Class IIb level of evidence, favoring the benefit of IV TPA over risk. One should really read and familiarize themselves with these recommendations. Listed below is a simple mnemonic to remember the list of IV TPA restrictions (Table 10).

Before reviewing these restrictions, realized that there are several terms used to caution the use of IV TPA such as *not recommended*, *potentially harmful*, or *contraindicated*. Essentially, clinicians are encouraged to make individual decisions that are both patient and treatment-specific. Since few of these criteria are actual "contraindications," this category will be referred to as "IV TPA restrictions." Although IV TPA restrictive criteria have been summarized into different categories above, a single IV TPA restriction list is extremely practical. Again, this list represents the AHA/ASA scientific statement recommendations and the 2018 AHA/ASA guidelines for the discouraged use of IV TPA. These documents suggest that IV TPA is not recommended for brain CT evidence of an acute intracranial hemorrhage or > 1/3 MCA infarct, intracranial aneurysm ≥10mm, onset > 4.5 hours or unknown, suspected aortic dissection, certain laboratory values (PAPI: PT >15, aPTT > 40, platelets < 100,000/mm3 or INR >1.7), therapeutic (not prophylactic) low molecular weight heparin (LMWH) within the previous 24 hours, suspected infective endocarditis, history of intracranial hemorrhage, intra-axial intracranial neoplasm, structural G.I. malignancy or recent bleeding event within 21 days, history of intracranial or spinal surgery, or ischemic stroke or head trauma in the previous three months. These can be summarized by the mnemonic 'NOT TPA CLIENTS™' (Table 10).

TABLE 10. IV TPA Restrictions: **NOT TPA CLIENTS**™

N	Non-Enhanced Contrast CT >1/3 MCA
O	Onset of Symptoms >4.5 Hrs or UNKNOWN
T	Ten, Intracranial Aneurysm ≥10mm
T	Tumor, Intra-Axial or GI (or GI Bleed <21d)
P	Prior Ischemic Stroke Within 3 Months
A	Aortic Dissection (Suspected)
C	Coagulopathy: Coumadin (if INR >1.7) and Coumadin Analogs (Direct Thrombin Inhibitors or Direct Factor Xa Inhibitors) PT >15, aPTT >40, PLTS <100,000 & INR >1.7
L	Low Molecular Weight Heparin <24 Hours (Full Treatment Dose, Not Prophylactic Dose)
I	Intracranial Hemorrhage - Acute or 3 Month History
E	Endocarditis, Infectious (Suspected)
N	Noncompressible Vessel Puncture Within 7 Days (Safety and Efficacy of IV TPA Uncertain)
T	Trauma, Severe Head Within 3 Months
S	Surgery, CNS (Intracranial or Spine) Within 3 Months

23.5 Neuroimaging and IV TPA

Another IV TPA restriction is **hypodense brain tissue**. Hypodense brain tissue was discussed in Chapter 21 (Stroke Imaging). As explained in that chapter, early ischemic changes (EICs) can be identified on noncontrast brain CTs but this terminology is often confusing. For this reason, only two terms should be utilized when interpreting ischemic changes on noncontrast brain CTs: *hypodense* and *isodense*. One should identify **hypodense brain tissue** which represents core infarct or **isodense, swollen brain tissue** which represents ischemic penumbra (Box 2). Again, isodense focal swelling represents a separate process than parenchymal hypoattenuation. Isodense brain tissue swelling represents threatened brain tissue or reversible ischemic penumbra.[14,15] Hypodense brain tissue, however, is representative of irreversibly damaged brain tissue or core infarct.[16]

BOX 2. Imaging Characteristic of Ischemic Penumbra and Core Infarct

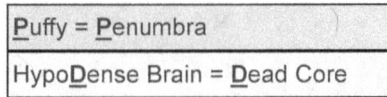

Both the earlier 2013 and new 2018 AHA/ASA guidelines recommended IV TPA even with the presence of EICs (brain swelling) on CT but also cautioned that hypodensity on CT can increase the risk of intracranial hemorrhage.[17] This makes sense because isodense brain tissue represents ischemic penumbra and parenchymal hypodensity represents core infarct. The 2018 AHA/ASA guidelines state, "There remains insufficient evidence to identify a threshold of acute CT hypoattenuation severity or extent that affects treatment response to IV alteplase. The extent severity of acute hypoattenuation or early ischemic changes should not be used as a criterion to withhold therapy for such patients who otherwise qualify." Nevertheless, they also state, "However, administering IV alteplase to patients whose CT brain imaging exhibits extensive regions of clear hypoattenuation is **not recommended**. These patients have a poor prognosis despite IV alteplase and severe hypo-attenuation defined as **obvious hypodensity represents irreversible injury**."

So what does all this really mean? It seems as if the 2018 AHA/ASA guidelines may be lumping hypodense brain tissue and early ischemic changes together when they state, "The extent severity of acute hypoattenuation or early ischemic changes should not be used as a criterion to withhold therapy for such patients who otherwise qualify." I somewhat agree with this statement because swollen, isodense brain tissue represents salvageable ischemic penumbra whereas hypodense brain tissue represents irreparably damaged core infarct. If early ischemic changes mean isodense and swollen brain tissue which is representative of salvageable ischemic penumbra, then their presence should not be used as criteria to withhold thrombolytic therapy. However, hypodense brain tissue represents irreparably damaged core infarct and for this reason, I agree with the guidelines when they state, "However administering IV alteplase to patients whose CT brain imaging exhibits extensive regions of clear hypoattenuation is not recommended. These patients have a poor prognosis despite IV alteplase and severe hypo-attenuation defined as obvious hypodensity represents irreversible injury." Thus, IV TPA administration is "not recommended" when extensive regions of clear hypoattenuation are present on noncontrast brain CT. Again, hypodense brain tissue that represents more than one-third of the MCA territory is an increased risk for symptomatic intracranial hemorrhage and represents irreversible injury (core infarct). This confusion can be eliminated by no longer categorizing both isodense and hypodense brain tissue as EICs. Again, instead of using the term EICs to describe acute ischemic changes on brain CT, one should **only use the terms *isodense* or *hypodense* brain tissue**.

23.6 IV TPA Limitations

IV TPA represents one of the greatest medical discoveries of the 21st century and may even contend as one of the greatest drugs in history. Despite these accolades, IV TPA still has limitations. These limitations are presented not as criticism for TPA but as a platform to enhance its use. Perhaps the greatest limitation of IV TPA is its relatively low rate of use in ischemic stroke patients. Why is that the case? Typically, most ischemic stroke patients do not present to the emergency department within three hours. So what can be done to improve this? One step would be to improve community awareness so stroke patients understand these time limitations. In fact, the new 2018 AHA/ASA guidelines state, "Public health leaders, along with medical professionals and others, should design and implement public education programs focused on stroke systems and the need to seek emergency care (by calling 911) in a rapid manner. These programs should be sustained over time and designed to reach racially/ethnically, age, and sex diverse populations."[5]

Another method would be to extend the time window for IV TPA. For this reason, recent studies such as the European Cooperative Acute Stroke Study (ECASS) 3 investigated extending the time window for IV TPA treatment.[18] In this trial, ischemic stroke patients received a benefit up to 4.5 hours after symptom onset. Specifically, the ECASS III study demonstrated 52% functional recovery when the treatment window for IV TPA was extended to 4.5 hours versus 45% functional recovery in patients receiving placebo. In other words, for one patient to benefit from the use of IV TPA between 3-4.5 hours, 14 patients will require treatment (Figure 2). The next chapter (Wake-Up Stroke) will discuss experimental stroke protocols that can potentially allow IV TPA to be administered for up to 24 hours!

Like every other aspect of stroke therapy, the sooner IV TPA is administered, the better it works. As stated by the new 2018 AHA/ASA guidelines, "In patients eligible for IV alteplase, benefit of therapy is time-dependent, and treatment should be initiated as quickly as possible."[5] TPA administration within 1.5 hours of symptom onset produced more favorable outcomes compared to administration within 1.5 to 3 hours, which was also shown to work better than administration within a 3 to 4.5-hour time frame.[6-11] A large meta-analysis of 6,756 patients from nine randomized trials investigating IV TPA further demonstrated the faster IV TPA is administered, the greater its proportional benefits. Furthermore, this meta-analysis emphasized the need for preventing delays in acute stroke treatment.[19] Clearly, the earlier IV TPA can be given the better its clinical benefits.

Despite its lower efficacy when given after three hours, the 2018 AHA/ASA guidelines also recommend IV TPA be administered between 3 to 4.5 hours after a stroke. Note that this recommendation is neither endorsed nor approved by the FDA and has a higher mortality rate. Also, the ECASS III trial excluded patients that were older than 80 years, taking anticoagulants, suffering a severe stroke (NIHSS greater than 25), and had a history of both diabetes and prior stroke. These were the initial exclusion criteria for IV TPA between three and 4.5 hours which can be remembered by the mnemonic 'EXPAND' (Table 11).

TABLE 11. Previous* Criteria for IV TPA Administered between 3 - 4.5 hours: **EXPAND**

E	Eighty, ≤80
X	X-Rays, CT ≤1/3 MCA
P	Prior Stroke and Diabetes History Excluded
A	Anticoagulant - Excluded Regardless of INR Value
N	NIHSS Score <25
D	Diabetes and Prior Stroke History Excluded

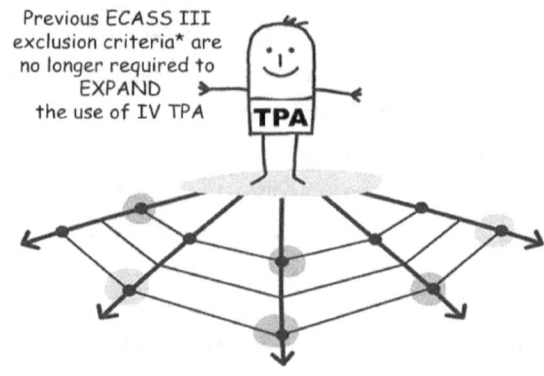

*Excluding a significant infarct (>1/3 MCA) and severe stroke symptoms (NIHSS >25), the new 2018 AHA/ASA guidelines have removed the previous ECASS III exclusion criteria for the administration of IV TPA 3 to 4.5 hours after symptom onset.

However, as stated in the 2018 AHA/ASA guidelines, careful analysis indicates that these exclusion criteria from the ECASS III Trial "may not be justified in practice."[5] The 2018 AHA/ASA guidelines allow the extended use of IV TPA between 3 and 4.5 hours for AIS patients who are > age 80, taking warfarin with an INR ≤ 1.7, had a prior stroke and are diabetic. These same guidelines do however state, "The benefit of IV alteplase between 3 and 4.5 hours from symptom onset for patients with very severe stroke symptoms (NIHSS > than 25) is uncertain." Excluding a significant infarct (>1/3 MCA) and severe stroke symptoms (NIHSS > than 25), the new 2018 AHA/ASA guidelines have pretty much eliminated the previous ECASS III exclusion criteria for the administration of IV TPA 3 to 4.5 hours from symptom onset.

Even with the extended treatment window of 4.5 hours, fewer than 5% of all ischemic stroke patients receive IV TPA. In addition, relatively large systemic doses of IV TPA are required to circulate throughout the entire body to reach comparably small vessels in the brain. Another significant limitation is IV TPA's relative ineffectiveness in large vessel occlusion (LVO) stroke (Figure 3). For example, LVOs such as occlusions of the internal carotid artery and the M1 segment of the middle cerebral artery have lower rates of recanalization than more distal vessel occlusions such as M2, M3, or M4 segments. Essentially, the effectiveness of IV TPA diminishes as vessel size increases. For example, IV TPA achieves early recanalization in less than 30% of patients with large vessel occlusion.[20] In addition to vessel size, IV TPA is also limited by clot burden. Specifically, longer thrombus length is indirectly related to IV TPA effectiveness, with thrombus lengths exceeding 10 mm predictive of unsatisfactory thrombolytic efficacy.[21-23]

FIGURE 3. IV TPA Limitations

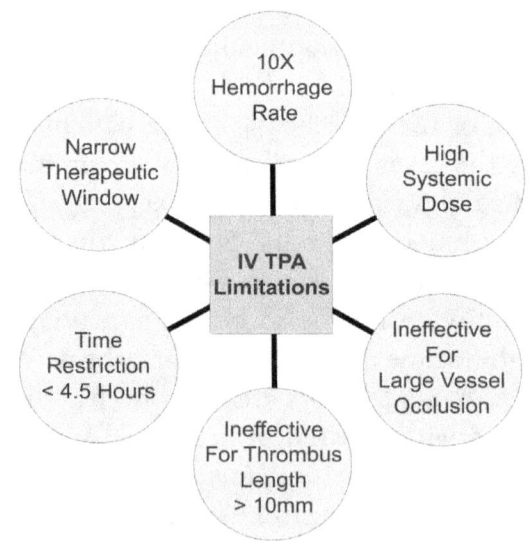

23.7 Cerebral Microbleeds (CMBs)

Cerebral microbleeds (CMBs) are small perivascular hemosiderin deposits that appear as dark lesions on MRI hemosiderin-sensitive imaging sequences. As discussed in Chapter 6 (Hemorrhagic

Stroke), CMBs can be caused by at least two pathological mechanisms: cerebral amyloid angiopathy (CAA) and hypertensive microangiopathy. AIS patients otherwise eligible to receive IV TPA have a high prevalence of CMBs, ranging from 18% to 68%.[24] This raises the question of whether IV TPA can safely be administered to patients with CMBs. Some evidence suggests that there is increased concern for symptomatic intracerebral hemorrhage in patients with >10 CMBs identified on MRI. The 2018 AHA/ASA guidelines state: "In otherwise eligible patients who have had a previously demonstrated small number (1-10) of CMBs on MRI, administration of IV alteplase is reasonable."[5] However, if the patient has > 10 CMBs, then an appropriate risk-benefit discussion and patient-level decision-making are recommended (Table 12). The 2018 AHA/ASA guidelines state: "In otherwise eligible patients who have had a previously demonstrated high burden of CMBs (> 10) on MRI, treatment with IV alteplase may be associated with an increased risk of sICH, and the benefits of treatment are uncertain. Treatment may be reasonable if there is the potential for substantial benefit."[5]

23.8 Pre-existing Antithrombotic Therapy and IV TPA

A new 2018 AHA/ASA guideline recommendation states: "The risk of antithrombotic therapy within the first 24 hours following treatment with IV alteplase (with or without EVT) is **uncertain**. Use might be considered in the presence of **concomitant conditions** for which such treatment given in the absence of IV to alteplase is known to provide substantial benefit or withholding such treatment is known to cause substantial risk." A retrospective, single-center study from South Korea found no increased risk of ICH with early initiation of antiplatelet or anticoagulant therapy (less than 24 hours) after IV alteplase or EVT compared with initiation after 24 hours.[25] Note that this recommendation is directed at patients with concomitant conditions (i.e., coronary stent) for which withholding antiplatelet therapy can cause substantial risk.

This recommendation is not intended for patients not currently taking antiplatelets to improve recanalization and generate better outcomes after IV TPA administration. In fact, a recent randomized trial demonstrated no benefit from 300 mg of intravenous aspirin administration 90 minutes after IV TPA treatment.[26] This trial was halted due to futility and an increased risk of intracerebral hemorrhage. The primary endpoint of this trial was a good outcome which was achieved in 54% of patients receiving aspirin and IV TPA (treatment group) compared with 57% of patients who received only IV TPA. Furthermore, this trial demonstrated a significantly increased risk of symptomatic hemorrhage in the early-aspirin group (relative risk, 3.4). This study concluded that the early initiation of antiplatelet therapy in conjunction with IV TPA is both ineffective and dangerous. Thus, one should wait at least 24 hours prior to initiating antiplatelet therapy after IV TPA treatment. Recall that in Chapter 18 (Platelets, Stents and Stroke), dual platelet inhibition for recurrent stroke was recommended 24 hours **after** the administration of IV TPA.

TABLE 12. Summary of 2018 AHA/ASA IV TPA / CMB Recommendations

Summary of 2018 AHA/ASA IV TPA / CMB Recommendations	
CMBs Identified on MRI	Recommendation
≤10	IV TPA Reasonable
>10	IV TPA Risks and Benefits Uncertain

CMB - Cerebral Microbleed, MRI - Magnetic Resonance Imaging, TPA - Tissue Plasminogen Activator

23.9 Conclusion

The therapeutic goal in AIS is the restoration of the ischemic penumbra by recanalization of an occluded blood vessel. The NINDS trial was a milestone study that demonstrated the efficacy of IV TPA in the recanalization of occluded blood vessels, so long as it was administered within the first three hours after stroke onset. Then, data from the ECASS III trial demonstrated that the benefits of IV TPA can be extended for up to 4.5 hours in select patients. This chapter reviewed the older inclusion and exclusion criteria for IV TPA. Furthermore, it discussed the recent 2015 AHA/ASA scientific statement and newer 2018 AHA/ASA guidelines regarding these criteria. By making these criteria more adaptable, the goal is to increase the number of patients who would benefit from IV TPA. Time is the enemy of the brain. The faster stroke patients are treated, the more beneficial their outcomes. It is essential to eliminate any potential delays in treatment. Delays in the administration of IV TPA not only result in worse functional outcome but also increase the risk of intracerebral hemorrhage.

IV TPA administration may be one of the greatest medical treatment discoveries of the 21st century. However, only a minority of AIS patients (less than 5%) in the United States receive it. Despite this and other limitations, IV TPA remains the standard of treatment for non-LVO AIS. Any AIS patient eligible for IV TPA should receive it. The AHA/ASA's recent scientific statement on IV TPA criteria also highlighted several areas of high priority for future study. Among these was neuroimaging to identify patients who may benefit from IV TPA based on tissue viability rather than arbitrary time points. This is especially relevant to AIS patients who present with wake-up strokes or strokes with an unclear time of onset. Wake-up stroke will be discussed in the next chapter and the role of physiologic imaging will be discussed throughout this text. As will be presented again and again, all ischemic stroke treatment rests on the ability to reperfuse threatened brain tissue (ischemic penumbra) which is dependent on collateral circulation.

While IV TPA is the only FDA approved pharmacological treatment for acute ischemic stroke, it is not the only FDA approved treatment for this cerebrovascular event. Subsequent chapters will discuss the only other FDA approved treatment for acute ischemic stroke: **endovascular treatment (EVT)**. IV TPA and EVT should always be considered as a continuum in the spectrum of ischemic stroke treatment since they have the same therapeutic goals—**the recanalization of an occluded vessel and the reperfusion of threatened brain tissue**. For this reason, both these treatment options should be considered in all AIS patients, particularly those with large vessel occlusion.

Abbreviations list

AHA, American Heart Association; AIS, acute ischemic stroke; ASA, American Stroke Association; CMBs, cerebral microbleeds; EVT, endovascular treatment; FDA, Food and Drug Administration; IV TPA, intravenous administration of recombinant tissue plasminogen activator; LMWHs, low molecular weight heparins; LVO, large vessel occlusion; MCA, middle cerebral artery; MRI, magnetic resonance imaging; NINDS, National Institute of Neurologic Disorders and Stroke; NNT, number needed to be treated; STEMI, ST–segment–elevation myocardial infarction.

References

1. The National Institute of Neurological Disorders and Stroke rt-PA Stroke Study Group. (1995). Tissue plasminogen activator for acute ischemic stroke. *N Engl J Med*, 333, 1581-87.
2. Keeley EC, Boura JA, Grines CL. (2003). Primary angioplasty versus intravenous thrombolytic therapy for acute myocardial infarction: a quantitative review of 23 randomised trials. *Lancet*, Jan 4, 361(9351), 13–20.
3. McAlister FA, Straus SE, Guyatt GH, Haynes RB. (2000). Evidence-Based Medicine Working Group. Users' guides to the medical literature: XX. Integrating research evidence with the care of the individual patient. *Jama*, 283, 2829–36.

4. Nasr DM, Brinjikji W, Cloft HJ, Rabinstein AA. (2013). Utilization of intravenous thrombolysis is increasing in the United States. *Int J Stroke*, 8, 681–88.
5. Powers WJ, Rabinstein AA, Ackerson T, Adeoye OM, Bambakidis NC, Becker K, Biller J, Brown M, Demaerschalk BM, Hoh B, et al. (2018) Guidelines for the Early Management of Patients With Acute Ischemic Stroke: A Guideline for Healthcare Professionals From the American Heart Association/American Stroke Association. *Stroke*, Epub 2018 Jan 24.
6. The Thrombolysis in Myocardial Infarction (TIMI) trial: phase I findings: TIMI Study Group. (1985). *N Engl J Med*, 312, 932–36.
7. Brott T, Haley EC, Levy DE, Barsan WG, Reed RL, Olinger CP, Marler JR. (1988). The investigational use of tPA for stroke. *Ann Emerg Med*, 17, 1202– 05. doi: http://dx.doi.org/10.1016/S0196-0644(88)80069-6.
8. Haley EC Jr, Brott TG, Sheppard GL, Barsan W, Broderick J, Marler JR, Kongable GL, Spilker J, Massey S, Hansen CA, Torner JC—TPA Bridging Study Group. (1993). Pilot randomized trial of tissue plasminogen activator in acute ischemic stroke: the TPA Bridging Study Group. *Stroke*, 24, 1000–04, doi: 10.1161/01.STR.24.7.1000.
9. Brott TG, Haley EC Jr, Levy DE, Barsan W, Broderick J, Sheppard GL, Spilker J, Kongable GL, Massey S, Reed R, Marler JR. (1992). Urgent therapy for stroke, part I: pilot study of tissue plasminogen activator administered within 90 minutes. *Stroke*, 23, 632–40, doi: 10.1161/01.STR.23.5.632.
10. Sundt TM Jr, Grant WC, Garcia JH. (1969). Restoration of middle cerebral artery flow in experimental infarction. *J Neurosurg*, 31, 311–21, doi: 10.3171/jns.1969.31.3.0311.
11. Crowell RM, Olsson Y, Klatzo I, Ommaya A. (1970). Temporary occlusion of the middle cerebral artery in the monkey: clinical and pathological observations. *Stroke*, 1, 439–48, doi: 10.1161/01.STR.1.6.439.
12. Brott T, Lu M, Kothari R, et al. (1998). Hypertension and its treatment in the NINDS rt-PA Stroke Trial. *Stroke*, 29(8), 1504–09.
13. Fiehler J, Albers GW, Boulanger JM, et al. (2007). Bleeding risk analysis in stroke imaging before thrombolysis (BRASIL): pooled analysis of T2*-weighted magnetic resonance imaging data from 570 patients. *Stroke*, 38(10), 2738–44.
14. Muir KW, Baird-Gunning J, Walker L, Baird T, McCormick M, Coutts SB. (2007). Can the ischemic penumbra be identified on noncontrast CT of acute stroke? *Stroke*, 38, 2485–90.
15. Butcher KS, Lee SB, Parsons MW, Allport L, Fink J, Tress B, Donnan G, Davis SM—EPITHET Investigators. (2007). Differential prognosis of isolated cortical swelling and hypoattenuation on CT in acute stroke. *Stroke*, 38, 941–47.
16. Dzialowski I, Hill MD, Coutts SB, Demchuk AM, Kent DM, Wunderlich O, von Kummer R. (2006). Extent of early ischemic changes on computed tomography (CT) before thrombolysis: prognostic value of the Alberta Stroke Program Early CT Score in ECASS II. *Stroke*, 37, 973–78.
17. Jauch EC, Saver JL, Adams HP Jr, Bruno A, Connors JJ, Demaerschalk BM, Khatri P, McMullan PW Jr, Qureshi AI, Rosenfield K, Scott PA, Summers DR, Wang DZ, Wintermark M, Yonas H;—on behalf of the American Heart Association Stroke Council; Council on Cardiovascular Nursing; Council on Peripheral Vascular Disease; Council on Clinical Cardiology. (2013). Guidelines for the early management of patients with acute ischemic stroke: a guideline for healthcare professionals from the American Heart Association/American Stroke Association. *Stroke*, 44, 870–947.
18. Hacke W, Kaste M, Bluhmki E, et al. (2008). Thrombolysis with alteplase 3 to 4.5 hours after acute ischemic stroke. *N Engl J Med*, 359(13), 1317-29.
19. Emberson J, Lees KR, Lyden P, Blackwell L, Albers G, Bluhmki E, et al. (2014). Effect of treatment delay, age, and stroke severity on the effects of intravenous thrombolysis with alteplase for acute ischaemic stroke: A meta-analysis of individual patient data from randomised trials. *Lancet*, 384, 1929-35.
20. Smith WS, for the Multi MERCI Investigators. (2006). Safety of mechanical thrombectomy and intravenous tissue plasminogen activator in acute ischemic stroke. Results of the multi mechanical embolus removal in cerebral ischemia (MERCI) trial, Part I. *Am J Neuroradiol*, 27, 1177-82.
21. *AJNR Am J Neuroradiol*, (2013). Oct, 34(10), 1908-13.

22. Rohan V, Baxa J, Tupy R, Cerna L, Sevcik P, Friesl M, Polivka J Jr, Polivka J, Ferda J. (2014). Length of occlusion predicts recanalization and outcome after intravenous thrombolysis in middle cerebral artery stroke. *Stroke*, Jul, 45(7), 2010-17.
23. Riedel CH, Zimmermann P, Jensen-Kondering U, Stingele R, Deuschl G, Jansen O. (2011). The importance of size: successful recanalization by intravenous thrombolysis in acute anterior stroke depends on thrombus length. *Stroke,* Jun, 42(6), 1775-7.
24. Viswanathan A, Chabriat H. (2006). Cerebral microhemorrhage. *Stroke*, 37, 550–55.
25. Jeong HG, Kim BJ, Yang MH, Han MK, Bae HJ, Lee SH. (2016). Stroke outcomes with use of antithrombotics within 24 hours after recanalization treatment. *Neurology,* 87, 996–1002.
26. Zinkstok SM and Roos YB. (2012). Early administration of aspirin in patients treated with alteplase for acute ischaemic stroke: A randomised controlled trial. *Lancet*, Jun 28.

Chapter 24

Wake-Up Stroke

24.1 Introduction

Wake-up stroke (WUS) occurs when a patient goes to sleep normally and awakens with stroke symptoms. WUS can account for more than 25% of acute ischemic stroke (AIS) patients.[1,2] Currently, acute stroke management is fundamentally determined by the time of symptom onset.[3] IV TPA remains the only FDA-approved drug for the treatment of ischemic stroke.[4] However, the use of IV TPA is predicated on the exact time of symptom onset. Wake-up stroke without a last known normal (LKN) or symptom onset time deprives the acute stroke provider of this valuable data, resulting in a therapeutic conundrum. Until recently, no therapeutic guidelines existed for this substantial group of stroke patients.

While the pathophysiologic mechanism of wake-up stroke is not entirely understood, most AIS occur during morning hours between 6 AM and 12 PM.[5,6] Yet, wake-up stroke patients still lack a distinct time of symptom onset. Currently, IV TPA can be administered up to 3 hours and its use may be extended up to 4.5 hours.[7,8] The lack of an exact time of symptom onset requires some other form of surrogate data to replace it. In this instance, researchers have turned to advanced neuroimaging techniques.[9]

24.2 Neuroimaging and Wake-Up Stroke

While many researchers consider neuroimaging modalities as a surrogate marker for symptom duration, they are far more valuable. Neuroimaging modalities provide a precise determination of brain function and physiology. They are vastly more accurate than arbitrary time points that do not account for individual patient physiology. In a sense, neuroimaging allows an arbitrary time window to be replaced by a precise "tissue" window. Further, WUS patients have more severe NIHHS scores, prolonged hospital admissions, and worse outcomes.[10] For these reasons, neuroimaging does not only serve as a surrogate marker for missing LKN data; it also supplies other valuable information such as the presence of a large vessel occlusion, the size of a core infarct, and the presence of threatened but still viable brain tissue (ischemic penumbra). This is of primary concern for WUS patients since they have a higher prevalence of large vessel disease.[11]

Realize that time from symptom onset is arbitrary because the presence of an ischemic penumbra or core infarct depends on multiple patient-specific factors including collateral flow, ischemic pre-conditioning, cerebral blood flow pressure, serum glucose, body temperature, and oxygen delivery capacity. The only way to determine if significant collaterals or ischemic penumbra exist is through neuroimaging as discussed in Chapter 21 (Stroke Imaging). The treatment of all stroke including WUS is based on the determination of the presence of threatened but still viable brain tissue (ischemic penumbra). Recall that the presence of hemorrhage or a greater than one-third the MCA territory hypodensity is considered restrictive criteria (contraindicated and not recommended, respectively) for the administration of IV TPA. In a similar manner, endovascular treatment cannot be performed unless a significant core infarct is excluded and the presence of threatened brain or an ischemic penumbra is determined. The risk of endovascular treatment may not be justified without determining that the benefit of potentially salvageable brain tissue (ischemic penumbra) exists.

24.3 Wake-Up Stroke (WUS) Clinical Trials

Neuroimaging is required to determine the presence of an occluded vessel, small core infarct, and significant ischemic penumbra. This determination is becoming more important for the treatment of all AIS, whether the occlusion involves a small or large vessel. In fact, investigators seeking WUS treatment options clearly demonstrated this point when researching the applications of neuroimaging for the treatment of WUS with either IV TPA or EVT. The researchers of the MR WITNESS Trial discussed their findings at the International Stroke Conference (ISC) 2016.[12] Essentially the trial tested the safety and ability to use IV TPA utilizing MRI diffusion-weighted imaging (DWI)-positive and fluid-attenuated inversion recovery (FLAIR)-negative mismatch. If this sounds familiar, it should. Chapter 21 (Stroke Imaging) described a cerebral blood flow (CBF) and a cerebral blood volume (CBV) mismatch pattern. Here, we are discussing an MRI mismatch pattern between DWI-positive images and FLAIR-negative images instead of a CTP mismatch pattern between CBF and CBV. A DWI MRI detects *cytotoxic* edema within the brain which occurs when there is lack of Brownian motion within a neuron. This occurs very quickly, minutes after a neuron has been affected by stroke. However, a FLAIR sequence represents *vasogenic* edema which takes hours to appear bright after it is affected by stroke. Thus, if a DWI sequence and a FLAIR sequence are both bright, this a matched defect representing irreparably damaged brain tissue. However, if the DWI sequence is bright and the FLAIR sequence is not, this is a mismatch which represents salvageable brain tissue or ischemic penumbra.

Patients were included in the MR WITNESS Trial if they met the TPA criteria discussed in Chapter 23, had no stroke symptoms 4.5-24 hours earlier, could get IV TPA within 4.5 hours of the time of symptom discovery, and their MRI study demonstrated a DWI-positive and FLAIR-negative mismatch. To remember these criteria, use the mnemonic 'MINT' (Table 1). The results from the MR WITNESS Trial in terms of functional independence were worse than the ECASS 3 trial. Recall in that trial, 14 patients required treatment (NNT) for one patient to benefit from the treatment (Figure 1). While this may not sound encouraging, one should remember that the treatment of stroke is an evolving process. Any process that advances the outcome of this devastating disease should be applauded. The MR WITNESS Trial requires a standing ovation because it demonstrates that the administration of IV TPA is dependent on tissue viability determined by neuroimaging and not by arbitrary time points. Rather than relying on arbitrary time points, shouldn't we be using this standard for any stroke patient that has neuroimaging evidence of ischemic penumbra and whose symptom duration is greater than 4.5 hours?

TABLE 1. MR WITNESS Trial Criteria: **MINT**

M	MRI Mismatch
I	IV TPA Within 4.5 Hours of Symptom Discovery
N	No Stroke Symptoms 4.5 – 24 Hours Earlier
T	TPA Criteria Met

Despite the findings of the MR WITNESS Trial, the 2018 AHA/ASA guidelines discourage the use of neuroimaging criteria for IV TPA treatment determination for wake-up ischemic stroke patients. Specifically, these guidelines state: "Use of imaging criteria to select ischemic stroke patients who awoke from stroke or have unclear time of onset for treatment IV alteplase is not recommended outside a clinical trial."[13] However, the guidelines encourage the use of imaging criteria to select appropriate EVT candidates.

FIGURE 1. MR WITNESS Trial Number Needed to Treat (NNT)

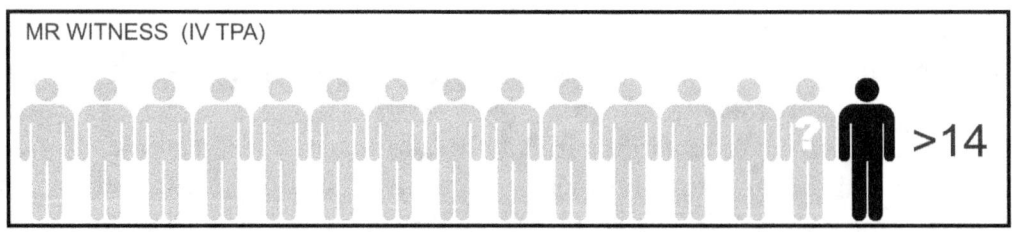

MR WITNESS Trial demonstrated that >14 people require treatment for one beneficial result

24.3.1 The DAWN Trial

The MR WITNESS Trial investigated the use of IV TPA in patients who presented with stroke symptoms between 4.5-24 hours earlier. On the other hand, the **D**WI or Computerized Tomography Perfusion **A**ssessment of Clinical Mismatch in the Triage of **W**ake-Up and Late Presenting Strokes Undergoing **N**eurointervention with Trevo (**DAWN**) Trial compared the outcomes of using the Trevo thrombectomy device plus medical management versus medical management alone.[14] Inclusion criteria included patients who presented 6 to 24 hours from last known normal and had an NIHSS >10, an anterior circulation large vessel occlusion documented by CTA or MRA, and a clinical-imaging mismatch between the neurologic deficit and infarct size. The DAWN Trial used either MRI or CTP selection criteria to determine the presence of viable penumbra. This trial was halted on its 31st month after enrolling 206 of its 500 anticipated patients.

The DAWN Trial demonstrated that EVT significantly decreased functional disability and improved functional independence at 90 days when compared to medical management (IV TPA) alone (48.6% versus 13.1%). This is a relative risk reduction in functional disability of 73%! This means that for every 2.8 treated patients, one additional patient was functionally independent at 90 days (Figure 2). This data demonstrates that EVT treatment within 24 hours in patients selected with sophisticated neuroimaging is more effective than patients whose treatment was previously determined by an arbitrary, less than six-hour time window. This again stresses the importance of either physiologic or functional imaging (which is patient-specific) over arbitrary time points.

For example, a patient who presents within three hours of stroke onset with no ischemic penumbra and a large core infarct would receive no benefit from either IV TPA or EVT. However, a patient who presents at 22 hours with a large vessel occlusion (LVO), small core infarct, and a significant ischemic penumbra would receive significant benefit from EVT therapy. Because the need to treat number (NNT) was only 2.8, there is tremendous potential for stroke patients to live an independent lifestyle without severe functional disability! The DAWN Trial currently has the largest successful treatment effect demonstrated by any endovascular stroke trial. The reduction in functional disability achieved in patients treated up to 24 hours is a tremendous message of hope for the thousands of stroke patients who present past the six-hour treatment window. Again, the DAWN Trial underscores the necessity of advanced neuroimaging (and not arbitrary time points) to determine EVT candidacy.

FIGURE 2. Dawn Trial Number Needed to Treat (NNT)

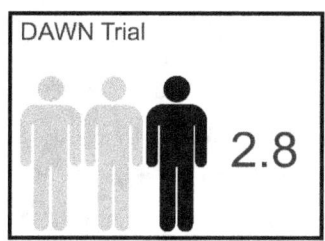

The DAWN Trial demonstrated 2.8 people require treatment for one beneficial result

In addition to the MR WITNESS and DAWN Trials, there are other trials and chief among them is the DEFUSE 3 Trial which is yet another endovascular trial demonstrating the effectiveness of EVT after six hours. This will be further discussed in the next chapter (Chapter 25, Endovascular Treatment). Like the DAWN Trial, the DEFUSE 3 Trial investigated the role of physiologic imaging in the determination of threatened brain tissue instead of using the time of symptom onset. Both the DAWN Trial and the DEFUSE 3 Trial stress the importance of physiologic imaging rather than arbitrary time points to determine brain tissue viability. As stated earlier, neuroimaging is the most critical factor to determine brain tissue viability in the therapeutic management of ischemic stroke.[15]

24.4 Conclusion

So where does this leave us with WUS? It is unlikely that stroke centers will adopt the DWI-FLAIR mismatch criteria discussed above in order to offer IV TPA treatment to wake-up stroke patients as reflected in the 2018 AHA/ASA guidelines.

However, EVT candidacy can be determined by advanced neuroimaging which is supported by the data from the DAWN and DEFUSE 3 Trials. Ongoing trials are investigating IV thrombolytic administration in WUS patients. However, the clinical conundrum of WUS underscores the importance of neuroimaging in the determination of brain tissue viability. It is not coincidental that this chapter on WUS follows the IV TPA chapter and precedes the EVT chapter. In many ways, WUS may represent the Rosetta Stone of the stroke arena. This is because it underscores the importance of utilizing neuroimaging to determine the degree of threatened brain tissue (ischemic penumbra) versus irreparably damaged brain tissue (core infarct) for each patient, rather than using arbitrary time points.

Advanced neuroimaging determines whether there is salvageable brain tissue or ischemic penumbra and nothing else can make this distinction. No clinical evaluation can discriminate between a completed stroke (core infarct) and salvageable brain tissue (ischemic penumbra). Certainly, multimodality neuroimaging techniques will play a crucial role in the determination of proper WUS patient selection. By quickly and accurately identifying threatened brain tissue (ischemic penumbra), neuroimaging will optimize and streamline future therapeutic strategies. While it may be difficult to offer IV TPA treatment to WUS patients, this is not the case for EVT. In fact, as will be discussed in the next chapter (and demonstrated by the results of the DAWN and DEFUSE 3 Trials), collateral circulation and not time is the true determinant of EVT candidacy.

Abbreviations list

AIS, acute ischemic stroke; CBF, cerebral blood flow; CBV, cerebral blood volume; CTA, computed tomography angiography; CTP, CT perfusion; DWI, diffusion-weighted imaging; EVT, endovascular treatment; FDA, Food and Drug Administration; FLAIR, fluid-attenuated inversion recovery; IV TPA, intravenous administration of recombinant tissue plasminogen activator; LKN, last known normal; LVO, large vessel occlusion; MCA, middle cerebral artery; MRA, magnetic resonance angiography; MRI, magnetic resonance imaging; NIHSS, National Institutes of Health Stroke Scale; NNT, number needed to treat; WUS, wake-up stroke.

References

1. Mackey J, Kleindorfer D, Sucharew H, Moomaw CJ, Kissela BM, Alwell K, et al. (2011). Population based study of wakeup strokes. *Neurology*, 76, 16627.
2. Moradiya Y, Janjua N. (2013). Presentation and outcomes of "wakeup strokes" in a large randomized stroke trial: Analysis of data from the international stroke trial. *J Stroke Cerebrovasc Dis*, 22, e28692.
3. Saver JL. (2006). Time is brain--quantified. *Stroke*, Jan, 37(1), 263-66.
4. Stroke Study Group. (1995). Tissue plasminogen activator for acute ischemic stroke. The National Institute of Neurological Disorders and Stroke rt-PA. *N Engl J Med*, Dec 14, 333(24), 1581-87.
5. Marler JR, Price TR, Clark GL, Muller JE, Robertson T, Mohr JP, Hier DB, Wolf PA, Caplan LR, Foulkes MA. (1989). Morning increase in onset of ischemic stroke. *Stroke*, Apr, 20(4), 473-76.
6. Elliott WJ. (1998). Circadian variation in the timing of stroke onset: a meta-analysis. *Stroke*, May, 29(5), 992-96.
7. Hacke W, Kaste M, Bluhmki E, Brozman M, Dávalos A, Guidetti D, et al. (2008). Thrombolysis with alteplase 3 to 4.5 hours after acute ischemic stroke. *N Engl J Med*, 359, 131729.
8. Marler JR, Tilley BC, Lu M, Brott TG, Lyden PC, Grotta JC, et al. (2000). Early stroke treatment associated with better outcome: The NINDS rtPA stroke study. *Neurology*, 55, 164955.
9. Kang DW, Kwon JY, Kwon SU, Kim JS. (2012). Wake-up or unclear-onset strokes: Are they waking up to the world of thrombolysis therapy? *Int J Stroke*, 7, 311-20.
10. Jiménez-Conde J, Ois A, Rodríguez-Campello A, Gomis M, Roquer J. (2007). Does sleep protect against ischemic stroke? Less frequent ischemic

strokes but more severe ones. *J Neurol*, 254, 7828.

11. Kim BJ, Lee SH, Shin CW, Ryu WS, Kim CK, Yoon BW. (2011). Ischemic stroke during sleep: Its association with worse early functional outcome. *Stroke*, 42, 19016.

12. Schwamm LH. IV Altephase in MR-Selected Patients With Stroke of Unknown Onset and Feasible: Results of the Multicenter MR WITNESS Trial (NCT01282242). *Stroke Service*, Massachusetts General Hospital, Harvard Medical School.

13. Powers WJ, Rabinstein AA, Ackerson T, Adeoye OM, Bambakidis NC, Becker K, Biller J, Brown M, Demaerschalk BM, Hoh B, et al. (2018) Guidelines for the Early Management of Patients With Acute Ischemic Stroke: A Guideline for Healthcare Professionals From the American Heart Association/American Stroke Association. *Stroke,* Epub 2018 Jan 24.

14. Nogueira RG, Jadhav AP, Haussen DC, et al. (2017). Thrombectomy 6 to 24 hours after stroke with a mismatch between deficit and infarct. *N Engl J Med*, 11 Nov.

15. Malhotra K, Liebeskind DS. (2015). Imaging in endovascular stroke trials. *J Neuroimaging*, 25, 51727.

Chapter 25

Endovascular Treatment

25.1 Introduction

Endovascular treatment (EVT) is one of the most important and powerful treatment modalities in any field of medicine. EVT has a number needed to treat (NNT) of 5.1 for patients to recover independent functional outcome. It also has an NNT of 2.6 for patients to reduce disability by at least one level on the modified Rankin scale (mRS) (Figure 1 and Table 1).[1] This chapter will review the major trials that proved EVT's efficacy and led to the subsequent American Heart Association and American Stroke Association (AHA/ASA) EVT guidelines in both 2015 and 2018. It will also discuss other insights that have been gained from these trials and subsequent added research. The treatment of acute ischemic stroke (AIS) is an ever-evolving process and in this regard, the role of IV TPA and EVT will also be explored.

FIGURE 1. Endovascular Number Needed to Treat (NNT)

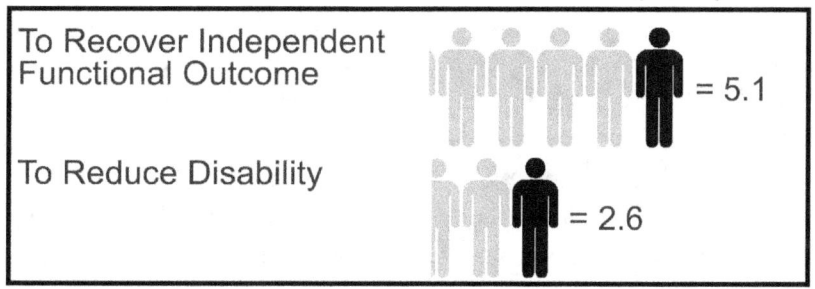

NNT = Number of people requiring treatment for one beneficial result

TABLE 1. Modified Rankin Scale (mRS)

Modified Rankin Scale	Description
0	No symptoms
1	No significant disability. Able to carry out all usual activities, despite some symptoms
2	Slight disability. Able to look after own affairs without assistance, but unable to carry out all previous activities
3	Moderate disability. Requires some help, but able to walk unassisted
4	Moderately severe disability. Unable to attend to own bodily needs without assistance, and unable to walk unassisted
5	Severe disability. Requires constant nursing care and attention, bedridden, incontinent
6	Dead

25.2 Initial Endovascular Trials

The first trial to demonstrate the clinical benefit of EVT was the PROACT II Trial.[2] The PROACT II Trial demonstrated that intra-arterial recombinant pro-urokinase (a thrombolytic agent) with IV heparin was superior to IV heparin alone for both recanalization and improved functional outcome measured at three months. Interestingly, the enrollment of this trial (1994) began at the same time the approval process for IV TPA was being conducted over 20 years ago. For many years thereafter, arguments would persist regarding whether EVT was warranted. It wasn't until 2013 that any other significant EVT trials were completed. During that year, three randomized controlled trials namely the **MR RESCUE**, **SYNTHESIS**, and **IMS III** Trials demonstrated no significant difference in functional outcome between EVT and medical management. Analyzing these trials today, there are several reasons why they failed to support the obvious benefits of EVT. Chief among these reasons are the lack of large vessel occlusion (LVO) confirmation on initial neuroimaging and the use of suboptimal endovascular devices. Both the IMS III and SYNTHESIS Trials did not evaluate LVO prior to randomization. Furthermore, antiquated technology (non-stent retriever) resulted in lower and slower revascularization rates.[3, 4]

In short, inadequate patient selection and the use of suboptimal endovascular devices were relevant factors that contributed to the failure of these earlier trials. These same trials demonstrated no clinical benefit of EVT, particularly in patients with large core infarcts present on initial CT imaging and where procedures were performed after 300 minutes (5 hours). Learning from these mistakes, it is critical to understand the enormous significance of proper neuroimaging, up-to-date technology, and enhanced workflow to improve recanalization time. Specifically, LVO AIS must be promptly diagnosed by advanced neuroimaging and immediately treated with optimal device technology. When it comes to LVO AIS patients, **we need to find them fast and fix them fast!** Additionally, proper patient selection for EVT candidacy must be performed to both exclude a significant core infarct and determine the presence of a significant ischemic penumbra.[5]

25.3 2015 Endovascular Trials

In 2015, a paradigm shift in the treatment of acute ischemic stroke (AIS) occurred when the results of the **MR CLEAN** (Multicenter Randomized Clinical trial of Endovascular treatment for Acute ischemic stroke in the Netherlands), **ESCAPE** (Randomized Assessment of Rapid Endovascular Treatment of Ischemic Stroke), **EXTEND IA** (A multicenter, randomized, controlled study to investigate EXtending the time for Thrombolysis in Emergency Neurological Deficits with Intra-Arterial therapy), **SWIFT PRIME** (Stent-retriever thrombectomy after intravenous t-PA vs. t-PA alone in stroke), and **REVASCAT** (Thrombectomy within 8 hours after symptom onset in ischemic stroke) trials were published.[6-10] These trials advocated rapid patient triage, sophisticated or innovative neuroimaging, and optimal stent retriever technology. Every trial concluded stent retriever-based EVT was safe, technically successful, and significantly reduced functional disability when compared to IV TPA alone. Additionally, these studies further highlighted the ability to select EVT candidates based upon LVO, small core infarct size, and ischemic penumbra status.

The MR CLEAN Trial was the first and largest of the five trials that demonstrated the superiority of EVT for LVO treatment. This trial was performed in the Netherlands and randomized 500 patients with radiographic-confirmed proximal arterial occlusion of the anterior circulation. It demonstrated that stent retriever-based EVT substantially improved functional outcome (as measured by the modified Rankin scale-figure) at 90 days when compared to standard IV TPA alone (36.2% versus 19.1%) (Table 2). Stent retrievers were used in 81.5% of the endovascular treatment arm, with a TICI 2b/3 score obtained in 59% of patients (Figure 2). The TICI score grades the degree of perfusion after recanalization from 0 (no perfusion) to 3 (complete perfusion) (Table 3). No significant difference in symptomatic intracranial hemorrhage or mortality rate was noted. Preliminary results of this trial led to the premature termination of the remaining four EVT trials.

TABLE 2. Functional Independence: 2015 EVT Trials Versus IV TPA

Functional Independence in 2015 EVT Trials VS IV TPA		
	Endovascular Treatment	IV TPA Alone
ESCAPE	53.0%	29.3%
EXTEND-IA	71.0%	40.0%
MR CLEAN	32.6%	19.1%
REVASCAT	43.7%	28.2%
SWIFT PRIME	60.0%	35.0%

TABLE 3. The TICI Grading System

TICI Score	Description
0	No perfusion
1	Perfusion past the initial obstruction, but limited distal branch filling with little or slow distal perfusion
2a	Perfusion of less than half of the vascular distribution of the occluded artery
2b	Perfusion of half or greater of the vascular distribution of the occluded artery
3	Full perfusion with filling of all distal branches

While multiple reperfusion scores exist, the TICI score is the most frequently utilized reperfusion assessment tool. It is currently the reperfusion assessment tool of choice in determining clinical outcome and all recent endovascular trials have utilized it. Furthermore, good TICI scores corresponded to good functional outcomes. The 2018 AHA/ASA guidelines state, "The technical goal of the thrombectomy procedure should be reperfusion to a modified Thrombolysis in Cerebral Infarction (mTICI) 2b/3 angiographic result to maximize the probability of a good functional clinical outcome."[11]

Stent retrievers permit quicker recanalization rates and improved functional outcomes in AIS LVO patients. These devices accomplish such by emitting radial force along the length of the thrombus while their stent-like struts grab it. In the **SWIFT Trial** (Solitaire flow restoration device versus the Merci Retriever in patients with acute ischemic stroke), a stent retriever (the Solitaire® device) was compared to the Merci® device (an older non-stent retriever device). This study demonstrated that stent retrievers had a higher recanalization rate (61% versus 24%) and improved independent functional outcome (58% versus 33%) compared to the Merci® device.[12] In a similar fashion, the **TREVO 2 Study** (Trevo® versus Merci® retrievers for thrombectomy revascularization of large vessel occlusions in acute ischemic stroke) demonstrated another stent retriever (Trevo®) also had better recanalization rates when compared to the Merci® device used in the SWIFT Trial.[13]

FIGURE 2. Stent Retriever Technology

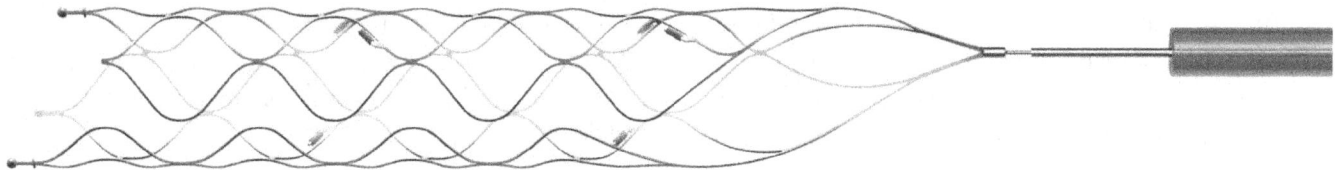

The Solitaire® Platinum Revascularization Device. Image courtesy Medtronic.

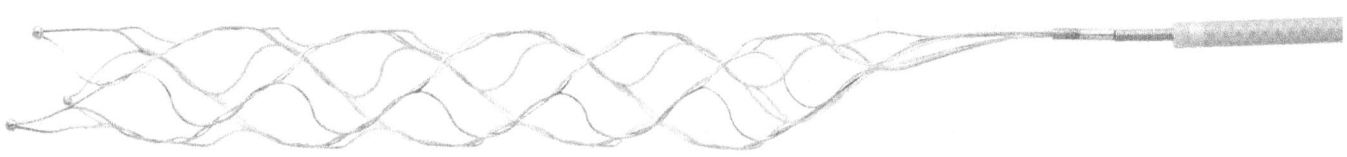

Trevo® XP ProVue Retriever. Image courtesy Stryker Neurovascular.

Copyright © 2013 Stryker

The MR CLEAN Trial provided significant insights not just for EVT but also for stroke management in general. One of its greatest insights was the authors' recommendation to assess vessel patency with neuroimaging performed *before or simultaneously* with IV TPA administration. Furthermore, they demonstrated that the presence of salvageable brain tissue (i.e. ischemic penumbra) is also beneficial for all AIS patients and not just for EVT patients. This philosophy was substantiated by a separate, multicenter analysis which demonstrated that core infarct and ischemic penumbra volume determination was beneficial for the outcome of all AIS patients (IV TPA patients in addition to EVT patients).[14] Moreover, the investigators attributed the lack of proper neuroimaging as a critical reason for the failure of the 2013 trials.

If the lack of proper neuroimaging was a critical reason for prior EVT trial failure, shouldn't it be used today? If LVO, small core infarct, and ischemic penumbra status confirmation are beneficial for IV TPA and EVT AIS patients, shouldn't neuroimaging be consistently utilized? The remainder of this text will tackle these important questions. For now, realize that these insights have changed the diagnosis and treatment of AIS. This study stressed neuroimaging was required to determine treatment. Recall that this trial accepted patients with an NIHSS score ≥ 2. This makes sense because the NIHSS is only one component of stroke assessment. Additionally, LVO, core infarct, and ischemic penumbra status confirmation will determine what therapy should be initiated. This is a paradigm shift in the diagnosis and treatment of AIS to a tissue-based model which is an image determinant model rather than an arbitrary time model (Figure 3). An easy way to remember these factors is with the mnemonic 'BLT' (Table 4).

FIGURE 3. Paradigm Shift in Acute Ischemic Stroke (AIS) Diagnosis and Treatment

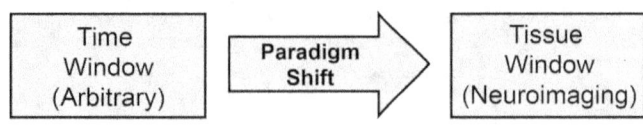

The MR CLEAN Trial also identified the use of suboptimal endovascular devices as another factor for trial failure (Table 5). This is reflected in the 2018 AHA/ASA guidelines which state, "The use of mechanical thrombectomy devices other than stent retrievers as first-line devices for mechanical thrombectomy may be reasonable in some circumstances, but stent retrievers remain the first choice."[11] Finally, the researchers stressed the importance of time efficiency. This concept is also reiterated in the 2018 AHA/ASA guidelines which state, "As with IV alteplase, reduced time from symptom onset to reperfusion with endovascular therapies is highly associated with better clinical outcomes. To ensure benefit, reperfusion to TICI grade 2b/3 should be achieved as early as possible within the therapeutic window."[11] The MR CLEAN Trial demonstrated that the same factors that hampered the earlier EVT trials were the same factors that must be optimized to effectively treat LVO AIS. These factors include advanced neuroimaging, time reduction, and advanced device technology. The MR CLEAN Trial represented a paradigm shift in the management of AIS, the likes of which have not been seen for 20 years.

TABLE 4. Acute Ischemic Stroke (AIS) Diagnosis and Treatment Factors: **BLT**

B	Binary Process
L	LVO Status Confirmation
T	Threatened Brain Status Confirmation

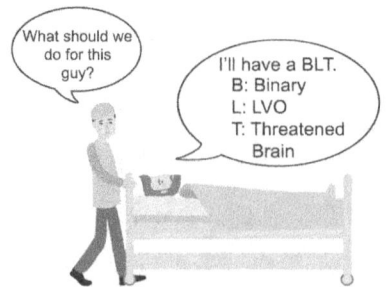

TABLE 5. Different Devices Used in EVT Trials

Different Devices Used In EVT Trials	
IMS III	Any FDA Approved Device (Only 5 Stentrievers)
MR CLEAN	82% Stentrievers
ESCAPE	79% Stentrievers
EXTEND-IA	Solitaire
REVASCAT	Solitaire
SWIFT PRIME	Solitaire

The ESCAPE or the **E**ndovascular treatment for **S**mall **C**ore and **A**nterior circulation **P**roximal occlusion with **E**mphasis on minimizing CT to recanalization times Trial emphasized rapid door-to-imaging time and rapid imaging-to-groin puncture time. Again, this trial underscores the goal of all LVO AIS treatment: *Find them fast and fix them fast*. However, it also analyzed specific steps to accomplish this goal (Box 1). The critical analysis of the rate determining steps prescribed for EVT is an essential requirement for the success of any stroke center (see Chapter 29, Stroke Efficiency). This trial also emphasized the use of advanced neuroimaging criteria such as ASPECTS, CTA, CTP, and multiphase CTA. EVT candidacy was determined by a small core infarct as measured by ASPECTS of 6-10 or a small CT perfusion (CTP) core infarct (↓CBF and ↓CBV). Salvageable brain was identified by determining the presence of moderate-to-good collateral circulation defined as 50% or more of middle cerebral artery (MCA) pial arterial circulation visualized on multiphase CTA. The ESCAPE trial also examined proximal anterior circulation (internal carotid artery and proximal MCA occlusions) and divided these occlusions into an EVT arm and a control group (IV TPA only). This trial demonstrated an improved functional independence (mRS 0-2) of 53% versus 29.3%, respectively (Table 2).

BOX 1. Analysis of Time Reduction Goals

| Emergency Dept. → Neuroimaging |
| Neuroimaging → Groin Puncture |

The SWIFT PRIME Trial examined LVO treated within six hours of symptom onset. Patient inclusion required ASPECTS ≥ 6 or an infarct size ≤ 40-50 mL and excluded large core infarct. Patients were divided into an endovascular arm and control group (IV TPA only) with improved functional independence (mRS 0-2) of 60% versus 35%, respectively. The EXTEND-IA trial compared EVT performed between six and eight hours of symptom onset to IV TPA alone, with improved functional independence (mRS 0-2) of 71% versus 40% favoring EVT. The REVASCAT trial examined 206 patients receiving EVT with LVO, NIHSS score ≥6, ≤ 8 hours from symptom onset, and an ASPECTS ≥7 (≥8 in patients 80-85 years old). Significant improvement in functional independence (mRS 0-2) was observed in the EVT arm (43.7%) versus the control arm (28.2%). No trial demonstrated a statistical difference in mortality and symptomatic intracranial hemorrhage between the EVT and control groups. These trials are summarized in Tables 2 and 6.

25.4 The AHA/ASA Guidelines

The 2015 EVT trial results led to both the updating of 2015 AHA/ASA guidelines and further recommendations.[15] Before discussing either the guidelines or recommendations, other important issues require consideration. First, these guidelines were endorsed by multiple disciplines that include the American Association of Neurologic Surgeons, the American Society of Neuroradiology, and the Cerebrovascular Section of the Congress of Neurological Surgeons. The multidisciplinary issues related to AIS require uniformity amongst various disciplines (neurology, neuroradiology and neurosurgery).

TABLE 6. Summary of 2015 EVT Trials

Summary of 2015 EVT Trials					
	MR CLEAN	ESCAPE	REVASCAT	EXTEND-IA	SWIFT PRIME
Time Period	≤6 Hours	≤12 Hours	≤8 Hours	≤6 Hours	≤6 Hours
Imaging Criteria	LVO determined by CTA or MRA (No specific ischemic penumbra criteria)	LVO determined by CTA or multi-phase CTA or determined by 1) ASPECTS >6 2) Moderate to good collateral circulation	Excluded if ASPECTS value <7 or <6 on MRI	CT perfusion	Excluded if ASPECTS value <6
Type of Endovascular Treatment	IA TPA, EVT or both	EVT	EVT	EVT	EVT

CT - Computerized Tomography, CTA - Computed Tomography Angiography, EVT - Endovascular Treatment, IA TPA - Intra-arterial therapy tissue plasminogen activator, MRA - Magnetic Resonance Angiogram, MRI - Magnetic Resonance Imaging

TABLE 7. AHA/ASA Recommendations for EVT: **ATLAS**

A	Age ≥18 Years
T	Treatment Initiated (Groin Puncture) Within 6 Hours
L	LVO (ICA or MCA M1 Segment)
A	ASPECTS ≥6
S	Score: NIHSS ≥6, Prestroke mRS 0-1

ASPECTS - Alberta Stroke Program Early CT Score,
EVT - Endovascular Treatment, LVO - Large Vessel Occlusion, NIHSS - National Institutes of Health Stroke Scale, mRS - Modified Rankin Scale

The guidelines were created to provide current recommendations for the EVT of AIS. However, as affirmed by the American Academy of Neurology, these guidelines serve as an *educational tool*, not as inclusion or exclusion criteria. These recommendations included treating patients ≥18 years, a pre-stroke mRS score of 0-1, an LVO (ICA or MCA), an ASPECTS ≥ 6, and a NIHSS score ≥ 6, with treatment to be initiated (groin puncture) within six hours. An easy way to remember these recommendations is with the mnemonic 'ATLAS' (Table 7). Again, these guidelines are an *educational tool* only and do not represent inclusion or exclusion criteria. Before examining each of these in detail, a few general concepts must be discussed. First, EVT should not impede the initiation of IV TPA when appropriate. More importantly, IV TPA should not delay the initiation of EVT. An AIS patient with a confirmed LVO must receive EVT as soon as possible. The net clinical benefit of EVT diminishes with time, so EVT must be performed as soon as possible.

25.5 Additional Recommendations

After the publication of the 2015 EVT trials, several meta-analyses evaluated them and provided even greater insights. First, the clinical benefits of EVT significantly declined with increasing time between symptom onset and arterial puncture. For every 9-minute delay in symptom onset to EVT reperfusion time, 1 in 100 treated patients suffered a worse functional outcome. Functional independence (mRS 0-2) of 64.1% was achieved with symptom onset to reperfusion times of 180 minutes but decreased to 46.1% when symptom onset to reperfusion time was increased to 480 minutes.[16] For every 4-minute delay in emergency department door to EVT reperfusion time, 1 in every 100 treated patients suffered a worse functional outcome (Box 2). Worsening functional independence at three months correlated to both increased emergency department door to reperfusion time and neuroimaging to reperfusion times.

BOX 2. Time Delay and Functional Outcome

Event	Delay	Functional Outcome
Symptom Onset to Reperfusion	9 Minutes	Worse
ED to Reperfusion	4 Minutes	Worse

EVT has critical time points that directly affect functional outcome. These points will be discussed in greater detail in Chapter 29 (Stroke Efficiency). In a normal sequence of events, an LVO AIS patient presents to the emergency department, receives neuroimaging which confirms LVO status and EVT candidacy, receives IV TPA, and is transported to the Neurointerventional (NI) lab to undergo groin puncture and reperfusion (Figure 4). Any factor that delays the sequential order of these steps results in a worse functional outcome. For example, a patient suspected of having an LVO should be transported from the emergency department to neuroimaging and receive a full complement of neuroimaging that includes a noncontrast brain CT, CTA, and CTP, or a noncontrast brain CT and dual-phase CTA.

FIGURE 4. Endovascular Treatment (EVT) Critical Time Points

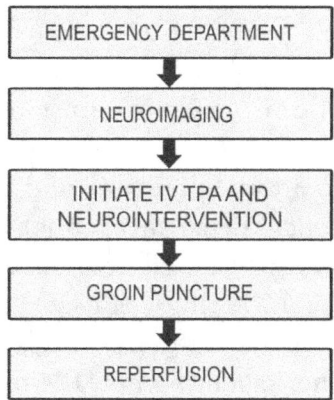

AIS patients should not receive a noncontrast brain CT, be transported back to the emergency room for further stroke reassessment, and then sent back to radiology for further neuroimaging (Figure 5). Instead, a rapid, binary assessment of stroke must be initially performed. The precise quantification (exact NIHSS score) may be completed before treatment. This process will be further discussed in Chapter 29 (Stroke Efficiency). Other more rapid and reliable screening processes can be performed to identify suspected LVO AIS patients so they may receive additional neuroimaging immediately after initial brain CT. The delays caused by inefficient neuroimaging translate into worse functional outcomes. Efficient neuroimaging reduces AIS diagnosis and treatment time which improves functional outcome. Efficient neuroimaging identifies EVT candidates quicker and allows AIS LVO patients to be recanalized faster.

FIGURE 5. Inefficient and Efficient Neuroimaging

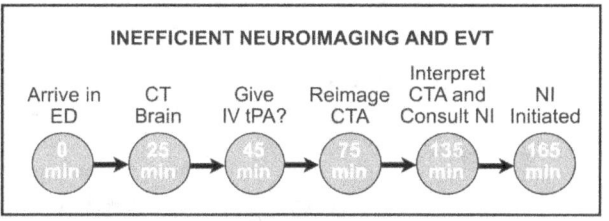

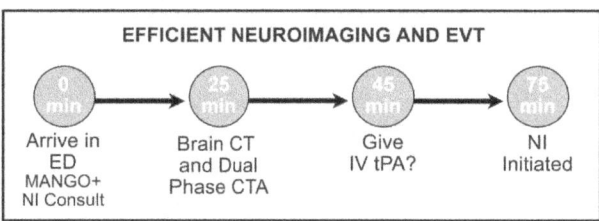

Every stroke center should optimize EVT by reducing treatment time. After an extensive meta-analysis of all five EVT trials, Saver et al. recommended the following critical time points: 50 minutes from brain neuroimaging to arterial puncture, 75 minutes from emergency department door to arterial puncture, and 110 minutes from emergency department door to reperfusion (Figure 6).[16] Every effort should be made to achieve these critical time points.

A meta-analysis of the EVT trials demonstrated several other salient points. The following recommendations are presented for consideration.

Age. Stroke can occur at any age. Unfortunately, none of the EVT trials investigated patients younger than 18 years (Table 8). In the MR CLEAN trial, 16% of patients were 80 years or older. The clinical benefit of EVT was shared by this group (≥ 80) without a significant variance in symptomatic internal hemorrhage or mortality. Similar results were seen in the ESCAPE Trial.

Treatment time and groin puncture. AIS symptom duration is a poor surrogate for brain tissue viability. Symptom duration should not determine EVT candidacy.

Everyone has a unique collateral circulation, and thus a unique tolerance to AIS. Rather than picking an arbitrary time point, research continues to stress the importance of physiologic imaging such as CT, MR perfusion imaging, or dual-phase CTA in determining tissue viability. However, a meta-analysis of the five EVT trials also demonstrate improved functional outcome when arterial puncture was initiated within 7.3 hours after symptom onset.[16] While this observation confirms the 2015 EVT AHA/ASA guidelines recommending initiation of arterial puncture within six hours after symptom onset, it also supports modifying this recommendation to extend treatment from 6 to 7.3 hours after onset. At the very least, the improved benefit of EVT beyond six hours after symptom onset supports the role of neuroimaging in identifying both LVO and ischemic penumbra and discourages the use of arbitrary time points. This point is further exemplified by the results of the DEFUSE 3 and DAWN Trials which now allow EVT for up to 16 and 24 hours in select AIS patients, respectively.[17,18] Thus, neuroimaging and not symptom duration shall determine EVT candidacy which should be extended up to 24 hours when appropriate.

Large vessel occlusions not analyzed. Most LVOs treated in these trials include internal carotid artery (ICA) and middle cerebral artery (MCA) occlusions involving the M1 segment. M2 segment occlusions were infrequently performed and anterior and posterior cerebral artery occlusions were rarely treated. These trials demonstrated no statistical evidence to support the treatment of patients with M2 occlusions.[1]

TABLE 8. Age Limit in EVT Trials

Age Limit in EVT Trials	
MR CLEAN	>18
ESCAPE	>18
EXTEND - IA	>18
REVASCAT	18 - 80
SWIFT PRIME	18 - 80

FIGURE 6. Recommended EVT Critical Time Points

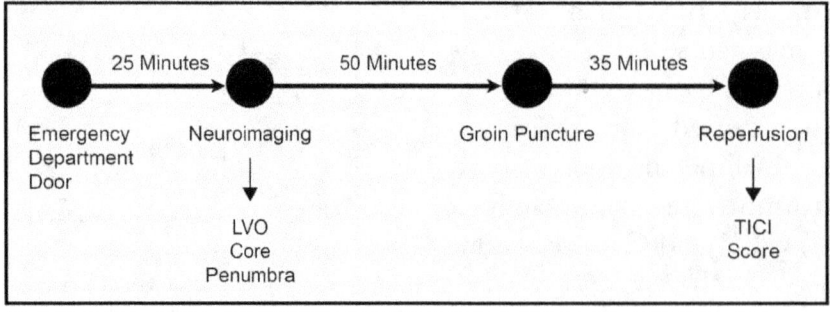

Adapted from: Saver, Jeffrey L., et al. "Time to Treatment With Endovascular Thrombectomy and Outcomes From Ischemic Stroke: A Meta-analysis." *JAMA* 316.12 (2016): 1279-1289

Recently, newer research also endorses EVT for M2 occlusions.[19] The 2018 AHA/ASA guidelines echo these sentiments by stating, "Although the benefits are uncertain, the use of mechanical thrombectomy with stent retrievers may be reasonable for carefully selected patients with AIS in whom treatment can be initiated (groin puncture) within six hours of symptoms onset and who have causative occlusion of the MCA segment 2 (M2) or MCA segment three (M3) portion of the MCAs."[11]

Basilar artery occlusion (BAO) was also excluded from these trials. LVO should be diagnosed with noninvasive imaging prior to EVT. The EVT trial results and AHA/ASA guidelines only apply to anterior circulation AIS and excludes the posterior circulation. However, stroke management from both a clinical and imaging perspective must include assessment of the large vessels of the posterior circulation (vertebral and basilar arteries). Thus, EVT for any patient with significant symptoms and an accessible LVO, despite its location, is completely reasonable. The 2018 AHA/ASA guidelines support this concept by stating, "Although the benefits are uncertain, the use of mechanical thrombectomy with stent retrievers may be reasonable for carefully selected patients with AIS in whom treatment can be initiated (groin puncture) within 6 hours of symptom onset and who have causative occlusion of the anterior cerebral arteries, *vertebral* arteries, *basilar* artery, or posterior cerebral arteries."[11] An easy way to remember the large vessels of the brain is with the mnemonic 'BAMBI' (Table 9).

TABLE 9. Large Vessels of the Brain: **BAMBI**

B	Basilar Artery
A	Anterior Cerebral Artery
M	Middle Cerebral Artery
B	Both Vertebral Arteries
I	Internal Carotid Artery

Like anterior circulation research, a smaller randomized trial also demonstrated a strong relationship between basilar artery recanalization and improved functional outcome.[20] Further, recanalization rates of over 75% have been reported with new generation endovascular devices.[21] A recent meta-analysis of 45 studies (n=2056) of BAO demonstrated a need to treat (NNT) number of 3 and 2.5 to decrease death or dependency and death alone, respectively (Figure 7).[22]

FIGURE 7. EVT Number Needed to Treat Basilar Artery Occlusion

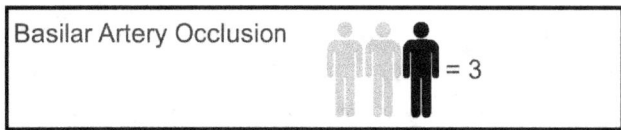

NNT = Number of people requiring treatment for one beneficial result

ASPECTS ≥ 6. Higher baseline ASPECT scores predict a favorable EVT outcome.[23,24] While ASPECT scoring of 6 or higher can exclude the presence of a large core infarct, shouldn't other indicators also be considered? There are other methods that can determine core infarct size such as CT and MR perfusion imaging. Also, assessment of collateral circulation with dual-phase CTA can be performed.

NIHSS score ≥ 6. The MR CLEAN trial included patients with NIHSS scores as low as 2. Higher NIHSS scores can correlate with more severe strokes and a higher probability of LVO. However, LVO can still present with lower or even zero NIHSS scores, provided adequate collaterals exist.[25] Since the NIHSS score cannot reliably exclude all LVO and because the MR CLEAN trial included patients with NIHSS scores as low as 2, how relevant is the NIHSS quantification of stroke? Shouldn't any NIHSS score be sufficient for EVT candidacy so long as the remainder of the inclusion criteria are met (LVO, small core infarct, and significant ischemic penumbra)? Of course, they should! This is reflected in the 2018 AHA/ASA guidelines which state: "Although the benefits are uncertain, the use of mechanical thrombectomy with stent retrievers may be reasonable for carefully selected patients with AIS in whom treatment can be initiated (groin puncture) within 6 hours of symptom onset and who have a pre-stroke mRS score >1, ASPECTS < 6 or NIHSS score < 6 and causative occlusion of the internal carotid artery (ICA) or proximal MCA (M1)."[11]

This again underscores the importance of a binary approach to AIS treatment and proper neurovascular imaging. Proper neuroimaging is required for all stroke patients and not just EVT patients. A multicenter analysis demonstrated the value of core and penumbra volume determination to functional outcome of *both* EVT and IV TPA patients.[13] This continues to underscore the importance of proper neuroimaging in all AIS patients and not only for EVT candidacy determination. However, the current 2018 AHA/ASA guidelines do not yet recommend imaging criteria for IV TPA candidacy and state: "Use of imaging criteria to select ischemic stroke patients who awoke with stroke or have unclear time of onset for treatment IV alteplase is not recommended outside a clinical trial."[11]

Some practitioners elect to perform CTA based on stroke severity since LVO is more frequently encountered with severe strokes. However, patients with mild clinical stroke syndromes still have a significant percentage of LVO (approximately 10% with an NIHSS score <6) and it is precisely these patients who are at risk of clinical deterioration.[26] This point cannot be overemphasized. Many centers erroneously consider only patients with severe stroke symptoms as candidates for EVT. However, based on LVO imaging, the full spectrum of baseline NIHSS scores have been treated (including NIHSS scores of zero). Due to exclusion criteria, very few patients with an NIHSS score of <6 were enrolled in these trials. But those who were (and had documented LVOs) had a consistent treatment response despite their lower NIHSS scores. Thus, when dealing with a patient with documented LVO and a low NIHSS score, one must consider the real risk of subsequent deterioration despite the low NIHSS score.[26] The 2018 AHA/ASA guidelines again state: "Although its benefits are uncertain, the use of mechanical thrombectomy with stent retrievers may be reasonable for patients with AIS in whom treatment can be initiated (groin puncture) within 6 hours of symptom onset and who have prestroke mRS score > 1, ASPECTS < 6, **NIHSS score < 6,** and causative occlusion of the internal carotid artery (ICA) or proximal MCA (M1)."[11]

Neuroimaging. All EVT trials required proof of LVO using noninvasive imaging, predominantly CTA. LVO status confirmation by CTA is considered standard procedure and includes extracranial and intracranial vasculature. One exception to this rule would be an unequivocally hyperdense artery (hyperdense MCA sign indicating an M1 occlusion or a hyperdense basilar artery sign indicating a basilar artery occlusion) which has a high sensitivity and specificity for LVO.[27] AIS patients with a hyperdense MCA or basilar artery should be transferred to the neurointerventional lab immediately as long as the ASPECT score ≥ 6. Centers that cannot perform CT or MR perfusion can usually perform dual-phase CTA. Adequate collaterals demonstrated by dual-phase CTA are a sufficient indicator of viable tissue (ischemic penumbra) and therefore, EVT candidacy. Also, dual-phase CTA can identify large vessel occlusions and thrombus length. Both factors should be considered in any patient receiving IV TPA since longer thrombus lengths (greater than 10 mm) and LVO usually do not respond to IV TPA alone. Both LVO and thrombus length are independent predictors of functional outcome. In fact, all the recent EVT trials discussed above used noninvasive arterial imaging (CTA or MRA of the intracranial and extracranial arteries) to confirm LVO status. Neuroimaging must always be utilized because symptom duration is a poor surrogate of tissue viability.

In terms of additional imaging, the MR CLEAN trial utilized the simple strategy of a noncontrast brain CT to exclude intracerebral hemorrhage and CTA to identify LVO. It is important to note, however, that the mean ASPECT score was 9, which is identical to other trials utilizing more selective imaging. While ASPECTS is theoretically simple and proven reliable, it is more difficult to apply it in clinical practice compared to an automated process such as CTP imaging. While ASPECTS was designed to reduce interobserver variability, this continues to be a major speed bump in noncontrast brain CT interpretation. CTP has been demonstrated to provide well-defined estimates of irreversibly damaged brain tissue that correlates to follow-up imaging.[28]

Furthermore, CTP has been demonstrated to reliably and rapidly provide objective assessment of both irreparably damaged core infarct and salvageable ischemic penumbra.[29] However, core infarct status can also be determined by ASPECTS alone.

General Anesthesia. Growing research indicates that general anesthesia (GA) reduces the clinical benefit of EVT compared to conscious sedation (CS).[30-32] Recently, a pooled analysis of the five 2015 EVT trials demonstrated worse functional outcomes in AIS patients receiving GA in conjunction with EVT.[33] Statistically significant differences in independent functional outcome (mRS 0-2) were determined in medical treatment (26.5%), EVT associated with GA (35.9%), and EVT performed on CS patients (50%). Furthermore, statistically significant differences were also identified in excellent functional outcome (mRS 0-1) for medical treatment (12.9%), EVT associated with GA (19%), and EVT performed on CS patients (30%). In addition, a significant reduction in mortality was demonstrated in the CS group (13.6% versus standard of care 18.9%), which was not identified in the GA group (18.3%). No statistically significant differences in pneumonia or vessel perforation rates were identified between the GA and CS patient groups. Pending further randomized trial results, this study concluded that general anesthesia should be avoided whenever possible.

While the exact reasons for worse outcomes with GA remain unknown, existing evidence suggests that these may be related to peri-procedural hemodynamics. A post hoc analysis of 60 patients receiving GA in the MR CLEAN Trial (which associated worse outcomes with GA) determined medications used for induction lowered blood pressure in a majority of patients who also required subsequent blood pressure-elevating medications.[34] These investigators determined that reductions in mean arterial pressure were associated with worse outcome. Future studies will compare GA and CS, emphasizing fast GA technique and strict blood pressure control (maintaining SBP > 140 mmHg).

Some EVT cases require GA and EVT performed with GA remains more effective than IV TPA alone. The current recommendations from an expert consensus statement of the Society of Neurointervention Surgery and the Neurocritical Care Society recommend GA in patients with severe agitation, low level of consciousness (GCS <8), loss of airway protective reflexes, respiratory compromise, and in selected posterior circulation stroke cases (Table 10).[35] However, the recent 2018 AHA/ASA guidelines pulled away from the consensus in this field by stating that since there is limited prospective randomized data and because only two small RCTs demonstrated no superiority of either treatment, "either method of procedural sedation is reasonable."[11] The GOLIATH trial, which is a larger trial, is currently underway to further investigate this issue.

TABLE 10. General Anesthesia Recommendations for EVT Patients: **GRAPE**

G	GCS <8, Low Level of Consciousness
R	Respiratory Compromise
A	Agitation, Severe
P	Posterior Circulation Stroke
E	Endangered Airway

25.6 DAWN and DEFUSE 3 Trials

As if the five back-to-back 2015 EVT trials and subsequent research that followed were not enough, the DAWN and DEFUSE 3 Trials represented even greater breakthroughs in stroke treatment. Doctors Nogueira and Albers, the lead authors of both of these trials, and their research teams should be considered nothing short of visionaries. The DAWN (**D**WI or CTP **A**ssessment with Clinical Mismatch in the Triage of **W**ake-Up and Late Presenting Strokes Undergoing **N**eurointervention with Trevo) Trial compared functional outcomes of using the Trevo thrombectomy device plus medical management versus medical management alone.[17] Inclusion criteria covered patients who presented 6 to 24 hours from last known normal and had an NIHSS >10, an anterior circulation large vessel occlusion documented by CTA or MRA, and a clinical-imaging mismatch between the neurologic deficit and infarct size. Recall the previously accepted time window for stroke treatment was within six hours after the first onset of symptoms. Additionally, approximately 60% of patients had their first stroke symptoms after awakening, meaning the time of stroke onset was unknown. Prior to the DAWN Trial, unknown symptom onset was a contraindication to either endovascular or thrombolytic treatment.

Patients enrolled in this trial met criteria for a mismatch between the severity of clinical deficits (measured by the NIHSS) and the volume of infarct, which was measured using diffusion-weighted magnetic resonance imaging or CTP. The mismatch was defined according to age: patients ≥ 80 years old had an infarct volume < 21 mL and an NIHSS score ≥ 10, whereas patients < 80 years old required either an NIHSS score ≥ 10 and an infarct volume less < 31 mL or an NIHSS score ≥ 20 with an infarct volume between 31 to 51 mL. This trial was halted before the maximum sample size was reached due to a pre-specified interim analysis which suggested a high probability of success.

The DAWN Trial demonstrated that EVT significantly decreased functional disability and improved functional independence at 90 days when compared to medical management (IV TPA) alone (48.6% versus 13.1%). That is, only 13% of medically managed patients were functionally independent three months after symptom onset compared to 49% of patients who received EVT. This is a relative risk reduction in functional disability of 73%! This means that for every 2.8 treated patients, one additional patient was functionally independent at 90 days (Figure 8).

FIGURE 8. DAWN Trial Number Needed to Treat (NNT)

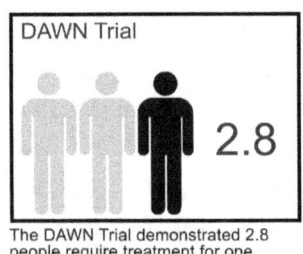

The DAWN Trial demonstrated 2.8 people require treatment for one beneficial result

This data demonstrates that EVT treatment within 24 hours in patients selected with advanced neuroimaging is more effective than patients whose treatment was previously determined by an arbitrary, less than six-hour time window. Unfortunately, the 13% rate of functional independence in the control group demonstrates that patients with severe LVO stroke who do not receive EVT will likely have a poor outcome.

These results stress the importance of neuroimaging (which is patient-specific) over arbitrary time points (not patient-specific). This trial demonstrates the use of a "tissue window" in determining if EVT eligibility is as good as, if not better than, the use of arbitrary time points. That is because this trial used advanced neuroimaging to determine the presence of threatened but salvageable brain tissue (ischemic penumbra) and ultimately EVT candidacy. In fact, Dr. Jovin, one of the senior authors of this trial, stated, **"The concept of time as the main or only selection criteria for endovascular patients is shattered."** The reduction in functional disability achieved in patients treated up to 24 hours is a tremendous message of hope for the thousands of stroke patients who present past the six-hour treatment window. By expanding the proportion of eligible patients that can receive EVT, the DAWN Trial is a huge step forward in stroke treatment. This trial and the DEFUSE 3 Trial (discussed below) led to new 2018 AHA/ASA EVT recommendations.

The DEFUSE 3 (Endovascular Therapy Following Imaging Evaluation for Ischemic Stroke 3) was a prospective randomized phase III multicenter-controlled trial that investigated anterior circulation LVO AIS patients treated with EVT plus standard medical therapy between 6 and 16 hours after stroke onset versus standard medical therapy alone. The purpose of this trial was to assess the safety and efficacy of EVT in patients selected by advanced neuroimaging within this extended time window. Prior to randomization, patients who met the inclusion criteria underwent either CTP/CTA or magnetic resonance diffusion-weighted imaging/perfusion weighting imaging/angiography (DWI/PWI/MRA). The DEFUSE Trial investigators also developed the RAPID™ (iSchemaView) software which enabled them to utilize CT perfusion or MRI diffusion and perfusion to identify patients with salvageable, ischemic penumbra (Target Mismatch Profile). Specifically, this software allowed the investigators to discern irreversibly damaged brain tissue (core infarct) from threatened but salvageable brain tissue (ischemic penumbra). Incidentally, the DAWN Trial used the same automated RAPID™ software to also select patients likely to have salvageable brain tissue in an extended time window.

The DEFUSE 3 Trial had multiple inclusion and exclusion criteria which can further be subdivided into clinical and neuroimaging inclusion and exclusion criteria.

Clinical inclusion criteria include:

- acute anterior circulation ischemic stroke
- age 18 to 90 years
- NIHSS ≥ 6
- EVT can be initiated (groin puncture) between six and 16 hours from stroke onset
- mRS ≤ 2 prior to qualifying stroke
- necessary consent

Neuroimaging and inclusion criteria include:

- ICA or MCA-M1 occlusion
- core infarct < 70 cc
- ratio of ischemic penumbra to a core infarct ≥ 1.8
- Penumbra ≥ 15 cc

The clinical inclusion criteria can be recalled by the mnemonic 'ANT MAN' (Table 11).

TABLE 11. Clinical Inclusion Criteria for DEFUSE 3 Trial: **ANTMAN**

A	Acute Anterior Circulation Ischemic Stroke
N	NIHSS ≥6
T	Time - EVT Initiated 6 -16 hours from Stroke Onset (Groin Puncture)
M	mRS ≤2 Prior to Qualifying Stroke
A	Age 18 - 90 Years
N	Necessary Consent

EVT - Endovascular Treatment, mRS - Modified Rankin Scale, NIHSS - National Institutes of Health Stroke Scale

The neuroimaging inclusion criteria can be recalled by the mnemonic 'CORP' (Table 12).

TABLE 12. Neuroimaging Inclusion Criteria for DEFUSE 3 Trial: **CORP**

C	Core Infarct <70 cc
O	Occlusion of ICA or MCA (M1)
R	Ratio of Penumbra to a Core Infarct ≥ 1.8
P	Penumbra ≥ 15 cc

There are several DEFUSE 3 exclusion criteria which can be remembered with the mnemonic 'A MESSI SPAGHETTI PLATE' (Table 13).

A shorter version of these exclusion criteria can be remembered by the mnemonic 'PUMP GAS' (Table 14). Once patients with salvageable brain tissue were identified, they were randomized to mechanical thrombectomy versus standard medical treatment and their clinical outcomes were assessed after three months. The DEFUSE 3 Trial demonstrated 45% of patients receiving EVT within the 16-hour time frame achieved functional independence 90 days after treatment, compared with 17% in the control group.

TABLE 14. DEFUSE 3 Abbreviated Exclusion Criteria: **PUMP GAS**

P	Pregnancy
U	Unable to Undergo Brain Imaging
M	Minimal Life Expectancy (< 6 Months)
P	Platelet Count < 50,000/μL
G	Glucose < 50 mg/dL or > 400 mg/dL
A	Abnormality of Bleeding
S	Seizures at Onset

In addition, EVT was also associated with improved survival: 14% of those receiving EVT died within 90 days of the study, compared with 26% in the control group. Patients who received EVT also had a reduction in severe functional outcome by about 50%. These results are astounding considering the fact that the stroke community recently considered these patients untreatable!

TABLE 13. Exclusion Criteria for DEFUSE 3 Trial: **A MESSI SPAGHETTI PLATE**

A	ASPECTS <6
M	Multiple Vascular Territory Occlusions
E	Evidence of ICA Dissection that is Flow Limiting or Aortic Dissection
S	Significant Mass Effect with Midline Shift
S	Stent that Precludes Safe EVT
I	Intracranial Process (Hemorrhage, Neoplasm or AVM)
S	Seizures at Stroke Onset if Baseline NIHSS Cannot be Obtained
P	Pregnancy
A	Allergic to Iodine
G	Glucose <50 mg/dL or >400 mg/dL
H	Hypertension that is Severe and Sustained (SBP >185 mmHg or DBP >110 mmHg)
E	Expectancy of Life <6 Months, Severe or Terminal Illness
T	TPA Given 3-4.5 Hours After LKN and Any of the Following: Age >80, Current Anticoagulant Use, History of Diabetes or Prior Stroke
T	TPA Given >4.5 Hours After LKN
I	Interference of Neurologic or Functional Evaluation by Pre-Existing Disease
P	Platelet Count <50,000/µL
L	Limited Scanning, Unable to Obtain CTP or MRI
A	Abnormality of Labs (INR >3) or Bleeding Abnormality
T	Tried EVT Prior to 6 Hours from Stroke Onset
E	Embolus Presumed Septic, Endocarditis - Suspicion of Bacterial

ASPECTS - Alberta Stroke Program Early CT Score, AVM - Arteriovenous Malformation, CTP - Computed Tomography Perfusion, DBP - Diastolic Blood Pressure, EVT - Endovascular Treatment, ICA - Internal Carotid Artery, INR - International Normalized Ratio, LKN - Last Known Normal, MRI - Magnetic Resonance Imaging, NIHSS - National Institutes of Health Stroke Scale, SBP - Systolic Blood Pressure, TPA - Tissue Plasminogen Activator (or Alteplase IV r-tPA)

There are a few points concerning these trials worth mentioning. First, the DEFUSE 3 Trial eligibility criteria were determined prior to the recent 2018 AHA/ASA guidelines. Some of DEFUSE 3 exclusions were based upon prior IV TPA restriction criteria. For example, age greater than 80, current anticoagulant use, history of diabetes or prior stroke, and NIHSS >25 were the ECASS III exclusion criteria for the administration of IV TPA between 3 and 4.5 hours. These criteria, as well as pregnancy, are no longer exclusion criteria for IV TPA administration and will likely be modified. However, the 2018 AHA/ASA guidelines currently state to follow the DAWN or DEFUSE 3 eligibility criteria for AIS within 6 to 16 hours and the DAWN eligibility criteria for AIS within 6 to 24 hours of last known normal. Next, approximately 40% of DEFUSE 3 participants would not have met the narrower DAWN eligibility criteria (DAWN participants had smaller core infarcts than those in DEFUSE 3). Specifically, larger core infarct lesions were allowed in DEFUSE 3 if salvageable brain tissue (ischemic penumbra) was present. Less severe stroke in DEFUSE 3 participants was also determined by

NIHSS inclusion criteria (≥10 in DAWN versus ≥ 6 in DEFUSE 3). Additionally, general anesthesia, a controversial EVT subject matter, was only used in 26 (28%) DEFUSE 3 patients.

The results from both the DAWN and DEFUSE 3 Trials lead to powerful conclusions. Clearly, the treatment windows for large vessel occlusion can be extended beyond six hours for appropriate patients determined by neuroimaging. This is because both trials demonstrated that collateral circulation varies from patient to patient, meaning stroke treatment can have very different timelines among different individuals. This unique physiology and not arbitrary time points should determine EVT candidacy. Indeed, both trials demonstrated that individual collateral circulation determines endovascular candidacy and not arbitrary time points. Both studies demonstrated that a significant number of LVO AIS patients' ischemic penumbra can be maintained by collateral circulation for many hours after symptom onset. In fact, it is estimated that approximately 40% of LVO AIS patients arrive in the emergency department more than six hours after onset of symptoms. However, as shown by the medical (non-EVT treatment) arms of both these trials, these collaterals can only function for a limited period of time. If these patients' large vessel occlusions are not recanalized and their ischemic penumbra is not reperfused, they will have large debilitating strokes.

So how does this change our treatment of acute ischemic stroke? New 2018 American Heart Association/American Stroke Association Guidelines for mechanical thrombectomy were issued at the International Stroke Conference 2018 following the presentation of DEFUSE 3 by its principal investigator, Dr. Greg Albers. Essentially, mechanical thrombectomy is *recommended* in anterior circulation, large vessel occlusion (LVO) acute ischemic stroke (AIS) patients that present within 6 and 16 hours of last known normal and meet "other" DAWN and DEFUSE 3 eligibility criteria. For anterior circulation LVO AIS patients who present within 6 to 24 hours after last known normal and meet "other" DAWN criteria, mechanical thrombectomy is *reasonable*. The new insights drawn by both the DAWN and DEFUSE 3 Trials can be remembered by the mnemonic 'TITAN' (Table 15).

So, what are these "other" criteria? Recall that the DAWN Trial demonstrated that EVT could be extended to 24 hours after last known well based upon a disproportionately severe clinical deficit in comparison with the size of a stroke on imaging.[17] In the DEFUSE 3 Trial, patients who met the inclusion criteria underwent either CT perfusion/CT angiography (CTP/CTA) or magnetic resonance (MR) diffusion-weighted imaging/perfusion-weighted imaging/angiography (DWI/PWI/MRA) studies prior to randomization. Essentially, both trials used advanced neuroimaging to discriminate irreparably damaged brain tissue (core infarct) from threatened but salvageable brain tissue (ischemic penumbra). Thus, both DAWN and DEFUSE 3 eligibilities are generally determined by advanced neuroimaging in addition to the more specific criteria listed above (Tables 11-14).

TABLE 15. DAWN and DEFUSE 3 Trial Insights: **TITAN**

T	Time Window No Longer Determines Eligibility	
I	Imaging Determines Eligibility	
T	Thrombectomy *Recommended* Between 6-16 Hours, *Reasonable* at 6-24 Hours*	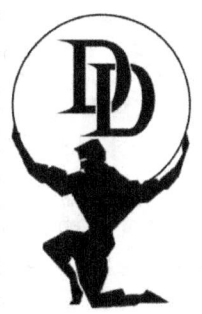
A	Always Accelerate Treatment	
N	No EVT if Eligible Leads to Bad Outcomes	

*EVT is *recommended* for LVO AIS patients within 6 and 16 hours of last known normal (LKN) and meet "other" DAWN or DEFUSE 3 eligibility criteria.
EVT is *reasonable* 6 to 24 hours after LKN and meet "other" DAWN criteria.

Neuroimaging has tremendous implications. Both the DAWN and DEFUSE 3 Trials confirmed every AIS patient has a unique collateral circulation that determines the course of their infarct evolution. If they are fortunate to have significant collaterals, mechanical thrombectomy can be performed for up to one day after last known normal. These findings destroy the antiquated notion of a time window that, until now, has been the cornerstone of stroke treatment. However, both the DAWN and DEFUSE 3 Trials demonstrate that a time window was only a surrogate marker for patient-specific collateral circulation. These trials demonstrate that real-time assessment of individual collateral circulation of the patient must be made at the time of presentation. Consider how many patients who may have benefited from this approach were tragically excluded due to surrogate time markers. Because both trials relied on perfusion imaging to determine EVT candidacy, it is likely that perfusion imaging or image-based assessment of the collateral circulation will become the standard for imaging from 6 to 24 hours for LVO AIS patients.

Despite the new "tissue window" philosophy which both of these trials endorse, "time is brain" remains a valid concept. This does not mean we should continue using time windows as surrogate markers to determine threatened brain tissue viability (ischemic penumbra); rather, we should keep in mind that despite the degree of individual collateral circulation, time during any stroke is **extremely precious**. The benefit of EVT can only be obtained as long as there is salvageable brain tissue (ischemic penumbra) left to rescue. Mechanical thrombectomy requires to be performed as quickly as possible and is consistently demonstrated to have better outcomes the earlier it is initiated. Both trials demonstrated EVT was most beneficial the earlier it was performed. The new 2018 AHA/ASA guidelines endorse this concept by stating, "As with IV alteplase, reduced time from symptom onset to reperfusion with endovascular therapies is highly associated with better clinical outcomes. To ensure benefit, reperfusion to TICI grade 2b/3 should be achieved as early as possible within the therapeutic window."[11]

Both the DAWN and DEFUSE 3 Trials have led to a paradigm shift from a "time window" to a "tissue window" basis for stroke treatment. These two trials represent tremendous steps forward in LVO AIS treatment because the message they convey changes our understanding of LVO AIS, enabling the treatment of a greater number of eligible patients with EVT. The profound results of both the DAWN and DEFUSE 3 Trials led to changes in the 2018 ASA/AHA guidelines for imaging and mechanical thrombectomy (Tables 15, 16, and 17).

TABLE 16. Summary of 2018 AHA/ASA Imaging Recommendations

	Summary of 2018 AHA/ASA Imaging Recommendations
Initial Imaging	Noncontrast brain CT within 20 minutes of arrival in the ED in at least 50% of patients who may be IV TPA and/or EVT candidates
<6 Hours From LKN EVT Eligible AIS Patients	Noninvasive intracranial vascular study should not delay IV TPA (if eligible)
	Reasonable to perform CTA for suspected LVO without serum creatinine concentration so long as no history of renal impairment
	MR or CT perfusion studies not recommended to determine EVT candidacy <6 hours from symptom onset
	Reasonable to utilize collateral flow status to determine EVT candidacy
6-24 Hours from LKN	Advanced neuroimaging (CTP, DWI - MRI or MR perfusion) to determine perfusion – core mismatch and maximum core size is recommended to help determine EVT candidacy

CT - Computerized Tomography, CTA - Computed Tomography Angiography, DWI - Diffusion-Weighted Magnetic Resonance Imaging, ED - Emergency Dept., EVT - Endovascular Treatment, LKN - Last Known Normal, LVO - Large Vessel Occlusion, TPA - Tissue Plasminogen Activator, MR - Magnetic Resonance, MRI - Magnetic Resonance Imaging

TABLE 17. Summary of 2018 AHA/ASA Endovascular Treatment (EVT) Recommendations

Time Period	Recommendation
<6 Hours	EVT **should be** performed if the following criteria are met: **ATLAS** (A) Age ≥18 years, (T) Treatment initiated (groin puncture) within 6 hours of symptom onset, (L) LVO - Large Vessel Occlusion (ICA or MCA M1 segment), (A) ASPECTS ≥6 NIHSS score ≥6, (S) Score: Pre-stroke mRS score 0-1. EVT may be **reasonable** for MCA M2 or M3 segment occlusions. EVT may be **reasonable** for ACA, the vertebral artery, basilar artery or PCA occlusion. EVT may be **reasonable** for pre-stroke mRS score >1, ASPECTS <6, NIHSS score <6 and ICA or MCA M1 segment occlusion.
6-16 Hours from LKN	EVT is **recommended** for anterior circulation LVO that meet other DAWN or DEFUSE 3 eligibility criteria.
6-24 Hours from LKN	EVT is **reasonable** for anterior circulation LVO that meet other DAWN eligibility criteria.

ACA - Anterior Cerebral Artery, ASPECTS - Alberta Stroke Program Early CT Score, EVT - Endovascular Treatment, ICA - Internal Carotid Artery, LVO - Large Vessel Occlusion, MCA - Middle Cerebral Artery, mRS - Modified Rankin Scale, NIHSS - National Institutes of Health Stroke Scale, PCA - Posterior Cerebral Artery

TABLE 18. Summary of DAWN and DEFUSE 3 Eligibility Criteria

Trial Inclusion	Criteria	mRS Score	Age	NIHSS	Infarct	LVO	Exclusion Criteria
DAWN	LKN 6-24 hrs	0-1	≥80	≥10	≤20cc	ICA or MCA M1	Imaging Exclusion Criteria: MIAMI VICE***
	Clinical: Mismatch	0-1	<80	≥10	≤30cc		
		0-1	<80	≥20	31-50cc		
DEFUSE 3	Clinical: ANTMAN*	≤2	18-90	≥6	<70cc	ICA or MCA M1	A MESSI SPAGHETTI PLATE****
	Imaging: CORP**	≤2					

*ANTMAN = (A) Acute anterior circulation ischemic stroke, (N) NIHSS >6, (T) Time - EVT initiated 6-16 hours from stroke onset (groin puncture), (M) mRS ≤2 prior to qualifying stroke, (A) Age 18-90 Years, (N) Necessary Consent.

**CORP = (C) Core infarct <70cc, (O) Occlusion of ICA or MCA (M1), (R) Ratio of penumbra to a core infarct ≥1.8, (P) Penumbra ≥15cc.

***MIAMI VICE = (M) mass effect with midline shift, (I) intracranial stent in same vascular territory, (A) aortic dissection (suspected), (M) multiple vascular territory occlusions, (I) intracranial tumor, (V) vasculitis (suspected), (I) intracranial hemorrhage, (C) carotid dissection, severe stenosis or occlusion, (E) excessive tortuosity of cervical vessels

****A MESSI SPAGHETTI PLATE = (A) ASPECTS <6, (M) Multiple vascular territory occlusions, (E) Evidence of ICA dissection that is flow limiting or aortic dissection, (S) Significant mass effect with midline shift, (S) Stent that precludes safe EVT, (I) Intracranial process (hemorrhage, neoplasm or AVM), (S) Seizures at stroke onset if baseline NIHSS cannot be obtained, (P) Pregnancy, (A) Allergic to iodine, (G) Glucose <50 mg/dL or >400 mg/dL, (H) Hypertension that is severe and sustained (SBP >185 mmHg or DBP >110 mmHg, (E) Expectancy of life <6 months, severe or terminal illness, (T) TPA given 3-4.5 hours after LKN and any of the following: age >80, current anticoagulant use, history of diabetes or prior stroke, (T) TPA given >4.5 hours after LKN, (I) Interference of neurologic or functional evaluation by pre-existing disease, (P) Platelet count <50,000/μl, (L) Limited scanning, unable to obtain CTP or MRI, (A) Abnormality of labs (INR >3) or bleeding abnormality, (T) Tried EVT prior to 6 hours from stroke onset, (E) Embolus presumed septic, endocarditis - suspicion of bacterial.

ICA - Internal carotid artery, LKN - Last known normal, MCA - Middle cerebral artery, TPA - Tissue plasminogen activator

Again, they state, " In selected patients with AIS within 6 to 16 hours of last known normal who have LVO in the anterior circulation and meet other DAWN or DEFUSE 3 eligibility criteria, mechanical thrombectomy is *recommended*." The word "recommended" is changed to "reasonable" and DEFUSE 3 is removed from the recommendation (since this trial included patients within 6 to

16 hours of last known normal) if patients present within 6 to 24 hours of last known normal. Thus the recommendation for this group of patients states, "in selected patients with AIS within 6 to 24 hours of last known normal who have an LVO in the anterior circulation and meet other DAWN eligibility criteria, mechanical thrombectomy is *reasonable*." The DAWN and DEFUSE 3 eligibility criteria are summarized below (Table 18).

25.7 Large Vessel Occlusion (LVO) and IV TPA

Recently, two large meta-analyses have suggested that IV TPA prior to EVT has no effect on the outcome of LVO AIS patients.[36,37] Other studies have supported this data indicating no benefit of IV TPA prior to EVT.[38,39] Despite increasing data that IV TPA given prior to EVT may have no significant impact on functional outcome, a randomized clinical trial is required to demonstrate the benefit of EVT alone compared to EVT with prior IV TPA. There is no current evidence not to administer IV TPA prior to EVT or that bridging IV TPA is effective for LVO AIS treatment prior to EVT. The MR CLEAN NO-IV Trial will examine the effect of EVT alone compared to IV TPA and EVT on functional outcome in LVO AIS patients. Until then, the current 2018 AHA/ASA guidelines state, "Patients eligible for IV alteplase should receive IV alteplase even if EVTs are being considered."[11]

25.8 Conclusion

EVT quite simply is one of the most effective treatment approaches of modern medicine which has dramatically demonstrated superiority over a very short period of time. Virtually all studies that demonstrate its efficacy were published in the *New England Journal of Medicine*, which has the highest impact factor of all medical journals. These results have led the AHA/ASA to change their stroke guidelines in 2015 and again in 2018. The key concepts derived from the positive EVT trials are to diagnose and treat LVO AIS patients as quickly as possible (find them fast and fix them fast). All AIS therapy is benefited by expediting treatment. Just like IV TPA, reduced time from symptom onset to treatment (EVT recanalization) is associated with better functional outcome. Any substantial delays in treatment, as well as inefficient imaging, should be strongly discouraged.

Determining EVT candidacy requires advanced neuroimaging modalities. Both CTP and dual-phase CTA can effectively identify patients with salvageable ischemic penumbra who would potentially benefit from EVT. EVT is vastly superior to IV TPA alone, with no significant difference in mortality or symptomatic intracerebral hemorrhage rate. EVT must always be considered for LVO AIS stroke treatment irrespective of intravenous thrombolysis eligibility. Finally, the results of both the DAWN and DEFUSE 3 Trials were astounding and stress the importance of patient-specific physiologic imaging over arbitrary chronologic measurements.

Abbreviations list

AHA/ASA, American Heart Association and American Stroke Association; AIS, acute ischemic stroke; ASPECTS, Alberta Stroke Program Early CT Score; BAO, basilar artery occlusion; CS, conscious sedation; CTA, computed tomography angiography; CTP, CT perfusion; DWI/PWI/MRA, magnetic resonance diffusion-weighted imaging/perfusion weighting imaging/angiography; EVT, endovascular treatment; GA, general anesthesia; ICA, internal carotid artery; IV TPA, intravenous administration of recombinant tissue plasminogen activator; LVO, large vessel occlusion; MCA, middle cerebral artery; mRS, modified Rankin scale; NI, neurointerventional; NIHSS, National Institutes of Health Stroke Scale; NNT, number needed to treat.

References

1. Goyal M, Menon BK, van Zwam WH, et al, HERMES collaborators. (2016). Endovascular thrombectomy after large-vessel ischaemic stroke: a meta-analysis of individual patient data

from five randomised trials. *Lancet*, 387(10029), 1723-31.
2. Furlan A et al. (1999). Intra-arterial prourokinase for acute ischemic stroke. The PROACT II study: a randomized controlled trial. Prolyse in Acute Cerebral Thromboembolism. *JAMA*, 282, 2003-11.
3. Mocco J, Fiorella D, Fargen KM, et al. (2015). Endovascular therapy for acute ischemic stroke is indicated and evidence based: a position statement. *J Neurointerv Surg*, 7, 79–81.
4. Khalessi AA, Fargen KM, Lavine S, Mocco J. (2013). Commentary: Societal statement on recent acute stroke intervention trials: results and implications. *Neurosurgery*, 73, E375–79.
5. Goyal M, Menon BK, Coutts SB, et al. (2011). Effect of baseline CT scan appearance and time to recanalisation on clinical outcomes in endovascular thrombectomy of acute ischemic strokes. *Stroke*, 42, 93–97.
6. Berkhemer OA, Fransen PS, Beumer D, van den Berg LA, Lingsma HF, Yoo AJ, et al. (2015). A randomized trial of intraarterial treatment for acute ischemic stroke. *N Engl J Med*, 372, 1120.
7. Campbell BC, Mitchell PJ, Kleinig TJ, Dewey HM, Churilov L, Yassi N, et al. (2015). Endovascular therapy for ischemic stroke with perfusion imaging selection. *N Engl J Med*, 372, 100918.
8. Goyal M, Demchuk AM, Menon BK, Eesa M, Rempel JL, Thornton J, et al. (2016). Randomized assessment of rapid endovascular treatment of ischemic stroke. *N Engl J Med*, 372, 101930.
9. Jovin TG, Chamorro A, Cobo E, de Miquel MA, Molina CA, Rovira A, et al. (2015). Thrombectomy within 8 hours after symptom onset in ischemic stroke. *N Engl J Med*, 372, 2296306.
10. Saver JL, Goyal M, Bonafe A, Diener HC, Levy EI, Pereira VM, et al. (2015). Stent retriever thrombectomy after intravenous tPA vs. tPA alone in stroke. *N Engl J Med*, 372, 228595.
11. Powers WJ, Rabinstein AA, Ackerson T, Adeoye OM, Bambakidis NC, Becker K, Biller J, Brown M, Demaerschalk BM, Hoh B, et al. (2018) Guidelines for the Early Management of Patients With Acute Ischemic Stroke: A Guideline for Healthcare Professionals From the American Heart Association/American Stroke Association. *Stroke*, Epub 24 Jan.
12. Saver JL, Jahan R, Levy EI, et al., for the SWIFT Trialists. (2012). Solitaire flow restoration device versus the Merci Retriever in patients with acute ischaemic stroke (SWIFT): a randomised, parallel-group, non-inferiority trial, *Lancet*, 380, 1241–49.
13. Nogueira RG, Lutsep HL, Gupta R, et al., for the TREVO 2 Trialists. (2012). Trevo versus Merci retrievers for thrombectomy revascularisation of large vessel occlusions in acute ischaemic stroke (TREVO 2): a randomised trial. *Lancet*, 380, 1231–40.
14. Zhu G, Michel P, Aghaebrahim A, Patrie JT, Xin W, Eskandari A, et al. (2013). Computed tomography workup of patients suspected of acute ischemic stroke: Perfusion computed tomography adds value compared with clinical evaluation, noncontrast computed tomography, and computed tomography angiogram in terms of predicting outcome. *Stroke*, 44, 1049-55.
15. Powers WJ et al. (2015). American Heart Association/American Stroke Association Focused Update of the 2013 Guidelines for the Early Management of Patients with Acute Ischemic Stroke Regarding Endovascular Treatment: A Guideline for Healthcare Professionals from the American Heart Association /American Stroke Association. *Stroke*, 46, 3020-35.
16. Saver, JL, et al. (2016). Time to Treatment With Endovascular Thrombectomy and Outcomes From Ischemic Stroke: A Meta-analysis. *JAMA*, 316(12), 1279-89.
17. Nogueira RG, Jadhav AP, Haussen DC, et al. (2017). Thrombectomy 6 to 24 hours after stroke with a mismatch between deficit and infarct. *N Engl J Med*, 11 Nov.
18. Albers GW, Marks MP, Kemp S, et al. (2018). Thrombectomy for Stroke at 6 to 16 Hours with Selection by Perfusion Imaging. *N Engl J Med*, 24 Jan.
19. Salahuddin H, Ramaiah G, Slawski DE, et al. (2017). Mechanical thrombectomy of M1 and M2 middle cerebral artery occlusions. *Jrnl of NeuroInt Surg*, Pub Online First: 13 July 2017.
20. Macleod, MR, et al. (2005). Results of a multicentre, randomised controlled trial of intra-arterial urokinase in the treatment of acute posterior circulation ischaemic stroke. *Cerebrovas Dis*, 20.1, 12-17.
21. Improved clinical outcome after acute basilar artery occlusion since the introduction of

endovascular thrombectomy devices. (2013). *Cerebrovas Dis,* 36, 394-400.

22. Kumar G, Shahripour RB, Alexandrov AV, Nagel S, Kellert L, Mohlenbruch M, Bosel J, Rohde S, Ringleb P. (2014). Recanalization of acute basilar artery occlusion improves outcomes: A meta-analysis. *Jrnl of NeuroInt Surg.*

23. Almekhlafi MA, Davalos A, Bonafe A, Chapot R, Gralla J, Pereira VM, et al. (2014). Impact of age and baseline nihss scores on clinical outcomes in the mechanical thrombectomy using solitaire FR in acute ischemic stroke study. *AJNR,* 35, 1337-40.

24. Spiotta AM, Vargas J, Hawk H, Turner R, Chaudry MI, Battenhouse H, et al. (2014). Impact of the aspect scores and distribution on outcome among patients undergoing thrombectomy for acute ischemic stroke. *Jrnl of neurointerv Surg.*

25. Kim JT, Park MS, Chang J, Lee JS, Choi KH, Cho KH. (2013). Proximal arterial occlusion in acute ischemic stroke with low NIHSS scores should not be considered as mild stroke. *PLoS One,* 8(8), e70996.

26. Coutts, SB., et al. (2012). CT/CT Angiography and MRI Findings Predict Recurrent Stroke After Transient Ischemic Attack and Minor Stroke. *Stroke,* 43.4, 1013-17.

27. Riedel, CH., et al. (2012). Thin-slice reconstructions of nonenhanced CT images allow for detection of thrombus in acute stroke. *Stroke,* 43.9, 2319-23.

28. Alber GW., et al. (2016). Ischemic core and hypoperfusion volumes predict infarct size in SWIFT PRIME. *Ann of neuro,* 79.1,: 76-89.

29. Campbell, BCV, et al. (2011). Imaging selection in ischemic stroke: feasibility of automated CT-perfusion analysis. *Intl Jrnl of Stroke,* 10.1 , 51-54.; Lansberg MG., et al. (2011). RAPID automated patient selection for reperfusion therapy. *Stroke,* 42.6, 1608-14.

30. Abou-Chebl A, Lin R, Hussain MS, Jovin TG, Levy EI, Liebeskind DS, Yoo AJ, Hsu DP, Rymer MM, Tayal AH, Zaidat OO, Natarajan SK, Nogueira RG, Nanda A, Tian M, Hao Q, Kalia JS, Nguyen TN, Chen M, Gupta R. (2010). Conscious sedation versus general anesthesia during endovascular therapy for acute anterior circulation stroke: preliminary results from a retrospective, multi-center study. *Stroke,* Jun, 41(6), 1175-79.

31. Jumaa MA, Zhang F, Ruiz-Ares G, Gelzinis T, Malik AM, Aleu A, Oakley JI, Jankowitz B, Lin R, Reddy V, Zaidi SF, Hammer MD, Wechsler LR, Horowitz M, Jovin TG. (2010). Comparison of safety and clinical and radiographic outcomes in endovascular acute stroke therapy for proximal middle cerebral artery occlusion with intubation and general anesthesia versus the non-intubated state. *Stroke,* Jun, 41(6), 1180-84.

32. Nichols C, Carrozzella J, Yeatts S, Tomsick T, Broderick J, Khatri PJ. (2010). Is periprocedural sedation during acute stroke therapy associated with poorer functional outcomes? *Neurointerv Surg,* Mar, 2(1), 67-70.

33. Campbell, B. (2017). Oral presentation. *Int Stroke Conference* 2017.

34. Berkhemer OA, van den Berg LA, Fransen PSS, et al. (2016). The effect of anesthetic management during intra-arterial therapy for acute stroke in MR CLEAN. *Neurology,* 87, 656–64.

35. Talke PO, Sharma D, Heyer EJ, Bergese SD, Blackham KA, Stevens RD. (2014). Republished: Society for neuroscience in anesthesiology and critical care expert consensus statement: Anesthetic management of endovascular treatment for acute ischemic stroke. *Stroke,* 45, e138-50.

36. Broeg-Morvay A, Mordasini P, Bernasconi C, et al. (2016). Direct mechanical intervention versus combined intravenous and mechanical intervention in large artery anterior circulation stroke: a matched-pairs analysis. *Stroke,* 47, 1037–44.

37. Tsivgoulis G, Katsanos AH, Mavridis D, et al. (2016). Mechanical thrombectomy improves functional outcomes independent of pretreatment with intravenous thrombolysis. *Stroke,* 47, 1661–64.

38. Weber R, Nordmeyer H, Hadisurya J, et al. (2016). Comparison of outcome and interventional complication rate in patients with acute stroke treated with mechanical thrombectomy with and without bridging thrombolysis. *J Neurointerv Surg,* Pub Online First: 22 Feb 2016.

39. Rai AT, Boo S, Buseman C, et al. (2017). Intravenous thrombolysis before endovascular therapy for large vessel strokes can lead to significantly higher hospital costs without improving outcomes. *Jrnl of NeuroInt Surg,* Pub Online First: 06 Jan 2017.

Chapter 26

Collateral Circulation

26.1 Introduction

The concept of collateral circulation has been discussed throughout this book but this dedicated chapter is presented for one simple reason: **Collateral circulation by far is the most unappreciated concept related to acute ischemic stroke (AIS).** Collateral flow represents blood flow diverted to areas of the brain compromised by arterial occlusion. Every aspect of current AIS treatment is dependent on cerebral collateral circulation. This is because threatened brain tissue (ischemic penumbra) can only survive temporarily with collateral flow until it can be rescued with reperfusion therapy (IV TPA and/or EVT). The history of cerebral collateral circulation is over a century old, yet physician awareness of collateral status and how it relates to stroke is severely lacking.[1] Cerebral collateral circulation differs among AIS patients and variations require patient-specific assessment of the collateral circulation, ischemic penumbra, and core infarct. Additionally, these physiologic differences that vary from individual to individual can only be determined by advanced neuroimaging and not by arbitrary time points. For this reason, EVT candidacy must be based on image confirmation of collateral flow to salvageable brain tissue (ischemic penumbra).

Previous chapters have discussed intravenous thrombolysis (IV TPA) and endovascular treatment (EVT). These are the only FDA-approved methods for AIS treatment. Recanalization is the goal of all AIS treatment whether it is done via IV TPA or EVT. The restoration of blood flow to the brain preserves the ischemic penumbra and halts its degradation into an irreparable core infarct. However, revascularization encompasses two distinct processes. These include recanalization of a proximal vessel occlusion with either IV TPA or EVT and reperfusion of the downstream arterial territory. While recanalization reestablishes anterograde tissue reperfusion, reperfusion of downstream regions within the brain (distal to the region of vascular occlusion) can be maintained by cerebral collateral circulation.

The collateral circulation of the brain can be divided into primary and secondary conduits. Primary conduits are formed by the Circle of Willis and connect the anterior with the posterior circulation as well as the right and left anterior circulation (Figure 1). Secondary connections include non-Circle of Willis related collateral circulation. Examples include the ophthalmic artery which supplies collateral circulation from the external carotid artery to the internal carotid artery and leptomeningeal collaterals which are small pial arterioles connecting the vascular territories of the middle cerebral artery (MCA) with those of the anterior cerebral artery (ACA). Leptomeningeal collaterals are frequently encountered in intracranial artery occlusions such as an MCA M1 occlusion (Figures 2, 3, and 4).

Several important collateral circulation concepts are illustrated by Figure 3 below. In vitro experiments have shown that neuronal death occurs minutes after vascular occlusion if there is poor or no collateral circulation. This is represented by the core infarct (Figure 3). However, animal experiments have also demonstrated that leptomeningeal collaterals can occur seconds after vascular occlusion.[2] These collaterals can perfuse the region of threatened brain tissue surrounding the core infarct called the ischemic penumbra.

FIGURE 1. Collateral Circulation (Primary Connection) Via the Circle of Willis

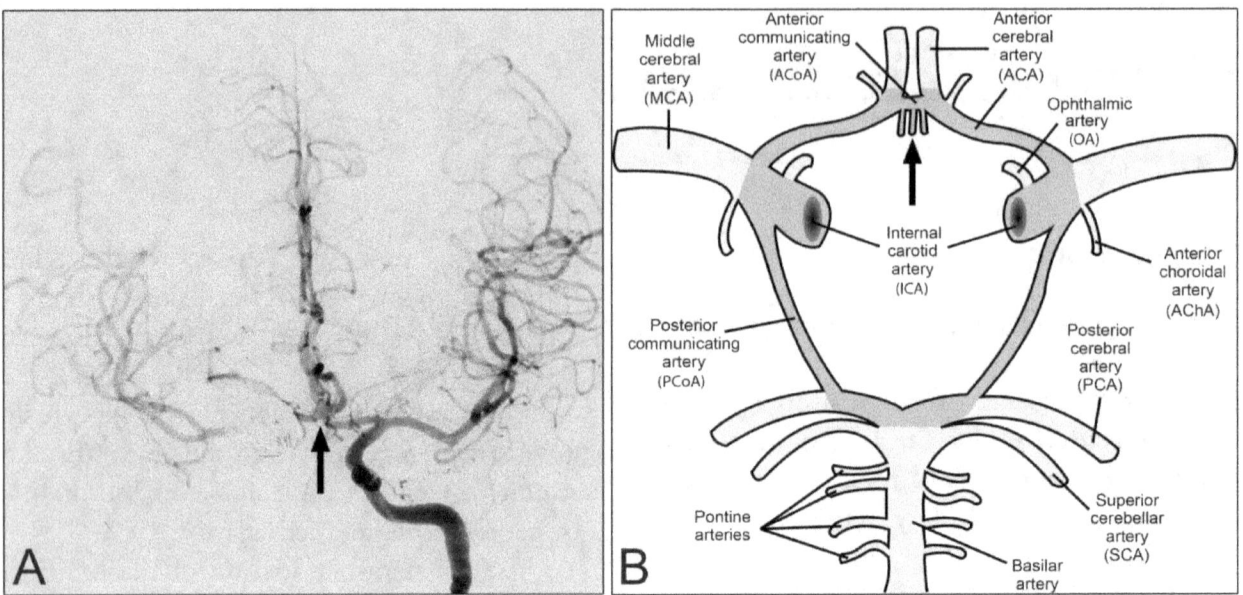

A) Contrast injection of the left internal carotid artery (ICA) demonstrates arterial flow from the left anterior circulation across the anterior communicating artery (arrow) to the right anterior circulation. (B) Diagram of circle of Willis illustrates collateral circulation across the anterior communicating artery (arrow).

FIGURE 2. Collateral Circulation (secondary connection) Via Leptomeningeal Collaterals

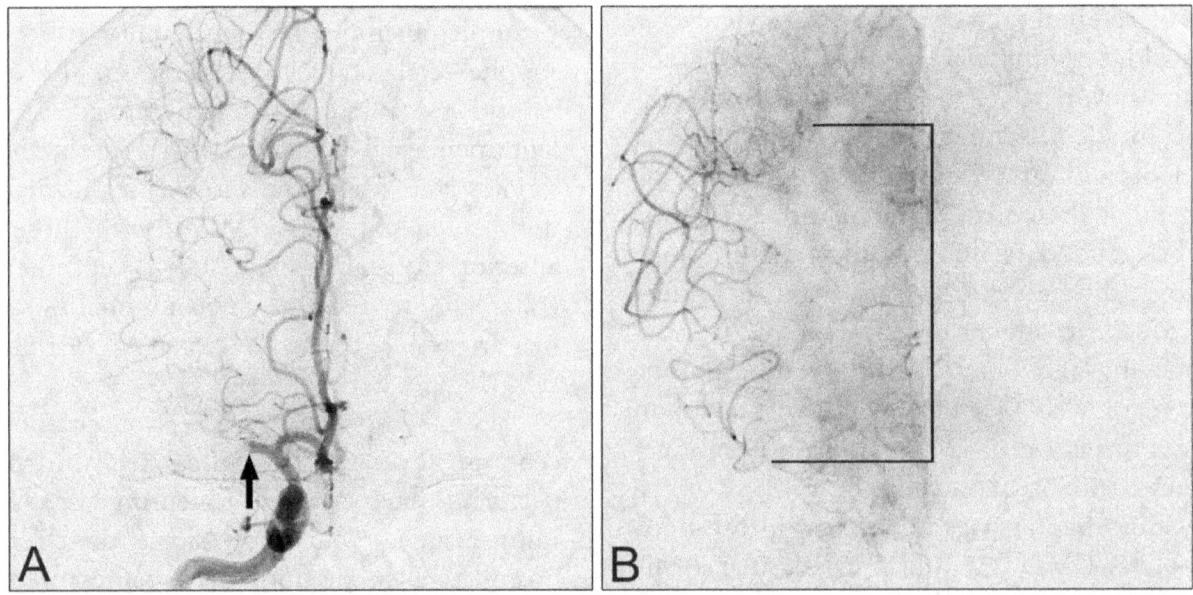

(A) Early arterial phase of right internal carotid artery injection demonstrates complete right MCA proximal M1 occlusion (arrow). (B) Late arterial phase demonstrates leptomeningeal collaterals from the right anterior cerebral artery (ACA) distribution which reestablished retrograde flow into the right middle cerebral artery (MCA) distribution.

FIGURE 3. Leptomeningeal Collateral Circulation

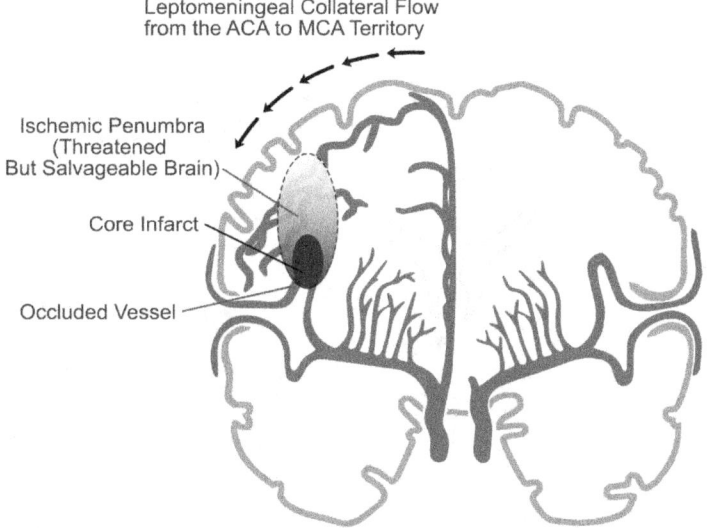

ACA= anterior cerebral artery, MCA = middle cerebral artery
Diagrammatic representation of right MCA M2 segment occlusion and surrounding core infarct (black oval). Due to leptomeningeal collateral circulation, there is preservation of ischemic penumbra (gray oval).

26.2 Collateral Circulation

The severity of AIS neurologic deficits at presentation and following reperfusion treatment is dependent upon collateral circulation.[3,4] Multiple studies have demonstrated that the success of IV TPA administration, EVT, the volume of final infarct, and hemorrhagic risk after reperfusion therapy are all related to collateral circulation status (Table 1).[5-25] Success of IV TPA administration and EVT depend on good collateral circulation whereas poor collaterals lead to larger infarct volumes and a higher risk of symptomatic hemorrhage after reperfusion therapy (Table 1).

Collateral circulation describes the network of arterial channels that reroute blood flow to regions of the brain when the primary vessels that usually supply it are occluded (Figure 4). As mentioned earlier, stroke intervention should not be dictated by arbitrary time points; rather, the patient's individual collateral status determines the ability to maintain a viable penumbra. Collateral status differs from patient to patient. It is the collateral status of each individual patient, determined by distinctive physiologic characteristics, which determines the ability to maintain a viable penumbra. A viable penumbra (and not arbitrary time points) establishes treatment potential (Figure 4). Every patient has a unique amount of time to maintain an ischemic penumbra because collateral circulation is patient-specific. While the ischemic penumbra exists, there is still viable brain tissue that can be salvaged by reperfusion. This is the true determinant of AIS treatment candidacy and not arbitrary time points.

TABLE 1. AIS Factors Associated with Collateral Circulation: **HAVE**

H	Hemorrhage Risk Increases with Poor Collaterals	
A	Administration of IV TPA Better with Good Collaterals	
V	Volume of Infarct Increases with Poor Collaterals	
E	EVT Success Better with Good Collaterals	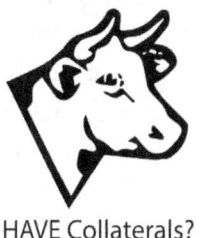 HAVE Collaterals?

TPA - Tissue Plasminogen Activator, EVT - Endovascular Treatment

FIGURE 4. Collateral Circulation and Arterial Occlusion

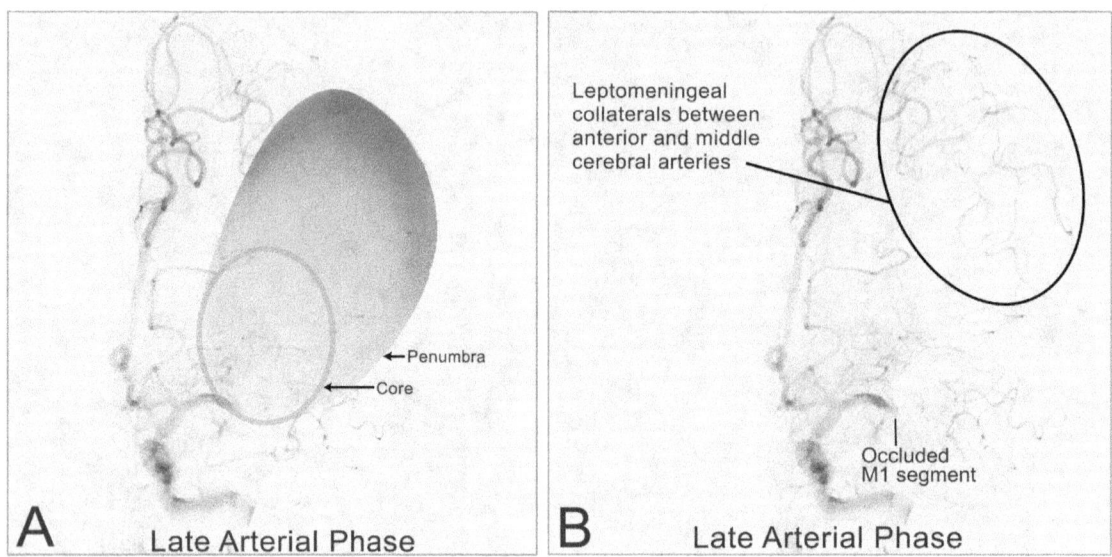

(A) Complete occlusion of left MCA M1 segment. Core infarct (Core) surrounded by ischemic penumbra (Penumbra). (B) Leptomeningeal collaterals from ACA preserve flow to the ischemic penumbra due to occluded left MCA M1 segment.

Neuroimaging has consistently demonstrated that patients with large core infarcts and poor collateral status have poor functional outcomes.[24, 26] This is because there is no significant ischemic penumbra or viable brain tissue to rescue. Alternatively, good collateral flow predicts better functional outcome and even suggests an extended time window for EVT.[27,28] Good cerebral collateral circulation can maintain the ischemic penumbra until recanalization can be performed. In fact, the presence of adequate collateral flow is an independent predictor of functional outcome following either IV TPA or EVT.[29-31] This is because there is significant ischemic penumbra or viable brain tissue to rescue. For this reason, the determination of collateral flow and viable penumbra tissue is a pivotal factor in acute stroke intervention. Again, this must be assessed on an individual basis utilizing advanced neuroimaging and not simply relying on arbitrary time points.

Collateral flow not only maintains penumbral tissue but also aids in recanalization. Twenty-five years ago, Ringelstein et al. proposed that collateral flow would increase the retrograde delivery of IV TPA to the distal end of an occlusive clot.[32] Since that time, this hypothesis was confirmed utilizing more sophisticated MRI imaging techniques.[30] This concept of collateral flow aiding in pharmacological recanalization in addition to maintaining the penumbra has been established by additional researchers.[4] Thus, the success of IV TPA is not because this drug dissolves a clot in an anterograde manner but because existing collaterals permit retrograde delivery of IV TPA to a clot. The same concept is further strengthened by the determination that the angiographic degree of collateralization was the **only predictor of functional outcome** in proximal middle cerebral artery occlusions treated by intra-arterial thrombolysis.[6]

26.3 Collateral Circulation Imaging

Due to its high temporal and spatial resolution, the gold standard for collateral circulation determination is **cerebral angiography**.[33-35] In clinical practice, however, therapeutic decisions are usually determined on the basis of noninvasive imaging (MRI, MRA, MRP, CTA or CTP). As stated earlier, the focus of this text is CT-based imaging because it is usually associated with lower cost, greater availability, and faster imaging. In this regard, ASPECTS, dual phase CTA and CTP have been extensively discussed in Chapter 21 (Stroke Imaging). Chapter 21 discussed ASPECTS as it relates to core assessment. However, ASPECTS not only correlates to core size but also assesses collateral circulation.[36] Multiphase and dual-phase CTA can directly visualize collateral circulation and correlate with angiographic leptomeningeal collaterals.[37] As demonstrated in the ESCAPE Trial, collateral flow evaluated by multiphase CTA was pivotal in determining clinical outcome.[38] Intermediate or good collateral circulation correlated with good functional outcome. Assessment of maintained or elevated cerebral blood volume (CBV) by CTP also correlated with good functional outcome.

No optimum imaging screening protocol to determine collateral circulation has been recognized. Certainly, advanced neuroimaging and techniques used to diagnose and treat AIS will continually evolve into advanced software driven tools to provide precise quantitative measurements of collateral circulation. In addition to CT based imaging, both conventional and emerging MRI-based imaging techniques can also assess collateral status. Currently, diffusion-weighted imaging stroke volume and cortical lesion pattern are predictive of the degree of collateral flow. For example, cortical lesion patterns on diffusion-weighted MRI are indicative of poor collaterals.[39] One emerging MRI-based imaging technique that is particularly appealing is *arterial spin labeling (ASL)*. ASL is a noncontrast perfusion imaging technique that measures cerebral blood flow based on magnetic labeling of arterial water. This technique may visualize collateral flow within cortical vessels which correlates to improved functional outcome.[40] In addition, ASL can provide anatomical detail similar to cerebral angiography without the use of exogenous contrast agents.[41]

Currently, CT-based neuroimaging techniques such as dual phase CTA can be utilized to rapidly and simultaneously assess both LVO and collateral status. Individual collateral status that is patient-specific can no longer be ignored. **This collateral status which differs among patients is the true determinant of stroke treatment and not arbitrary time points.** Previous chapters have discussed both the administration of IV TPA and EVT. This discussion demonstrated that 514 patients had to be treated with IV TPA and 37 patients with EVT in order to prevent one patient from death or dependency.[16, 42-49]

Patient selection in these previous randomized trials was determined by arbitrary time points and neglected the variability of patient-specific collateral circulation. Thus, these trials led to the exclusion of thousands of patients who would have potentially benefited from tissue-based therapy rather than therapy based on arbitrary time points. Furthermore, this logic would also exclude all patients with wake-up stroke and those with unknown symptom onset which can account for one-third of all AIS patients. Clearly, the dynamics that affect AIS progression and the rate of brain cell death vary from patient to patient. Arbitrary time points alone can no longer be considered sufficient to determine AIS patient candidacy. Neuroimaging must continue to play an increasing role in refining EVT candidacy. Both the DAWN and DEFUSE 3 trials have demonstrated that the progression of irreparably damaged brain tissue (core infarct) is less dependent on time and more dependent on individual collateral circulation.[50] EVT candidacy must be determined on a patient-specific basis utilizing advanced neuroimaging to identify salvageable ischemic penumbra rather than depending on arbitrary time points. This point is reiterated in the 2018 AHA/ASA guidelines which state: "It may be reasonable to incorporate collateral flow status into clinical decision-making in some candidates to determine eligibility for mechanical thrombectomy."[51]

Regardless of collateral circulation status, reperfusion treatment must always be initiated as early as possible because of its transient nature. Early and decisive action is integral to improve functional outcome. However, do not confuse this "time is brain" concept with AIS candidacy determined by arbitrary time windows. Again, reperfusion treatment is dependent upon individual, patient-specific collateral circulation which must be determined at presentation with advanced neuroimaging. Although patient-specific, collateral circulation is limited, meaning reperfusion treatment should be initiated as soon as possible. Again, the importance of collateral status does not negate optimization of acute stroke algorithms such as the reduction of onset to treatment times, which is always of paramount importance.[52]

26.4 Conclusion

Collateral circulation constitutes an important, if not the most important aspect of acute stroke intervention that, for whatever reason, remains largely unappreciated. AIS imaging protocols must include noninvasive methods of collateral flow assessment. The determination of patient-specific collateral status improves the ability to effectively treat AIS and increases the therapeutic time window for EVT. However, this does not negate the fact that optimization of AIS algorithms to reduce treatment time onset remains of paramount importance.[52] While many MRI investigational techniques continue to expand the ability to assess collateral status and determine treatment, they are not yet ready for widespread implementation. Furthermore, even existing conventional MRI techniques such as diffusion-weighted imaging currently cannot be performed as efficiently as CT based imaging. For this reason, CT based imaging is still the favored imaging modality. Collateral circulation is an essential determinant in the treatment of every AIS patient.

Abbreviations list

ACA, anterior cerebral artery; AIS, acute ischemic stroke; ASL, arterial spin labeling; ASPECTS, Alberta Stroke Program Early CT Score; CBV, cerebral blood volume; CTA, computed tomography angiography; CTP, computed tomography perfusion; EVT, endovascular treatment; IV TPA, intravenous thrombolysis; LVO, large vessel occlusion; MCA, middle cerebral artery; MRA, magnetic resonance angiography; MRI, magnetic resonance imaging; MRP, magnetic resonance perfusion.

References

1. Mount LA, Taveras JM. (1957). Arteriographic demonstration of the collateral circulation of the cerebral hemispheres. *AMA Arch NeurPsych,* 78, 235–53.
2. Morita Y, Fukuuchi Y, Koto A, Suzuki N, Isozumi K, Gotoh J, et al. (1997). Rapid changes in pial arterial diameter and cerebral blood flow caused by ipsilateral carotid artery occlusion in rats. *Keio J Med,* 46(3), 120–7.
3. Roberts HC, Dillon WP, Furlan AJ, Wechsler LR, Rowley HA, Fischbein NJ, et al. (2002). Computed tomographic findings in patients undergoing intra-arterial thrombolysis for acute ischemic stroke due to middle cerebral artery occlusion: results from the PROACT II trial. *Stroke,* 33(6), 1557–65.
4. Marks MP, Lansberg MG, Mlynash M, Olivot JM, Straka M, Kemp S, et al. (2014). Diffusion and Perfusion Imaging Evaluation for Understanding Stroke Evolution 2 Investigators. Effect of collateral blood flow on patients undergoing endovascular therapy for acute ischemic stroke. *Stroke,* 45(4), 1035–39.
5. Galimanis A, Jung S, Mono M-L, Fischer U, Findling O, Weck A, et al.(2012). Endovascular therapy of 623 patients with anterior circulation stroke. *Stroke,* 43(4), 1052–57.
6. Kucinski T, Koch C, Eckert B, Becker V, Krömer H, Heesen C, et al.(2003). Collateral circulation is an independent radiological predictor of outcome after thrombolysis in acute ischaemic stroke. *Neuroradiology,* 45(1), 11–18.
7. Toni D, Fiorelli M, Bastianello S, Falcou A, Sette G, Ceschin V, et al. (1997). Acute ischemic strokes improving during the first 48 hours of onset: predictability, outcome, and possible mechanisms. A comparison with early deteriorating strokes. *Stroke,* 28(1), 10–14.
8. Rosenthal ES, Schwamm LH, Roccatagliata L, Coutts SB, Demchuk AM, Schaefer PW, et al. (2008). Role of recanalization in acute stroke outcome: rationale for a CT angiogram-based "benefit of recanalization" model. *AJNR Am J Neuroradiol,* 29(8), 1471–75.
9. Tan JC, Dillon WP, Liu S, Adler F, Smith WS, Wintermark M. (2007). Systematic comparison of perfusion-CT and CT-angiography in acute stroke patients. *Ann Neurol,* 61(6), 533–43.
10. Tan IYL, Demchuk AM, Hopyan J, Zhang L, Gladstone D, Wong K, et al. (2009). CT angiography clot burden score and collateral score: correlation with clinical and radiologic outcomes in acute middle cerebral artery infarct. *AJNR Am J Neuroradiol,* 30(3), 525–31.

11. Bang OY, Saver JL, Kim SJ, Kim GM, Chung CS, Ovbiagele B, et al. (2011). Collateral flow predicts response to endovascular therapy for acute ischemic stroke. *Stroke*, 42(3), 693–99.
12. Gerber JC, Petrova M, Krukowski P, Kuhn M, Abramyuk A, Bodechtel U, et al. (2016). Collateral state and the effect of endovascular reperfusion therapy on clinical outcome in ischemic stroke patients. *Brain Behav*, 6(9), e00513.
13. Leng X, Lan L, Liu L, Leung TW, Wong KS. (2016). Good collateral circulation predicts favorable outcomes in intravenous thrombolysis: a systematic review and meta-analysis. *Eur J Neurol*, 23(12), 1738–49.
14. Leng X, Fang H, Leung TWH, Mao C, Miao Z, Liu L, et al. (2016). Impact of collaterals on the efficacy and safety of endovascular treatment in acute ischaemic stroke: a systematic review and meta-analysis. *J Neurol Neurosurg Psychiatry*, 87(5), 537–44.
15. Liebeskind DS, Jahan R, Nogueira RG, Zaidat OO, Saver JL—SWIFT Investigators. (2014). Impact of collaterals on successful revascularization in Solitaire FR with the intention for thrombectomy. *Stroke*, 45(7), 2036–40.
16. Goyal M, Demchuk AM, Menon BK, Eesa M, Rempel JL, Thornton J, et al.—ESCAPE Trial Investigators. (2015). Randomized assessment of rapid endovascular treatment of ischemic stroke. *N Engl J Med*, 372(11), 1019–30.
17. Tan BYQ, Wan-Yee K, Paliwal P, Gopinathan A, Nadarajah M, Ting E, et al. (2016). Good Intracranial Collaterals Trump Poor ASPECTS (Alberta Stroke Program Early CT Score) for Intravenous Thrombolysis in Anterior Circulation Acute Ischemic Stroke. *Stroke*, 47(9), 2292–98.
18. Ovbiagele B, Buck BH, Liebeskind DS, Starkman S, Bang OY, Ali LK, et al. (2008). Prior antiplatelet use and infarct volume in ischemic stroke. *J Neurol Sci*, 264(1-2), 140–44.
19. Boers AM, Jansen IG, Berkhemer OA, Yoo AJ, Lingsma HF, Slump CH, et al.—MR CLEAN trial investigators†. (2016). Collateral status and tissue outcome after intra-arterial therapy for patients with acute ischemic stroke. *J Cereb Blood Flow Metab*, Jan 1, X16678874.
20. Christoforidis GA, Vakil P, Ansari SA, Dehkordi FH, Carroll TJ. (2017). Impact of pial collaterals on infarct growth rate in experimental acute ischemic stroke. *AJNR Am J Neuroradiol*, 38(2), 270–75.
21. Son JP, Lee MJ, Kim SJ, Chung JW, Cha J, Kim GM, et al. (2017). Impact of Slow Blood Filling via Collaterals on Infarct Growth: Comparison of Mismatch and Collateral Status. *Stroke*, 19(1), 88–96.
22. Vagal A, Menon BK, Foster LD, Livorine A, Yeatts SD, Qazi E, et al. (2016). Association Between CT Angiogram Collaterals and CT Perfusion in the Interventional Management of Stroke III Trial. *Stroke*, 47(2), 535–38.
23. Leng X, Fang H, Leung TWH, Mao C, Xu Y, Miao Z, et al. (2016). Impact of Collateral Status on Successful Revascularization in Endovascular Treatment: A Systematic Review and Meta-Analysis. *Cerebrovasc Dis*, 41(1-2), 27–34.
24. Bang OY, Saver JL, Kim SJ, Kim GM, Chung CS, Ovbiagele B, et al.—UCLA-Samsung Stroke Collaborators. (2011). Collateral flow averts hemorrhagic transformation after endovascular therapy for acute ischemic stroke. *Stroke*, 42(8), 2235–39.
25. Liebeskind DS, Tomsick TA, Foster LD, Yeatts SD, Carrozzella J, Demchuk AM, et al.—IMS III Investigators. (2014). Collaterals at angiography and outcomes in the Interventional Management of Stroke (IMS) III trial. *Stroke*, 45(3), 759–64.
26. Hill MD, Demchuk AM, Goyal M, Jovin TG, Foster LD, Tomsick TA, et al.–IMS3 Investigators. (2014). Alberta Stroke Program early computed tomography score to select patients for endovascular treatment: Interventional Management of Stroke (IMS)-III Trial. *Stroke*, 45, 444-49.
27. Ribo M, Flores A, Rubiera M, Pagola J, Sargento-Freitas J, Rodriguez-Luna D, et al. (2011). Extending the time window for endovascular procedures according to collateral pial circulation. *Stroke*, 42, 3465–69.
28. Hwang YH, Kang DH, Kim YW, Kim YS, Park SP, Liebeskind DS. (2015). Impact of time-to-reperfusion on outcome in patients with poor collaterals. *AJNR Am J Neuroradiol*, 36, 495–500.
29. Nicoli F, Scalzo F, Saver JL, et al, for the UCLA Stroke Investigators. (2014). The combination of baseline magnetic resonance perfusion-weighted imaging-derived tissue volume with severely prolonged arterial-tissue delay and

diffusion-weighted imaging lesion volume is predictive of MCA-M1 recanalization in patients treated with endovascular thrombectomy. *Neuroradiology*, 56, 117–27.

30. Nicoli F, Lafaye de Micheaux P, Girard N. (2013). Perfusion-weighted imaging-derived collateral flow index is a predictor of MCA M1 recanalization after IV thrombolysis. *AJNR Am J Neuroradiol*, 34, 107–14.

31. Zhang S, Zhang X, Yan S, et al. (2016). The velocity of collateral filling predicts recanalization in acute ischemic stroke after intravenous thrombolysis. *Sci Rep*, 6, 27880, Kim SJ, Son JP, Ryoo S, et al. (2014). A novel magnetic resonance imaging approach to collateral flow imaging in ischemic stroke. *Ann Neurol*, 76, 356–69.

32. Ringelstein EB, Biniek R, Weiller C, et al. (1992). Type and extent of hemispheric brain infarctions and clinical outcome in early and delayed middle cerebral artery recanalization. *Neurology*, 42, 289–98.

33. McVerry F, Liebeskind DS, Muir KW. (2012). Systematic review of methods for assessing leptomeningeal collateral flow. *AJNR Am J Neuroradiol*, 33(3), 576–82.

34. Martinon E, Lefevre PH, Thouant P, Osseby GV, Ricolfi F, Chavent A. (2014). Collateral circulation in acute stroke: assessing methods and impact: a literature review. *J Neuroradiol*, 41(2), 97–107.

35. Raymond SB, Schaefer PW. (2017). Imaging Brain Collaterals: Quantification, Scoring, and Potential Significance. *Top Magn Reson Imaging*, 26(2), 67–75.

36. Choi JY, Kim EJ, Hong JM, Lee SE, Lee JS, Lim YC, et al. (2011). Conventional enhancement CT: a valuable tool for evaluating pial collateral flow in acute ischemic stroke. *Cerebrovasc Dis*, 31, 346–52.

37. Kim SJ, Noh HJ, Yoon CW, Kim KH, Jeon P, Bang OY, et al. (2012). Multiphasic perfusion computed tomography as a predictor of collateral flow in acute ischemic stroke: comparison with digital subtraction angiography. *Eur Neurol*, 67, 252–55.

38. Menon BK, d'Esterre CD, Qazi EM, Almekhlafi M, Hahn L, Demchuk AM, et al. (2015). Multiphase CT angiography: a new tool for the imaging triage of patients with acute ischemic stroke. *Radiology*, 275, 510–20.

39. Souza LC, Yoo AJ, Chaudhry ZA, Payabvash S, Kemmling A, Schaefer PW, et al. (2012). Malignant CTA collateral profile is highly specific for large admission DWI infarct core and poor outcome in acute stroke. *AJNR Am J Neuroradiol*, 33, 1331–36.

40. Zaharchuk G. (2011). Arterial spin label imaging of acute ischemic stroke and transient ischemic attack. *Neuroimaging Clin N Am*, 21, 285–301.

41. Robson PM, Dai W, Shankaranarayanan A, Rofsky NM, Alsop DC. (2010). Time-resolved vessel-selective digital subtraction MR angiography of the cerebral vasculature with arterial spin labeling. *Radiology*, 257, 507–15.

42. National Institute of Neurological Disorders and Stroke rt-PA Stroke Study Group. (1995). Tissue plasminogen activator for acute ischemic stroke. *N Engl J Med*, 333(24), 1581–88.

43. Hacke W, Kaste M, Bluhmki E, Brozman M, Dávalos A, Guidetti D, et al.—ECASS Investigators. (2008). Thrombolysis with alteplase 3 to 4.5 hours after acute ischemic stroke. *N Engl J Med*, 359(13), 1317–29.

44. Jovin TG, Chamorro A, Cobo E, de Miquel MA, Molina CA, Rovira A, et al.—REVASCAT Trial Investigators. (2015). Thrombectomy within 8 hours after symptom onset in ischemic stroke. *N Engl J Med*, 372(24), 2296–306.

45. Saver JL, Goyal M, Bonafe A, Diener HC, Levy EI, Pereira VM, et al.—SWIFT PRIME Investigators. (2015). Stent-retriever thrombectomy after intravenous t-PA vs. t-PA alone in stroke. *N Engl J Med*, 372(24), 2285–95.

46. Berkhemer OA, Fransen PS, Beumer D, van den Berg LA, Lingsma HF, Yoo AJ, et al.—MR CLEAN Investigators. (2015). A randomized trial of intraarterial treatment for acute ischemic stroke. *N Engl J Med*, 372(1), 11–20.

47. Campbell BCV, Mitchell PJ, Kleinig TJ, Dewey HM, Churilov L, Yassi N, et al.;—EXTEND-IA Investigators. (2015). Endovascular therapy for ischemic stroke with perfusion-imaging selection. *N Engl J Med*, 372(11), 1009–18.

48. Bracard S, Ducrocq X, Mas JL, Soudant M, Oppenheim C, Moulin T, et al.—THRACE investigators. (2016). Mechanical thrombectomy after intravenous alteplase versus alteplase alone after stroke (THRACE): a randomised controlled trial. *Lancet Neurol*, 15(11), 1138–47.

49. Mocco J, Zaidat OO, von Kummer R, Yoo AJ, Gupta R, Lopes D, et al.—THERAPY Trial Investigators*. (2016). Aspiration Thrombectomy After Intravenous Alteplase Versus Intravenous Alteplase Alone. *Stroke*, 47(9), 2331–38.
50. Nogueira RG, Jadhav AP, Haussen DC, et al. (2017). Thrombectomy 6 to 24 hours after stroke with a mismatch between deficit and infarct. *N Engl J Med*, 11 Nov; Albers GW, Marks MP, Kemp S, et al. (2018). Thrombectomy for Stroke at 6 to 16 Hours with Selection by Perfusion Imaging. *N Engl J Med*, 24 Jan.
51. Powers WJ, Rabinstein AA, Ackerson T, Adeoye OM, Bambakidis NC, Becker K, Biller J, Brown M, Demaerschalk BM, Hoh B, et al. (2018). Guidelines for the Early Management of Patients With Acute Ischemic Stroke: A Guideline for Healthcare Professionals From the American Heart Association/American Stroke Association.. *Stroke,* Epub 24 Jan 2018.
52. Soulleihet V, Nicoli F, Trouve J, et al. (2014). Optimized acute stroke pathway using Medical Advanced Regulation for Stroke (M.A.R.S.) and repeated public awareness campaigns. *Am J Emerg Med,* 32, 225–32.

Chapter 27

Prehospital Stroke Assessment

27.1 Introduction

Chapter 25 (Endovascular Treatment) emphasized the rapid diagnosis and treatment of large vessel occlusion (LVO) acute ischemic stroke (AIS). It reviewed the tremendous superiority of endovascular treatment (EVT) versus IV TPA alone. Primary stroke centers (PSCs) can adequately treat most stroke patients but cannot perform EVT. For this reason, LVO AIS patients **must** be transported directly to comprehensive stroke centers (CSCs) which can perform EVT. A CSC has the same capabilities as a PSC but can also provide 24/7 EVT, cerebrovascular neurosurgery, and neurocritical care. The detection and treatment of LVO AIS have far-reaching implications that extend beyond the walls of the hospital. Because only EVT-capable hospitals (CSCs) can adequately care for LVO AIS, these patients must be appropriately screened by EMS personnel before reaching the hospital. This way, EMS personnel can bring LVO AIS patients directly to CSCs that can perform EVT and avoid PSCs that cannot. CSCs are usually the largest and best-equipped hospitals within a geographic region that provide intensive care and specialized techniques including EVT for stroke treatment.

The mantra for LVO AIS patients is to **find them fast and fix them fast!** Without effective LVO screening, EMS personnel can inappropriately transport an LVO AIS patient to a non-CSC which cannot perform EVT. This LVO AIS patient will then have to be transferred to a hospital that can perform EVT. You might ask, why would EMS take an LVO AIS patient to a hospital that cannot perform EVT? The answer is, without effective screening for LVO, this happens daily. PSCs can treat most AIS but generally do not provide catheter-based procedures (EVT). Patients suspected of having an LVO should go to a CSC that can provide adequate care in a timely manner.

However, every day LVO patients are transferred to CSCs after they are first incorrectly transported to PSCs which cannot perform EVT. This preventable treatment delay can potentially result in ischemic penumbra decaying into irreparably damaged, core infarct.[1] A recent analysis of a national database (from University Health System Consortium, Clinical Database/Resource Manager) determined the effect of hospital transfer on outcomes after EVT.[2] This study reviewed 8,533 inpatient admissions that received EVT from 118 institutions and demonstrated lower rates of mortality in patients who presented as direct admits to endovascular centers compared to patients who presented as transfers (14.9% vs 18.6%). Furthermore, patients presenting directly to CSCs had faster time to revascularization compared to patients presenting as transfers. Both the SWIFT PRIME and ESCAPE trials demonstrated delayed EVT times in transferred patients. Similarly, a recent meta-analysis demonstrated that LVO AIS patients requiring interhospital transfer (from PSC to CSC) required, on average, an additional 142 minutes.[3] Many other studies now associate these transfer delays with significant worse outcome.[4,5] The bottom line is, an LVO AIS patient must go directly to a CSC first or suffer a significant possibility of a worse functional outcome.

Getting LVO AIS patients to the correct facility (CSC) the first time is the reason why EMS prehospital screening is essential. EMS assessment must be based upon a rapid and reliable protocol that can screen for LVO. EMS must effectively screen suspected LVO AIS patients so they can be transported to CSCs and immediately receive EVT. Similarly, a patient with a non-LVO AIS should be delivered to a PSC. LVO AIS patients who are directly transported to CSCs have tremendously improved median arrival-to-groin puncture times.[6] So how should EMS personnel be instructed to adequately screen for LVO? A recent abstract published in the AHA journal *Circulation* discussed this point.[7] It states that while prehospital stroke scales that perform LVO screening such as the Cincinnati Prehospital Stroke Severity Scale (CPSSS), the Los Angeles Prehospital Stroke Screen (LAPSS), the Los Angeles Motor Scale (LAMS), and the Rapid Arterial Occlusion Evaluation Scale (RACE) are available, most have low sensitivity for the detection of LVO. It recommends a better and more accurate prehospital scale is necessary to deliver LVO AIS patients to the closest CSC, concluding that a new scale is required to improve prehospital LVO screening. The American Heart Association (AHA)/American Stroke Association (ASA) 2018 guidelines for the early management of patients with acute ischemic stroke also state, "better stroke identification tools are needed in the prehospital setting."[8] These same guidelines further state, "**implementation of a stroke protocol to be used by EMS personnel is strongly encouraged**."

Many of the concerns raised by this article and the AHA/ASA are addressed by a newer assessment tool for LVO called 'VAN.'[9] VAN is an acronym that stands for **vision**, **aphasia**, and **neglect**. VAN is performed by first assessing motor strength. Motor assessment is carried out by asking the patient to hold up both arms, palms up for 10 seconds. Note that this exam is focusing on motor strength only (not coordination or positional sense). No drift or weakness indicates this patient is VAN negative. That is, the patient has been determined not to have an LVO within 10 seconds. If, however, the patient has any weakness, the examiner goes to the remainder of the VAN assessment which includes vision, aphasia, and neglect analysis.

To examine vision, the examiner looks for a visual or optic field cut within all four visual quadrants. The examiner checks for double vision and asks the patient to track the examiner's finger movement to the right and then to the left with their eyes. The examiner then asks the patient if there are any complaints of new onset of blindness. If the patient has a field cut, double vision, uneven tracking, or complaints of new blindness, then the vision portion of the VAN assessment (in conjunction with motor weakness) is positive. If the vision assessment is positive or any other component of the VAN assessment is positive (in conjunction with motor weakness), the patient is suspected to have an LVO. The examiner has completed the VAN assessment and this suspected LVO AIS patient should be transferred to a CSC. If the patient demonstrates no field cut, denies double vision or new onset of blindness, the vision portion of the VAN assessment is deemed negative. The examiner should go on to the next portion of the VAN assessment which is aphasia.

To examine aphasia, the examiner determines if the stroke patient has expressive aphasia, receptive aphasia, global aphasia, or is asymptomatic (no aphasia). To determine if there is expressive aphasia, the examiner asks the stroke patient to name two objects, such as a watch and a pen. To test for receptive aphasia, the examiner asks the patient to follow two commands such as blinking or making a fist. If the stroke patient has both an expressive and receptive aphasia, this is referred to as global aphasia. If the aphasia assessment is positive (expressive, receptive, or global aphasia) or any other component of the VAN assessment is positive (in conjunction with motor weakness), the patient is suspected to have an LVO. The examiner has completed the VAN assessment and this patient should be transferred to a stroke center that can perform EVT (CSC). If the patient demonstrates no aphasia, the aphasia portion of the VAN assessment is negative and the examiner should go on to the next portion of the VAN assessment which is neglect.

To examine neglect, the examiner tests to see if the stroke patient is unable to sense either side of their face, arms, or legs at the same time, is unable to identify their own extremity, or is ignoring one side of the body. In addition, under the VAN assessment, forced gaze to one side or the inability to track to one side was included as a neglect criterion. If the neglect assessment is positive or any other component of the VAN assessment is positive (with motor weakness), the patient is suspected to have an LVO. The examiner has completed the VAN assessment and this patient should be transferred to a stroke center that can perform EVT. If the patient demonstrates no form of neglect (which again also includes gaze preference or the inability to track to one side), the neglect portion of the VAN assessment is negative. If the patient demonstrates no neglect and no vision abnormalities or aphasia, the VAN assessment is completed and is negative. That is, this patient is not suspected of having an LVO.

To summarize, the VAN assessment is positive if a stroke patient has weakness (measured by raising both arms palms up for 10 seconds) plus any one component of the VAN assessment (vision, aphasia, or neglect). If any components of the VAN assessment are positive (in conjunction with motor weakness), this patient is suspected of having an LVO and should be taken to a CSC that can perform EVT. The VAN assessment is considered negative if the patient has no weakness (as described above) or has weakness, but the remainder of the VAN assessment including vision, aphasia, or neglect are all negative. That is, this patient is not suspected of having LVO and is not required to be taken to a stroke center that can perform EVT.

What is the VAN assessment really testing? As we learned earlier, neglect is typically a parietal lobe function whereas aphasia is generally a left-sided brain function. Gaze preference results from damage to the frontal gaze center (frontal lobe). Motor strength is controlled by the motor cortex located in the posterior portion of the frontal lobe. The primary visual cortex is located posteriorly in the occipital lobe. Essentially, the VAN assessment is testing for stroke (or any other process for that matter) that can affect two or more cortical distributions. When we compare small vessel occlusions against large vessel occlusions, small vessel occlusions normally occur in distal vessels and usually affect one cortical distribution, typically resulting in one cortical symptom. Because large vessel occlusions tend to be more proximal occlusions, they can affect multiple vascular distributions downstream. This results in multiple cortical distribution deficits (Figure 1).

FIGURE 1. Cortical Regions and Associated Deficits

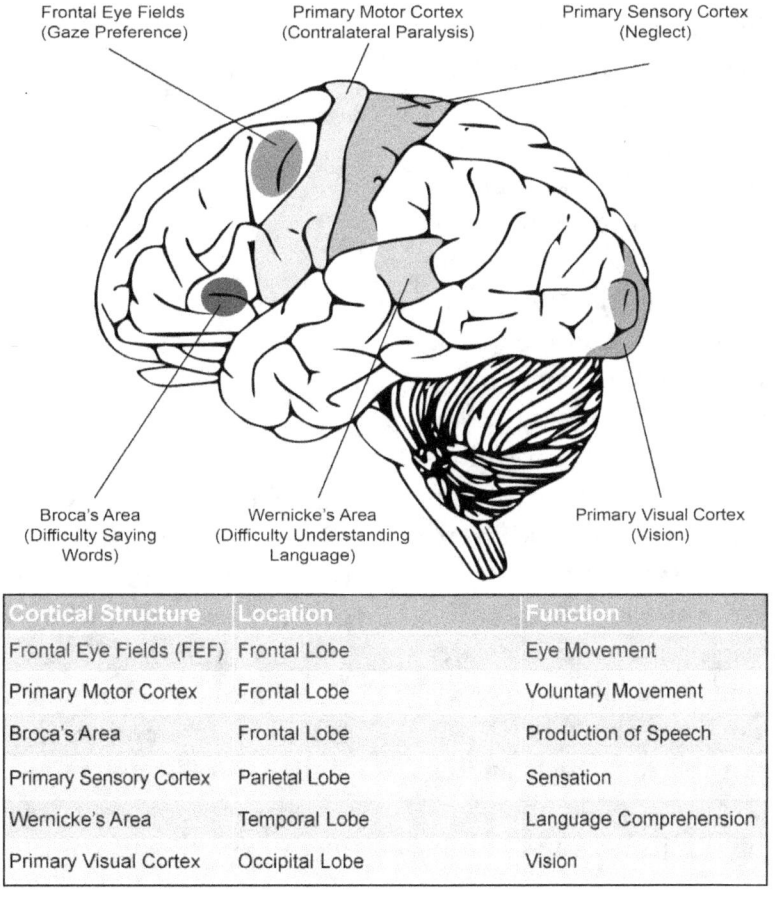

Cortical Structure	Location	Function
Frontal Eye Fields (FEF)	Frontal Lobe	Eye Movement
Primary Motor Cortex	Frontal Lobe	Voluntary Movement
Broca's Area	Frontal Lobe	Production of Speech
Primary Sensory Cortex	Parietal Lobe	Sensation
Wernicke's Area	Temporal Lobe	Language Comprehension
Primary Visual Cortex	Occipital Lobe	Vision

FIGURE 2. Lacunar Infarct

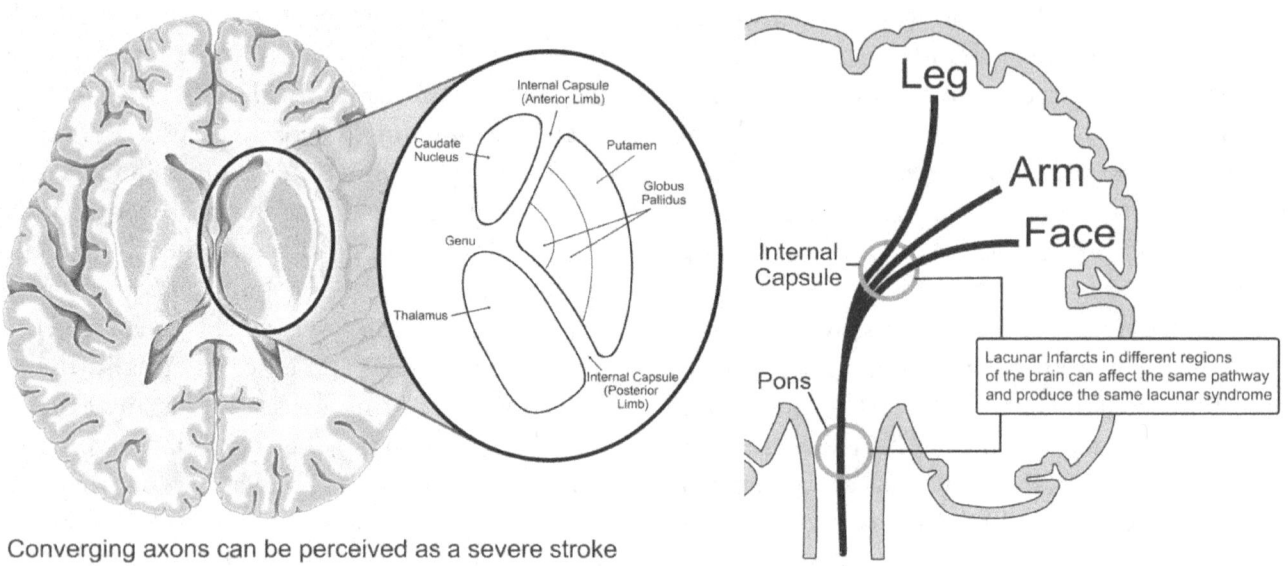

Converging axons can be perceived as a severe stroke

As discussed earlier, lacunar infarcts are a form of small vessel disease. However, if a lacunar infarct occurs within the internal capsule where multiple axons converge from multiple regions of the cortex, this can be perceived as a severe stroke caused by an LVO (Figure 2). Nonetheless, these tend to cause either pure motor or sensory symptoms because a lacunar infarct involving the internal capsule includes axons of neurons within similar regions of the cortex. A pure motor hemiparesis or a pure sensory stroke lacks visual, aphasia, or other deficits which are tested by the VAN assessment. That is, a pure motor hemiparesis or pure sensory stroke lacks multiple cortical distributions and the absence of these additional cortical symptoms would present as a VAN-negative assessment.

How does the VAN assessment compare to other LVO screening tools? The best way to answer this question is to analyze the brain regions specifically evaluated by these screening tools (Figure 3). Areas of the brain that are typically examined are the frontal gaze center, motor cortex, sensory cortex, visual cortex, and language centers of the brain. One language center is Broca's area which is located in the left frontal lobe. Strokes affecting this region result in expressive aphasia. The region of the brain responsible for understanding language is along the left superior temporal region and strokes affecting this region can result in receptive or Wernicke's aphasia. Finally, hemineglect most commonly results from right-sided (nondominant), parietal lobe stroke.

FIGURE 3. Brain Regions Commonly Evaluated by LVO Screening Tools

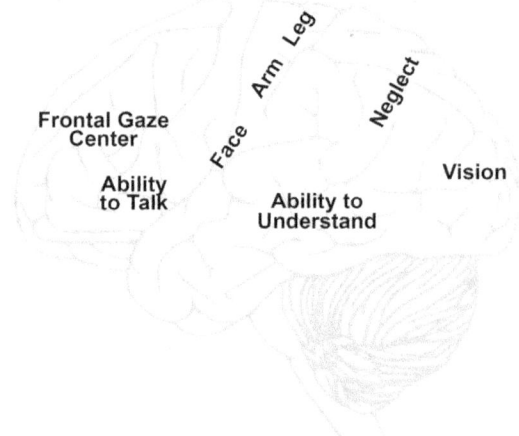

The Rapid Arterial Occlusion Evaluation Scale (RACE) score examines the frontal gaze center, the ability to talk, the ability to understand, neglect, vision, and the motor cortex (face, arm, and leg distributions) (Figure 4). The Texas Stroke Intervention Prehospital Stroke Severity Scale or LEGS score examines the frontal gaze center, the ability to talk, the ability to understand, vision, and the motor cortex (leg distribution) (Figure 5). Note that this does not include the face or arm regions of the motor cortex. The Los Angeles Motor Scale or LAMS score examines the face and arm distributions of the motor cortex (Figure 6). The Cincinnati Prehospital Stroke Severity Scale or CPSSS score examines the frontal gaze center, the ability to talk, the ability to understand, and the motor cortex (arm distribution) (Figure 7). The 3-item stroke scale or 3I-SS assesses the frontal gaze center and the motor cortex (arm and leg distributions) (Figure 8). The VAN assessment examines the frontal gaze center, the ability to talk, the ability to understand, neglect, vision, and the motor cortex (arm distribution) (Figure 9). Comparing the VAN assessment to most LVO screening tools mentioned above (excluding the RACE score), it examines many more cortical regions for stroke deficits (Figure 10).

FIGURE 4. Rapid Arterial Occlusion Evaluation Scale (RACE)

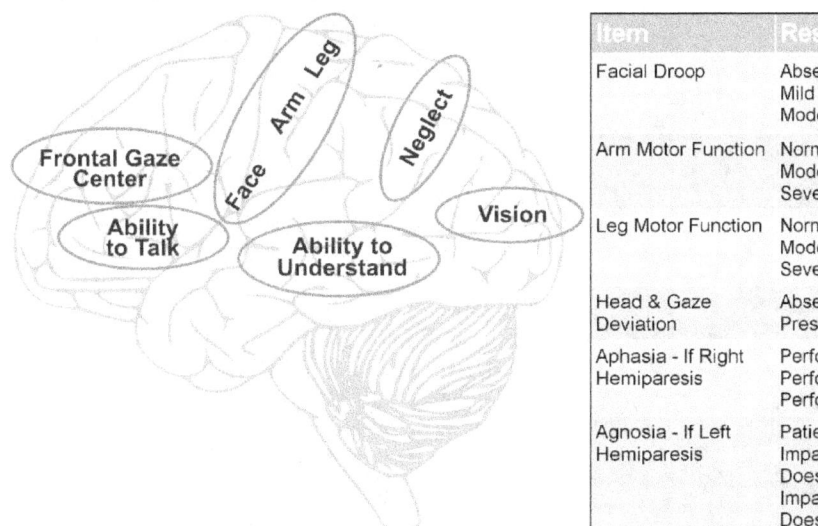

Item	Result	Score
Facial Droop	Absent	0
	Mild	1
	Moderate to Severe	2
Arm Motor Function	Normal to Mild	0
	Moderate	1
	Severe	2
Leg Motor Function	Normal to Mild	0
	Moderate	1
	Severe	2
Head & Gaze Deviation	Absent	0
	Present	1-2
Aphasia - If Right Hemiparesis	Performs Both Tasks Correctly	0
	Performs One Task Correctly	1
	Performs Neither Correctly	2
Agnosia - If Left Hemiparesis	Patient Recognizes Arm and Impairment	0
	Does Not Recognize Arm or Impairment	1
	Does Not Recognize Arm	2

FIGURE 5. The Texas Stroke Intervention Pre-Hospital Stroke Severity Scale (LEGS)

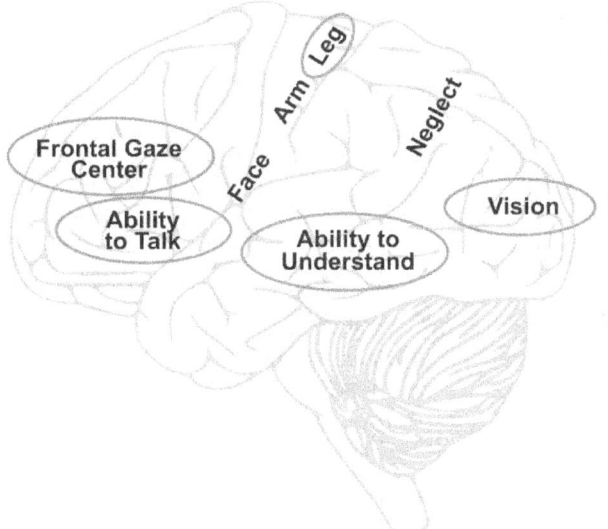

Item		Score	Symptom Severity
Leg Strength			
	Right	0	No drift
		1	Drift
		2	Some effort against gravity
		3	No effort against gravity
		4	No movement
	Left	0	No drift
		1	Drift
		2	Some effort against gravity
		3	No effort against gravity
		4	No movement
Eyes/Visual Fields		0	No visual field deficit
		1	Either upper or lower visual field deficit
		2	Both upper or lower visual field deficit
		3	Blind in both eyes
Gaze		0	No gaze paralysis
		1	Partial gaze paralysis
		2	Forced deviation to one side
Speech/ Language		0	Normal
		1	Mild loss of fluency or comprehension
		2	Incomprehensible
		3	Mute/comatose

FIGURE 6. The Los Angeles Motor Scale (LAMS)

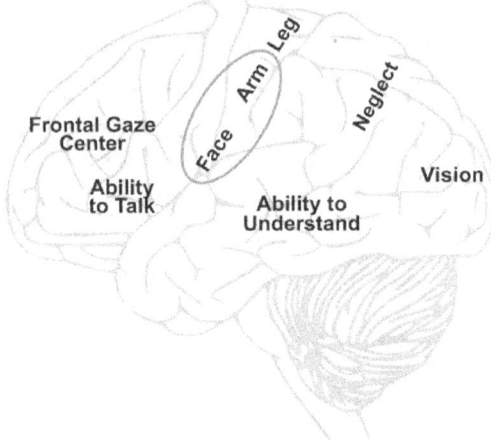

Deficit	Severity	Score
Facial Droop	Absent	0
	Present	1
Arm Drift	Absent	0
	Drifts down on one side	1
	Falls rapidly on one side	2
Grip Strength	Normal	0
	Weak grip on one side	1
	No grip on one side	2

FIGURE 7. The Cincinnati Prehospital Stroke Severity Scale (CPSSS)

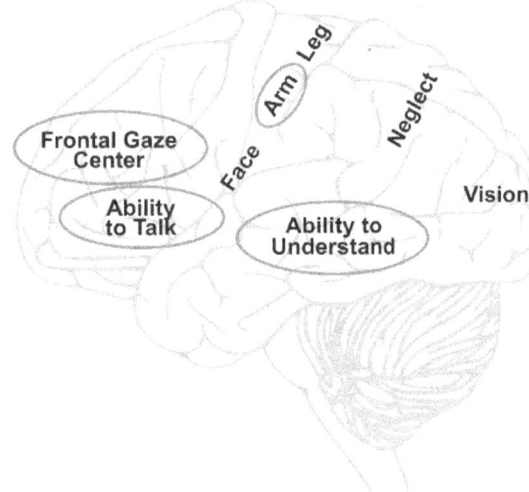

Item	Severity	CPSSS Score
Conjugate Gaze Deviation	Absent	0
	Present	2
LOC or Commands		
	a) Answers both correctly	0
	Answers one or both incorrectly, or	1
	b) Follows both commands correctly	0
	Follows one or both commands incorrectly	1
Arm Strength (both arms 10 seconds)	Does not fall to bed	0
	Falls to bed	1
Score Total		0-4

FIGURE 8. The 3-Item Stroke Scale (3I-SS)

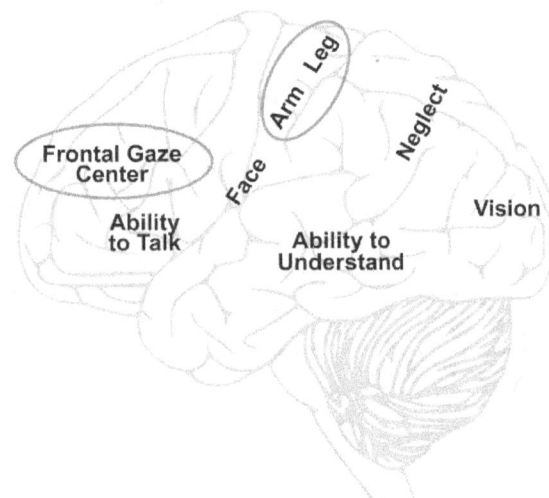

Item	Severity	Score
Disturbance of consciousness	No	0
	Mild	1
	Severe	2
Gaze and head deviation	Absent	0
	Incomplete gaze/head deviation	1
	Forced gaze/head deviation	2
Hemiparesis	Absent	0
	Moderate	1
	Severe	2
Score (Total)		0 - 6

FIGURE 9. The VAN Assessment

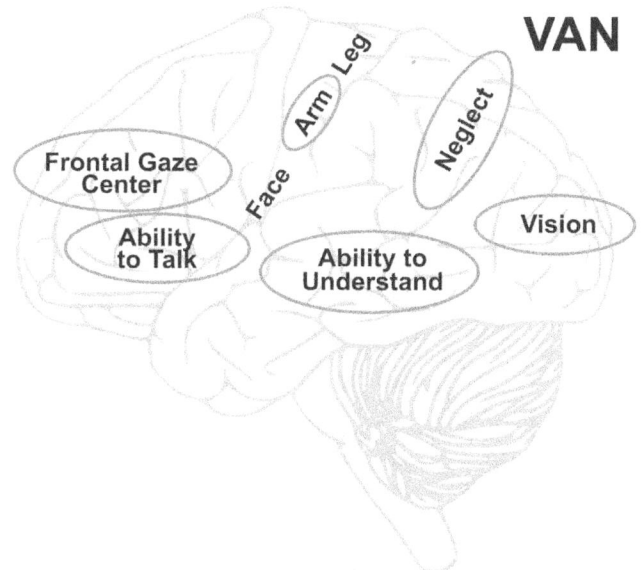

Unlike the other LVO screening tools, the VAN assessment does not require calculating an assessment score or a subjective rating of symptom severity. By eliminating the severity of symptoms, the VAN assessment reduces examiner subjectivity. In fact, the VAN study demonstrated 100% interobserver reliability among VAN trained nurses and stroke physicians.[9] The mantra for LVO is to **find them fast and fix them fast!** How can EMS personnel screen for LVO accurately and quickly when most other prehospital screening tools for LVO apart from VAN involve subjectivity and scoring charts? For this reason, the simplicity and accuracy of VAN as a prehospital LVO screening tool cannot be surpassed. However, this screening can be made even simpler by using the mnemonic 'MANGO™' (Table 1).

Before proceeding, one point must be made very clear. That is, MANGO™ is simply a mnemonic based on the VAN assessment tool. As such, its purpose is to make the VAN assessment tool easier to remember and perform and is in no way meant to discount the excellent work performed by Dr. Taleb et al.[9] Any discussion pertaining to this mnemonic is based upon the excellent work of Dr. Taleb and his colleagues.

The MANGO™ mnemonic reminds one to utilize weakness as the key symptom for LVO assessment. Motor strength is examined by asking the patient to hold up both arms, palms up for 10 seconds. Note that this exam is focusing on motor strength only and not coordination or positional sense. If there is no weakness, or the 'M' portion of the MANGO™ assessment is negative, the stroke patient is not suspected to have an LVO. That is, they have been determined not to have an LVO within 10 seconds. If, however, there is weakness or the 'M' portion of the MANGO™ assessment is positive, then complete the remainder of the MANGO™ mnemonic.

TABLE 1. LVO Screening Mnemonic: **MANGO**™

M	Motor Weakness

A	Aphasia
	    Expressive (name 2 objects)
	    Receptive (follow 2 commands)

N	Neglect
	    Unable to feel both sides at the same time, or
	    Unable to identify own arm, or
	    Ignoring one side

G	Gaze Preference, Inability to Track or Double Vision
O	Optic Field Cut or New Blindness

FIGURE 10. The VAN Assessment Compared to Other LVO Screening Tools

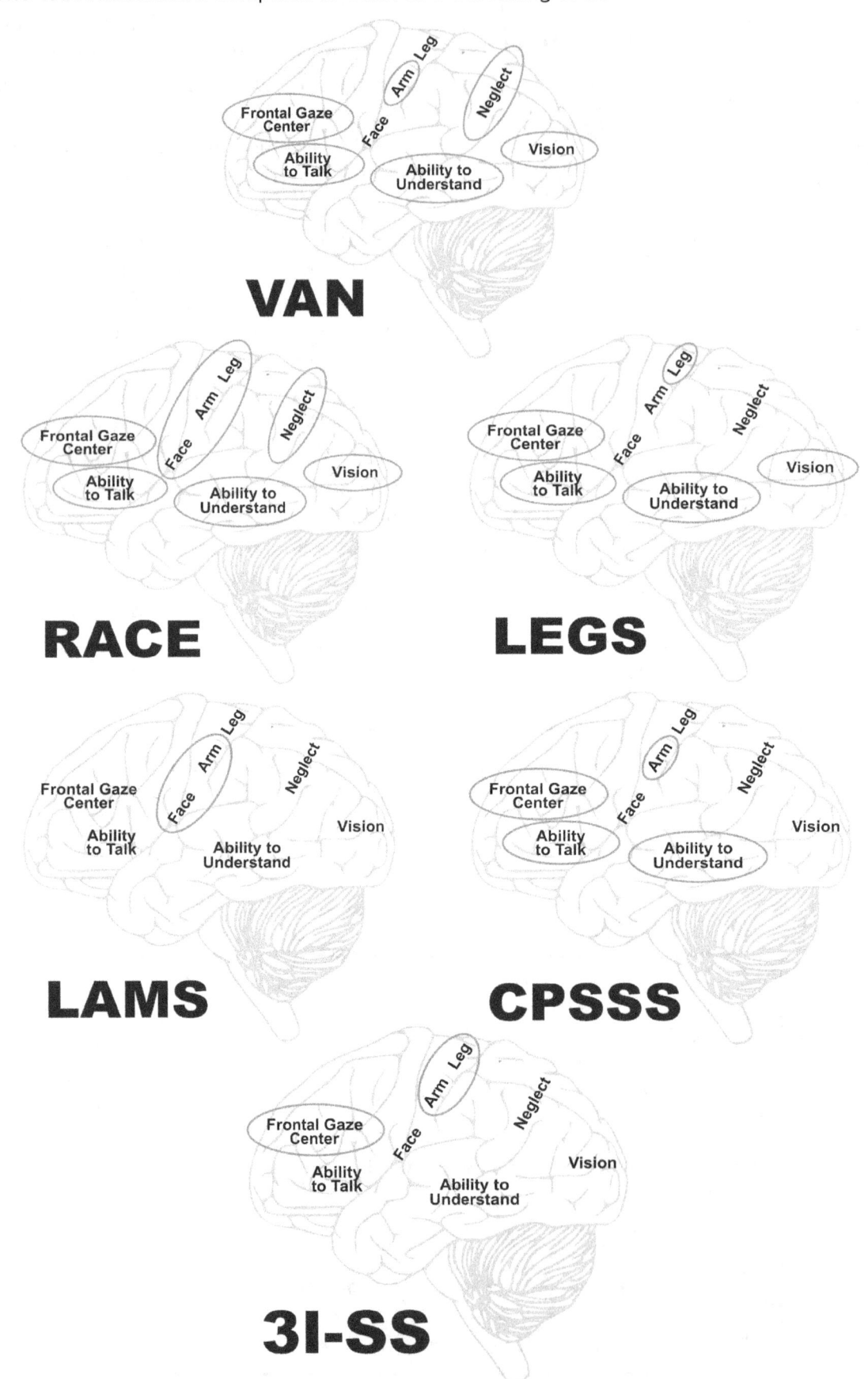

If any one of the remaining categories (aphasia, neglect, gaze preference or inability to track, optic field cut or new blindness) tests positive, then an LVO is suspected and this patient should be taken to a CSC. To summarize, an LVO is suspected if there is weakness or the 'M' or "motor weakness" portion of the MANGO™ mnemonic is positive, and any remaining component of the MANGO™ mnemonic is also positive. An LVO is not suspected if the 'M' or "motor weakness" portion of the MANGO™ mnemonic is negative (no motor weakness) or the 'M' or "motor weakness" portion of the MANGO™ mnemonic is positive and all remaining components (A-N-G-O) of the MANGO™ mnemonic are negative (Figure 11).

FIGURE 11. MANGO™ Algorithm and Prehospital Acute Ischemic Stroke (AIS) Assessment

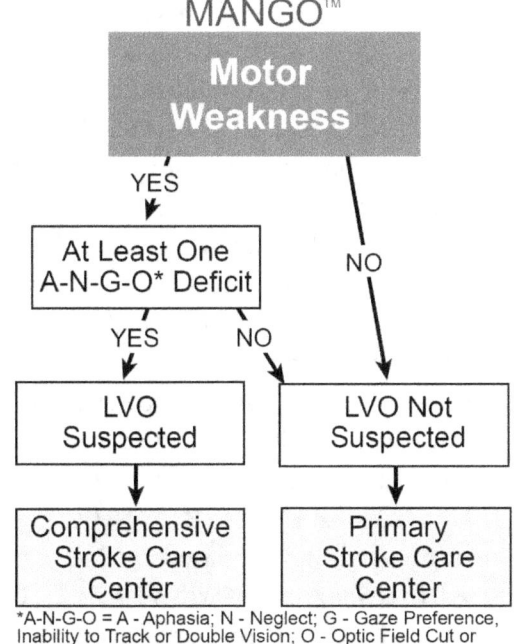

*A-N-G-O = A - Aphasia; N - Neglect; G - Gaze Preference, Inability to Track or Double Vision; O - Optic Field Cut or New Blindness

Again, the MANGO™ mnemonic reminds one that weakness is the key symptom for LVO assessment. If there is no motor weakness or the 'M' portion of the MANGO™ assessment is negative, the stroke patient is not suspected to have an LVO. If, however, there is motor weakness or the 'M' portion of the MANGO™ mnemonic is positive, then complete the remainder of the MANGO™ mnemonic. If any of the remaining categories (aphasia, neglect, gaze preference, inability to track, double vision, optic field cut or new blindness) tests positive, then this stroke patient is suspected of having an LVO and should go to a CSC (Figure 11).

27.2 2018 AHA/ASA Prehospital Stroke Assessment Recommendations

As of February 2018, the 2018 AHA/ASA evidence committee determined there is insufficient evidence to recommend any particular LVO screening tool or a threshold stroke severity that would warrant patient triage to a CSC. This has led to the recommendation which states, "When several IV alteplase-capable hospital options exist within a defined geographic region, the benefit of bypassing the closest to bring the patient to one that offers a higher level of stroke care, including mechanical thrombectomy, is uncertain. Further research is needed."[8] Essentially, the 2018 American Heart Association/American Stroke Association Guidelines state there is insufficient evidence to recommend one prehospital screening scale over another to triage LVO AIS patients to a CSC. This new recommendation is based upon the known impact of delays in IV alteplase administration on outcomes, and because additional research is necessary.[10] Further studies such as the RACECAT Trial that will be performed in Barcelona, Spain are needed to address this issue.

However, other factors also require consideration. These include the relative ineffectiveness of IV TPA for LVO AIS patients and the significant loss of EVT candidacy when LVO AIS patients are incorrectly taken to a non-CSC. These issues are somewhat addressed in the description section of the above recommendation which states, "For prehospital patients with **suspected LVO** by a stroke severity scale, the Mission: Lifeline Severity-Based Stroke Triage Algorithm for EMS recommends **direct transport to a comprehensive stroke center** if the travel time to the comprehensive stroke center is <15 additional minutes compared with the travel time to the closest primary stroke center or acute stroke-ready hospital. However, at this time, there is insufficient evidence to recommend 1 scale over the other or a specific threshold of additional travel time for which bypass of a primary stroke center or acute stroke-ready hospital is justifiable."[8]

While this discussion section of the AHA/ASA "recommends direct transport" of suspected LVO AIS patients to CSCs over PSCs, it seems to depart from their recommendation which states that the benefit of bringing a patient to a CSC and bypassing a closer PSC is uncertain. One reason formulating AIS triage recommendations is difficult is because the AHA/ASA guidelines state that in regard to the use of prehospital LVO screening, *"at this time, there is insufficient evidence to recommend one scale over the other."* This being said, the AHA/ASA acknowledges that there are regional differences in LVO prehospital screening and recognizes at least six different prehospital LVO screening tools.[11-16] So while there is currently insufficient evidence to recommend one prehospital LVO screening tool over the other, we should not abandon prehospital LVO screening. In fact, since the publication of the 2018 AHA/ASA guidelines, recent studies have validated the use of a new prehospital LVO AIS screening tool. In addition, further studies have also demonstrated that portable devices may quickly and accurately detect severe stroke in the prehospital setting and can effectively field triage LVO AIS patients to CSCs.

This newer research will be discussed shortly. However, the current 2018 AHA/ASA guidelines state that the benefit of bringing a patient to a CSC and bypassing a closer PSC is uncertain. At any rate, what is certain and what is perhaps the underlying premise for all AIS treatment is the strong correlation between time to treatment and benefit. IV TPA is relatively ineffective in the treatment of LVO AIS. LVO stroke accounts for only 11% of all AIS but is responsible for nearly all AIS related deaths, 90% of its societal cost, and 80% of significant functional disability. Thus, LVO AIS patients must be identified and treated in a timely manner. This means all AIS (non-LVO and LVO) suspected patients must receive proper prehospital screening so suspected LVO AIS patients can be identified and taken to the correct hospital (a CSC) the first time. The 2018 AHA/ASA guidelines further state, "Given the known impact of delays to IV alteplase on outcomes, the known impact of delays to mechanical thrombectomy on outcome, and the anticipated delays in transport for mechanical thrombectomy in eligible patients originally triaged to a nonendovascular center, the Mission: Lifeline algorithm **may be a reasonable guideline** in some circumstances."[8] Again, there is a strong correlation between time to treatment and benefit. This benefit is reduced and potentially lost if LVO AIS patients are initially taken to PSCs that are incapable of properly caring for them.

Again, the 2018 AHA/ASA guidelines conclude that there is insufficient evidence to recommend one prehospital LVO screening scale over another. They also recognize that prehospital LVO screening scales vary from region to region. Prehospital LVO screening tools are being used and will continue to be used to triage suspected LVO AIS patients to CSCs. At the time of their publication, I would agree with the 2018 AHA/ASA guidelines which state that in terms of prehospital LVO screening, *"at this time, there is insufficient evidence to recommend one scale over the other."* However, subsequent to their publication and specifically as of April 2018, there has been validation of a simple, reliable and accurate prehospital LVO AIS screening tool. On the other hand, even if we ignore this recent research, I would still respectfully disagree with the current 2018 AHA/ASA guidelines. This is because the 2018 AHA/ASA guideline recommendations are based on "all comers," whether AIS patients are non-LVO or LVO AIS patients. Even based on this assumption, probability models have demonstrated AIS patients will have better outcomes when the time of transport between PSCs and CSCs is from 10 to 30 minutes.[17] By the way, this analysis was performed by some of the same researchers that conducted the ESCAPE Trial. Again, this analysis includes both non-LVO and LVO AIS patients. However, as transport time between a PSC and CSC increases (45 minutes or longer), it makes more sense to take all (LVO and non-LVO) AIS patients to PSCs initially. Thus, based on probability alone, it would be reasonable to transport all AIS-suspected (non-LVO and LVO) patients to CSCs if this could be done in a timely manner (≤ 30 minutes).

The 2018 AHA/ASA guidelines also state: "Customization of the guideline to optimize patient outcomes will be needed to account for local and regional factors, including the availability of endovascular centers, door in-door out times for nonendovascular stroke centers, intrahospital transport times, and DTN and door-to-puncture times."[5] As discussed above, based on probability alone and evaluating "all comers" (both non-LVO and LVO AIS patients), patients will have better outcomes if taken directly to a CSC when the transport time between PSCs and CSCs is from 10 to 30 minutes.[17] Again, as the transport time between a PSC and CSC increases (45 minutes or longer), it makes more sense to take all (LVO and non-LVO) AIS patients to PSCs initially. Thus, based entirely on probability, it would be reasonable to transport all AIS-suspected (non-LVO and LVO) patients to CSCs if this can be done in a timely manner (≤ 30 minutes). This complies with the 2018 AHA/ASA guidelines which allow "customization of the guideline to optimize patient outcomes."[8]

However, a practice which transports "all comers" based on the distance of PSCs or CSCs is flawed for many reasons. LVO AIS patients need to be transported to CSCs and non-LVO AIS patients to PSCs where they can receive appropriate treatment. It makes no sense to transport an LVO AIS patient to a PSC where they cannot be properly treated nor does it make sense to transport a non-LVO AIS patient to a CSC when they can be properly treated at a PSC. Thus, effective prehospital field triage is dependent on simple, reliable, and accurate LVO AIS screening. Again, the AHA/ASA has determined that there is insufficient evidence to recommend one prehospital LVO screening scale over another. However, that does not negate the fact that prehospital LVO screening tools are currently being used to identify suspected LVO AIS patients and properly transport them to a CSC.[16] Additionally, researchers also demonstrated LVO AIS screening tools can be effectively used to directly transfer suspected LVO AIS patients to CSCs provided "EMS assessment was reliable and accurate."[18]

A simple, reliable, and accurate prehospital LVO screening tool is not just vital to ensure that LVO AIS patients are properly transported to CSCs to receive EVT. It is equally important to ensure non-LVO AIS patients also receive rapid and effective treatment at PSCs. Non-LVO AIS patients who inappropriately bypass PSCs have potential delays in thrombolysis and can overburden CSCs with patients that can receive appropriate care at a PSC. Again, there is a strong correlation between time to treatment and benefit. One of this chapter's objectives is to describe a simple, reliable, and accurate prehospital LVO AIS assessment tool. By reliably screening suspected LVO AIS patients, we are no longer dealing with a triage model purely based on probability. This would permit the effective triage of AIS patients to an appropriate stroke center. Non-LVO AIS patients would be transported to PSCs and rapidly receive thrombolysis and LVO AIS patients would be transported to CSCs to receive EVT. More importantly, LVO AIS patients would not be transported to PSCs where they cannot be effectively treated and non-LVO AIS patients would not overburden CSCs.

At the time of the AHA/ASA 2018 Guidelines publication (February 2018), the evidence review committee concluded that accuracy of any prehospital LVO screening was inadequate. Their uncertainty as to where to transport a suspected LVO AIS patient (CSC or PSC) was based on their belief that before February 2018, no simple, reliable, and accurate LVO AIS screening tool existed. Fortunately, a simple, accurate, and reliable prehospital LVO AIS screening tool has recently been described and validated. The components of this exam are also included in the MANGO™ mnemonic. So how is this possible if the study on which the MANGO™ mnemonic is based upon states that its components require validation?[9] More importantly, how can the MANGO™ mnemonic claim to be a reliable prehospital LVO AIS screening tool when the 2018 AHA/ASA guidelines specifically state no such LVO AIS prescreening tool exists?

The 2018 AHA/ASA guidelines were published in February 2018. Two months later in April 2018, new research was published which provided both retrospective and prospective validation of components within the MANGO™ mnemonic.[19] The "ACT FAST" algorithm whose components are contained within the MANGO™ mnemonic consists of assessing for (1) unilateral arm weakness <10 seconds, (2) aphasia if the right arm is weak or gaze preference/hemineglect if the left arm is weak, and (3) the exclusion of stroke mimics (Table 2). It is important to understand that as simple as this approach may seem, this algorithm has been demonstrated to show **higher specificity and reliability than all other pre-existing screening tools for LVO AIS recognition**.

Perhaps no field in medicine continues to evolve as rapidly as the management of AIS. For example, in 2013, EVT for LVO AIS was declared ineffective. Then remarkably in 2015, five separate endovascular trials demonstrated the superiority of EVT versus IV TPA alone. Next, a couple years later, the DEFUSE 3 and DAWN Trials demonstrated that in appropriately selected patients, EVT was effective within 16 and 24 hours, respectively. So while the recent 2018 AHA/ASA guidelines stated no effective LVO AIS screening tools existed at the time of its publication, current research (published only two months after the publication of the 2018 AHA/ASA guidelines) now suggests otherwise. Now that a simple, reliable, and accurate prehospital LVO AIS screening tool has been validated, it's important to revisit issues that were discussed earlier.

TABLE 2. Components of ACT-FAST Algorithm

RIGHT BRAIN	LEFT BRAIN
Right gaze preference	Left gaze preference
Neglect	Aphasia

First, prior to the ACT-FAST prehospital LVO AIS screening tool, the clinical evaluation of LVO AIS (as rightfully called out by the 2018 AHA/ASA guidelines) hasn't been that great.[20,21] In fact, only three prehospital LVO AIS screening tools (RACE, LAMS and the Cincinnati Stroke Triage Assessment Tool) have published validation studies with specificities of ≤ 70% for determining LVO using image confirmation as the reference standard.[22-26] In addition to the low specificity, these prehospital LVO AIS screening tools were subjective and required calculation. The components of the ACT-FAST prehospital LVO AIS screening tool, which are also included within the MANGO™ mnemonic, are simple to perform, have a high specificity for LVO AIS recognition, are objective, and require no calculation.[19]

Note that the MANGO™ mnemonic also contains all the components of both the earlier discussed VAN study and the more recently published ACT-FAST Algorithm. Both of these studies raise similar points and complement each other in many regards. First, both the VAN and ACT-FAST Algorithms evaluate multiple cortical distributions and as such, may render false positives by other cortical processes such as hemorrhage or tumor. Further, both of these studies demonstrated nonphysician LVO AIS assessment was not only possible but also extremely accurate. In the VAN study, appropriately trained emergency department nurses had 100% correlation with their stroke physician counterparts for LVO AIS assessment.[9] In the ACT-FAST study, excellent LVO AIS assessment correlation was achieved with minimally trained paramedics and their stroke physician counterparts.[19] Both studies clearly demonstrated **appropriately trained nonphysicians (emergency department nurses and paramedics) could accurately screen for LVO AIS**. Analysis of both of these studies allows one to conclude that **a simple, accurate and reliable prehospital LVO AIS screening tool does exist and has been validated**. These tools would enable the effective triage of LVO AIS patients to CSCs and non-LVO AIS patients to PSCs.

Both the VAN study and ACT-FAST Algorithm complement each other in several regards (Table 3). First, the VAN study was a single center study which evaluated 62 stroke patients making this a relatively small pilot study. However, the ACT-FAST Algorithm retrospectively evaluated

565 consecutive patients. Next, one criticism of the ACT-FAST Algorithm is that it was not designed to assess posterior circulation LVO. However, the posterior circulation was addressed in the VAN study and is clearly represented in the MANGO™ mnemonic. Also note that while the authors of the ACT-FAST Algorithm state it was not designed to assess the posterior circulation, gaze preference can also be encountered when the paramedian pontine reticular formation (PPRF) is affected by posterior circulation LVO (refer to Chapter 14). However, the "O" in the MANGO™ mnemonic represents "optic field cut or new blindness" and clearly examines the posterior circulation. Thus, the MANGO™ mnemonic can identify *suspected* LVO patients whose diagnosis can be confirmed by imaging upon admission.

TABLE 3. Synopsis of VAN and ACT-FAST LVO Screening

	VAN	ACT-FAST
Validated	NO	YES
Cerebral Circulation	Anterior and Posterior	Anterior

Even if we ignored the significance of the VAN and ACT-FAST screening tools, MANGO™-positive patients should still be transported directly to CSCs based on probability alone and assuming we accept the 2018 AHA/ASA statement that a reliable prehospital LVO screening tool is unavailable. Why? As stated above, based on probability alone, both non-LVO and LVO AIS patients theoretically would do better if transported to CSCs within 30 minutes. However, by utilizing the MANGO™ mnemonic, we would reduce the burden of "all comers" (both non-LVO and LVO AIS patients) that would flood CSCs and improve the ability to transport non-LVO and LVO AIS patients to their correct facilities (PSCs and CSCs, respectively). Also, recall that MANGO™ false positives are caused by intracranial processes affecting two or more cortical distributions such as brain tumors or hemorrhages. A valid argument can be made that CSCs are better equipped at treating these entities. As will be discussed further in Chapter 29 (Stroke Efficiency), the MANGO™ mnemonic also serves as an LVO screening tool that can be used both in the prehospital and hospital-based setting. Thus, it allows the synchronous and efficient evaluation of suspected LVO AIS patients, thereby reducing LVO image confirmation time and improving outcome.

27.3 EMS and Stroke

Prehospital stroke evaluation is an essential element for effective LVO screening, diagnosis, and treatment. Hospitals or stroke centers that do not have regular interactions with their EMS providers are doing their community a disservice. Approximately 35% to 70% of stroke patients are transported to the emergency department by ambulance. Thus, EMS providers are typically the first medical professionals to assess a stroke patient. The prehospital assessment and identification of stroke, as well as supportive care during transport to the hospital and appropriate routing of stroke patients to a designated stroke center, are all essential. The last point regarding the delivery of stroke patients in an effective manner to the closest and most appropriate hospital cannot be overemphasized.

The adoption of LVO AIS protocols requires collaboration among individual hospital systems, EMS providers, and regional and state guidelines. For example, in the state of Rhode Island, physicians were able to successfully implement an LVO protocol by generating consensus across healthcare systems and adopting a single stroke severity score.[27] Using this prehospital screening tool, patients suspected of having an LVO were directly transported to a CSC if transport time is ≤ 30 minutes and to a primary stroke center (PSC) for transportation times > 30 minutes. For LVO suspected patients who presented to a PSC, their guidelines also required rapid neuroimaging to confirm LVO status.

Currently, there are two methods of prehospital destination decision-making for suspected AIS patients. The first involves transporting the patient to the closest stroke center to receive IV thrombolysis regardless of stroke center status (drip and ship model). Once at the hospital, the patient is screened for an LVO and if necessary, transported to the nearest endovascular center for EVT. Yet, this method is questionable for several reasons that were discussed earlier. The second model involves transferring the patient directly to the nearest CSC to receive IV TPA and EVT if necessary. Again, the 2018 American Heart Association/American Stroke Association Guidelines for acute ischemic stroke management recommend, "When several IV alteplase-capable hospital options exist within a defined geographic region, the benefit of bypassing the closest to bring the patient to one that offers a higher level of stroke care, including mechanical thrombectomy, is uncertain. Further research is needed." However, as discussed earlier and based on probability alone, a strong argument can be made to transport all AIS patients to CSCs if this can be done in a timely manner (≤30 minutes). This argument is only strengthened by a reliable prehospital LVO AIS screening tool which can be recalled by the MANGO™ mnemonic.

However, critics of LVO AIS prehospital screening tools will continue to emphasize potentially slower IV thrombolysis times but **recall that IV TPA is limited both by an LVO and clot length**. Furthermore, 30 to 40 percent of LVO AIS patients initially taken to PSCs and then transported to a CSC for EVT are no longer EVT candidates (due to the progression of ischemic penumbra into a core infarct). Currently, EVT reperfusion is typically not achieved until a median of 4 hours and 45 minutes from stroke onset.[28] Every minute during a typical LVO ischemic stroke results in the death of nearly two million neurons.[29] Improvements in systems of care that can appropriately deliver suspected LVO AIS patients directly to endovascular-capable hospitals (CSCs) are desperately needed.

27.4 Future Considerations

Earlier, this chapter discussed the analogy between LVO AIS and myocardial infarction (MI). One tremendous advantage in the evaluation of acute MI is the EKG. By obtaining an EKG with a portable device, cardiac patients can be triaged with great accuracy in the prehospital setting. Currently, there is no stroke "EKG" that can appropriately identify and field triage a LVO AIS to a CSC. Again, the prehospital identification of LVO AIS by EMS is a prerequisite for effective triage to a CSC. Kellner et al. have described a portable device that can potentially field triage suspected LVO AIS patients.[30] The Volumetric Impedance Phase Shift Spectroscopy (VIPS) device (Cerebrotech Visor™, Cerebrotech Medical Systems) can be worn like a visor and uses low-energy radio waves to assess brain tissue infarct (Figure 12). Brain tissue abnormalities secondary to stroke alter these radio waves which are detected by the device. During this study, three separate readings taken by the device per patient required only **30 seconds!**

FIGURE 12. The Volumetric Impedance Phase Shift Spectroscopy (VIPS) Device

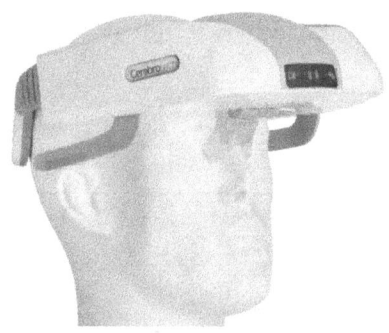

This study demonstrated the VIPS device could distinguish severe stroke (defined in the study as LVO, severe intra or extracranial stenosis with a concomitant NIHSS ≥6, ICH ≥60 cc, and a large arterial distribution infarct) from mild stroke with a sensitivity of 93% and a specificity of 92%. It further demonstrated low false negative and false positive rates of only 7% and 8% respectively, indicating this device can quickly provide a high sensitivity and specificity for the detection of severe stroke. The ability to accurately determine the presence of an LVO AIS in the prehospital setting is intriguing but the practicality of this device's widespread use by EMS, economics and devices using similar technology must be considered. In addition, another company (Neural Analytics, Los Angeles, CA) is developing a similar device using transcranial Doppler-based technology. However, these types of devices require further evaluation with prospective, randomized control trials prior to their implementation.

27.5 Conclusion

The importance of rapidly and accurately screening for LVO AIS cannot be overstated. To appropriately screen LVO AIS patients, paramedics and emergency technicians require an effective prehospital stroke screening tool. While many prehospital screening tools exist, no single scale has emerged as a consensus leader but recently published research may soon solve this dilemma. Additionally, newer portable devices have emerged that may provide high sensitivity and specificity for severe stroke detection. The ability of a portable device to accurately detect severe stroke would be a game changer. However, these devices require further investigation prior to their implementation. Massive efforts to validate prehospital stroke screening tools and produce portable stroke detecting devices only underscore the immense importance of LVO AIS field triage.

Currently, there are multiple prehospital stroke evaluation scales yet the majority remain suboptimal because they are complex, subjective, time-consuming, and frequently require calculations. However, the VAN LVO evaluation is a simple screening protocol that has been utilized successfully in several communities. While the study of the VAN evaluation was limited in subject size, this limitation was addressed by a more recent and larger study (ACT-FAST Algorithm). As discussed earlier, in many regards these two studies appear to complement each other's limitations. Prehospital evaluation of both the anterior and posterior circulation can be remembered with the mnemonic 'MANGO™.' By performing this mnemonic, EMS personnel can effectively screen for LVO AIS patients and transport them directly to a CSC. Here, they can receive appropriate neuroimaging to verify LVO, collateral circulation, and/or salvageable ischemic penumbra status. The prehospital identification of LVO AIS can greatly improve stroke care by the direct transport of a suspected LVO AIS patient to a CSC, which would reduce treatment time and improve functional outcome.

PSCs and CSCs must facilitate excellent working relationships to better serve their communities. LVO stroke accounts for only 11% of all AIS but is responsible for nearly all AIS related deaths, 90% of its societal cost, and 80% of significant functional disability. While there are multiple methods available to screen LVO AIS, most have several disadvantages related to subjectivity and scoring. The MANGO™ mnemonic can effectively perform prehospital LVO screening. All suspected LVO AIS patients should receive image confirmation at CSCs that can provide EVT. Effectively utilizing prehospital screening tools in conjunction with sophisticated neuroimaging can rapidly determine LVO status and EVT candidacy. This method allows us to **find them fast and fix them fast!**

Abbreviations list

AIS, acute ischemic stroke; CPSSS, Cincinnati Prehospital Stroke Severity Scale; CSCs, comprehensive stroke centers; CTA, computed tomography angiography; CTP, CT perfusion; EVT, endovascular treatment; LAMS, Los Angeles Motor Scale; LAPSS, Los Angeles Prehospital Stroke Screen; LEGS, Texas Stroke Intervention Pre-Hospital Stroke Severity Scale; LVO, large vessel occlusion; PSCs, primary stroke centers; RACE, Rapid Arterial Occlusion Evaluation Scale; VAN, vision, aphasia, and neglect; VIPS, Volumetric Impedance Phase Shift Spectroscopy; 3I-SS, 3-Item Stroke Scale.

References

1. Mokin M, Gupta R, Guerrero WR, et al. (2016). ASPECTS decay during inter-facility transfer in patients with large vessel occlusion strokes. *Journal of NeuroInterventional Surgery,* Pub. Online First: 22 April 2016.

2. Rinaldo L, Brinjikji W, McCutcheon BA, Bydon M, Cloft H, Kallmes DF, Rabinstein AA. (2016). Hospital transfer associated with increased mortality after endovascular revascularization for acute ischemic stroke. *J Neurointerv Surg*, 16 Dec.
3. Saver JL, Goyal M, van der Lugt A, Menon BK, Majoie CB, Dippel DW, et al. (2016). HERMES Collaborators. Time to treatment with endovascular thrombectomy and outcomes from ischemic stroke: a meta-analysis. *JAMA*, 316, 1279–1288.
4. Mohamad NF, Hastrup S, Rasmussen M, Andersen MS, Johnsen SP, Andersen G, et al. (2016). Bypassing primary stroke centre reduces delay and improves outcomes for patients with large vessel occlusion. *European Stroke Journal*, 1, 85–92.
5. Froehler MT, Saver JL, Zaidat OO, Jahan R, Aziz-Sultan MA, Klucznik RP, et al. (2017). STRATIS Investigators. Interhospital transfer before thrombectomy is associated with delayed treatment and worse outcome in the STRATIS Registry (Systematic Evaluation of Patients Treated With Neurothrombectomy Devices for Acute Ischemic Stroke). *Circulation*, 136, 2311–2321.
6. Zaidi SF, Shawver J, Espinosa Morales A, Salahuddin H, Tietjen G, Lindstrom D, Parquette B, Adams A, Korsnack A, Jumaa MA. (2016). Stroke care: initial data from a county-based bypass protocol for patients with acute stroke. *J Neurointerv Surg*, 24 Jun.
7. Sequeira D, Martin-Gill C, Guyette FX, Jadhav AP. 2015 Abstract 12493: Comparison of Prehospital Stroke Scales. *Circulation*, 132, A12493.
8. Powers WJ, Rabinstein AA, Ackerson T, Adeoye OM, Bambakidis NC, Becker K, Biller J, Brown M, Demaerschalk BM, Hoh B, et al. (2018). Guidelines for the Early Management of Patients With Acute Ischemic Stroke: A Guideline for Healthcare Professionals From the American Heart Association/American Stroke Association. *Stroke*, Epub 24 Jan.
9. Taleb MS., et al. (2016). Stroke vision, aphasia, neglect (VAN) assessment—a novel emergent large vessel occlusion screening tool: pilot study and comparison with current clinical severity indices. *NeuroInterv Surg*, 16(7), 525-33.
10. Saver JL, Fonarow GC, Smith EE, Reeves MJ, Grau-Sepulveda MV, Pan W, Olson DM, Hernandez AF, Peterson ED, Schwamm LH. (2013). Time to treatment with intravenous tissue plasminogen activator and outcome from acute ischemic stroke. *JAMA*, 309, 2480–88.
11. Katz BS, McMullan JT, Sucharew H, Adeoye O, Broderick JP. (2015). Design and validation of a prehospital scale to predict stroke severity: Cincinnati Prehospital Stroke Severity Scale. *Stroke*, 46, 1508–12.
12. Lima FO, Silva GS, Furie KL, Frankel MR, Lev MH, Camargo ÉC, Haussen DC, Singhal AB, Koroshetz WJ, Smith WS, Nogueira RG. (2016). Field assessment stroke triage for emergency destination: a simple and accurate prehospital scale to detect large vessel occlusion strokes. *Stroke*, 47, 1997–2002.
13. Perez de la Ossa N, Carrera D, Gorchs M, Querol M, Millan M, Gomis M, Dorado L, Lopez-Cancio E, Hernandez-Perez M, Chicharro V, Escalada X, Jimenez X, Davalos A. (2014). Design and validation of a prehospital stroke scale to predict large arterial occlusion: the rapid arterial occlusion evaluation scale. *Stroke*, 45, 87–91.
14. Hastrup S, Damgaard D, Johnsen SP, Andersen G. (2016). Prehospital acute stroke severity scale to predict large artery occlusion: design and comparison with other scales. *Stroke*, 47, 1772–76.
15. Singer OC, Dvorak F, du Mesnil de Rochemont R, Lanfermann H, Sitzer M, Neumann-Haefelin T. (2005). A simple 3-item stroke scale: comparison with the National Institutes of Health Stroke Scale and prediction of middle cerebral artery occlusion. *Stroke*, 36, 773–76.
16. Nazliel B, Starkman S, Liebeskind DS, Ovbiagele B, Kim D, Sanossian N, Ali L, Buck B, Villablanca P, Vinuela F, Duckwiler G, Jahan R, Saver JL. (2008). A brief prehospital stroke severity scale identifies ischemic stroke patients harboring persisting large arterial occlusions. *Stroke*, 39, 2264–67
17. Holodinsky JK, Williamson TS, Kamal N, Mayank D, Hill MD, Goyal M. (2017). Drip and Ship Versus Direct to Comprehensive Stroke Center: Conditional Probability Modeling. *Stroke*, Jan, 48(1), 233-38.
18. Zhao H, Coote S, Pesavento L, Churilov L, Dewey HM, Davis SM, et al. (2017). Large vessel occlusion scales increase delivery to endovascular centers without excessive harm from misclassifications. *Stroke*, 48, 568– 573.

19. Zhao H, Pesavento L, Coote S, Rodrigues E, Salvaris P, Smith K, Bernard S, Stephenson M, Churilov L, Yassi N, Davis SM and Campbell B. (2018). Ambulance Clinical Triage for Acute Stroke Treatment: Paramedic Triage Algorithm for Large Vessel Occlusion. *Stroke*, Apr, 49(4), 945-951.
20. Turc G, Maïer B, Naggara O, Seners P, Isabel C, Tisserand M, et al. (2016). Clinical scales do not reliably identify acute ischemic stroke patients with large-artery occlusion. *Stroke*, 47, 1466–1472.
21. Michel P. (2017). Prehospital scales for large vessel occlusion: closing in on a moving target. *Stroke*, 48, 247–249.
22. de la Ossa NP, Carrera D, Gorchs M, Querol M, Millan M, Gomis M, et al. (2014). Design and validation of a prehospital stroke scale to predict large arterial occlusion the rapid arterial occlusion evaluation scale. *Stroke*, 45, 87–91.
23. Perez de la Ossa N, Ribo M, Jimenez X, Abilleira S. (2016). Prehospital scales to identify patients with large vessel occlusion. *Stroke*, 47, 2877–2878.
24. Noorian A, Sanossian N, Liebeskind DS, Starkman S, Eckstein M, Stratton S, et al. (2016). Field validation of prehospital LAMS score to identify large vessel occlusion ischemic stroke patients for direct routing to emergency neuroendovascular centers. *Stroke*, 47, A83–A83.
25. Noorian AR, Sanossian N, Shkirkova K, Liebeskind DS, Eckstein M, Stratton S, et al. (2017). Paramedic-administered LAMS identifies ischemic stroke with large vessel occlusion and intracranial hemorrhage for routing to comprehensive stroke centers and compares favorably to other screening methods. *Stroke,* 48:A118.
26. McMullan JT, Katz B, Broderick J, Schmit P, Sucharew H, Adeoye O. (2017). Prospective prehospital evaluation of the Cincinnati stroke triage assessment tool. *Prehosp Emerg Care*, 21, 481–488.
27. Jayaraman MV, Iqbal A, Silver B, Siket MS, Amedee C, McTaggart RA, Paolucci G, Rhodes J, Potvin J, Tucker M, Alexander-Scott N. (2017). Developing a statewide protocol to ensure patients with suspected emergent large vessel occlusion are directly triaged in the field to a comprehensive stroke center: how we did it. *J Neurointerv Surg*, Mar, 9(3), 330-32.
28. Goyal M, Menon BK, Van Zwam WH, et al. (2016). Endovascular thrombectomy after large-vessel ischaemic stroke: a meta-analysis of individual patient data from five randomised trials. *Lancet,* 387, 1723-31.
29. Saver JL. (2006). Time is brain—quantified. *Stroke*, 37, 263-66.
30. Kellner, CP et al. (2018). The VITAL study and overall pooled analysis with the VIPS non-invasive stroke detection device. *J Neurointerv Surg*, Mar, 6.

Chapter 28

Hospital-Based Stroke Assessment

28.1 Introduction

While based on a relatively straightforward premise, the treatment of acute ischemic stroke (AIS) can be difficult. **The paramount goal of AIS treatment is to restore perfusion to the ischemic penumbra.** Initially, an AIS patient has a central core of irreparably damaged brain tissue (core infarct) surrounded by a zone of an ischemic penumbra (Figure 1). Every patient has a distinct, individual timeframe during which threatened brain tissue (ischemic penumbra) may be salvaged to restrict core infarct size (Figure 2).[1] However, the presence of core infarct and ischemic penumbra can only be determined with neuroimaging.

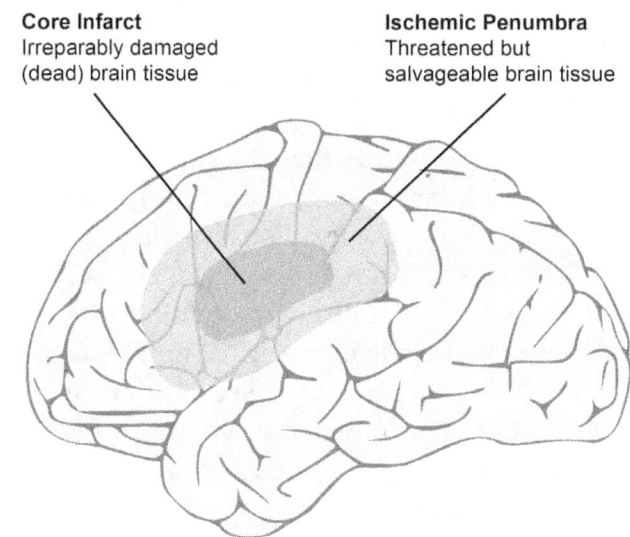

FIGURE 1. Core Infarct Versus Ischemic Penumbra

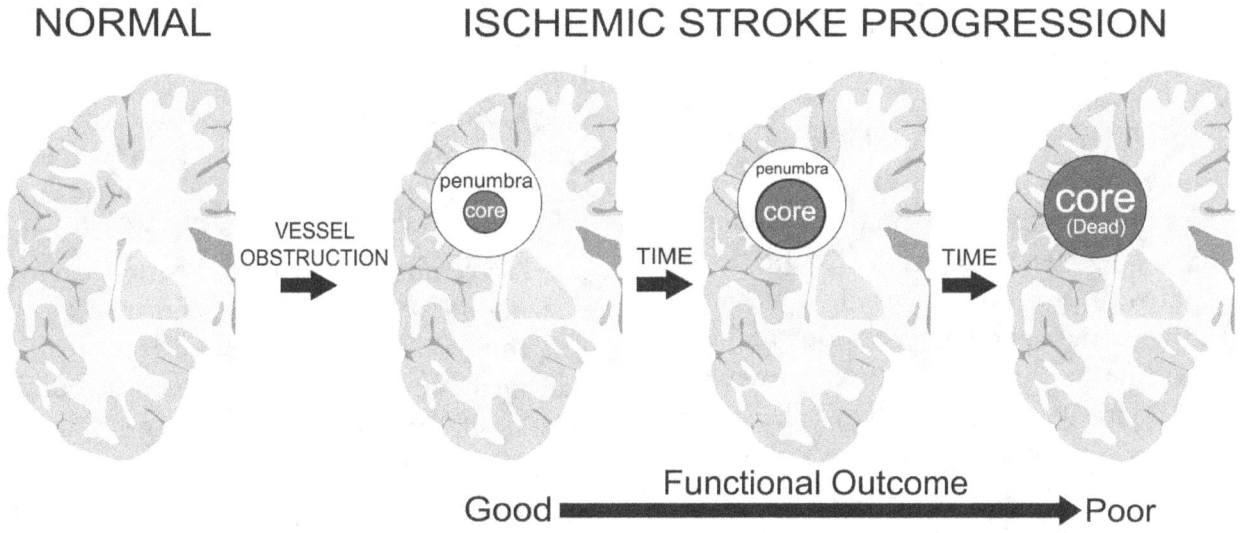

FIGURE 2. Progression of Ischemic Penumbra into Core Infarct

28.2 Acute Ischemic Stroke (AIS) Assessment

Since AIS patients have distinct individual physiology, arbitrary time points should not determine treatment decisions.[2] Instead, the rapid and reliable identification of AIS patients who possess salvageable brain tissue (ischemic penumbra) should be emphasized. Practical, reliable, and fast protocols must be utilized to identify potential AIS treatment candidates. These protocols must focus on the immediate cause of an AIS, namely **arterial occlusion**. Once an arterial occlusion has been verified, core infarct and ischemic penumbra must also be assessed. The previous chapter (Chapter 27, Prehospital Stroke Assessment) discussed multiple points of confusion regarding different AIS prehospital screening tools. Complicated and subjective AIS assessment systems continue to exacerbate both prehospital and hospital stroke assessment. A simple prehospital and hospital-based AIS assessment protocol is desperately needed.

The diagnosis and management of stroke can be an immensely complex problem. Most complex problems require immense resources and capital to solve. Stroke is no exception. For example, instead of ordering just a noncontrast brain CT, what if a CTA and CTP were necessary to manage every suspected AIS patient? This can be done (and some centers do engage in this practice) but isn't it more practical to perform additional neuroimaging only on those AIS patients suspected of having a large vessel occlusion (LVO)? By following practical protocols, AIS can be efficiently managed without expending enormous resources or capital. Another limited resource (particularly in rural hospitals) is that of subspecialist physicians (neurosurgeons, neurointerventionalists, and neurologists). Many hospitals do not have subspecialist coverage. However, every hospital has an Emergency Department, a Radiology Department, and nurses. This infrastructure is all that is necessary to allow any hospital to independently diagnose and treat most AIS patients.

Emergency department physicians can manage thousands of different disease processes. What makes the management of AIS any different? My emergency department physician colleagues consistently give the same response: **AIS is too complex.** They consider the diagnosis and treatment of AIS to be a dynamic and constantly evolving process. They also require a consistent yet concise algorithm to manage AIS just like any other disease process. Emergency department physicians are an incredible resource because they are always in the hospital and they evaluate every AIS patient. Incidentally, many emergency department physicians currently diagnose and treat AIS (including IV TPA administration) independently. The protocols that follow not only aid in the diagnosis and treatment of AIS but also enhance its understanding.

AIS is an immensely complex subject matter. However, as the title of this text states, it can be simplified. When an AIS stroke patient presents with symptoms, this information must be processed to yield a diagnosis to determine if the patient is having a stroke and if so, what region of the brain and vascular territories have been affected? When an AIS patient presents to the Emergency Department, a history is obtained, a physical exam is performed, and labs are drawn. Essentially, there are five general diagnostic categories to consider when examining a potential AIS patient. These include: (1) LVO AIS < 6 hours of symptom onset, (2) LVO AIS 6 - 24 hours of symptom onset, (3) non-LVO mild AIS, (4) transient ischemic attack (TIA), and (5) stroke mimic or no stroke. Understanding these five categories, rapid screening protocols, and neuroimaging permit any hospital to diagnose and treat most AIS. The emphasis of time cannot be overstated in AIS management. Each one of these categories and their respective protocols will now be reviewed. Before proceeding, realize that no optimal clinical or imaging protocol for the diagnosis and treatment of AIS currently exists.

28.3 Large Vessel Occlusion Acute Ischemic Stroke (LVO AIS) Must Be Prioritized

This text extensively reviewed the pathophysiology of the different subtypes of AIS. However, from a more practical and efficient context, the treatment of AIS must be divided into LVO and non-LVO AIS. This is because LVOs are by far the most devastating form of AIS and require our utmost attention. LVO AIS represents only 11% of all AIS but this small fraction is responsible for all AIS related deaths, 90% of AIS costs, and 80% of functional disability. This minority of AIS patients account for the overwhelming majority of AIS death, cost, and functional dependency. LVO AIS patients must be identified and treated quickly. **Thus, stroke protocols must prioritize LVO status.** By using efficient and practical protocols, LVO AIS can be effectively diagnosed and treated with very little resources or subspecialty physician requirements. However, Neurology (if available) should be consulted for the evaluation of every potential AIS patient.

Diagnostic and treatment protocols for AIS must prioritize LVO status. In the cardiac world, ST–segment–elevation myocardial infarction (STEMI) and non-STEMI patients are treated differently. In a similar fashion, LVO and non-LVO stroke must be treated differently (Figure 3). In the cardiac realm, non-STEMI heart disease receives medical treatment whereas a STEMI patient requires cardiac intervention (without IV thrombolytic). Similarly, LVO AIS patients must be identified quickly, receive IV TPA, mobilized to the neurointerventional suite, and treated promptly (Figure 3). In the cardiac domain, STEMI status is determined by an EKG. In the stroke arena, LVO status is confirmed by neuroimaging. However, to suggest that every suspected stroke patient should receive additional neuroimaging in a similar manner that every suspected MI receives an EKG would be problematic. In the stroke arena, a rapid protocol is required to confirm LVO, a small core infarct, and salvageable brain tissue (ischemic penumbra). Thus, a successful protocol requires two components. The first component **clinically** screens for suspected LVO AIS and the second component confirms the presence of an LVO, a small core infarct, and significant ischemic penumbra with **neuroimaging**.

FIGURE 3. LVO and Non-LVO Require Different Treatment Modalities

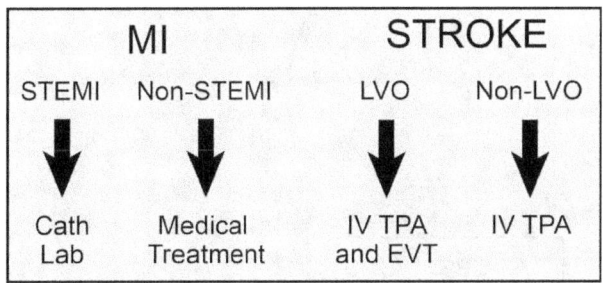

LVO - Large Vessel Occlusion; MI - Myocardial Infarction; STEMI - ST Elevation Myocardial Infarction

Neurology (if available) should be consulted and a noncontrast brain CT should be obtained for the evaluation of every potential AIS patient. The initial evaluation of all AIS patients should include the 'MANGO™' mnemonic to screen for LVO AIS (Table 1). All cases of stroke are important, but the most devastating form of AIS by far is LVO and thus requires our greatest attention. For this reason, LVOs must be diagnosed and treated quickly. The MANGO™ mnemonic stresses motor weakness as its key assessment for LVO screening (Table 1). This acts as a binary assessment for LVO AIS (Figure 4). Any AIS patient who is MANGO™-positive (motor weakness plus any other A-N-G-O component) is suspected of having an LVO which must be confirmed by advanced neuroimaging. An LVO is not suspected if the 'M' or "motor weakness" portion of the MANGO™ mnemonic is negative (no motor weakness), or the 'M' or "motor weakness" portion of the MANGO™ mnemonic is positive but each of the remaining components of the MANGO™ mnemonic are negative (Figure 4).

TABLE 1. LVO Screening Mnemonic: **MANGO**™

M	Motor Weakness
A	Aphasia Expressive (name 2 objects) Receptive (follow 2 commands)
N	Neglect Unable to feel both sides at the same time, or Unable to identify own arm, or Ignoring one side
G	Gaze Preference, Inability to Track or Double Vision
O	Optic Field Cut or New Blindness

FIGURE 4. MANGO™ Algorithm

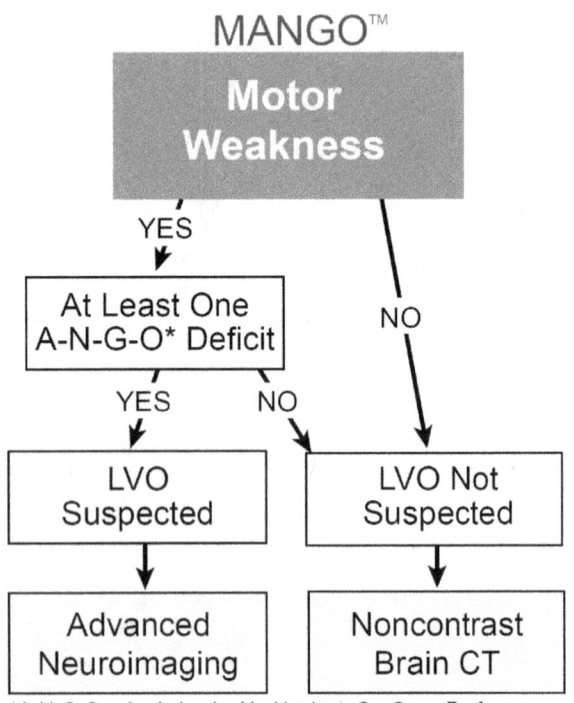

*A-N-G-O = A - Aphasia; N - Neglect; G - Gaze Preference, Inability to Track or Double Vision; O - Optic Field Cut or New Blindness

Any AIS patient who is MANGO™-positive (motor weakness plus any other A-N-G-O component) is suspected of having an LVO which must be confirmed by neuroimaging. False positives can be caused by any process that involves at least two cortical regions (neoplasm, hemorrhage) and can be excluded by neuroimaging. Neurointerventional consultation (if available) and neuroimaging must be initiated simultaneously for all MANGO™-positive suspected LVO AIS patients. The neuroimaging protocol consists of noncontrast brain CT and dual-phase CTA (< 6 hours from symptom onset) or a noncontrast brain CT and CTP/CTA (6-24 hours from symptom onset). Waiting for creatinine values before performing contrast CT studies is unnecessary.[3] Again, no optimal imaging protocol exists for the diagnosis and treatment of AIS but the recent 2018 American Heart Association/American Stroke Association Guidelines state, "An organized protocol for the emergency evaluation of patients with suspected stroke is recommended."[4]

28.4 Large Vessel Occlusion Acute Ischemic Stroke (LVO AIS) < 6 Hours From Symptom Onset

The 2018 AHA/ASA guidelines have different LVO AIS imaging and EVT recommendations based on time from symptom onset. From an EVT perspective, the AHA/ASA has retained older and developed new guidelines based on time from symptom onset. For LVO AIS patients presenting within six hours, these recommendations include treating patients ≥18 years having a prestroke mRS score of 0-1, an LVO (ICA or MCA), an ASPECTS ≥ 6, and an NIHSS score ≥ 6, with treatment to be initiated (groin puncture) within six hours. An easy way to remember these recommendations is with the mnemonic 'ATLAS' (Table 2).

In addition to understanding these EVT eligibility criteria, it is essential that one understands the role of neuroimaging in the determination of EVT candidacy. Combining both the imaging and EVT recommendations by the 2018 AHA/ASA guidelines directs the evaluation of LVO AIS patients.

TABLE 2. AHA/ASA Recommendations for EVT < 6 Hours From Symptom Onset: **ATLAS**

A	Age ≥18 Years
T	Treatment Initiated (Groin Puncture) Within 6 Hours
L	LVO (ICA or MCA M1 Segment)
A	ASPECTS ≥6
S	Score: NIHSS ≥6, Prestroke mRS 0-1

ASPECTS - Alberta Stroke Program Early CT Score, EVT - Endovascular Treatment, LVO - Large Vessel Occlusion, NIHSS - National Institutes of Health Stroke Scale, mRS - Modified Rankin Scale

Again, the 2018 AHA/ASA guidelines recognize three EVT time points: (1) < 6 hours, (2) 6-16 hours, and (3) 6-24 hours. Additionally, these guidelines make individual recommendations for each category. Thus, our imaging protocols must reflect these guidelines. From an imaging perspective, these guidelines can be broken down into LVO AIS patients that present (1) < 6 hours and (2) 6-24 hours (this second category also includes the 6-16-hour EVT timeframe).

Neuroimaging is necessary to determine LVO, core infarct, and ischemic penumbra status. This is precisely why neuroimaging is required in addition to performing the NIHSS. The literature shows performing neuroimaging improves AIS patient outcome regardless of IV TPA, EVT, or both IV TPA and EVT treatment. This is because neuroimaging answers questions the NIHSS cannot in terms of LVO, core infarct, and ischemic penumbra status. The sooner LVO, core infarct, and ischemic penumbra status are determined, the quicker LVO AIS patients are treated and the better their functional outcome.

The neuroimaging protocol for suspected LVO AIS patients with stroke symptoms < 6 hours from last known normal consists of a noncontrast brain CT and dual-phase CTA (Figure 5). This same imaging protocol can also be applied to those AIS patients with an NIHSS score ≥ 6 (the current AHA/ASA guideline NIHSS score recommendation for EVT candidacy). The first step of this protocol and the first imaging step in all suspected AIS patients is obtaining a noncontrast brain CT. The new 2018 American Heart Association/American Stroke Association Guidelines state, "All patients admitted to the hospital with suspected acute stroke should receive brain imaging evaluation on arrival at the hospital. In most cases, noncontrast CT (NCCT) will provide the necessary information to make decisions about acute management."[4] A brain CT is the workhorse of stroke imaging and is ordered on every AIS patient to exclude hemorrhage, greater than one-third middle cerebral artery territory infarct (hypodense brain tissue), or a stroke mimic. But can a noncontrast brain CT determine the presence of a large vessel occlusion, a small core infarct, and a significant ischemic penumbra?

In fact, a noncontrast brain CT can assess core infarct and ischemic penumbra. Hypodense brain tissue is indicative of irreversible, core infarct whereas isodense, swollen brain tissue is indicative of a salvageable, ischemic penumbra (Box 1). The ability to assess the CT imaging findings of AIS can also be difficult. For this reason, ASPECTS should be utilized to assess hypodense brain tissue on a brain CT scan. The mnemonic CHILI-6™ can aid in remembering the different structures that comprise ASPECTS (Table 3). Every noncontrast brain CT should receive an ASPECT score between 1 and 10. When calculating an ASPECT score, only hypodense brain tissue should be scored because it represents irreversible, core infarct. ASPECTS can also predict the risk of intracranial hemorrhage and functional outcome. ASPECTS is the imaging equivalent of the NIHSS score. An ASPECT score ≤ 7 has a 14-fold increased risk of symptomatic intracranial hemorrhage when compared to an ASPECT score > 7.[5] ASPECTS has greater sensitivity than the NIHSS in determining both functional outcome and the rate of symptomatic intracranial hemorrhage.[5] The 2018 AHA/ASA guidelines also incorporate ASPECTS into their recommendations (Table 2). For these reasons, employing ASPECTS in addition to performing the NIHSS is strongly encouraged.

BOX 1. Imaging Characteristic of Penumbra Versus Core

| Puffy = Penumbra |
| HypoDense Brain = Dead Core |

TABLE 3. ASPECTS Mnemonic: **CHILI-6**™

CH	Caudate Head
I	Internal Capsule
L	Lentiform Nucleus
I	Insular Cortex
6	M1 - M6 (GL and SGL)

GL - Ganglionic Level; SGL - Supraganglionic Level

FIGURE 5. Large Vessel Occlusion Acute Ischemic Stroke (LVO AIS) Management, <6 Hours

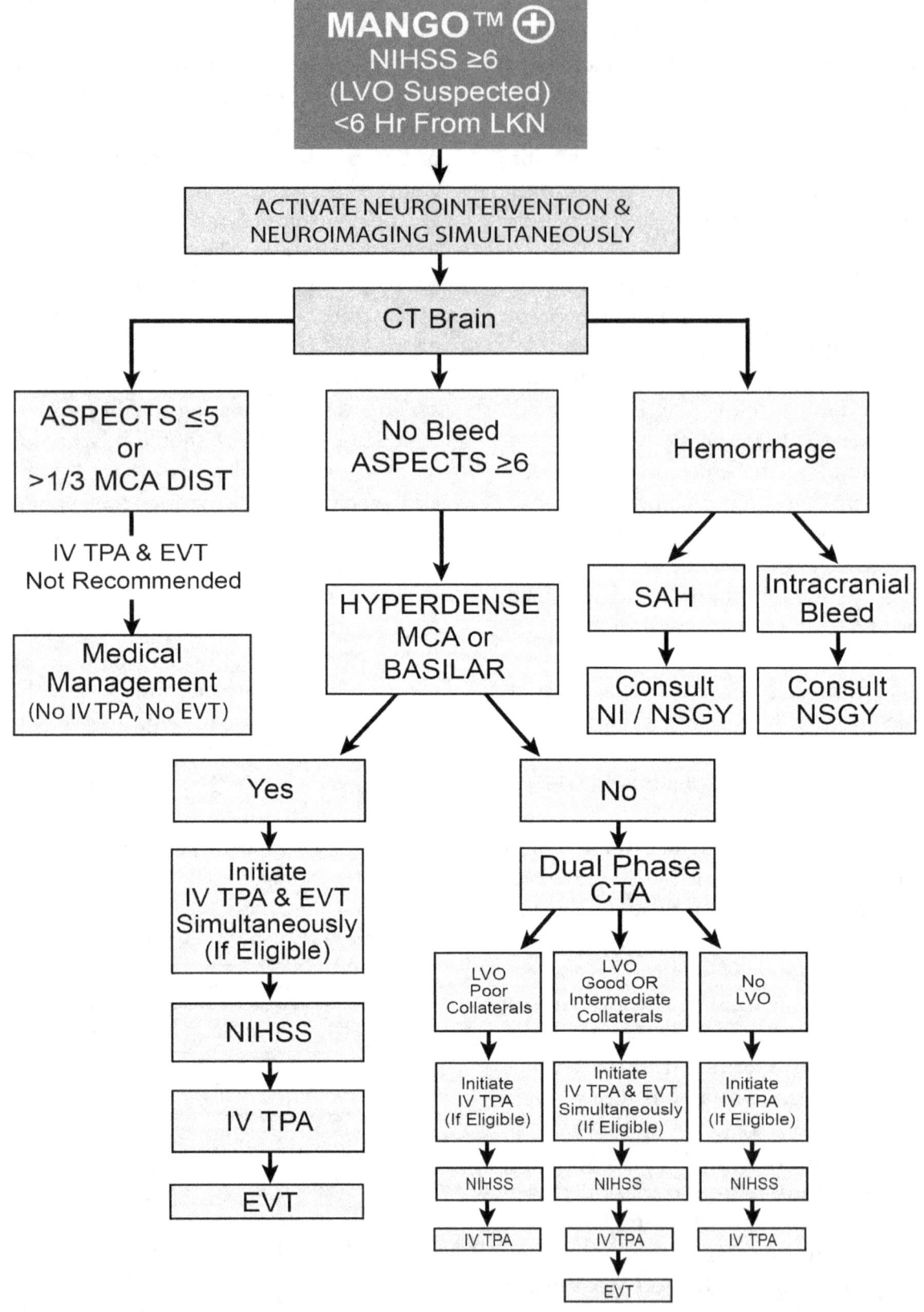

ASPECTS - Alberta Stroke Program Early CT Score, CTA - Computed Tomography Angiogram, CTP - Computed Tomography Perfusion, Dist - Distribution, EVT - Endovascular Treatment, LKN - Last Known Normal, LVO - Large Vessel Occlusion, MCA - Middle Cerebral Artery, NI - Neurointervention, NIHSS - National Institutes of Health Stroke Scale, NSGY - Neurosurgery, SAH - Subarachnoid Hemorrhage, TPA - Tissue Plasminogen Activator

What about a noncontrast brain CT's ability to determine the presence of an LVO? Actually, as discussed in Chapter 21, a hyperdense middle cerebral artery (MCA) sign or basilar artery sign should be considered in LVO unless proven otherwise. If either a hyperdense MCA or basilar artery sign is present, the suspected LVO AIS patient is MANGO™-positive and if ASPECTS ≥ 6, IV TPA administration and neurointervention should be initiated simultaneously, provided there are no IV TPA restrictions (Figure 5, Box 2 and Table 4). Thus, every noncontrast brain CT should be scrutinized for at least four important findings: (1) hemorrhage, (2) ASPECTS ≤ 5, (3) ASPECTS ≥ 6, and (4) hyperdense arteries (Box 2).

TABLE 4. IV TPA Restrictions: **NOT TPA CLIENTS**™

N	Non-Enhanced Contrast CT >1/3 MCA
O	Onset of Symptoms >4.5 Hrs or UNKNOWN
T	Ten, Intracranial Aneurysm ≥10mm
T	Tumor, Intra-Axial or GI (or GI Bleed <21d)
P	Prior Ischemic Stroke Within 3 Months
A	Aortic Dissection (Suspected)
C	Coagulopathy: Coumadin (if INR >1.7) and Coumadin Analogs (Direct Thrombin Inhibitors or Direct Factor Xa Inhibitors) PT >15, aPTT >40, PLTS <100,000 & INR >1.7
L	Low Molecular Weight Heparin <24 Hours (Full Treatment Dose, Not Prophylactic Dose)
I	Intracranial Hemorrhage - Acute or 3 Month History
E	Endocarditis, Infectious (Suspected)
N	Noncompressible Vessel Puncture Within 7 Days (Safety and Efficacy of IV TPA Uncertain)
T	Trauma, Severe Head Within 3 Months
S	Surgery, CNS (Intracranial or Spine) Within 3 Months

If no hyperdense MCA or basilar artery sign is present and ASPECTS ≥ 6, proceed with dual-phase CTA of the intracranial circulation and single-phase CTA of the extracranial arteries (Figure 5). Dual-phase CTA can confirm LVO status and location and much more. Once the presence of an LVO has been confirmed by dual phase CTA, the next step is to determine if the LVO AIS patient has a small core infarct and a significant ischemic penumbra. As discussed in Chapter 21, this can be accomplished with either functional or physiologic imaging (Figure 6). Physiologic imaging is a two-step process consisting of a CTP (confirms small core infarct and significant ischemic penumbra) and CTA (confirms LVO status). Functional imaging (dual-phase CTA), on the other hand, is a single-step process wherein multiphase or dual-phase CTA can confirm LVO and collateral status simultaneously (Figure 7).

FIGURE 6. Functional and Physiologic Neuroimaging to Assess Viable Brain Tissue

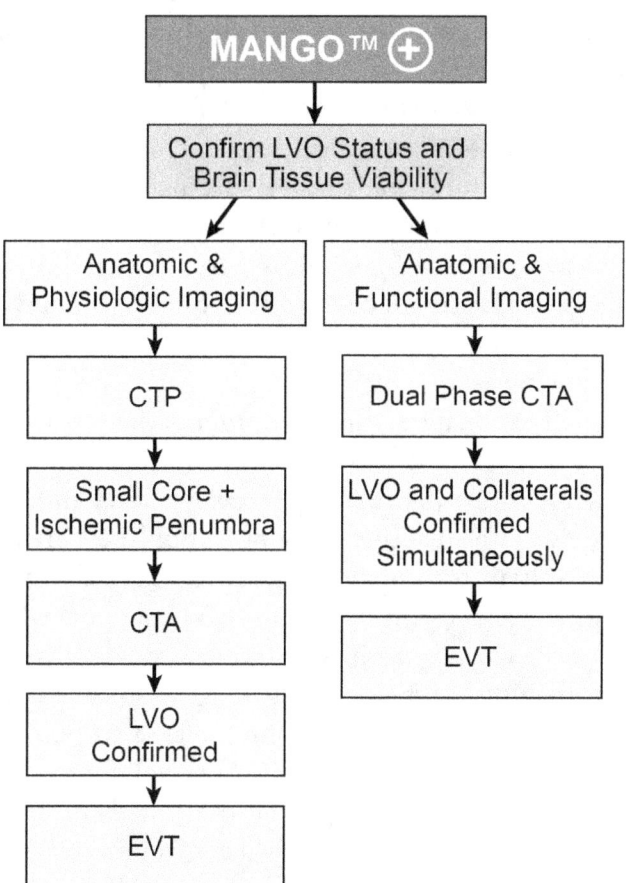

BOX 2. AIS Brain CT Surveillance

Intracerebral Hemorrhage	Intracerebral hemorrhage is a contraindication for both IV TPA and EVT. Medical therapy (unless neurosurgical intervention is required) is recommended.
ASPECTS* ≤5	This is indicative of significant core infarct. IV TPA and EVT is "not recommended" in these AIS patients or those with >1/3 MCA distribution infarct.
ASPECTS* ≥6	Potential candidate for both IV TPA or EVT depending upon screening protocols and further imaging (CTA/CTP or dual phase CTA). Both IV TPA and EVT should be considered if there is a LVO, a small core infarct and salvageable brain tissue (ischemic penumbra) or significant collaterals.
Hyperdense Arteries	A hyperdense MCA or basilar artery sign = LVO until proven otherwise. If ASPECTS ≥6, initiate IV TPA and neurointervention (if eligible).

* ASPECTS scored with hypodense (and not isodense) tissue only

Concerning LVO AIS patients that are otherwise eligible for EVT, the 2018 AHA/ASA guidelines state: "For patients who otherwise meet criteria for EVT, a noninvasive intracranial vascular study is recommended during the initial imaging evaluation of the acute stroke patient, but should not delay IV alteplase if indicated. For patients who qualify for IV alteplase according to the guidelines from professional medical societies, initiating IV alteplase before noninvasive vascular imaging is recommended for patients who have not had noninvasive vascular imaging as part of their initial imaging assessment for stroke. Noninvasive intracranial vascular imaging should then be obtained as quickly as possible."[4]

Let us analyze this recommendation further. First, the AHA/ASA recommend noninvasive intracranial vascular imaging. However, they immediately state that this imaging should be part of the "initial imaging assessment for stroke." They discourage delaying IV TPA for AIS patients who do not receive noninvasive intracranial vascular imaging as their initial imaging assessment. This recommendation has three very clear points. First, performing noninvasive intracranial vascular imaging should be part of the initial imaging assessment of AIS patients when appropriate. Appropriateness is determined by any AIS patient who is suspected of having an LVO. Again, any AIS patient who is MANGO™-positive (motor weakness plus any other A-N-G-O component) is suspected of having an LVO which must be confirmed by noninvasive intracranial vascular imaging (Figure 5).

Second, this recommendation also states that noninvasive intracranial vascular imaging should not delay initiating IV TPA. Moreover, noninvasive intracranial vascular imaging should not delay initiating EVT as well. In fact, nothing should delay any form of AIS treatment. Finally, the guidelines state that this imaging "be obtained as quickly as possible." Once an LVO, small core infarct, and significant ischemic penumbra have been confirmed, IV TPA administration and EVT should be initiated simultaneously, provided there are no IV TPA restrictions (Figure 5 and Table 4). IV TPA should be initiated on all eligible LVO AIS patients regardless of their NIHSS score because an LVO has just been confirmed by imaging. That is, every eligible LVO AIS stroke patient, despite their apparent stroke severity, should receive IV TPA.

FIGURE 7. Dual Phase CTA Efficiency

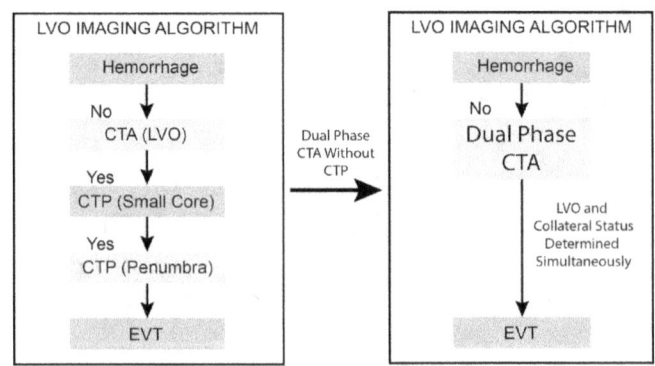

An NIHSS score can be calculated while IV TPA is being prepared and the patient is awaiting EVT. EVT should never be delayed to administer IV TPA. Instead, IV TPA should be administered as EVT is being initiated. Every stroke center should use the administration time of IV TPA (1 hour) as a metric to determine how quickly EVT candidates are transported to the neurointerventional (NI) suite for EVT. If IV TPA is completely administered before EVT is initiated (groin puncture), there is room for improvement. After imaging and IV TPA initiation, an NIHSS should be performed. The MANGO™ mnemonic in conjunction with neuroimaging protocols can aid in the effective diagnosis and treatment of LVO AIS (Figure 5). Again, **minutes matter in the diagnosis and treatment of stroke**. Based on the recommended critical time points for EVT discussed in Chapter 25, there are **25 minutes** available to complete neuroimaging (Figure 8). Make sure to get it right the first time! Don't perform a noncontrast brain CT only and then send an AIS patient (whose functional outcome is time-dependent) back for additional imaging (Figure 9). Again, treatment efficiency is precisely what the AHA/ASA guidelines recommend.

FIGURE 8. Recommended EVT Critical Time Points

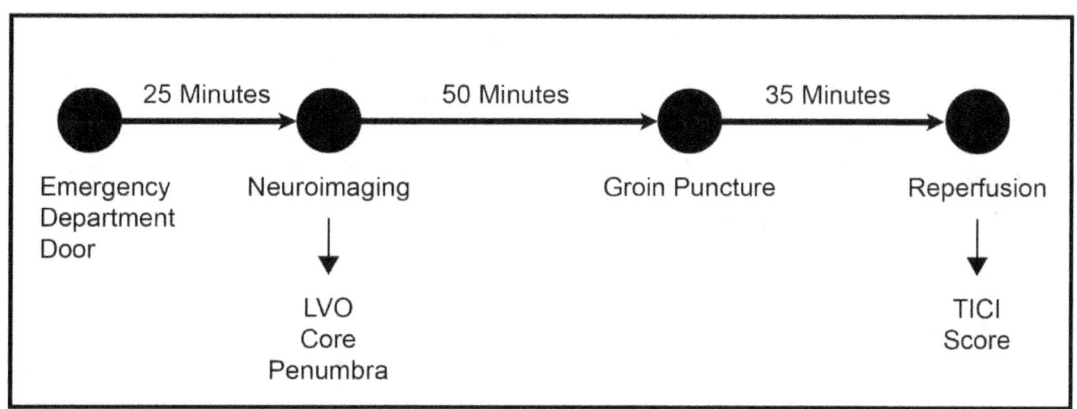

Adapted from: Saver, Jeffrey L., et al. "Time to Treatment With Endovascular Thrombectomy and Outcomes From Ischemic Stroke: A Meta-analysis." *JAMA* 316.12 (2016): 1279-1289

FIGURE 9. Inefficient and Efficient Neuroimaging

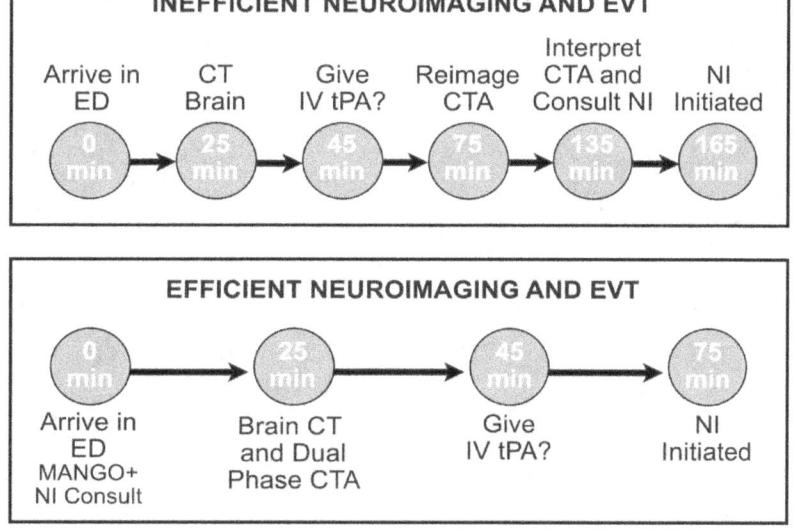

The next relevant 2018 AHA/ASA guideline recommendation for this category (LVO AIS patients that present < 6 hours) states, "Additional imaging beyond CT and CTA or MRI and magnetic resonance angiography (MRA) such as perfusion studies for selecting patients for mechanical thrombectomy in < 6 hours is not recommended."[4] Six randomized controlled trials (RCTs) demonstrated the clinical benefit of EVT when performed within six hours of stroke onset. The *majority* of these trials (four) used advanced neuroimaging to determine EVT eligibility while the *minority* of these trials (two) did not. In addition, the recently published DAWN and DEFUSE 3 Trials also employed advanced neuroimaging. The AHA/ASA conclude that because the minority of earlier RCTs did not use advanced neuroimaging, the use of these techniques "could lead to the exclusion of patients who would benefit from the treatment and are therefore not indicated at this time."[4] This really does not make any sense because the purpose of advanced neuroimaging (as exemplified by the DAWN and DEFUSE 3 Trials) is to determine individual collateral circulation and salvageable brain tissue (ischemic penumbra), which in turn determine EVT candidacy.

The strongest predictor of functional outcome in LVO AIS patients is the neuroimaging-based assessment of core infarct. For example, trials that used less selective neuroimaging (as the current AHA/ASA guidelines recommend) such as the THRACE, MR CLEAN and REVASCAT Trials had a worse treatment effect (worse functional outcome) than trials that used more selective imaging such as SWIFT PRIME, ESCAPE and EXTEND-IA. These last three trials that utilized more selective neuroimaging to determine a small core infarct size demonstrated a higher treatment effect than less selective neuroimaging-based trials (THRACE, MR CLEAN and REVASCAT). If the AHA/ASA endorse better treatment outcome, they should endorse advanced neuroimaging to determine the presence of a small core infarct and significant penumbra in addition to LVO to determine EVT candidacy. Again, the strongest predictor of functional outcome after EVT is the neuroimaging-based assessment of pre-procedure core infarct. In addition, trials that actively identified ischemic penumbra prior to treatment consistently demonstrated the highest rates of functional independence ever reported with mechanical thrombectomy (60% and 71%).[6]

One cannot assume that all LVO AIS patients presenting within six hours have salvageable brain tissue (ischemic penumbra). However, one can both adhere to these guidelines and determine the presence of adequate collaterals simply by obtaining a dual-phase CTA and not performing CT perfusion (Figure 5). In fact, the new AHA/ASA guidelines also state, "It may be reasonable to incorporate collateral flow status into clinical decision-making in some candidates to determine eligibility for mechanical thrombectomy."[4] In this protocol, we are imaging AIS patients suspected of having LVO. Thus, we are checking the "collateral flow status" in "some candidates" who are suspected of having LVO by dual-phase CTA "to determine eligibility for mechanical thrombectomy."[4]

I endorse dual-phase CTA because it requires no special software, no post-processing, is easy to interpret, and determines LVO and collateral status simultaneously (Figures 7 and 10). Simply put, dual-phase CTA is the **simplest and fastest imaging method to determine EVT candidacy**. Since it is easy to interpret, **non-specialist physicians and even non-physicians** can participate in LVO AIS management. If an LVO AIS patient is suspected (MANGO™ positive) and presents < 6 hours from symptom onset, perform dual-phase CTA to confirm LVO and collateral flow status simultaneously (Figures 5, 6, 7 and 10). Intermediate to good collaterals suggest a small core infarct and significant ischemic penumbra.

Thus, for suspected LVO AIS patients (MANGO™ positive) that present < 6 hours of last known normal, our imaging protocol (excluding MRI) is represented by Figure 5. Note that this conforms to the 2018 AHA/ASA guidelines as it (1) represents a noninvasive intravascular study that does not delay IV TPA administration, (2) does not involve CT or MR perfusion studies, and (3) reasonably incorporates collateral flow status into determining EVT eligibility.

FIGURE 10. Dual Phase CTA

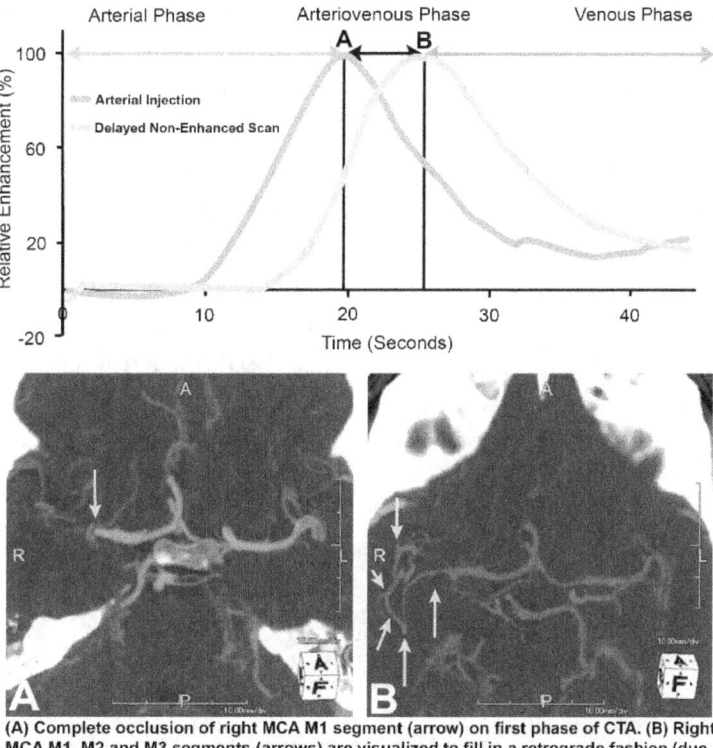

(A) Complete occlusion of right MCA M1 segment (arrow) on first phase of CTA. (B) Right MCA M1, M2 and M3 segments (arrows) are visualized to fill in a retrograde fashion (due to collateral supply from ACA leptomeningeal collaterals) in the second CTA phase.

28.5 Large Vessel Occlusion Acute Ischemic Stroke (LVO AIS) 6 – 24 Hours from Symptom Onset

The analysis of LVO AIS covered most of this protocol discussion. However, certain points should be refreshed and critical distinctions require further discussion. First, neurology (if available) should be consulted and a noncontrast brain CT should be obtained for the evaluation of every potential AIS patient. Additional imaging should also be obtained based on the 2018 AHA/ASA guidelines which recommend: "For patients who otherwise meet criteria for EVT, a noninvasive intracranial vascular study is recommended during the initial imaging evaluation of the acute stroke patient, but should not delay IV alteplase if indicated. For patients who qualify for IV alteplase according to the guidelines from professional medical societies, initiating IV alteplase before noninvasive vascular imaging is recommended for patients who have not had noninvasive vascular imaging as part of their initial imaging assessment for stroke. Noninvasive intracranial vascular imaging should then be obtained as quickly as possible."[4] That is, this same recommendation applies to all LVO AIS patients who meet EVT criteria within 24 hours of symptom onset.

Except for one, the same points regarding imaging and efficiency are just as relevant for LVO AIS patients who present 6-24 hours from symptom onset. That is, because this protocol involves LVO AIS patients who present 6-24 hours from symptom onset, **these patients are no longer eligible for IV TPA**. Since these patients cannot receive IV TPA, this entire imaging protocol needs to be performed at the onset because it cannot possibly delay IV TPA administration. This imaging protocol can also be applied to those AIS patients with an NIHSS score ≥ 6 (the current AHA/ASA guideline NIHSS score recommendation for EVT candidacy). However, in distinction to LVO AIS patients who present < 6 hours from symptom onset, the AHA/ASA guidelines state: "In selected patients with AIS within 6 to 24 hours of last known normal who have an LVO in the anterior circulation, **obtaining CTP, DWI/MRI, or MRI perfusion is recommended** to aid in patient selection for mechanical thrombectomy, but only when imaging and other eligibility criteria from RCTs showing benefit are being strictly applied in selecting patients for mechanical thrombectomy."[4] As described above, the 2018 new AHA/ASA guidelines also state, "It may be reasonable to incorporate collateral flow status into clinical decision-making in some candidates to determine eligibility for mechanical thrombectomy."[4]

To adhere to the recommendations above, this protocol (LVO AIS patients who present 6-24 hours from symptom onset) utilizes CTP to perform "perfusion" and determine "collateral flow status." Thus, this imaging protocol for LVO AIS patients that present 6-24 hours from symptom onset consists of a noncontrast brain CT, CTA, and CTP (Figure 11). Note that this conforms to the 2018 AHA/ASA guidelines as it (1) represents a noninvasive intravascular study, (2) does involve CTP, and (3) reasonably incorporates collateral flow status into determining EVT eligibility. Again, these patients are not eligible for IV TPA so this is not a consideration in this protocol.

FIGURE 11. Large Vessel Occlusion Acute Ischemic Stroke (LVO AIS) Management, 6-24 Hours

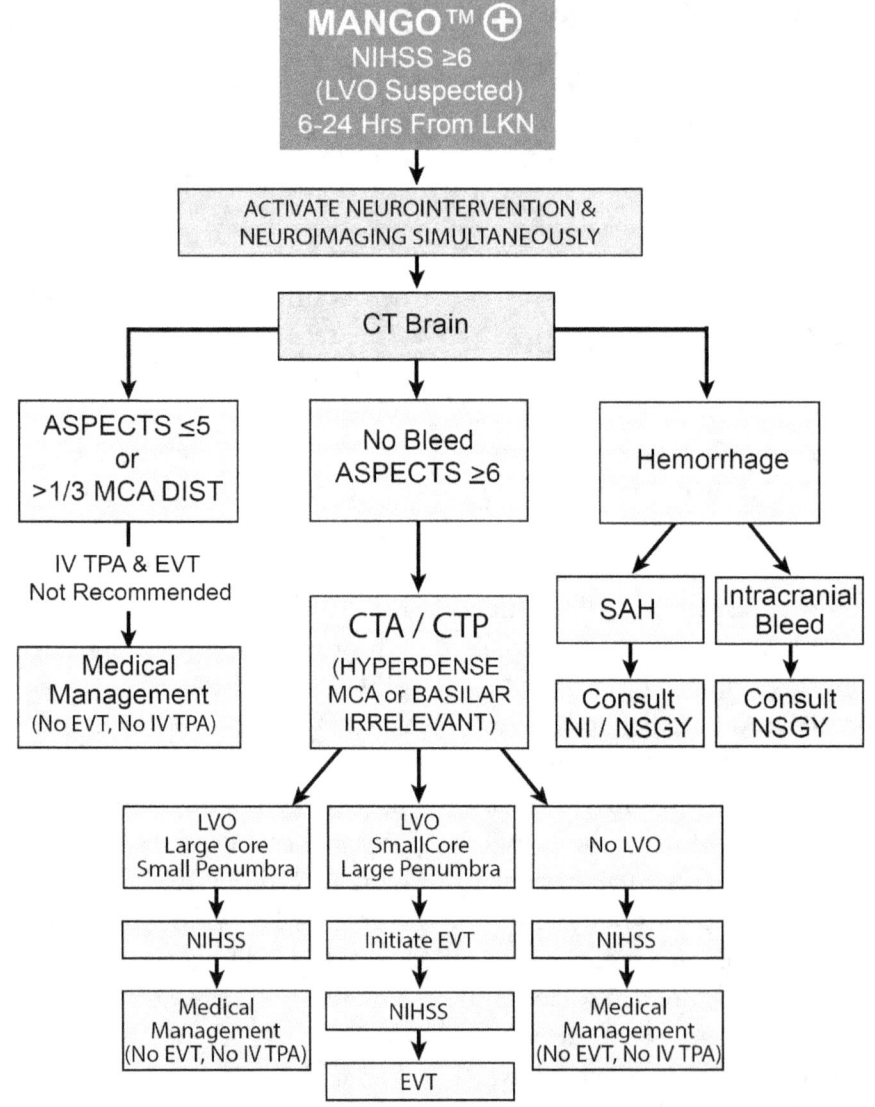

ASPECTS - Alberta Stroke Program Early CT Score, CTA - Computed Tomography Angiogram, CTP - Computed Tomography Perfusion, Dist - Distribution, EVT - Endovascular Treatment, LKN - Last Known Normal, LVO - Large Vessel Occlusion, MCA - Middle Cerebral Artery, NI - Neurointervention, NIHSS - National Institutes of Health Stroke Scale, NSGY - Neurosurgery, SAH - Subarachnoid Hemorrhage, TPA - Tissue Plasminogen Activator

As stated earlier, the 2018 AHA/ASA guidelines have different LVO AIS imaging and EVT recommendations based on time from symptom onset. Since the publication of the DAWN and DEFUSE 3 Trials, these recommendations have been modified for LVO AIS patients that present within 6 to 16 hours and 6 to 24 hours from symptom onset. Essentially, EVT is *recommended* in anterior circulation, large vessel occlusion (LVO) acute ischemic stroke (AIS) patients that present within 6 to 16 hours of last known normal and meet "other" DAWN or DEFUSE 3 eligibility criteria. EVT is *reasonable* for anterior circulation LVO AIS patients who present within 6 to 24 hours after last known normal and meet "other" DAWN criteria. These new recommendations are based on the DAWN and DEFUSE 3 Trials and can be remembered by the mnemonic 'TITAN' (Table 5). The 2018 AHA/ASA guidelines have three distinct EVT recommendations based on time from symptom onset: (1) less than 6 hours, (2) 6-16 hours, and (3) 6-24 hours, and make individual recommendations for each category (Table 6). The 2018 AHA/ASA guidelines have two distinct imaging recommendations based on time from symptom onset: (1) less than 6 hours and (2) 6-24 hours, and make individual recommendations for each category (Table 7).

TABLE 5. AHA/ASA EVT Recommendations 6-24 Hours from Symptom Onset: **TITAN**

T	Time Window No Longer Determines Eligibility
I	Imaging Determines Eligibility
T	Thrombectomy *Recommended* Between 6-16 Hours, *Reasonable* at 6-24 Hours*
A	Always Accelerate Treatment
N	No EVT if Eligible Leads to Bad Outcomes

*EVT is *recommended* for LVO AIS patients within 6 and 16 hours of last known normal (LKN) and meet "other" DAWN or DEFUSE 3 eligibility criteria.
EVT is *reasonable* 6 to 24 hours after LKN and meet "other" DAWN criteria.

TABLE 6. Summary of 2018 AHA/ASA Endovascular Treatment (EVT) Recommendations

Time Period	Recommendation
<6 Hours	EVT **should be** performed if the following criteria are met: **ATLAS** **(A)** Age ≥18 years, **(T)** Treatment initiated (groin puncture) within 6 hours of symptom onset, **(L)** LVO - Large Vessel Occlusion (ICA or MCA M1 segment), **(A)** ASPECTS ≥6 NIHSS score ≥6, **(S)** Score: Pre-stroke mRS score 0-1. EVT may be **reasonable** for MCA M2 or M3 segment occlusions. EVT may be **reasonable** for ACA, the vertebral artery, basilar artery or PCA occlusion. EVT may be **reasonable** for pre-stroke mRS score >1, ASPECTS <6, NIHSS score <6 and ICA or MCA M1 segment occlusion.
6-16 Hours from LKN	EVT is **recommended** for anterior circulation LVO that meet other DAWN or DEFUSE 3 eligibility criteria.
6-24 Hours from LKN	EVT is **reasonable** for anterior circulation LVO that meet other DAWN eligibility criteria.

ACA - Anterior Cerebral Artery, ASPECTS - Alberta Stroke Program Early CT Score, EVT - Endovascular Treatment, ICA - Internal Carotid Artery, LVO - Large Vessel Occlusion, MCA - Middle Cerebral Artery, mRS - Modified Rankin Scale, NIHSS - National Institutes of Health Stroke Scale, PCA - Posterior Cerebral Artery

TABLE 7. Summary of 2018 AHA/ASA Imaging Recommendations

Summary of 2018 AHA/ASA Imaging Recommendations	
Initial Imaging	Noncontrast brain CT within 20 minutes of arrival in the ED in at least 50% of patients who may be IV TPA and/or EVT candidates
<6 Hours From LKN EVT Eligible AIS Patients	Noninvasive intracranial vascular study should not delay IV TPA (if eligible)
	Reasonable to perform CTA for suspected LVO without serum creatinine concentration so long as no history of renal impairment
	MR or CT perfusion studies not recommended to determine EVT candidacy <6 hours from symptom onset
	Reasonable to utilize collateral flow status to determine EVT candidacy
6-24 Hours from LKN	Advanced neuroimaging (CTP, DWI - MRI or MR perfusion) to determine perfusion – core mismatch and maximum core size is recommended to help determine EVT candidacy

CT - Computerized Tomography, CTA - Computed Tomography Angiography, DWI - Diffusion-Weighted Magnetic Resonance Imaging, ED - Emergency Dept., EVT - Endovascular Treatment, LKN - Last Known Normal, LVO - Large Vessel Occlusion, TPA - Tissue Plasminogen Activator, MR - Magnetic Resonance, MRI - Magnetic Resonance Imaging

28.6 Neuroimaging and MANGO™

There are several interesting points regarding the study conducted by Taleb Mohammed S., et al., on which the MANGO™ mnemonic is based upon.[7] First, this LVO screening tool had a 100% negative predictive value. That is, no LVOs were missed. False positives were identified but anything (hemorrhage, tumor, etc.) that affects more than two cortical distributions will generate a false positive result. However, the concern is not overcalling stroke but undercalling it. In this regard, the fact that no LVOs were missed is impressive. In addition, this screening tool was 90% specific whereas the NIHSS was only 74% specific for LVO status. Further, **with proper training**, the interobserver reliability between trained nurses and stroke physicians was 100%. Finally, these trained nurses (who had 100% interobserver reliability with stroke physicians) initiated imaging and thus effectively managed emergent LVO AIS.

The MANGO™ mnemonic can increase the speed and accuracy of LVO screening and be performed by non-specialist physicians and nurses. In fact, it was performed by Emergency Department nurses with a 100% concordance to their stroke physician counterparts. These Emergency Department nurses not only screened patients for LVO; they also verified LVO status by ordering subsequent testing (CTA). Again, nurse assessment for LVO status in AIS patients had no variance when those same patients were assessed by stroke physicians.[7] This protocol, in conjunction with proper neuroimaging, would allow a hospital to effectively care for their own AIS patients utilizing limited resources and non-specialist physicians (Figure 9). However, Neurology (if available) should be consulted for the evaluation of every potential AIS patient.

28.7 Neuroimaging and the NIHSS

The NIHSS should be performed after neuroimaging but before either IV TPA administration or EVT. The greatest NIHSS examiner in the world cannot furnish anywhere near the diagnostic and treatment information provided by neuroimaging. This statement is intended to reinforce the concept that AIS can be effectively treated by non-specialist physicians in rural hospitals. Again, any hospital with neurology coverage should alert neurology for every suspected AIS and have neurology perform the NIHSS.

The treatment of stroke is a binary process based on the presence of stroke and not its exact quantification. The most recent comprehensive stroke center (CSC) recommendations by the American Heart Association/American Stroke

Association (AHA/ASA) state, "The NIHSS is recommended to be recorded in the first admitting note or in the first neurology consultation note, whichever comes first, or in a separate earlier note."[8] The AHA/ASA also recommend an NIHSS be performed prior to either IV TPA administration or EVT. They further state that "the NIHSS should be performed by a certified examiner." These recommendations also stress that "Ideally, the NIHSS should be administered before initial imaging is performed to establish a baseline and should therefore be administered to both ischemic and hemorrhagic stroke patients, **but we recognize that often, this is not done before imaging** in clinical practice." They further state, **"We also want to emphasize that imaging should not be delayed to perform the NIHSS."** The recent 2018 AHA/ASA guidelines state, "the use of a stroke severity rating scale, *preferably* the NIHSS is recommended."[4]

Both LVO AIS protocol discussed earlier support performing the NIHSS by a certified examiner before the administration of IV TPA or EVT, but after imaging. This is because the MR CLEAN Trial authors and other researchers recommend that vessel patency assessment with neuroimaging be performed *before or simultaneously* with IV TPA administration. Furthermore, they demonstrated that the presence of salvageable brain tissue (i.e. ischemic penumbra) is also beneficial for all AIS patients and not just for EVT patients. This philosophy was substantiated by a separate, multicenter analysis which demonstrated that core infarct and ischemic penumbra volume determination was beneficial for the outcome of all AIS patients (IV TPA patients in addition to EVT patients).[9] Trials that actively identified ischemic penumbra prior to treatment consistently demonstrated the highest rates of functional independence ever reported with mechanical thrombectomy (60% and 71%).[6]

This is just one protocol and certainly, the AHA/ASA recommendations can be interpreted in several different ways. However, the NIHSS is a core measure and necessary requirement for CSCs. Performing the NIHSS after imaging and before either IV TPA administration or EVT is acceptable. Nonetheless, many institutions prefer to perform the NIHSS as soon as possible and this is also acceptable. In this situation, once an AIS patient arrives at the ED, the NIHSS should be performed on a first come, first served basis whether by the ED physician, stroke neurologist, physician assistant, or nurse. However, the NIHSS should preferably be administered by a neurologist if it can be performed in a timely manner.

Unfortunately, not all hospitals have neurology coverage or 24/7 availability. Studies have demonstrated that the initial clinical diagnosis of AIS by ED physicians which were later validated by a board-certified neurologist had a sensitivity of 92%.[10] A more recently published study (2017) which included 15,721 patients again demonstrated the sensitivity and specificity of the clinical diagnosis of AIS by ED physicians to be high (91.3% and 92.7%).[11] Interestingly, missed AIS diagnosis was more common with milder, non-specific, or transient symptoms at presentation and far less common with severe LVO AIS. The AHA/ASA also recommend an NIHSS be performed prior to either IV TPA administration or EVT by a "certified examiner." Training and certification for the NIHSS is readily available (www.NIHSS.com) and some studies suggest that properly trained nurses can perform the NIHSS with reliability similar to a stroke-trained neurologist.[12] Again, these comments are intended for hospital systems that do not readily have neurology coverage. If available, the NIHSS should preferably be administered by a neurologist.

The NIHSS is a terrific tool for the quantification of stroke. However, like the complicated prehospital AIS scoring systems discussed in Chapter 27, it requires calculated scores and involves a subjective analysis. The treatment of stroke needs to be simple and objective. Nevertheless, even if the NIHSS was performed correctly 100% of the time, AIS intervention is still a binary process that does not require a 42-point scale. Simply put, are we going to treat an AIS patient with an NIHSS score of 1, 5, or 30 any differently? Of course, IV TPA eligibility and LVO status need to be determined, but neither IV TPA administration nor

EVT is NIHSS score dependent. The treatment of stroke depends largely on the presence of a debilitating stroke (binary issue) and not an NIHSS score. If a debilitating AIS exists, it requires treatment regardless of its NIHSS score. One of the greatest examples of this philosophy is the MR. CLEAN Trial that offered EVT to AIS patients with an NIHSS score ≥ 2.[13]

The NIHSS is an excellent clinical tool for the assessment of stroke. However, the assessment of arterial occlusion (the most important consideration for AIS diagnosis and treatment) is not part of this classification instrument. Thus, the NIHSS has a greater role in the quantification of stroke rather than the diagnosis and treatment of appropriate AIS treatment candidates. The AHA/ASA discourages using the NIHSS as the only criteria to withhold IV TPA in an otherwise eligible patient. This is because patients with LVO AIS may still have a low NIHSS score and certain stroke deficits are not detected by the NIHSS. Furthermore, the NIHSS cannot distinguish a completed core infarct from a potentially treatable ischemic penumbra. So, while the NIHSS is a great clinical rating instrument, it cannot reliably exclude the presence of an LVO and is unable to determine if a small core infarct and viable ischemic penumbra exist.

28.8 Rapidly Improving or Mild Stroke Symptoms

Neurology (if available) should be consulted and a noncontrast brain CT should be obtained for the evaluation of every potential AIS patient. The treatment of mild or minor stroke is difficult because currently, neither an accepted definition exists nor is there an NIHSS score cut-off point to direct thrombolytic therapy. Rather, it appears that the definition of minor ischemic stroke and its most appropriate treatment vary widely among physicians.[14] Minor stroke is commonly defined as an NIHSS score of 5 or less, but this definition requires further consideration because some deficits may be more disabling than others. Thus, an operational definition of mild or minor stroke cannot be determined based on an NIHSS score alone.

Similarly, the treatment of rapidly improving or minor stroke symptoms is also confusing for several reasons. First, rapidly improving or minor stroke symptoms have often been clumped into the same category. However, The National Institute of Neurological Disorders and Stroke (NINDS) Trial initially had separate exclusion criteria for minor stroke patients **or** patients who presented with major symptoms that rapidly improved.[15] Thus, these categories (minor stroke symptoms and rapidly improving stroke symptoms) must be considered separately.

The treatment of minor stroke is important for many reasons. First, more than half of all AIS patients initially present with mild ischemic stroke.[16] Second, a significant number of these patients do not receive IV TPA.[17] Lastly, while AIS patients with mild stroke will typically have a good functional outcome even without IV TPA administration, a significant number do not.[18]

A minor stroke is commonly defined as an NIHSS score ≤ 5. Yet, other studies have suggested using an NIHSS score ≤ 3 to define a minor stroke.[19] Despite these NIHSS score-based definitions, there are no specific NIHSS criteria for the recommended use of IV TPA in minor (or any other form of) ischemic stroke. Recently, one study consensus agreed on a minimal NIHSS score of 2-3 to warrant IV TPA administration in AIS patients.[20] Interestingly, a previous international survey reviewing the inclusion and exclusion criteria for IV TPA reached the same consensus on a minimal NIHSS score of 2-3 to warrant treatment.[21] Another study also demonstrated that patients who had an initial NIHSS score > 3 had 5.95 times the risk of having an unfavorable outcome.[22] A recent survey demonstrated most clinicians disapproved of IV TPA administration in patients with an NIHSS score ≤ 1.[17] Yet another survey indicated most physicians do not have a threshold NIHSS score below which they would not recommend IV TPA.[23] Rather, their decision was based on the perceived disability of the specific ischemic deficit.

Recall that the NIHSS score does not reflect certain signs and symptoms of posterior circulation stroke such as headache, vertigo, nausea, and truncal ataxia. In addition, the NINDS Trial also excluded minor stroke symptoms (isolated monoparesis with minor weakness, pure sensory syndrome, isolated facial weakness, and isolated dysarthria). Available data on AIS patients with very minor ischemic stroke (VMIS) defined by an NIHSS score of 0 or 1 is very limited.[20] However, a large retrospective analysis evaluated IV TPA administration in 5,910 mild stroke patients (NIHSS ≤ 5, including 109 patients with NIHSS = 0) and concluded that IV TPA treatment complications were similar for all NIHSS categories.[24] This meta-analysis of nine major IV TPA trials conducted by the Stroke Thrombolysis Trialists Collaboration concluded: "Irrespective of age or **stroke severity**, despite an increased rate of fatal intracranial hemorrhage during the first few days after treatment, alteplase significantly improves the overall odds of a good stroke outcome when delivered within 4.5 hours of stroke onset, with earlier treatment associated with bigger proportional benefits."[24]

Recent data from the Safe Implementation of Treatments in Stroke-International Stroke Thrombolysis Registry (SITS-ISTR) demonstrated good functional outcomes and similar risk of symptomatic intracerebral hemorrhage in **mild** stroke treated between 0-3 and 3-4.5 hours.[25] Similar results were also reported in the Get With the Guidelines-Stroke registry.[20] These results have led to a new 2018 AHA/ASA guideline recommendation which states: "For otherwise eligible patients with **mild** stroke presenting in the 3 to 4.5-hour window, treatment with IV alteplase may be reasonable. Treatment risks should be weighed against possible benefits."[4]

Another important minor stroke consideration is that the NIHSS is only one component that determines treatment. Rather than focusing on a specific NIHSS score, it may be helpful to determine what impact stroke deficits will have on quality of life. Based on this analysis, mild AIS can be divided into *mild but disabling* and *mild but nondisabling* AIS categories. For example, while an isolated language deficit will not result in a high NIHSS score, language difficulty would be disabling if an AIS patient worked as a teacher. Again, the NIHSS score is only one component that determines treatment. In fact, IV TPA administration is recommended in patients with mild but disabling symptoms regardless of their baseline NIHSS score.[26] Conversely, patients with no or low NIHSS scores (0 or 1) will likely do well regardless of treatment. However, even a low NIHSS score may adversely affect the quality of life of an AIS patient if the deficit is significant (i.e. an isolated hemianopia or an isolated aphasia). Because IV TPA carries a 1% risk of fatal intracranial hemorrhage, the risks and benefits of this procedure must be discussed with the patient and their family in order to arrive at a treatment decision. As stated in the AHA/ASA recommendation above, "Treatment risks should be weighed against possible benefits."[4]

Don't forget secondary stroke prevention applies to patients with both mild disabling and nondisabling stroke. The CHANCE Trial was reviewed in Chapters 17 and 18 and supports the use of dual antiplatelet therapy for recurrent stroke prevention (Box 3). Recall that prior to initiating antithrombotic therapy, cardioembolic mechanisms must be excluded. Also, dual antiplatelet therapy should not be initiated within 24 hours of IV TPA administration. These recommendations have been adopted by the new 2018 AHA/ASA stroke guidelines which state, "In patients presenting with **minor** stroke, treatment for 21 days with dual antiplatelet therapy (aspirin and clopidogrel) begun within 24 hours can be beneficial for early secondary stroke prevention for a period of up to 90 days from symptom onset."[4]

BOX 3. Ischemic Dual Antiplatelet Protocol

Drug	Loading Dose	Maintenance Dose
Clopidrogel*	300mg	75mg Daily After Loading Dose
Aspirin*	81mg	81mg Daily After Loading Dose

* Must exclude cardioembolic etiology and cannot be administered within 24 hrs of IV TPA bolus

In addition to a quantitative assessment of mild stroke, there is still the concern of rapidly improving deficits. Patients presenting with mild AIS or rapidly improving stroke symptoms (RISS) are often excluded from receiving IV TPA despite a significant incidence of poor functional outcome.[28] However, rapidly improving stroke symptoms may represent an unstable state that may be followed by even worse symptoms. One study demonstrated patients who had a 4-point improvement in their NIHSS score that were not treated with IV TPA were more likely to have a worse subsequent neurological outcome.[27] The 2018 AHA/ASA guidelines now recommend: "Because time from onset of symptoms to treatment has such a powerful impact on outcomes, treatment with IV alteplase should not be delayed to monitor for further improvement."[4] Due to the strong relationship of time to treatment outcome, observing mild or fluctuating deficits is no longer an encouraged practice by the current guidelines. In a similar manner, the US Food and Drug Administration no longer considers rapidly improving or minor stroke symptoms to be contraindications for IV TPA.

So how does one use this information to properly treat rapidly improving or mild stroke symptoms? The treatment of minor ischemic stroke and rapidly improving symptoms with IV TPA is supported by the 2018 AHA/ASA guidelines. Yet, difficulty persists concerning mild or minor stroke treatment because no operational definition exists. However, there appears to be a consensus on a minimal NIHSS score of 2 to 3 to warrant IV TPA treatment. Also, the risk of unfavorable outcome is significantly higher when patients with an initial NIHSS score higher than this limit are left untreated. Regardless of the NIHSS score, mild stroke with disabling symptoms requires treatment. The decision whether or not to administer IV TPA is determined by weighing the risk of symptomatic intracranial hemorrhage against the benefit of a good functional outcome. In this regard and pending patient-specific clinical judgment, higher initial NIHSS scores (≥2), disabling minor stroke symptoms, and rapidly improving symptoms (especially a 4-point improvement in the NIHSS score) may justify the use of IV TPA (Figure 12). Finally, secondary stroke prevention should be considered in all patients with rapidly improving or minor stroke symptoms (Figure 12).

28.9 Transient Ischemic Attack (TIA)

Neurology (if available) should be consulted and a noncontrast brain CT should be obtained for the evaluation of every potential AIS patient. A transient ischemic attack (TIA) results from the same pathophysiologic mechanism(s) as an AIS. That is, it can result from an occluded or compromised blood vessel that supplies oxygen to the brain. The key to understanding, diagnosing, and treating TIAs is to understand what TIAs are and what they are not. One must abstain from time-based definitions of TIAs such as "brief episodes of focal loss of brain function of *less than 24-hour duration*, thought to be due to ischemia that can usually be localized to that portion of the brain supplied by one vascular system."[28] This outdated definition is misleading and, quite frankly, dangerous.

Advances in neuroimaging have dramatically changed our understanding of TIAs. These advances have led to a *newer* tissue-based definition of TIAs that is endorsed by the American Heart Association, the American Stroke Council, and the American Academy of Neurology.[29] TIAs are now described as "a transient episode of neurologic dysfunction caused by focal brain, spinal cord, or retinal ischemia, *without evidence of acute infarction*." This newer definition of TIAs tremendously assists in distinguishing a TIA from AIS because MRI can be utilized to recognize tiny DWI-positive lesions as AIS, *regardless of whether symptoms are transient and regardless of the duration*. MRI DWI can discern AIS and enables better detection of smaller lesions that are representative of AIS and not TIA. Thus, MRI DWI can differentiate TIAs (no imaging findings) from actual AIS (DWI-positive imaging).

FIGURE 12. Rapidly Improving or Mild Stroke Symptom Assessment

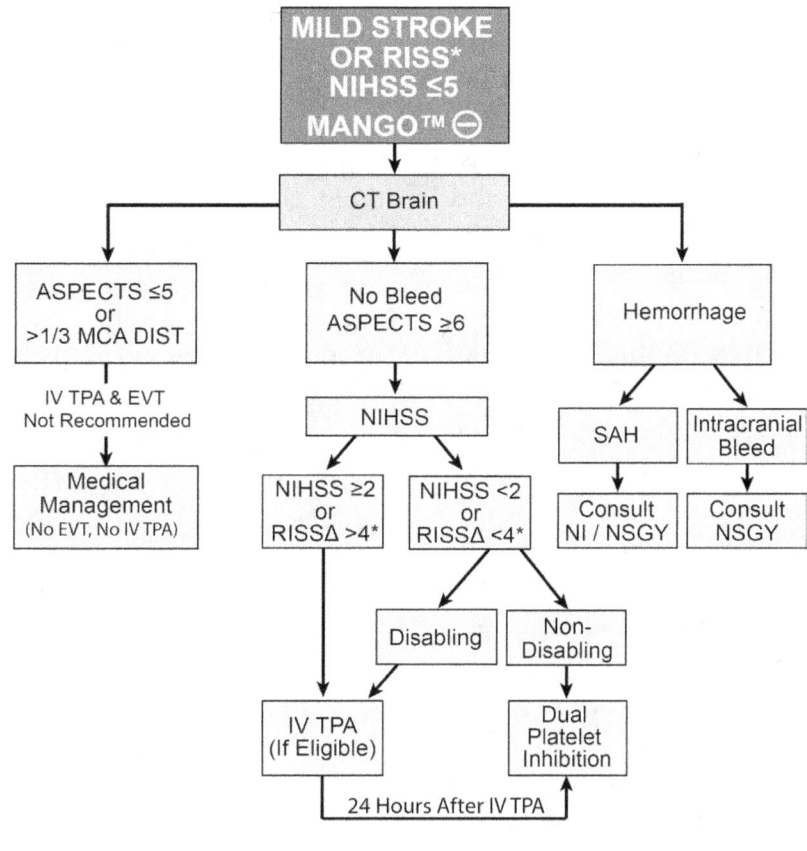

ASPECTS - Alberta Stroke Program Early CT Score, CT - Computed Tomography, Dist - Distribution,
EVT - Endovascular Treatment, LVO - Large Vessel Occlusion, MCA - Middle Cerebral Artery,
NI - Neurointervention, NIHSS - National Institutes of Health Stroke Scale, NSGY - Neurosurgery,
RISSΔ >4 - Rapidly Improving Stroke Symptoms with a change in NIHSS score >4 points,
SAH - Subarachnoid Hemorrhage, IV TPA - Intravenous Tissue Plasminogen Activator

Therefore, MRI DWI is required to effectively diagnose a TIA after obtaining a noncontrast brain CT. Patients with neurologic deficits that resolve in less than 24 hours but also have DWI-positive lesions on MRI have AIS and are at the highest risk of in-hospital recurrent stroke. However, simply by applying the newer tissue-based definition (TIA with no infarction), one can tremendously reduce the incidence of subsequent stroke to 0.4%. That is, MRI imaging can distinguish TIAs (no imaging findings) from ischemic stroke (positive DWI lesions) regardless of symptom duration. MRI DWI-positive lesions are considered ischemic stroke regardless of symptom duration and are at a higher risk for recurrent stroke. This allows the distinction between high-risk ischemic stroke (DWI-positive imaging) and low-risk TIA (no imaging findings) groups, with high-risk patients benefiting from specialized stroke centers and low-risk patients not requiring hospitalization (Figure 13).

FIGURE 13. Transient Ischemic Attack (TIA) Diagnostic and Treatment Protocol

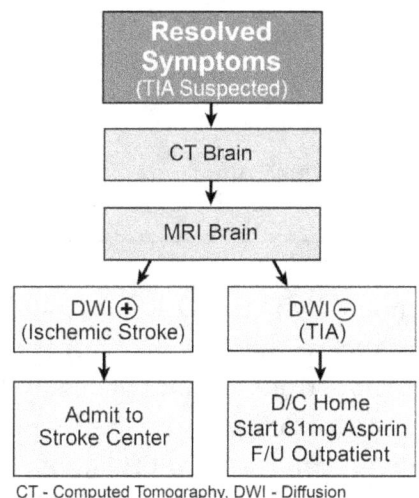

CT - Computed Tomography, DWI - Diffusion Weighted Imaging, D/C - Discharge, F/U - Follow-up
MRI - Magnetic Resonance Imaging, TIA - Transient Ischemic Attack

28.10 Stroke Mimic and No Stroke

Neurology (if available) should be consulted and a noncontrast brain CT should be obtained for the evaluation of every potential AIS patient. The term *stroke mimic* is used for manifestations of nonvascular disease processes that can mimic a stroke and thus confound its diagnosis. The ability to discern acute ischemic stroke (AIS) from other conditions that can mimic its presentation is necessary. This is because while mimics may produce stroke-like symptoms, they generally have very different therapeutic implications. Yet, stroke mimics continue to be often misdiagnosed as AIS and in some reports, up to 31% of the time.[30]

The most common stroke mimics include seizures, hypoglycemia, intracranial lesions, migraine headaches, vestibular dysfunction, encephalopathy, sepsis, and multiple sclerosis. These can be remembered by the mnemonic 'MIMICKERS™' (Table 8). Again, the recognition of stroke mimics is important because they have different therapeutic implications than AIS. Stroke mimics often lack cardiovascular risk factors such as hypertension, hyperlipidemia, and atrial fibrillation.[31]

TABLE 8. Stroke Mimickers: **MIMICKERS**™

M	Metabolic-Hypoglycemia or Hyperglycemia
I	Ictal-Seizures
M	Multiple Sclerosis
I	Intracranial Lesions (traumatic, infectious, hemorrhagic and neoplastic)
C	Classic and Specific Migraine Subtypes
K	Keep Balance? (Vestibular Dysfunction)
E	Encephalopathy
R	Regular Diastolic Pressure
S	Sepsis

The mnemonic 'MIMICKERS™' should be considered in the workup of every suspected AIS patient. Again, stroke mimics generally lack cardiovascular risk factors such as hypertension, hyperlipidemia, and atrial fibrillation. However, if one has difficulty discerning between a stroke mimic and AIS, remember the stroke mimic rule:

If the diagnosis of a stroke mimic cannot be confirmed before the IV TPA administration window closes (4.5 hours), assume the patient has an AIS and give IV TPA (Figure 14). Fortunately, the iatrogenic use of IV TPA given to stroke mimics has been demonstrated to be safe.[32-34] The stroke mimic (no stroke diagnostic/treatment) protocol is summarized below (Figure 14). This statement is supported by the 2018 AHA/ASA guidelines which state: "The risk of symptomatic intracranial hemorrhage in the stroke mimic population is quite low; thus, starting IV alteplase is probably recommended in preference over delaying treatment to pursue additional diagnostic studies."[4]

FIGURE 14. Stroke Mimic/No Stroke Diagnostic and Treatment Protocol

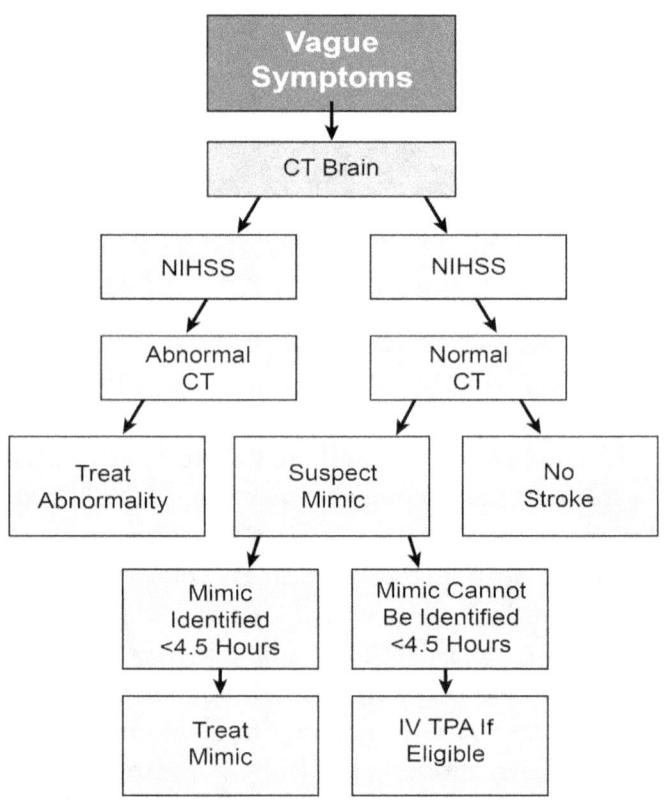

28.11 Conclusion

The effective diagnosis and treatment of AIS can be immensely complex. Hospital systems must function with limited resources while the diagnosis and treatment of AIS continues to evolve. Based on a relatively straightforward premise, the treatment of AIS can be difficult. The goal of AIS treatment is to restore perfusion to the ischemic penumbra. This is particularly relevant for LVO AIS which accounts for approximately 11% of all AIS but is responsible for all AIS related stroke death, 90% of societal cost, and 80% of poor functional outcome. This minority of AIS patients accounts for the overwhelming majority of AIS death, cost, and functional dependency. Thus, this is the most important AIS subtype that must be diagnosed and treated quickly.

While the diagnosis and treatment of AIS can be complex, it doesn't have to be. Effective clinical and imaging protocols are necessary for the proper diagnosis and management of AIS. This chapter reviewed five basic clinical and imaging protocols that quickly and efficiently diagnose and manage LVO AIS: (< 6 hours LKN), LVO AIS (6-24 hours LKN), non-LVO mild AIS, transient ischemic attack (TIA), and stroke mimic or no stroke. Furthermore, it demonstrated that these clinical and imaging protocols can allow a hospital to effectively care for AIS patients utilizing limited resources and non-specialist physicians. However, Neurology (if available) should be consulted for the evaluation of every potential AIS patient. These protocols are summarized in Figure 15.

Abbreviations list

AHA/ASA, American Heart Association/ American Stroke Association; AIS, acute ischemic stroke; ASPECTS, Alberta Stroke Program Early CT Score; CSCs, comprehensive stroke centers; CTA, computed tomography angiography; CTP, CT perfusion; DWI, diffusion-weighted imaging; EKG, electrocardiogram; EVT, endovascular treatment; IV TPA, intravenous administration of recombinant tissue plasminogen activator; LKN, last known normal; LVO, large vessel occlusion; LVO AIS, large vessel occlusion acute ischemic stroke; MI, myocardial infarction; MRI, magnetic resonance imaging; NCCT, noncontrast CT; NI, neurointerventional; NIHSS, National Institutes of Health Stroke Scale; RCTs, randomized controlled trials, RISS, rapidly improving stroke symptoms; STEMI, ST–segment–elevation myocardial infarction; TIA, transient ischemic attack; VMIS, very minor ischemic stroke.

Stroke Made Simple

FIGURE 15. Hospital-Based Acute Ischemic Stroke (AIS) Assessment

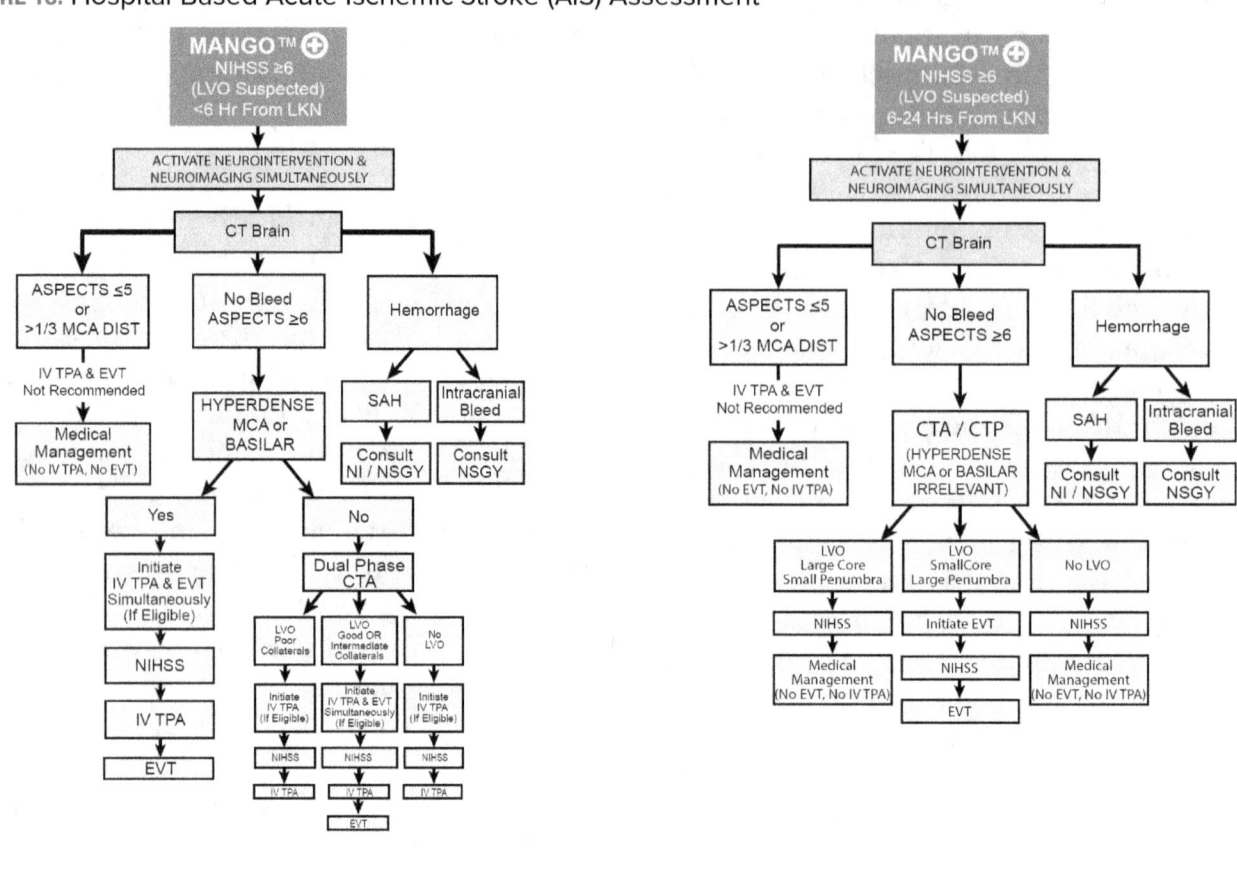

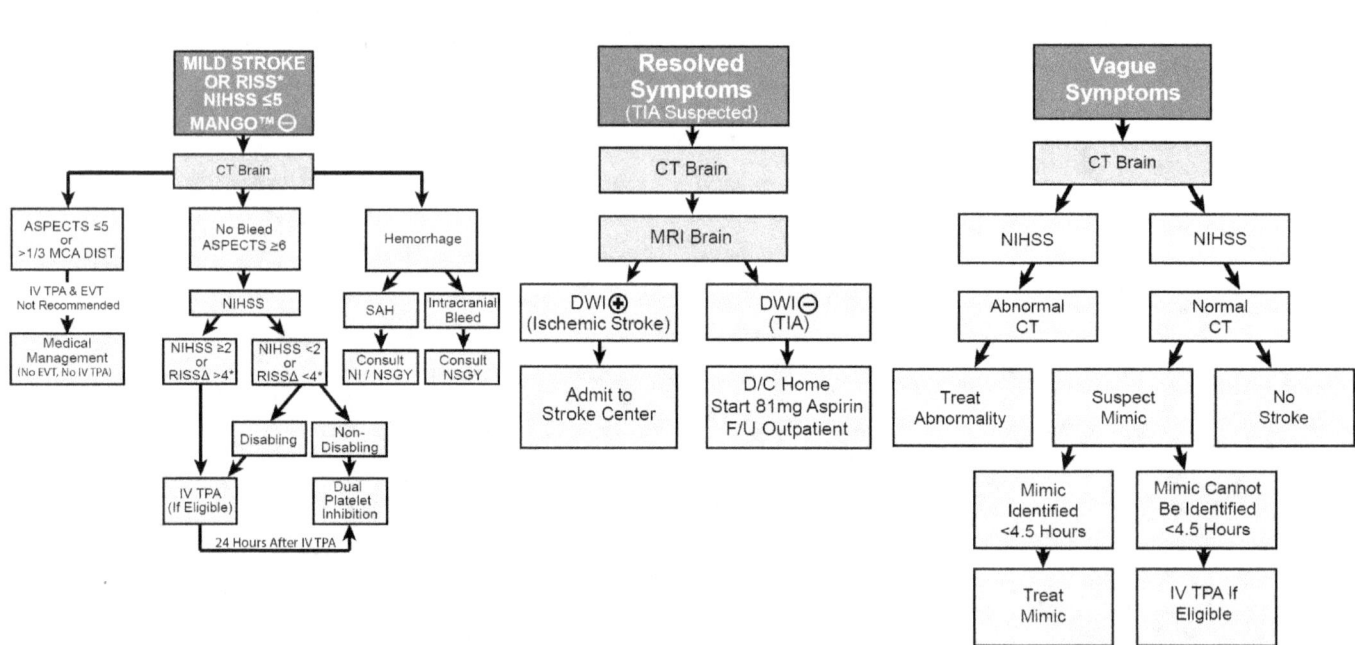

ASPECTS - Alberta Stroke Program Early CT Score, CTA - Computed Tomography Angiogram, CTP - Computed Tomography Perfusion, D/C - Discharge, Dist - Distribution, DWI - Diffusion Weighted Imaging, F/U - Follow-up, EVT - Endovascular Treatment, LKN - Last Known Normal, LVO - Large Vessel Occlusion, MCA - Middle Cerebral Artery, MRI - Magnetic Resonance Imaging, NI - Neurointervention, NIHSS - National Institutes of Health Stroke Scale, NSGY - Neurosurgery, RISS - Rapidly Improving Stroke Symptoms with a change in NIHSS score >4 points, SAH - Subarachnoid Hemorrhage, IV TPA - Intravenous Tissue Plasminogen Activator

References

1. Campbell BC, Christensen S, Tress BM, et al.—EPITHET Investigators. (2013). Failure of collateral blood flow is associated with infarct growth in ischemic stroke. *Jrnl of Cereb Blood Flow and Metab*, 33, 1168–72.
2. Hacke W, Kaste M, Fieschi C, et al. (1998). Randomised double-blind placebo-controlled trial of thrombolytic therapy with intravenous alteplase in acute ischaemic stroke (ECASS II). *Lancet*, 352, 1245–51.
3. Hinson JS, et al. (2016). Risk of Acute Kidney Injury After Intravenous Contrast Media Administration. *Ann Emerg Med*, 1-10.
4. Powers WJ, Rabinstein AA, Ackerson T, Adeoye OM, Bambakidis NC, Becker K, Biller J, Brown M, Demaerschalk BM, Hoh B, et al. (2018). Guidelines for the Early Management of Patients With Acute Ischemic Stroke: A Guideline for Healthcare Professionals From the American Heart Association/American Stroke Association. *Stroke*, Epub 24 Jan.
5. Barber PA, Demchuk AM, Zhang J, et al. (2000). Validity and reliability of a quantitative computed tomography score in predicting outcome of hyperacute stroke before thrombolytic therapy. ASPECTS Study Group. Alberta Stroke Programme Early CT Score. *Lancet*, 355, 1670–74.
6. Saver JL, Goyal M, Bonafe A, et al. (2015). Stent-retriever thrombectomy after intravenous t-PA vs. t-PA alone in stroke. *N Engl J Med*, 372, 2285-95; Campbell BCV, Mitchell PJ, Kleinig TJ, et al. (2015). Endovascular therapy for ischemic stroke with perfusion-imaging selection. *N Engl J Med*, 372, 1009-18.
7. Stroke vision, aphasia, neglect (VAN) assessment—a novel emergent large vessel occlusion screening tool: pilot study and comparison with current clinical severity indices. (2016). *NeuroInterv Surg*, 16(7), 525-33.
8. Leifer D, Bravata DM, Connors JJB, Hinchey JA, Jauch EC, Johnston SC, Latchaw R, Likosky W, Ogilvy C, Qureshi AI, et al. (2011). Metrics for measuring quality of care in comprehensive stroke centers: detailed follow-up to Brain Attack Coalition comprehensive stroke center recommendations: a statement for healthcare professionals from the American Heart Association/American Stroke Association. *Stroke*, Mar, 42(3), 849–77.
9. Zhu G, Michel P, Aghaebrahim A, Patrie JT, Xin W, Eskandari A, et al. (2013). Computed tomography workup of patients suspected of acute ischemic stroke: Perfusion computed tomography adds value compared with clinical evaluation, noncontrast computed tomography, and computed tomography angiogram in terms of predicting outcome. *Stroke*, 44, 1049-55.
10. Morgenstern LB, Lisabeth LD, Mecozzi AC, Smith MA, Longwell PJ, McFarling DA. (2004). A population-based study of acute stroke and TIA diagnosis. *Neurology*, 62, 895-900.
11. Tarnutzer AA, Lee SH, Robinson KA, Wang Z, Edlow JA, Newman-Toker DE. (2017). ED misdiagnosis of cerebrovascular events in the era of modern neuroimaging: A meta-analysis. *Neurology*, 88, 1468-77.
12. Dewey HM, Donnan GA, Freeman EJ, Sharples CM, Macdonell RA, McNeil JJ, et al. (1999). Interrater reliability of the National Institutes of Health Stroke Scale: rating by neurologists and nurses in a community-based stroke incidence study. *Cerebrovasc Dis*, 9, 323–27.
13. Berkhemer OA, Fransen PS, Beumer D, van den Berg LA, Lingsma HF, Yoo AJ, et al. (2015). A randomized trial of intraarterial treatment for acute ischemic stroke. *N Engl J Med*, 372, 1120.
14. van Swieten JC, Koudstaal PJ, Visser MC, Schouten HJ, van Gijn J. (1988). Interobserver agreement for the assessment of handicap in stroke patients. *Stroke*, 19, 604–7.
15. NINDS rt-PA Stroke Study Group. (1995). Tissue plasminogen activator for acute ischemic stroke. *N Engl J Med*, 333, 1581–87.
16. Reeves M, Khoury J, Alwell K, Moomaw C, Flaherty M, et al. (2013). Distribution of National Institutes of Health stroke scale in the Cincinnati/Northern Kentucky Stroke Study. *Stroke*, 44, 3211-13.
17. Smith EE, Fonarow GC, Reeves MJ, Cox M, Olson DM, et al. (2011). Outcomes in mild or rapidly improving stroke not treated with intravenous recombinant tissue-type plasminogen activator: findings from Get With The Guidelines-Stroke. *Stroke*, 42, 3110-15.
18. Nedeltchev K, Schwegler B, Haefeli T, Brekenfeld C, Gralla J, et al. (2007). Outcome of stroke with

mild or rapidly improving symptoms. *Stroke*, 38, 2531-35.
19. Fischer U, Baumgartner A, Arnold M, Nedeltchev K, Gralla J, De Marchis GM, et al. (2010). What is a minor stroke? *Stroke*, 41(4), 661–610; Park TH, Hong KS, Choi JC, Song P, Lee JS, Lee J, et al. (2013). Validation of minor stroke definitions for thrombolysis decision making. *J Stroke Cerebrovasc Dis,* 22, 482–90.
20. Romano JG, Smith EE, Liang L, Gardener H, Camp S, Shuey L, Cook A, Campo-Bustillo I, Khatri P, Bhatt DL, Fonarow GC, Sacco RL, Schwamm LH. (2015). Outcomes in mild acute ischemic stroke treated with intravenous thrombolysis: a retrospective analysis of the Get With the Guidelines-Stroke registry. *JAMA Neurol*, 72, 423–31.
21. Dirks M, Niessen LW, Koudstaal PJ, Franke CL, Van Oostenbrugge RJ, and Dippel DWJ. (2007). Intravenous thrombolysis in acute ischaemic stroke: from trial exclusion criteria to clinical contraindications. An international Delphi study. *Jrnl of Neurology, Neurosurg and Psych*, 78 (7). 685–89.
22. Initial Stroke Severity Is the Major Outcome Predictor for Patients Who Do Not Receive Intravenous Thrombolysis due to Mild or Rapidly Improving Symptoms. (2011). *ISRN Neurology*.
23. Logallo N, Kvistad CE, Naess H, Waje-Andreassen U, Thomassen L. (2014). Mild stroke: safety and outcome in patients receiving thrombolysis. *ActaNeurolScandSuppl*, 37-40.
24. Lindley RI, Wardlaw JM, Whiteley WN, Cohen G, Blackwell L, et al. (2015). Alteplase for acute ischemic stroke: outcomes by clinically important subgroups in the Third International Stroke Trial. *Stroke*, 46, 746-56.
25. Ahmed N, Wahlgren N, Grond M, Hennerici M, Lees KR, Mikulik R, Parsons M, Roine RO, Toni D, Ringleb P—SITS Investigators. (2010). Implementation and outcome of thrombolysis with alteplase 3-4.5 h after an acute stroke: an updated analysis from SITS-ISTR. *Lancet Neurol*, 9, 866–74.
26. Kohrmann M, Nowe T, Huttner HB et al. (2009). Safety and outcome after thrombolysis in stroke patients with mild symptoms. *Cerebrovascular Diseases*, 27(2), 160-16.
27. Smith EE, Abdullah AR, Petkovska I, Rosenthal E, Koroshetz WJ, and Schwamm LH. (2005). Poor outcomes in patients who do not receive intravenous tissue plasminogen activator because of mild or improving ischemic stroke," *Stroke*, 36 (11), 2497–99.
28. National Institute of Neurological Disorders and Stroke. Special report from the National Institute of Neurological Disorders and Stroke: classification of cerebrovascular diseases, III. *Stroke,* 21, 637–76. (1990).
29. *Stroke*, 40(6), 2276. (2009).
30. Kothari R, Barsan W, Brott T, et al. (1995). Frequency and accuracy of prehospital diagnosis of acute stroke. *Stroke*, 26, 937–41.
31. Merino JG, Luby M, Benson RT, et al. (2013). Predictors of acute stroke mimics in 8187 patients referred to a stroke service. *J Stroke Cerebrovasc Dis*, 22, 397-403.
32. Brunser AM, Illanes S, Lavados PM, et al. (2010). Exclusion criteria for intravenous thrombolysis in stroke mimics: An observational study.
33. Chernyshev OY, Martin-Schild S, Albright KC, et al (2010). Safety of tPA in stroke mimics and neuroimaging-negative cerebral ischemia. *Neurology*, 74, 1340–45.
34. Tsivgoulis G, Zand R, Katsanos AH, Goyal N, Uchino K, Chang J, Dardiotis E, Putaala J, Alexandrov AW, Malkoff MD, and Alexandrov AV. (2015). Safety of Intravenous Thrombolysis in Stroke Mimics. *Stroke,* 46, 1281-87.

Chapter 29

Stroke Efficiency

29.1 Introduction

Henry Ford invented the assembly line over 100 years ago. This permitted the synchronous production of an automobile and reduced assembly time by 90%. Prior to this innovation, automobile components were made one at a time from start to finish. These components were produced by highly trained craftsmen. While the quality was very high, production was extremely limited. This piecemeal production of car components was considered "standard practice" and incredibly inefficient. Prior to the assembly line, automotive production within the United States was craft-based, extending back to the Colonial era. The assembly line represented a paradigm shift in production efficiency.

The assembly line introduced mass production and replaced horse and buggies with gasoline engine powered automobiles. It allowed automobiles to be assembled 90% faster. As amazing as this process was, the result was even more phenomenal. Automobile cost was reduced such that every middle-class family and the average working individual could afford one. Cars allowed individuals to travel 10 times faster than they previously could with a horse and buggy. Automobiles allowed people to travel, businesses to grow, and civilization to flourish. They permitted people to live in remote and rural areas. The modern-day capitalist economy would not exist without the invention of the assembly line.

The current diagnosis and treatment of acute ischemic stroke (AIS) are not unlike the pre-assembly line production of automobiles. That is, highly trained physicians with different training backgrounds (emergency department physicians, neurologists, radiologists, and neurointerventionalists) typically evaluate AIS patients differently. For example, rarely do all these different physicians perform the National Institutes of Health Stroke Scale (NIHSS). Certainly, the NIHSS is not performed by EMS personnel, which raises another issue. In addition to variations in physician AIS evaluation, differences exist between prehospital and hospital evaluation of AIS. Emergency medical service (EMS) personnel evaluate AIS patients in the prehospital setting differently than emergency department physicians who evaluate them within the hospital. These differences disrupt synchronous and efficient AIS diagnosis and treatment. Ideally, physicians and non-physicians should evaluate AIS in a synchronous and efficient manner utilizing rapid, practical, and reliable protocols to improve stroke efficiency.

This text has consistently reinforced the concept that individual collateral circulation physiology rather than arbitrary time points determines AIS treatment. Each AIS patient should be treated individually based on distinct physiology and not arbitrary time points. This is because the unique collateral circulation of a 30-year-old is vastly different from the unique collateral circulation of a 90-year-old. Despite these differences in individual physiology, it is imperative to treat AIS as rapidly as possible. The ischemic clock is ticking whether someone has an ischemic penumbra that can be sustained for three or five hours. Effective AIS efficiency can mean the difference between a good and poor outcome. AIS efficiency has been discussed throughout this text but this chapter will critically analyze multiple steps in AIS diagnosis and treatment pathway that can be optimized.

There is an old game show called "Beat the Clock" which challenged contestants to perform random and bizarre tasks within a limited time. In a sense, every time we diagnose and treat an AIS patient, we are playing "Beat the Clock" because we only have a limited time to perform these tasks. However, unlike the game show, AIS diagnosis and treatment tasks are often the same. Similar sequences of events occur every time IV TPA is administered or endovascular treatment (EVT) is performed. If one knew what task was going to be performed on "Beat the Clock" and practiced these tasks repetitively, one would likely be a winner. By reviewing and critically evaluating the tasks involved in the diagnosis and treatment of AIS, our patients will more likely be winners, too.

Chapter 25 reviewed specific events and suggested time reduction goals to perform EVT more efficiently (Figure 1). These steps will be divided into four basic categories required for AIS management. These categories include AIS **screening**, **diagnosis**, **quantification**, and **treatment** (Figure 2). The sequence of the steps required for the administration of IV TPA and EVT will be reviewed and critically analyzed to improve efficiency. The more efficiently these steps can be performed, the greater the probability of having a good functional outcome.

FIGURE 2. Acute Ischemic Stroke (AIS) Treatment Steps

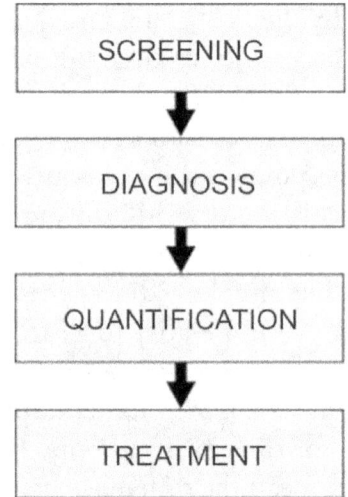

29.2 AIS Screening

AIS screening may be the most crucial step in its diagnosis and treatment. This step is so important that it has led others to state, "Effective and efficient prehospital triage of patients with emergent large vessel occlusion is now the holy grail of stroke care delivery innovation."[1] It is essential to separate large vessel occlusion (LVO) AIS from non-LVO AIS. This is because while LVO only accounts for approximately 11% of all AIS, it accounts for all AIS related stroke death, 90% of AIS societal cost, and 80% of poor functional outcome. Thus, this minority of AIS patients accounts for the overwhelming majority of AIS death, cost, and functional dependency.

The diagnosis of AIS stroke can no longer be considered a separate prehospital and hospital process. LVO screening should involve EMS personnel and physicians working together to develop rapid and effective protocols to screen for LVO AIS reliably. EMS and physicians must work together to prioritize AIS patients who are suspected of having an LVO in the prehospital setting before they reach the hospital. This is because suspected LVO AIS patients should be transported to a comprehensive stroke care center (CSC) to receive immediate and proper care. EVT nearly doubles functional outcome and is now the new standard of care for LVO AIS. Unfortunately, 30% of LVO AIS patients transferred from a primary stroke center (PSC) to a CSC arrive too late for EVT (ischemic penumbra decays into a core infarct).

FIGURE 1. Recommended EVT Time Points

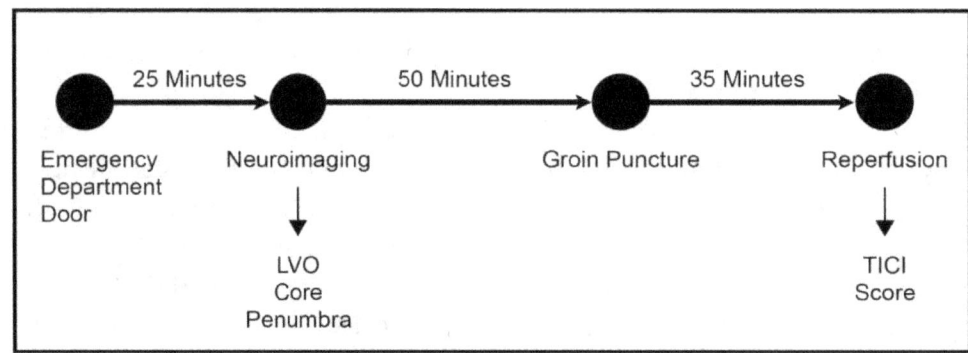

Adapted from: Saver, Jeffrey L., et al. "Time to Treatment With Endovascular Thrombectomy and Outcomes From Ischemic Stroke: A Meta-analysis." *JAMA* 316.12 (2016): 1279-1289

Rapid screening of suspected LVO AIS patients by EMS personnel allows these patients to be transported to a CSC, the right hospital the first time. The MANGO™ mnemonic is one way to adequately assess patients in the prehospital setting as it allows EMS personnel to "find them fast." More importantly, the MANGO™ mnemonic can also be used by physicians in the hospital setting to reliably identify suspected LVO AIS patients whose LVO status can be later confirmed by neuroimaging. Thus, the MANGO™ mnemonic serves as a bridge between the prehospital and hospital setting for LVO AIS screening. It accomplishes this feat by allowing non-specialist physicians and non-physicians to effectively and reliably screen for LVO AIS in the same rapid, reliable, synchronous, and efficient manner (Figure 3). Thus, the MANGO™ mnemonic is the first step in our synchronous and efficient AIS assembly line.

FIGURE 3. MANGO™ and LVO Screening

STROKE SCREENING

PRE-HOSPITAL (EMS) — MANGO™ — HOSPITAL (MD)

This process allows LVO AIS patients to be delivered to a CSC so they may be treated promptly. If possible, all suspected LVO AIS patients **must** go to a CSC in a timely fashion (≤30 minutes) (Figure 4). While the patient is being evaluated and if the patient or family members are able, complete a checklist that includes all the IV TPA restrictions (Table 1). In addition, the patient and/or family should be consented for EVT (mechanical thrombectomy and/or thromboaspiration) and conscious sedation or general anesthesia. By performing these two tasks, the patient is "lined up" for further potential treatment. Whether the patient has an LVO or non-LVO AIS, critical decisions must be made to reduce both AIS diagnosis and treatment time in order to improve functional outcome. As recognized by the 2018 AHA/ASA guidelines, reduced time from symptom onset to reperfusion with either IV TPA or EVT leads to better clinical outcomes.[2]

FIGURE 4. Prehospital Acute Ischemic Stroke (AIS) Assessment

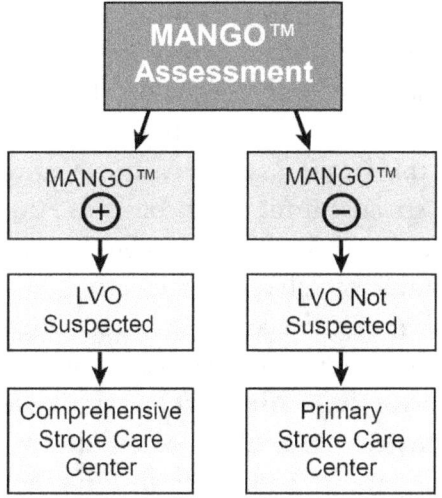

TABLE 1. IV TPA Restrictions: **NOT TPA CLIENTS**™

N	Non-Enhanced Contrast CT >1/3 MCA
O	Onset of Symptoms >4.5 Hrs or UNKNOWN
T	Ten, Intracranial Aneurysm ≥10mm
T	Tumor, Intra-Axial or GI (or GI Bleed <21d)
P	Prior Ischemic Stroke Within 3 Months
A	Aortic Dissection (Suspected)
C	Coagulopathy: Coumadin (if INR >1.7) and Coumadin Analogs (Direct Thrombin Inhibitors or Direct Factor Xa Inhibitors) PT >15, aPTT >40, PLTS <100,000 & INR >1.7
L	Low Molecular Weight Heparin <24 Hours (Full Treatment Dose, Not Prophylactic Dose)
I	Intracranial Hemorrhage - Acute or 3 Month History
E	Endocarditis, Infectious (Suspected)
N	Noncompressible Vessel Puncture Within 7 Days (Safety and Efficacy of IV TPA Uncertain)
T	Trauma, Severe Head Within 3 Months
S	Surgery, CNS (Intracranial or Spine) Within 3 Months

29.3 AIS Image Confirmation (Diagnosis)

Once an LVO AIS is suspected (MANGO™ +), its status must be confirmed with neuroimaging (Figure 5). Neuroimaging does not have to be complex. If done correctly, most non-specialist physicians and even non-physicians can properly evaluate it. This is yet another component of a synchronous and efficient stroke assembly line. Our goal is to enable non-specialist physicians and even non-physicians to be able to participate in the diagnosis and treatment of AIS. By simplifying this process, more individuals can participate in the stroke assembly line. Neuroimaging excludes stroke mimics and confirms AIS diagnosis. It also determines LVO, core infarct, ischemic penumbra, or collateral circulation status. No clinical exam can make these assessments. Let me repeat that statement: **Clinical examination by itself cannot determine LVO status, core infarct size, ischemic penumbra, or collateral circulation.** That means non-specialist physicians can utilize neuroimaging to determine AIS diagnosis and treatment (LVO, core infarct size, ischemic penumbra, or collateral circulation) and effectively manage AIS.

Neuroimaging efficiency can also be improved from a procedural and technical standpoint. First, suspected LVO AIS patients should receive all neuroimaging up front and simultaneously. That is, they should receive a noncontrast brain CT followed by additional neuroimaging (CTA/CTP or dual-phase CTA) concomitantly. Suspected LVO AIS patients should not receive a noncontrast brain CT, stop for additional examination such as an NIHSS score and decide whether to administer IV TPA, begin IV TPA if agreed upon, and then proceed again with additional imaging. This is a waste of time and therefore compromises brain tissue viability (Figure 6). Currently, in many stroke centers, a brain CT is performed and then patients are clinically assessed to determine their NIHSS score. After this assessment, patients may or may not receive IV TPA and additional imaging such as a CTA and CTP. Performing a brain CT first and waiting for hours in some cases to perform a CTA and CT perfusion is an incredible waste of valuable time and brain cells. In one study, investigators determined that obtaining a CTA immediately after a brain CT reduced the time necessary to initiate EVT by almost an hour and 30 minutes.[1] Saving an hour and a half equates to saving almost *200 million* neurons!

FIGURE 6. Inefficient vs. Efficient Neuroimaging

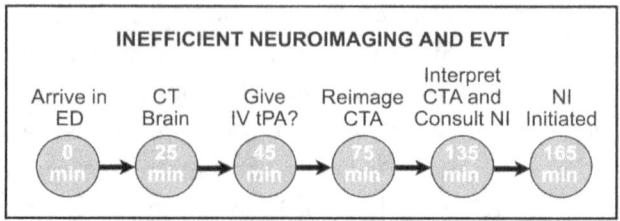

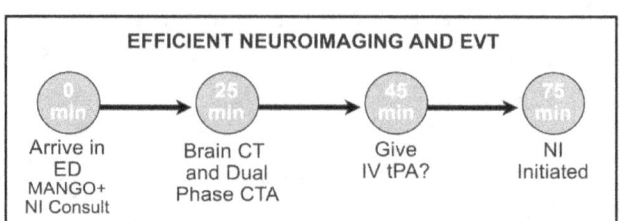

Neuroimaging is far more sensitive in the detection of stroke and the prediction of symptomatic intracranial hemorrhage and functional outcome than the NIHSS. If neuroimaging demonstrates any type of vascular occlusion and the patient is eligible, initiate IV TPA administration. IV TPA restrictions have already been determined during the initial emergency department screening. If LVO and ischemic penumbra status is confirmed, IV TPA administration should be initiated before or while the patient is being transported to the neurointerventional lab. This method decreases the required time to both perform EVT and administer IV TPA. An NIHSS should be performed after imaging **because imaging, and not an NIHSS score, determines diagnosis and treatment.** Understandably, the NIHSS score is a core measure which can be performed before treatment but after imaging.

LVO status is only one factor that determines EVT candidacy. Once LVO status has been confirmed, the next step is to determine the presence of viable brain tissue. Excluding MRI, this can be performed in one of two ways: a **CTP** which demonstrates a mismatch (low cerebral blood flow and sustained or elevated cerebral blood volume) or **dual phase CTA** (Figure 7). I endorse the use of dual phase CTA. This chapter is entitled *Stroke Efficiency* and dual-phase CTA is the quintessential example of this. This is because dual-phase CTA requires no special software, no post-processing, is easy to interpret, and determines LVO, clot length, and collateral status simultaneously.

Simply put, dual-phase CTA is the simplest and fastest way to determine EVT candidacy. This allows nonspecialized physicians and even non-physicians to interpret these images and participate in stroke management. Dual-phase CTA is just another factor that can support an efficient stroke assembly line. CTP and dual-phase CTA are diagrammatically summarized below (Figure 8).

FIGURE 5. Large Vessel Occlusion (LVO), Acute Ischemic Stroke (AIS) Management

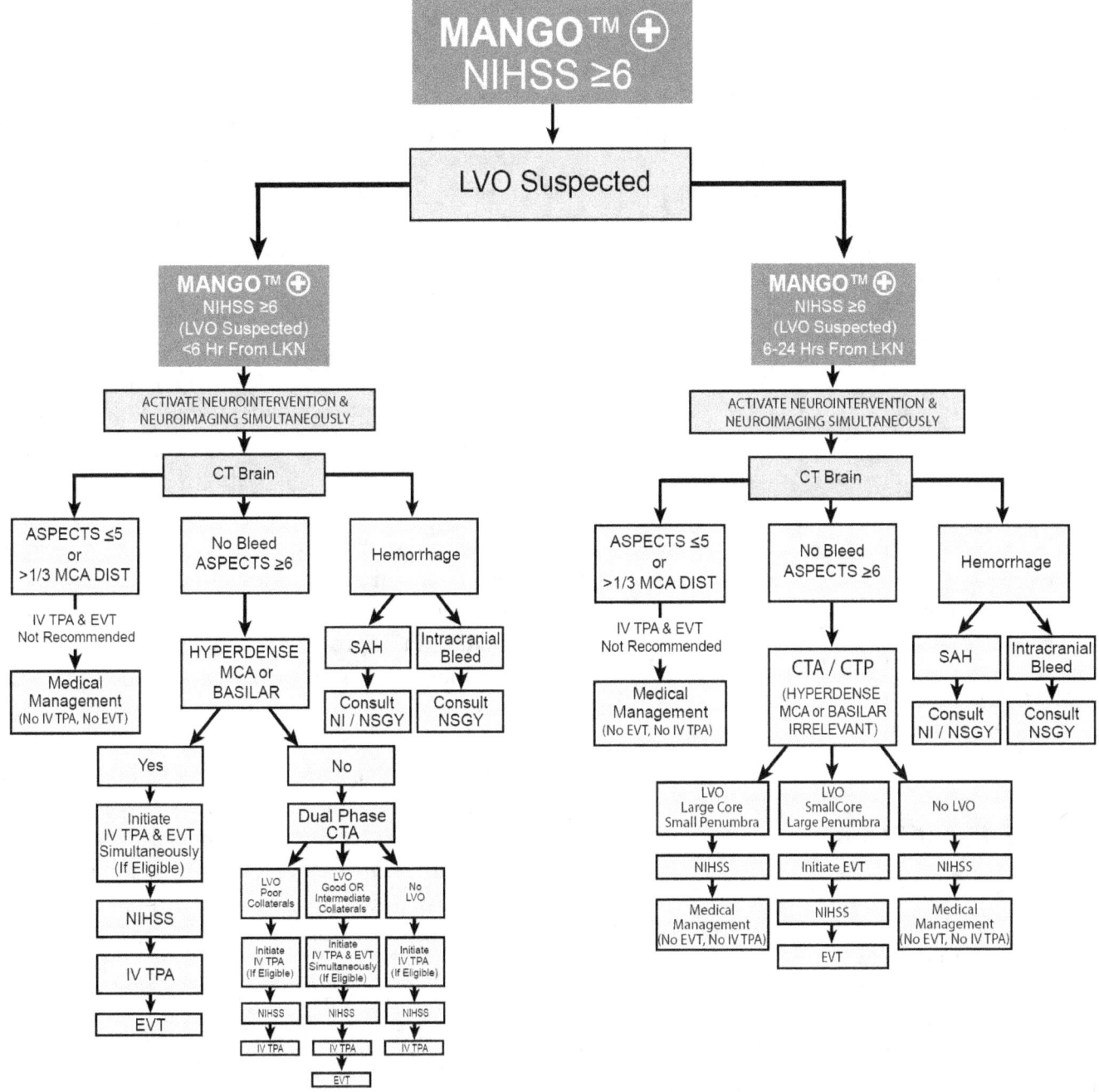

ASPECTS - Alberta Stroke Program Early CT Score, CTA - Computed Tomography Angiogram, CTP - Computed Tomography Perfusion, D/C - Discharge, Dist - Distribution, DWI - Diffusion Weighted Imaging, F/U - Follow-up, EVT - Endovascular Treatment, LKN - Last Known Normal, LVO - Large Vessel Occlusion, MCA - Middle Cerebral Artery, MRI - Magnetic Resonance Imaging, NI - Neurointervention, NIHSS - National Institutes of Health Stroke Scale, NSGY - Neurosurgery, SAH - Subarachnoid Hemorrhage, TPA - Tissue Plasminogen Activator

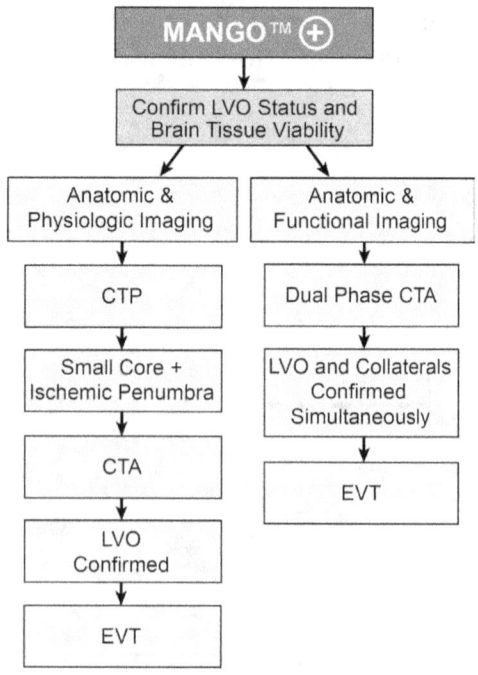

FIGURE 7. Functional and Physiologic Neuroimaging to Assess Viable Brain Tissue

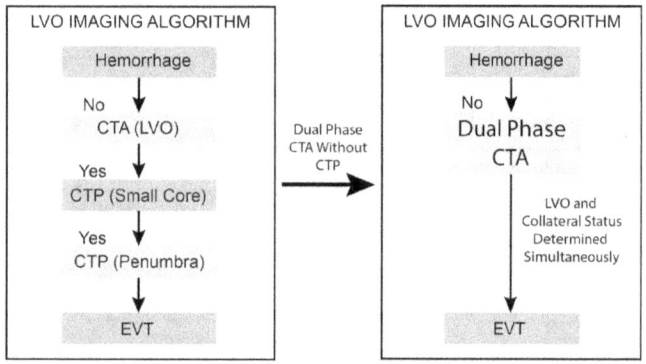

FIGURE 8. Dual-Phase CTA Efficiency

29.4 AIS Quantification

The NIHSS should be performed after neuroimaging but before either IV TPA administration or EVT. The greatest NIHSS examiner in the world cannot supply anywhere near the diagnostic and treatment information provided by neuroimaging. More importantly, the NIHSS score is only one component in the management of stroke. The NIHSS is a core measure and necessary requirement for CSCs which can be performed after imaging but before AIS treatment. The NIHSS is a terrific tool for the quantification of stroke. However, like the complicated prehospital AIS scoring systems discussed in Chapter 27, it requires calculated scoring and involves subjective analysis. **The treatment of stroke needs to be simple and objective**. Even if the NIHSS is performed correctly 100% of the time, AIS intervention is still a binary process that does not require a 42-point scale. The treatment of stroke is dependent on the presence of a disabling stroke (binary issue) and not an NIHSS score. As discussed earlier, the NIHSS score is only one component in the management of stroke.

Imaging, and not the NIHSS score, confirms stroke diagnosis and treatment because the assessment of arterial occlusion (the most important consideration for **all** AIS diagnosis and treatment) is not part of the NIHSS. Thus, the NIHSS has a greater role in the quantification of stroke rather than its diagnosis and treatment. This is because the NIHSS cannot distinguish a completed core infarct from a potentially treatable ischemic penumbra. So while the NIHSS is a great clinical rating instrument, it cannot reliably exclude the presence of an LVO. It is also unable to determine if a small core infarct and viable ischemic penumbra exist. Neuroimaging is required to determine LVO, core infarct, and ischemic penumbra status. Neuroimaging determines IV TPA and EVT candidacy and improves functional outcome for both treatments. This is precisely why neuroimaging must be performed before conducting an NIHSS. The literature shows neuroimaging improves AIS patient outcome regardless of IV TPA, EVT, or both IV TPA and EVT. This is because neuroimaging answers questions the NIHSS cannot in terms of LVO, core infarct, and ischemic penumbra status. The sooner LVO, core infarct, and ischemic penumbra status are determined, the quicker these patients can be treated and the better their functional outcomes. Again, neuroimaging (and not the NIHSS) confirms AIS diagnosis and treatment. An NIHSS score does not determine IV TPA administration or EVT candidacy.

29.5 AIS Treatment

After AIS diagnosis, treatment must be initiated. Currently, the only FDA approved treatment methods for AIS are IV TPA and EVT. If an LVO and sufficient collateral circulation are determined by dual phase CTA or other imaging methods, both IV TPA and EVT should be initiated immediately. There are two key rate-limiting steps in AIS treatment requiring efficiency analysis. These include IV TPA preparation for administration and preparation for neurointervention. Before IV TPA is administered, it must be prepared and delivered by the pharmacy. Also, before a patient can be transported to the neurointerventional suite, a team must be present and ready to perform EVT. Both steps can be incorporated into one single rate-limiting step by administering IV TPA after image confirmation while the patient is either being transported or waiting to be transported to the neurointerventional suite. In this manner, both IV TPA administration and EVT times can be improved, thus increasing the efficiency of our stroke assembly line.

29.5.1 Neurointerventional Activation

The LVO AIS protocol discussed in Chapter 25 recommended consulting the neurointerventional physician once an LVO AIS patient was suspected (Figures 5, 6 and 9). The algorithm demonstrates that this step occurs prior to any neuroimaging (Figures 5, 6 and 9). If neuroimaging confirms EVT candidacy, the neurointerventional team must be summoned. This step requires critical analysis as poor coordination can result in significant treatment delays and poor functional outcome. Unfortunately, most stroke centers that perform EVT do not have available in-house nurses and technologists 24/7. That is, the staff is typically on-call and takes 30 minutes to reach the hospital. After arrival, it usually takes another 30 minutes to prepare the patient for neurointervention. Thus, after EVT has been initiated, the patient may not be treated for at least another hour! There are different ways to solve this problem. Before discussing the solution, greater analysis of this problem is required.

There are generally three models that describe how the neurointerventional team (nurses and technologists) is activated for on-call cases (after hours and weekends). These include the Ever-Ready, Remote, and Transitional Models. The Ever-Ready Model is typically encountered in academic and large stroke centers. In this model, the neurointerventional team (consisting of nurses and technologists) is activated once the neurointerventional physician is consulted. The Ever-Ready Model has the advantage of having the neurointerventional team available to receive the LVO AIS patient as soon as LVO and ischemic penumbra status have been confirmed by imaging. However, this model has a severe disadvantage because it requires considerable resources for personnel to be available for all **potential** EVT cases. The team can be activated and arrive at the hospital awaiting to perform EVT, but neuroimaging may demonstrate the AIS patient is not an EVT candidate. In this model, the team is activated for every potential EVT case. Most community hospitals don't have the resources required to maintain the Ever-Ready Model. The major advantage of the Ever-Ready Model is its immediate activation and minimal time delay to perform EVT (Table 2). Its major disadvantage, however, is the tremendous resources required to maintain it. To be functional, this model would likely require separate teams of technologists and nurses covering both AM and PM shifts.

The Remote Model is the most frequently utilized neurointerventional team activation method. In this model, the neurointerventional team is mobilized only after EVT candidacy has been confirmed by LVO and collateral circulation status. However, in this model team members (nurses and technologists) typically require 30 minutes to arrive at the hospital. In addition, preparing the patient for treatment usually requires an additional 30 minutes. In the best-case scenario, this results in a one-hour delay to initiate EVT. Nevertheless, it is not uncommon to experience delays greater than two hours. The major advantage of the Remote Model is its efficient use of resources (Table 2). On the other hand, its major disadvantage is the increased time required for the neurointerventional team to arrive at the hospital and prepare the patient for EVT.

Both the Ever-Ready and Remote Models have their respective strengths and weaknesses

(Table 2). If the strengths of both these models could be harnessed and their weaknesses eliminated, a more practical and efficient model would emerge. This is precisely the goal of the most efficient model - the Transitional Model. The Transitional Model is a more practical method in which hospital staff already present within the hospital are trained to transport LVO AIS patients to the neurointerventional suite and prepare them for intervention once EVT candidacy is confirmed. By employing the Transitional Model, hospital staff can both transport the LVO AIS patient and prepare them for EVT while the nurses and technologists that comprise the on-call neurointerventional team are traveling to the hospital. Typically, the neurointerventional team arrives within 30 minutes. During this time, in-house hospital staff can transport the patient to the neurointerventional suite and prepare the patient for EVT. The new 2018 American Heart Association/American Stroke Association Guidelines state "Systems should be designed, executed and monitored to emphasize expeditious assessment and treatment."[2] If this isn't an endorsement for the Transitional Model, I don't know what is.

TABLE 2. Neurointerventional Activation Models

Model	Resources	Delay
Ever Ready	↑	↓
Remote	↓	↑
Transitional	↓	↓

The big question is, which hospital staff would transport and prepare the LVO AIS patient for EVT before the neurointerventional team arrives? One option is to have the neurointensive care unit (NICU) nurse or the nurse who will be accepting the patient after EVT to be part of this transition team. In this manner, this nurse would learn about the patient before receiving them in the NICU. In addition to this nurse, at least one more person from the hospital staff would be required to assist her. The logical choice would be the emergency department nurse who is already caring for the patient. That way, the emergency department and NICU nurses can prepare the patient while waiting for the neurointerventional team to arrive. This model would reduce both healthcare cost and EVT activation time. By improving stroke efficiency, functional outcome is also enhanced.

The Transitional Model represents the optimal model for most stroke centers. It reduces treatment time like the Ever-Ready Model and also increases the efficiency of resources like the Remote Model (Table 2). Proper organization would allow any stroke center to engage in the Transitional Model. Hospital systems can provide enormous benefits to their community by engaging in this relatively simple concept. The Transitional Model also highlights another important concept. That is, all EVT image-confirmed candidates must be transferred to the neurointerventional lab as soon as possible. All assessments must be performed in the neurointerventional lab. This includes all consultations, NIHSS scoring, and evaluation from other services such as anesthesia. Performing any assessment in a location other than the neurointerventional lab such as the emergency department only delays recanalization and reduces optimal functional outcome. Every four minutes that the patient is not in the neurointerventional lab can result in a worse functional outcome.

Just as the MANGO™ mnemonic served as a bridge between the prehospital and hospital setting for LVO AIS screening, the Transitional Model serves as a bridge to increase neurointerventional efficiency. It accomplishes this feat by allowing the emergency department which receives the LVO AIS patient to interact with both the neurointerventional team that will treat the patient and the NICU nurse who will care for the patient after EVT. The Transitional Model streamlines EVT initiation and thereby contributes to our synchronous and efficient AIS assembly line.

29.5.2 "FAST" Procedure

Chapter 25 (Endovascular Treatment) discussed the benefits of conscious sedation over general anesthesia when performing EVT.[3-5] In addition to not intubating AIS patients, other factors that could also increase EVT efficiency must be considered. For example, is an arterial line necessary for EVT considering that placing an arterial line sometimes takes longer than the endovascular procedure itself? Is a Foley catheter really required for a 30-minute procedure? In addition to time efficiency issues, the 2018 AHA/ASA guidelines state, "Routine placement of indwelling bladder catheters should not be performed because of the associated risk of catheter-associated urinary tract infections."[2] If all the neurointerventionalists performing these procedures in one hospital use similar supplies, wouldn't it be easier to set up for these procedures? These factors that can reduce EVT reperfusion times are summarized by the mnemonic 'FAST' (Table 3).

TABLE 3. EVT Accelerators: **FAST**

F	Foley Catheter, No Foley Catheter
A	A Line, No A Line
S	Stock, Use Similar Supplies
T	Tube, No Tube (Intubation)

29.6 Conclusion

The efficient diagnosis and treatment of AIS cannot be overemphasized. The four categories that were discussed include AIS screening, image confirmation (diagnosis), quantification with the NIHSS, and treatment. These categories can be recalled using the mnemonic 'SINC' (Table 4). LVO AIS screening is particularly important because LVO AIS is responsible for nearly all ischemic stroke-related deaths, 90% of societal cost, and 80% of significant functional disability. EMS personnel should bring suspected LVO AIS patients to a CSC provided they can be transported in a timely fashion (≤ 30 minutes). Here, time efficiency and taking an LVO AIS patient to the correct hospital the first time can mean the difference between a good or poor functional outcome. The remainder of this chapter reviewed the importance of efficient AIS diagnosis and treatment. Efficiency, non-specialist physician, and even non-physician AIS assessment were emphasized.

TABLE 4. Stroke Efficiency Categories: **SINC**

S	Screening
I	Image Confirmation
N	NIHSS Quantification
C	Carry Out Treatment

AIS efficiency can be tremendously improved by critically evaluating the four categories mentioned above. The beginning of this chapter discussed the importance of the automobile assembly line. This introduced the concept of a "team approach" to an industry that was once managed by highly trained craftsmen who worked individually. This analogy can be extended to highly trained physicians, each with different training backgrounds. Specialist physicians, non-specialist physicians, and non-physicians must work together in a multidisciplinary fashion for efficient AIS diagnosis and treatment.

This chapter also outlined the step-by-step processes that allow the diagnosis and treatment of AIS to be performed efficiently (Figure 9). This process was broken down into the four categories of screening, diagnosis (image confirmation), quantification, and treatment. During the screening portion of this process, the MANGO™ mnemonic is utilized to synchronize both EMS and emergency department (ED) screening for LVO AIS. In addition, IV TPA restrictions and consent for EVT should be obtained (Figure 9). This completes the screening category. During the diagnosis portion of this process, neurointervention and neuroimaging should be initiated simultaneously. This means a noncontrast brain CT followed by either a CTP/CTA or dual phase CTA should be performed. I endorse the use of dual phase CTA because it is more efficient. All imaging should be obtained at the same time whenever possible. This completes the diagnosis category. After diagnosis (image confirmation) is complete, quantification with the NIHSS should be performed. After quantification, treatment is initiated. If this involves EVT, the transitional model, no general anesthesia, no Foley, no A-line and the use of similar stock material are all recommended to reduce treatment time.

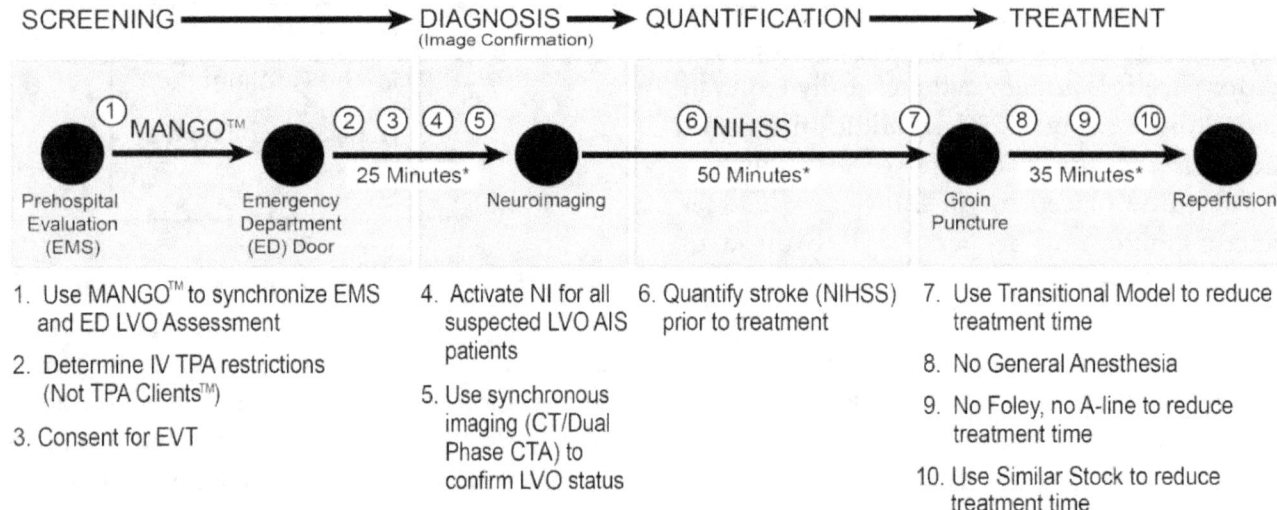

FIGURE 9. Stroke Efficiency and Endovascular Treatment (EVT)

MANGO™ = M - Motor Weakness, A - Aphasia; N - Neglect; G - Gaze Preference, Inability to Track or Double Vision, O - Ocular Field Cut or Blindness. AIS - Acute Ischemic Stroke, ED - Emergency Department, EMS - Emergency Medical Services, EVT - Endovascular Treatment, LVO - Large Vessel Occlusion, NI - Neurointervention, NIHSS - National Institute of Health Stroke Scale. * Adapted from: Saver, Jeffrey L., et al. "Time to Treatment With Endovascular Thrombectomy and Outcomes From Ischemic Stroke: A Meta-analysis." JAMA 316.12 (2016): 1279-1289

The assembly line reduced the time to produce a car by 90%. Shouldn't we strive to reduce stroke diagnosis and treatment time by 90% as well? The same philosophy that once interfered with the production of automobiles continues to confound both the diagnosis and treatment of AIS. The assembly line's efficiency resulted in the reduction of automobile cost. Shouldn't we work together in the same manner to reduce AIS health-related cost? The greatest aspect of the assembly line was its product, the automobile. It allowed most families and average working people to afford a car. Shouldn't we develop AIS protocols that are affordable and available to the American public? The automobile allowed people to live in remote and rural areas. Shouldn't we develop AIS protocols that can be employed by rural hospitals? The automobile allowed our civilization to flourish. Shouldn't we help our civilization flourish by maintaining the functionality of its citizens?

Abbreviations list

AIS, acute ischemic stroke; CSC, comprehensive stroke center; CT, computed tomography; CTA, computed tomography angiography; CTP, CT perfusion; ED, emergency department; EMS, emergency medical service; EVT, endovascular treatment; FDA, Food and Drug Administration; IV TPA, intravenous administration of recombinant tissue plasminogen activator; LVO, large vessel occlusion; NICU, neurointensive care unit; NIHSS, National Institutes of Health Stroke Scale; PSC, primary stroke center.

References

1. Taleb Mohammed S., et al. (2016). Stroke vision, aphasia, neglect (VAN) assessment—a novel emergent large vessel occlusion screening tool: pilot study and comparison with current clinical severity indices. *NeuroInterv Surg,* 16(7), 525-33.
2. Powers WJ, Rabinstein AA, Ackerson T, Adeoye OM, Bambakidis NC, Becker K, Biller J, Brown M, Demaerschalk BM, Hoh B, et al. (2018). Guidelines for the Early Management of Patients With Acute Ischemic Stroke: A Guideline for Healthcare Professionals From the American Heart Association/American Stroke Association. *Stroke,* Epub 24 Jan.
3. Abou-Chebl A, Lin R, Hussain MS, Jovin TG, Levy EI, Liebeskind DS, Yoo AJ, Hsu DP, Rymer MM, Tayal AH, Zaidat OO, Natarajan SK, Nogueira RG, Nanda A, Tian M, Hao Q, Kalia JS, Nguyen TN, Chen M, Gupta R. (2010). Conscious sedation versus general anesthesia during endovascular therapy for acute anterior

circulation stroke: preliminary results from a retrospective, multicenter study. *Stroke*, Jun, 41(6), 1175-79.

4. Jumaa MA, Zhang F, Ruiz-Ares G, Gelzinis T, Malik AM, Aleu A, Oakley JI, Jankowitz B, Lin R, Reddy V, Zaidi SF, Hammer MD, Wechsler LR, Horowitz M, Jovin TG. (2010). Comparison of safety and clinical and radiographic outcomes in endovascular acute stroke therapy for proximal middle cerebral artery occlusion with intubation and general anesthesia versus the nonintubated state. *Stroke*, Jun, 41(6), 1180-84.

5. Nichols C, Carrozzella J, Yeatts S, Tomsick T, Broderick J, Khatri PJ. (2010). Is periprocedural sedation during acute stroke therapy associated with poorer functional outcomes? *Neurointerv Surg*, Mar, 2(1), 67-70.

Chapter 30

Stroke Communication

This text discussed several principles related to acute ischemic stroke (AIS). However, none of these principles really matter if they are not effectively understood or applied. Stroke is a multidisciplinary endeavor requiring a team approach. For this team to function, it must utilize effective communication. The importance of consistent and reliable communication in the diagnosis and treatment of acute ischemic stroke (AIS) cannot be overemphasized.

Helen Keller was a remarkable woman who was born blind and deaf. Through enormous persistence and hard work, she learned to communicate by touch. This mode of communication, facilitated by sensation, was her form of language. In a sense, language is a symbol of reality. If one were to visualize an apple, one might think of a golden delicious apple, a Macintosh apple, a honey crisp apple, and so on. While Helen Keller never knew what an apple looked like, she was able to taste and smell it. So while she had never seen the color of an apple, she could conceptualize it. While her reality of an apple (based on taste and smell) varied from ours, Helen understood what the word for apple meant when it was impressed on her skin. That is, she could communicate with other people by using the same symbols of reality, *i.e. language*. If we cannot effectively communicate with each other, we are essentially deaf and blind. Tragically, this happens far too often in the world of stroke. For this reason, it is essential to adopt a universal vocabulary and use the same terms when dealing with stroke patients. A simple way to recall many of these terms is with the mnemonic 'CHOCOLATE' (Table 1).

Abbreviations list

AIS, acute ischemic stroke.

TABLE 1. Universal Stroke Vocabulary: **CHOCOLATE**

C	Core and Penumbra
H	NI**H**SS Score
O	Occlusion: LVO vs Non-LVO
C	CTA and CTP
O	Open Collaterals
L	Last Known Normal
A	ASPECTS
T	TICI Score
E	Embolic vs Thrombotic

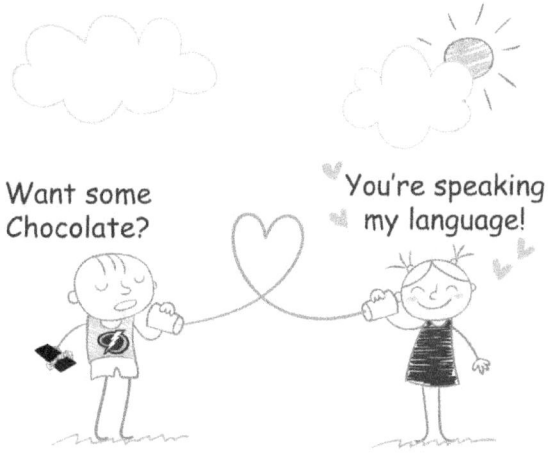

Chapter 31

Summary

"All things being equal, the simplest solution tends to be the best one."
— William of Ockham

31.1 Stroke

Stroke is an enormous problem facing both our nation and the world. Stroke can be classified as either ischemic or hemorrhagic stroke (Figures 1 and 2). Dedicated chapters (Chapter 6: Hemorrhagic Stroke, Chapter 7: Cerebral Aneurysms, Chapter 8: Vasculopathies, and Chapter 9: Cerebrovascular Malformations) discussed the various etiologies of hemorrhagic stroke such as hypertensive hemorrhage, cerebral amyloid angiopathy, aneurysmal subarachnoid hemorrhage (aSAH), perimesencephalic venous subarachnoid hemorrhage (PMVSAH), vasculitis, mycotic aneurysms, and hemorrhagic venous infarct. Cerebral aneurysms, vascular malformations, and vasculopathies were also reviewed.

FIGURE 1. Stroke Classification and Incidence

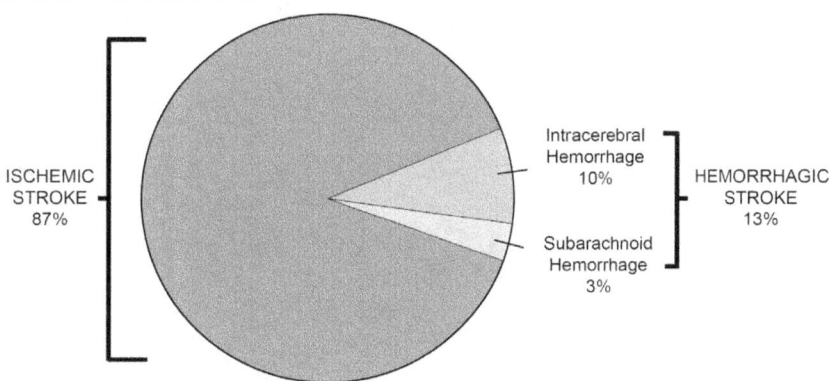

FIGURE 2. Classification of Stroke Subtypes

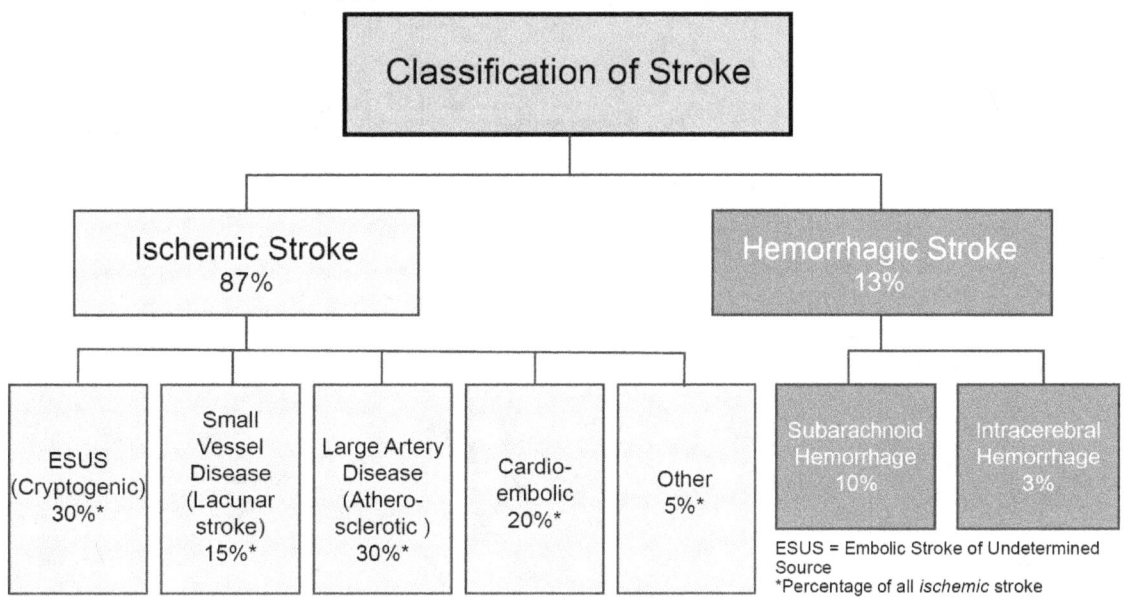

ESUS = Embolic Stroke of Undetermined Source
*Percentage of all *ischemic* stroke

31.2 Ischemic Penumbra and Core Infarct

The distinction between ischemic penumbra and core infarct determines the basis of all AIS treatment (Figure 3). The paramount goal of AIS treatment is the rapid restoration of cerebral perfusion to the ischemic penumbra. Without this potentially life-saving treatment, an ischemic penumbra can only last for so long before it transforms into an irreparably damaged core infarct (Figure 4). Conversely, there is no reason to treat patients with irreparable core infarct when there is no clinical benefit. Thus, health care professionals must be able to discern irreparably damaged (core infarct) from threatened but still salvageable (ischemic penumbra) brain tissue.

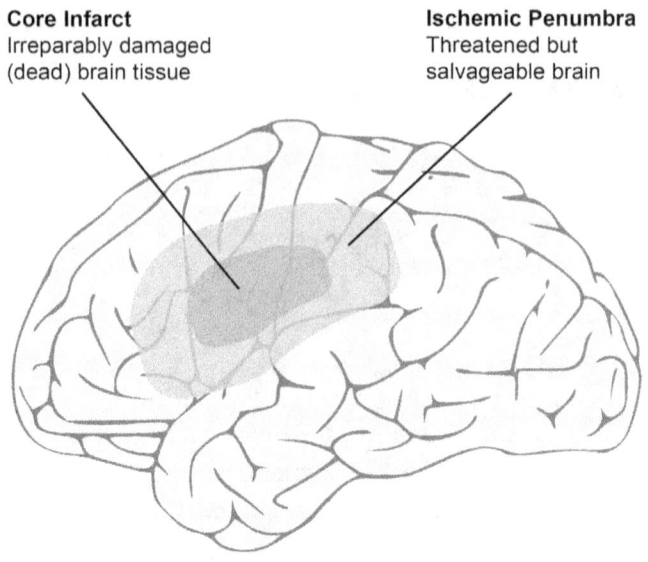

FIGURE 3. Core Infarct Versus Ischemic Penumbra

Core Infarct
Irreparably damaged (dead) brain tissue

Ischemic Penumbra
Threatened but salvageable brain

FIGURE 4. Progression of Ischemic Penumbra into Core Infarct

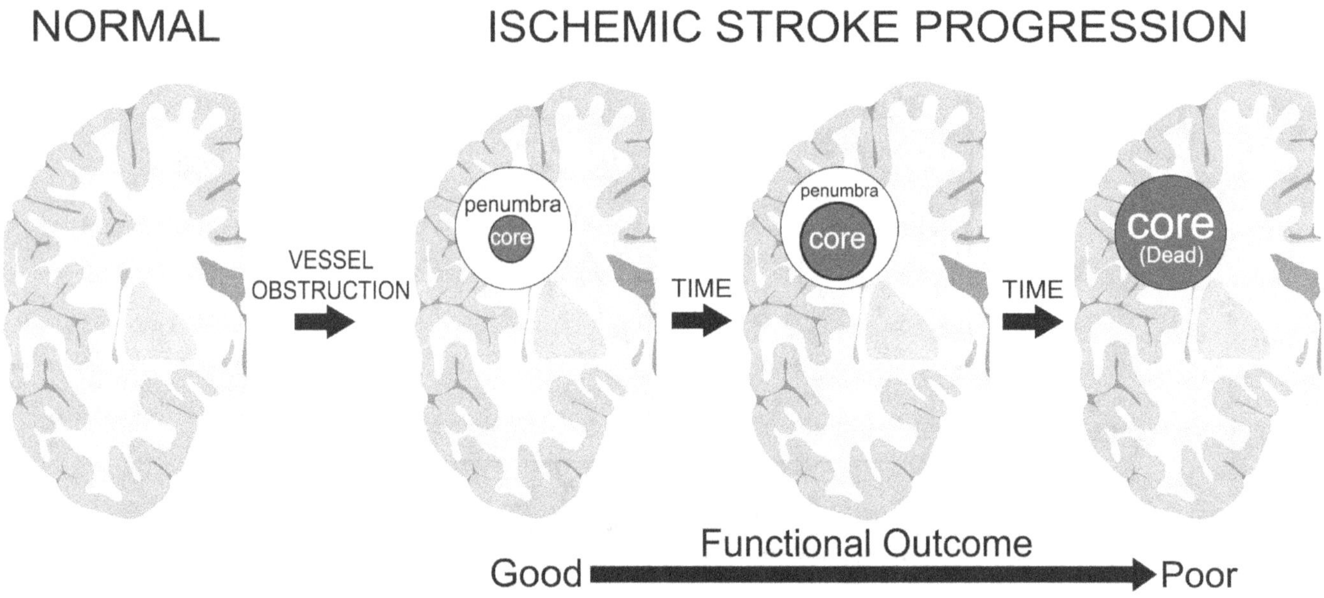

31.3 Cortical and Cerebrovascular Anatomy

Basic knowledge of neurologic and cerebrovascular anatomy is sufficient to diagnose and treat most AIS (Figure 5). The anterior circulation includes the segments and branches of the internal carotid artery, the middle cerebral artery, and the anterior cerebral artery (Figures 5, 6, 7 and 8). The posterior circulation includes both vertebral arteries, the posterior inferior cerebellar arteries (PICA), the basilar artery (BA), the anterior inferior cerebellar arteries (AICA), pontine perforators (PP), the superior cerebellar arteries (SCA), and the posterior cerebral arteries (PCA) (Figure 9).

Understanding these arterial territories, the regions of the cortex they supply and associated deficits help one determine a stroke plan (Figure 10 and Table 1).

FIGURE 5. Angiograms (AP) of Anterior and Posterior Circulation

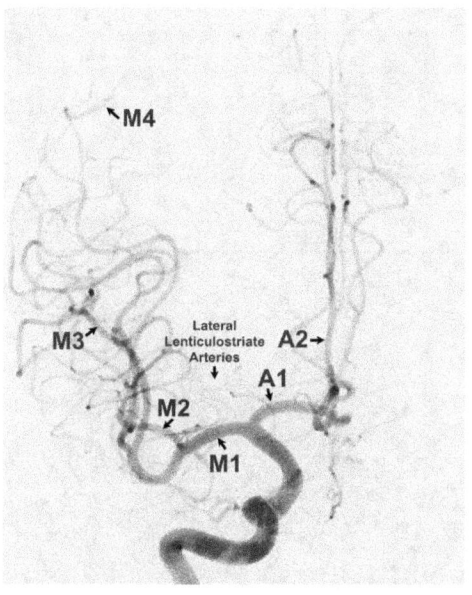
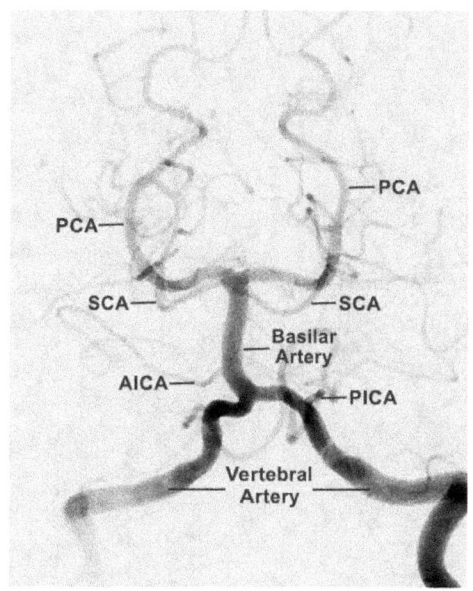

FIGURE 6. The 4 Segments of the Internal Carotid Artery (ICA)

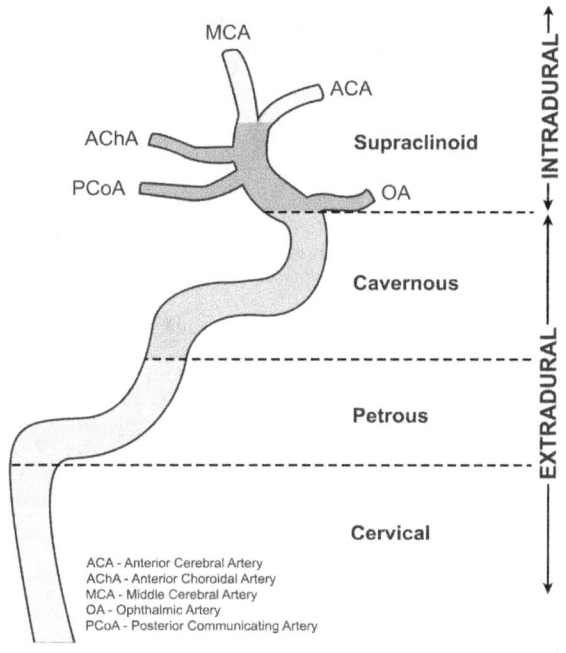

FIGURE 7. The 4 Segments of the Middle Cerebral Artery (MCA)

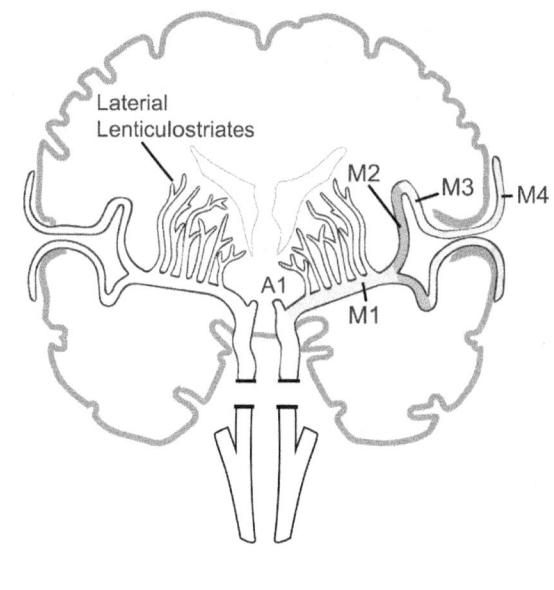

FIGURE 8. The Basic Anatomy of the Anterior Cerebral Artery (ACA)

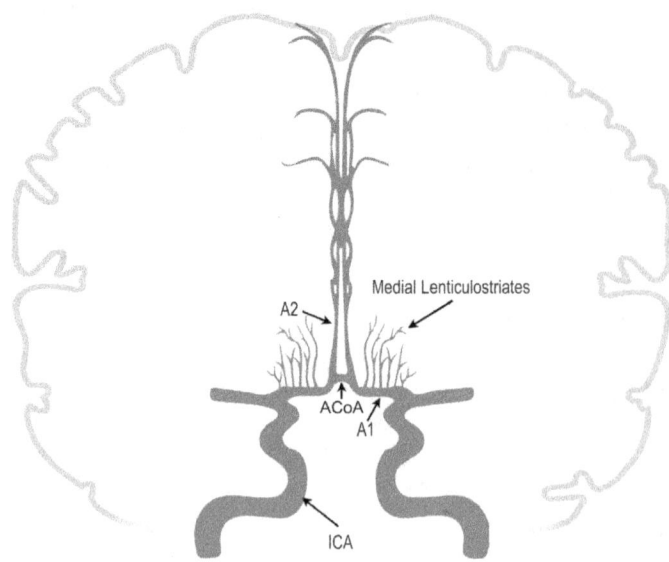

FIGURE 9. The Posterior Circulation

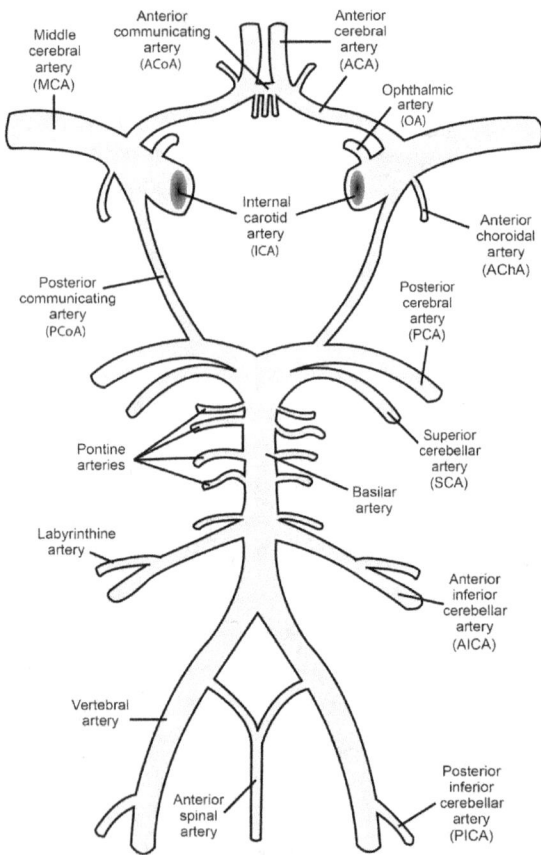
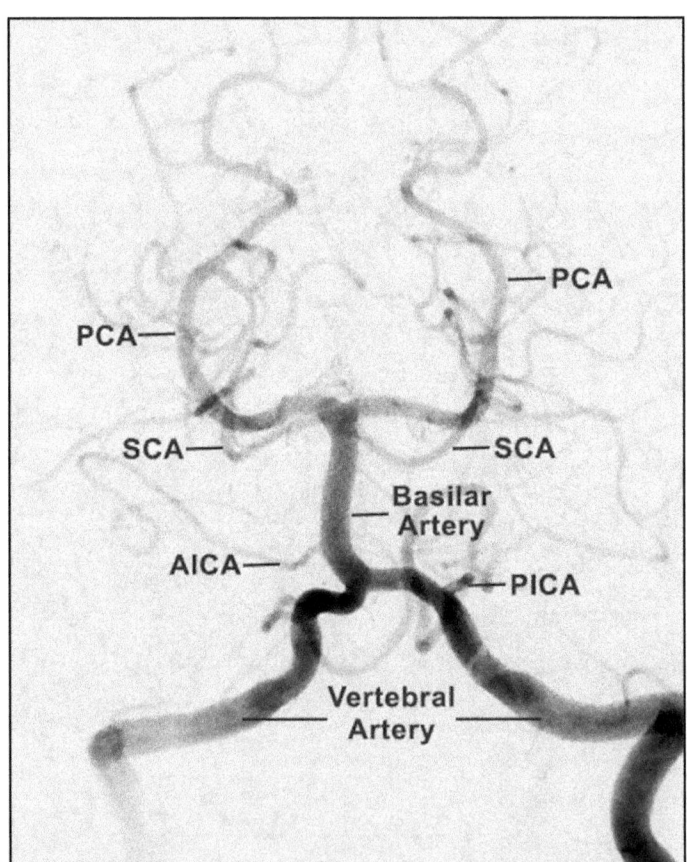

FIGURE 10. Cortical Regions and Associated Deficits

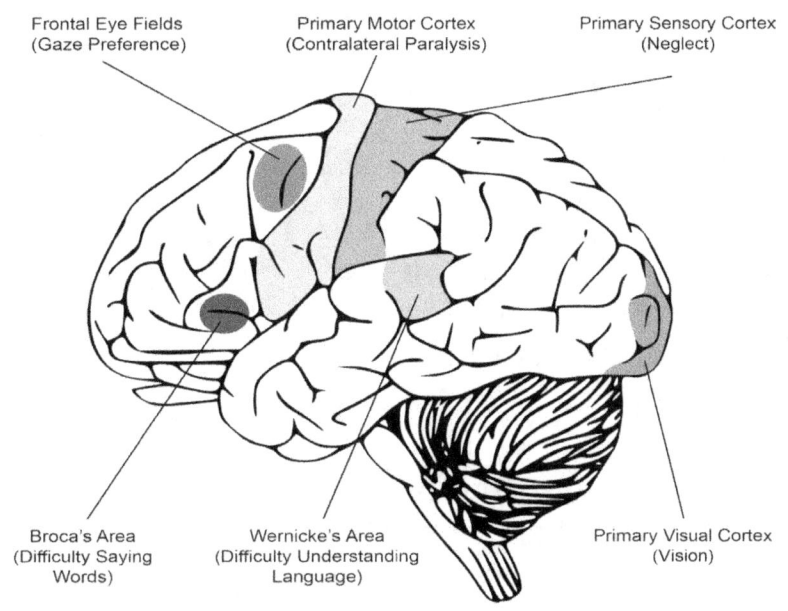

Cortical Structure	Location	Function
Frontal Eye Fields (FEF)	Frontal Lobe	Eye Movement
Primary Motor Cortex	Frontal Lobe	Voluntary Movement
Broca's Area	Frontal Lobe	Production of Speech
Primary Sensory Cortex	Parietal Lobe	Sensation
Wernicke's Area	Temporal Lobe	Language Comprehension
Primary Visual Cortex	Occipital Lobe	Vision

TABLE 1. The Stroke Plan: S-PLAN

S	Source (embolic or thrombotic)
P	Pathophysiology (etiology)
L	Location (of brain affected)
A	Artery (arterial territory involved)
N	Neuroimaging

Source	Pathophysiology	Location	Artery	Neuroimaging
• Embolic • Thrombotic	**C**: Cardioembolic (20%) **A**: Atherosclerotic large vessel disease (30%) **U**: Undetermined etiology - ESUS (30%) **S**: Small vessel disease or lacunar infarct (15%) **E**: Everything else or other (5%)	• Frontal • Parietal • Temporal • Occipital • Cerebellar • Thalamic • Brainstem	• ICA • MCA • ACA • Vertebral • Basilar • PICA • ACA • SCA	• CT • CTA • CTP • MRI • MRA • Angio

31.4 Posterior Circulation Stroke

Posterior circulation stroke can be classified into *cerebellar stroke, brainstem stroke, thalamic stroke,* and *occipital lobe stroke.* Cerebellar stroke can present as a variety of deficits but its five principal symptoms are gait abnormalities, ataxia, tremor, ocular motor abnormalities, and hypotonia (Tables 2 and 3). Proper neurologic examination of cerebellar function is necessary (Box 1). Cerebellar stroke that exclusively presents as vertigo poses an enormous diagnostic challenge.

TABLE 3. The Five Principal Signs of Cerebellar Dysfunction: **GATOR**

G	Gait
A	Ataxia
T	Tremor
O	Oculomotor Abnormalities
R	Relaxed Muscles or Hypotonia

TABLE 2. Cerebellar Stroke Symptoms: **DARK NIGHT DIVA**

D	**Dysmetria** - inability to judge distance and stop movement at a chosen point
A	**Ataxia** - uncoordinated movement
R	**Relaxed muscles**, hypotonia (floppy and weak muscles)
K	**Kinesia** - Dysdiadochokinesis, inability to perform rapidly altering movements (i.e. pronation and supination of hands). Dysrhythmokinesis, disorder of the rhythm of rapid alternating movements.
N	**Nystagmus**
I	**Intention tremor** - during movement and not at rest
G	**Gait abnormality** (one form of ataxia)
H	**Headache**
T	**Tipsy** - vertigo, falls to injured side
D	**Dysphonia** - slurred explosive speech
I	**Ipsilateral motor symptoms**
V	**Vomiting** and nausea
A	**Asynergia** - loss of motor coordination, jerky movements

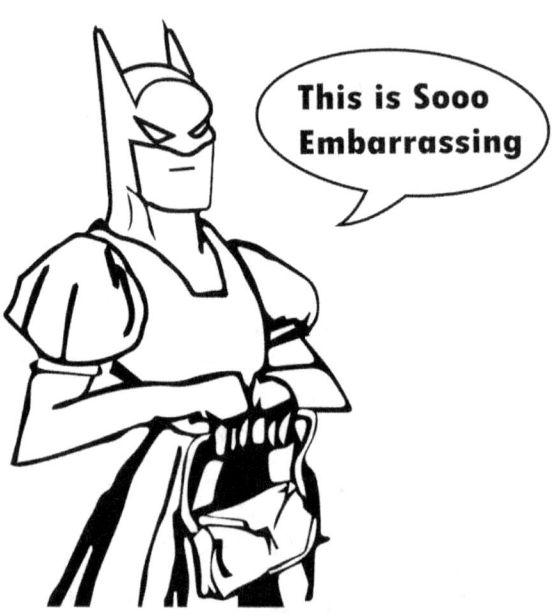

BOX 1. Cerebellar Examination: **HAL**

H: Head	Nystagmus Overshooting of eyes "Ahhh" "La, La, La"
A: Arms (Upper Extremities)	Thigh slapping Finger to nose Tap on a tune
L: Lower Extremities	Stand at rest Gait Heel-to-toe Heel-to-knee Heel-to-shin

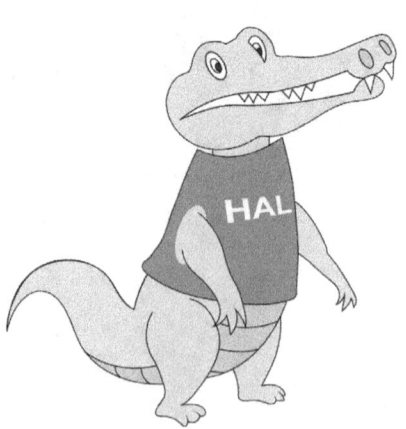

The four major forms of benign vertigo necessary to differentiate from cerebellar stroke include *benign paroxysmal positional vertigo (BPPV), migrainous vertigo, Ménière's disease* and *vestibular neuritis*. BPPV has symptom duration lasting for less than one minute whereas vestibular neuritis can present as hours or days of continuous vertigo (Table 4). These benign entities have differences in their presentation and physical exam compared to cerebellar stroke (Figure 11). Specific symptoms that suggest cerebellar stroke include direction-changing nystagmus, severe ataxia, the inability to walk, vascular risk factors and sudden, immediate symptoms (Table 5). Specific symptoms favoring neuroimaging (preferably DWI MRI and MRA) include the inability to walk, direction changing nystagmus. and any focal neurologic deficit (Table 6).

TABLE 4. Benign Paroxysmal Positional Vertigo (BPPV) and Vestibular Neuritis

Vertigo Cause	Symptoms	Exam
BPPV	Intense, less than 1 minute symptoms Positional exacerbation	Dix-Hallpike
Vestibular Neuritis	Hours or days of continuous vertigo Positional exacerbation	HINTS

TABLE 5. Clues to Cerebellar Infarction: **DIVAS**

D	Direction Changing Nystagmus
I	Inability to Walk
V	Vascular Risk Factors
A	Ataxia, Severe
S	Sudden Immediate Symptoms

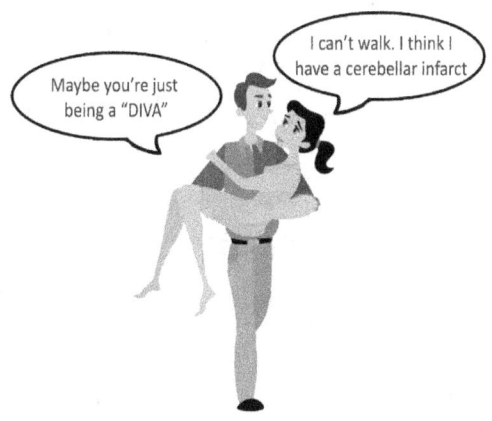

TABLE 6. Indications for Neuroimaging for Vertigo: **IDA**

I	Inability to Walk Without Support
D	Direction-Changing Nystagmus
A	Any Focal Neurologic Deficit

FIGURE 11. Vertigo Algorithm

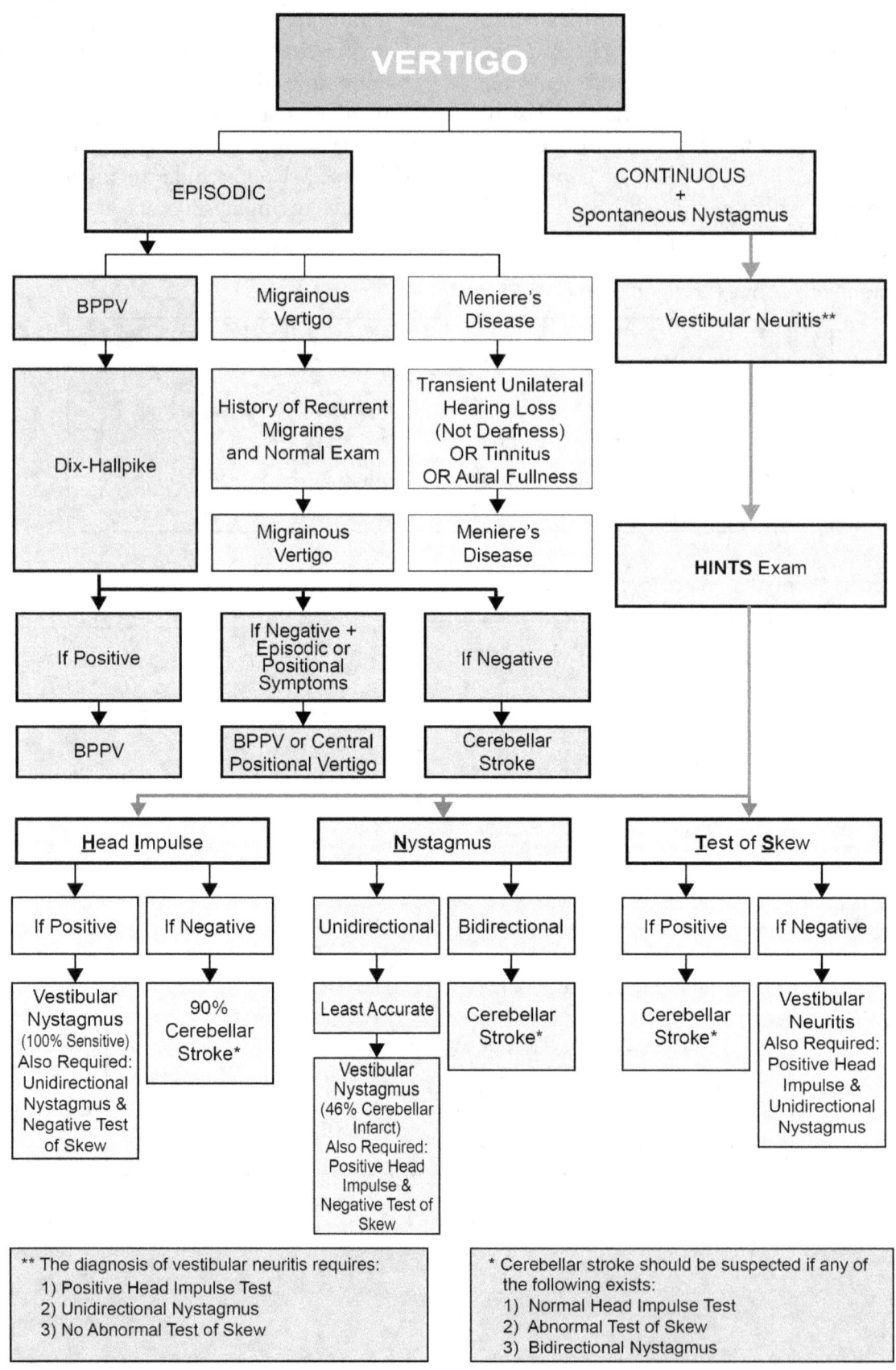

Thalamic stroke can cause any type of stroke symptom including motor weakness, aphasia, neglect, and cognitive or visual abnormalities. Because the thalamus has a distinct role in arousal and vigilance, loss of consciousness associated with AIS suggests thalamic involvement. The thalamus can also be divided into four distinct vascular regions, each of which has a specific constellation of symptoms (Figure 12 and Table 7). Thalamic lacunar infarct was also reviewed (Chapter 5, Ischemic Stroke).

The brainstem consists of the midbrain, the pons, and the medulla (Figure 13). Like the thalamus, the brainstem contains multiple cranial nerve nuclei and neural pathways. The neural pathways (located either medially or laterally) run up and down the brainstem in a cranial-caudal direction and the cranial nerves typically run perpendicular to them. The location of neural pathways and cranial nerves within the brainstem are summarized by "the four rules of the brainstem" (Figure 14). The intersection location of a cranial nerve and neural pathway can predict specific brainstem vascular syndromes within the pons and medulla (Figure 14). The midbrain (the most superior component of the brainstem) has a more complex, less predictable vascular supply but characteristic midbrain vascular syndromes exist (Figure 15). The occipital lobe is predominantly associated with vision and the visual pathway has many different regions of arterial supply throughout its course (Figure 16).

FIGURE 13. The Brainstem

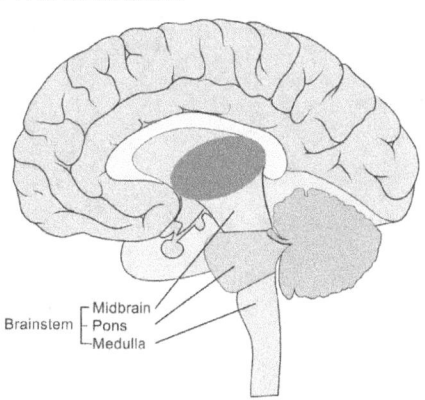

FIGURE 12. The Thalamic Vascular Supply

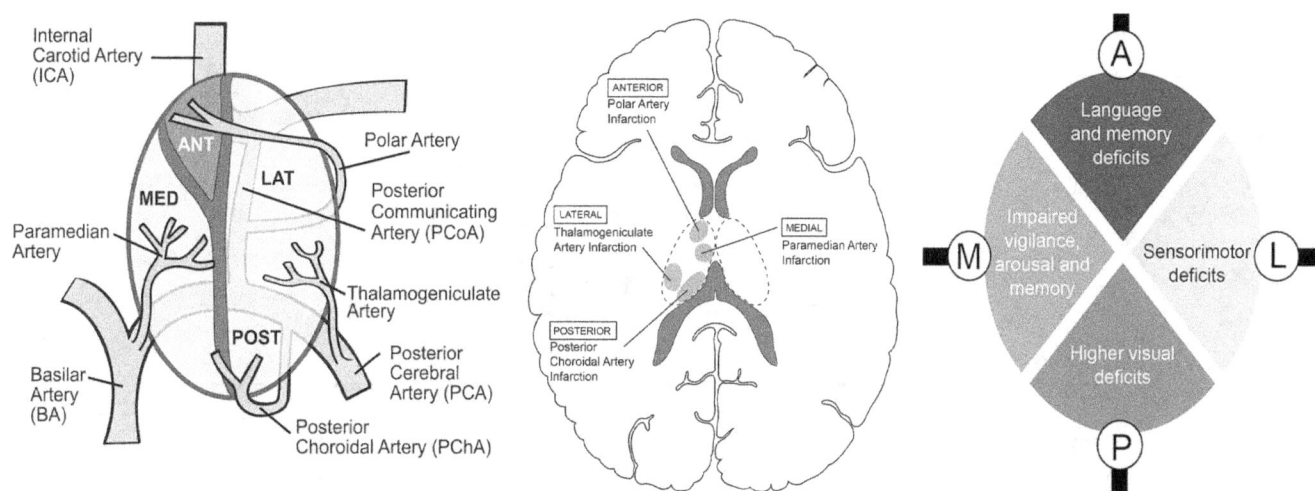

TABLE 7. Thalamic Deficits and Associated Regions

	Deficit	Region	Artery	Origin
L	Language, (Dominant) and Memory	Anterior	Polar Artery (Absent in 40%)	PCoA
M	Motor and Sensory	Lateral	Thalamogeniculate Artery	P2
A	Arousal, Vigilance and Memory	Medial	Paramedian Artery	P1
O	Optic or Visual	Posterior	Posterior Choroidal Artery	P2

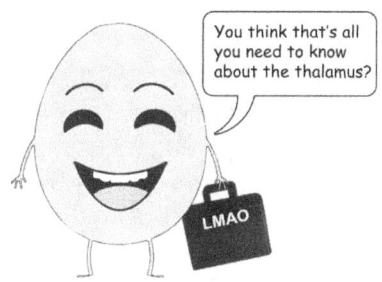

Stroke Made Simple

FIGURE 14. The Four Rules of the Brainstem

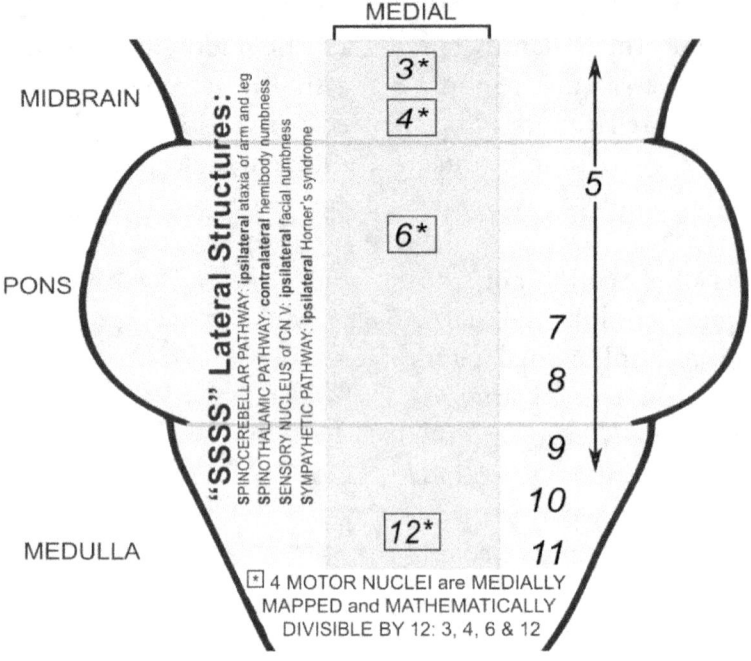

"MMMM" 4 MIDLINE STRUCTURES
MOTOR PATHWAY (corticospinal tract): **contralateral** hemibody (arm and leg) weakness
MEDIAL LEMNISCUS: **contralateral** hemibody numbness (loss of vibration and proprioception)
MEDIAL LONGITUDINAL FASCICULUS: **ipsilateral** internuclear ophthalmoplegia
MOTOR NUCLEUS AND NERVE: **ipsilateral** cranial neuropathy (3, 4, 6 or 12)

"SSSS" Lateral Structures:
SPINOCEREBELLAR PATHWAY: **ipsilateral** ataxia of arm and leg
SPINOTHALAMIC PATHWAY: **contralateral** hemibody numbness
SENSORY NUCLEUS of CN V: **ipsilateral** facial numbness
SYMPATHETIC PATHWAY: **ipsilateral** Horner's syndrome

4 MOTOR NUCLEI are MEDIALLY MAPPED and MATHEMATICALLY DIVISIBLE BY 12: 3, 4, 6 & 12

FIGURE 15. Midbrain Vascular Syndromes

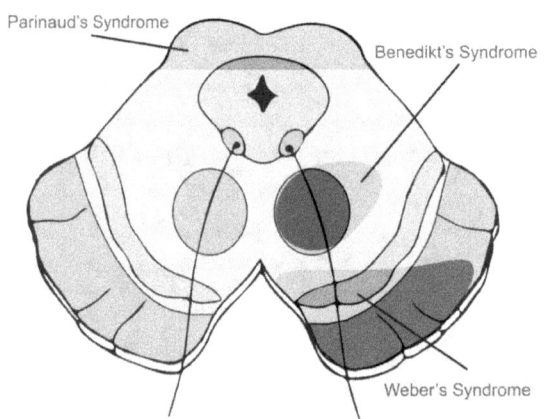

Syndrome	Structure	Cranial Nerve	Tracts	Deficits
Weber	Base	III	Corticospinal	Oculomotor palsy with crossed hemiplegia
Claude	Tegmentum	III	Red nucleus and brachium conjunctivum	Oculomotor palsy with contralateral cerebellar ataxia and tremor
Benedikt	Tegmentum	III	Red nucleus, corticospinal and brachium conjunctivum	Oculomotor palsy with contralateral cerebellar ataxia, tremor and corticospinal signs
Nothnagel	Tectum	Unilateral or Bilateral III	Superior cerebellar peduncle	Ocular palsies; paralysis of gaze and cerebellar ataxia
Parinaud	Dorsal		Supranuclear mechanism for upward gaze and other structures in periaqueductal gray matter	Paralysis of upward gaze and accommodation, fixed pupils

FIGURE 16. The Arterial Territories of the Visual Pathway

Ophthalmic Artery: Retina and extracranial optic nerve

Anterior Cerebral, Anterior Communicating and Hypophyseal Artery: Intracranial optic nerve and optic chiasm

Middle Cerebral Artery and Posterior Cerebral Artery: Optic Radiation

Posterior Communicating and Anterior Choroidal Arteries: Optic tract

Anterior and Posterior Choroidal Arteries: Lateral geniculate nucleus

Posterior Cerebral Artery: Primary visual cortex

31.5 TIAs, Stenting, Stroke Mimics, and Secondary Stroke Prevention

Transient ischemic attack (TIA), stenting, venous stroke, and stroke mimics were discussed. A newer image-based definition of TIAs differentiates high-risk AIS patients (with imaging findings) from low-risk TIA patients (without imaging findings) (Table 8). Carotid and vertebral artery dissection were also discussed. The CADISS Trial demonstrated no significant difference between anticoagulation (heparin or Lovenox® bridging to warfarin) and antiplatelet (aspirin, dipyridamole, or clopidogrel alone or in combination) treatment for recurrent stroke prevention or death. The 2018 AHA/ASA Guidelines recommend: "For patients with AIS and extracranial carotid or vertebral artery dissection, treatment with either antiplatelet or anticoagulant therapy for 3 to 6 months may be reasonable."[1] The indications for carotid endarterectomy, carotid stenting, intracranial angioplasty, and intracranial stenting were reviewed. Both the SAMMPRIS and VISSIT Trials concluded aggressive medical management is the safest treatment option for intracranial atherosclerotic disease.

TABLE 8. **TIA**

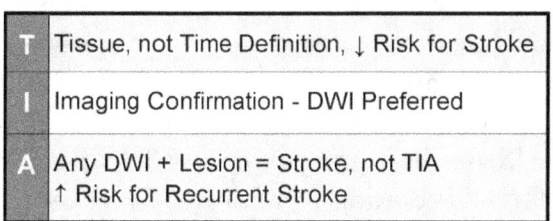

T	Tissue, not Time Definition, ↓ Risk for Stroke
I	Imaging Confirmation - DWI Preferred
A	Any DWI + Lesion = Stroke, not TIA ↑ Risk for Recurrent Stroke

The role of secondary stroke prevention examined platelet inhibition and microembolic disease. The CHANCE Trial demonstrated that the administration of clopidogrel and aspirin provided greater benefits than either the administration of aspirin or clopidogrel alone, leading to a new 2018 AHA/ASA guideline recommendation: "In patients presenting with minor stroke, treatment for 21 days with dual antiplatelet therapy (aspirin and clopidogrel) begun within 24 hours can be beneficial for early secondary stroke prevention for a period of up to 90 days from symptom onset."[1]

Stroke mimics must also be considered in the management of every potential AIS patient (Table 9). If one has difficulty discerning between a stroke mimic and AIS, remember the *stroke mimic rule*: **If the diagnosis of a stroke mimic** cannot be confirmed before or within the IV TPA treatment time window (4.5 hours), assume the patient has an AIS and administer IV TPA. The new 2018 AHA/ASA guidelines state that "the risk of symptomatic intracranial hemorrhage in the stroke population is quite low; thus, starting IV alteplase is probably recommended in preference over delaying treatment to pursue additional diagnostic studies."[1]

31.6 The Evolution of Acute Ischemic Stroke (AIS) Treatment

The chapters discussing the National Institutes of Health Stroke Scale (NIHSS), stroke imaging, collateral circulation, IV TPA, wake-up stroke, and endovascular treatment (EVT) focused on AIS diagnosis and treatment specifics. The paramount goal of AIS treatment is the rapid restoration of cerebral perfusion to the ischemic penumbra. Failing to do so will transform threatened brain tissue (ischemic penumbra) into irreparably damaged core infarct. Currently, recanalizing occluded blood vessels and restoring perfusion to the ischemic penumbra is the only way to treat AIS. The only two FDA-approved treatment options for AIS are the administration of IV TPA and/or EVT. The evolution of both these treatment options was presented (Box 2).

BOX 2. The Evolution of Acute Ischemic Stroke (AIS) Treatment

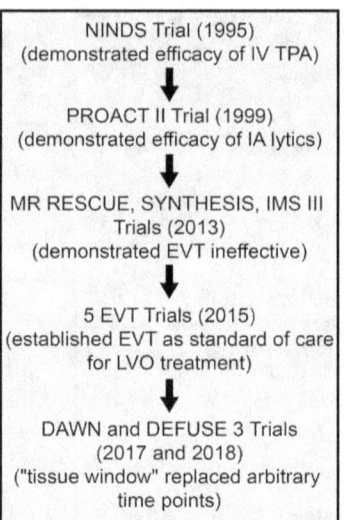

31.7 IV TPA

The decision to administer IV TPA is based on many factors and arbitrary time points (Tables 10 and 11). Imaging restrictions for IV TPA include hemorrhage or hypodense brain tissue that is >1/3 the MCA distribution. Hypodense brain tissue (core infarct) must be distinguished from isodense tissue swelling (ischemic penumbra) (Box 3). CTA and CTP imaging criteria for core infarct and ischemic penumbra were reviewed along with other imaging criteria (Box 4). IV TPA's previous 3-hour therapeutic window from stroke onset may be expanded up to 4.5 hours. Previous 3 to 4.5-hour ECASS III exclusion criteria according to the new 2018 AHA/ASA guidelines "may not be justified in practice" (Table 12).[1] The 2018 AHA/ASA guidelines allow the extended use of IV TPA between 3 and 4.5 hours for AIS patients who are > age 80, taking warfarin with an INR ≤ 1.7, had a prior stroke, and are diabetic. These same guidelines do however state, "The benefit of IV alteplase between 3 and 4.5 hours from symptom onset for patients with very severe stroke symptoms (NIHSS > 25) is uncertain." Excluding a significant infarct (>1/3 MCA) and severe stroke (NIHSS > 25), the current 2018 AHA/ASA guidelines have nearly eliminated the previous ECASS III exclusion criteria for the administration of IV TPA 3 to 4.5 hours from symptom onset.

TABLE 9. Stroke Mimics: **MIMICKERS**™

M	Metabolic-Hypoglycemia or Hyperglycemia
I	Ictal-Seizures
M	Multiple Sclerosis
I	Intracranial Lesions (traumatic, infectious, hemorrhagic and neoplastic)
C	Classic and Specific Migraine Subtypes
K	Keep Balance? (Vestibular Dysfunction)
E	Encephalopathy
R	Regular Diastolic Pressure
S	Sepsis

TABLE 10. IV TPA Inclusion Criteria: **CAN**

C	Clinical Diagnosis of Ischemic Stroke (Measure Role Neurologic Deficit)
A	Age > 18 (18-80 for 3-4.5 hrs)
N	Need to Initiate Treatment Within 4.5 Hours

TABLE 11. IV TPA Restrictions: **NOT TPA CLIENTS**™

N	Non-Enhanced Contrast CT >1/3 MCA
O	Onset of Symptoms >4.5 Hrs or UNKNOWN
T	Ten, Intracranial Aneurysm ≥10mm
T	Tumor, Intra-Axial or GI (or GI Bleed <21d)
P	Prior Ischemic Stroke Within 3 Months
A	Aortic Dissection (Suspected)
C	Coagulopathy: Coumadin (if INR >1.7) and Coumadin Analogs (Direct Thrombin Inhibitors or Direct Factor Xa Inhibitors) PT >15, aPTT >40, PLTS <100,000 & INR >1.7
L	Low Molecular Weight Heparin <24 Hours (Full Treatment Dose, Not Prophylactic Dose)
I	Intracranial Hemorrhage - Acute or 3 Month History
E	Endocarditis, Infectious (Suspected)
N	Noncompressible Vessel Puncture Within 7 Days (Safety and Efficacy of IV TPA Uncertain)
T	Trauma, Severe Head Within 3 Months
S	Surgery, CNS (Intracranial or Spine) Within 3 Months

BOX 3. Imaging Characteristic of Penumbra versus Core

Puffy = **P**enumbra
Hypo**D**ense Brain = **D**ead Core

BOX 4. Imaging Characteristic of Penumbra versus Core

Study	Ischemic Penumbra	Core Infarct
Brain CT	Isodense Tissue Swelling	Hypodensity
Multi- or Dual Phase CTA	Good or Intermediate Collaterals	Poor Collaterals
CTP	Mismatched (↓CBF - ↑CBV)	Matched (↓CBF - ↓CBV)

TABLE 12. Previous* Required Criteria for IV TPA from 3 - 4.5 hours: **EXPAND**

E	Eighty, ≤80	
X	X-Rays, CT ≤1/3 MCA	Previous ECASS III exclusion criteria* are no longer required to EXPAND the use of IV TPA
P	Prior Stroke and Diabetes History Excluded	
A	Anticoagulant - Excluded Regardless of INR Value	
N	NIHSS Score <25	
D	Diabetes and Prior Stroke History Excluded	

*Excluding a significant infarct (>1/3 MCA) and severe stroke symptoms (NIHSS >25), the new 2018 AHA/ASA guidelines have removed the previous ECASS III exclusion criteria for the administration of IV TPA 3 to 4.5 hours after symptom onset.

In addition to its narrow therapeutic window and low effectiveness for LVO AIS, there are other limitations associated with the use of IV TPA (Figure 17). Perhaps, the greatest limitation of IV TPA is that less than 5% of AIS patients receive it. Despite these limitations, IV TPA has a proven and effective role in AIS treatment and should be administered whenever possible (Figure 18).

FIGURE 17. Limitations of IV TPA

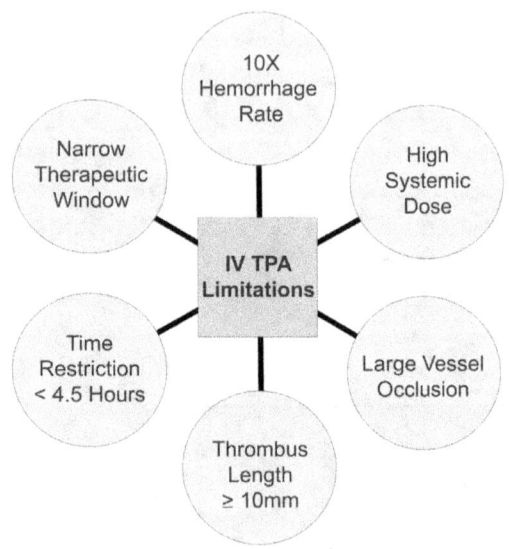

FIGURE 18. Need to Treat Number for IV TPA, EVT and STEMI Patients

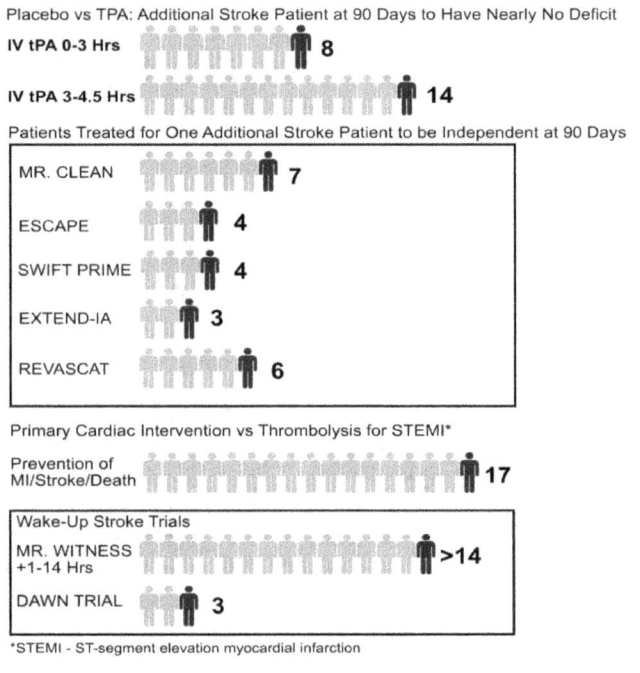

*STEMI - ST-segment elevation myocardial infarction

31.8 Endovascular Treatment (EVT)

Endovascular treatment (EVT) is one of the most important and powerful treatment modalities in any field of medicine (Table 13). The enormous success of the five 2015 EVT trials resulted in a paradigm shift in LVO AIS treatment, which is now the standard of care. Analysis of the five 2015 EVT trials demonstrated three essential components required for successful EVT. First, neuroimaging must demonstrate the presence of an LVO and salvageable brain tissue. Next, paradigm shifts in workflow are required to reduce recanalization times. Finally, stent retrievers improved recanalization rate and time. LVO AIS patients require rapid diagnosis and treatment consisting of rapid screening, imaging confirmation, and recanalization.

TABLE 13. EVT vs IV TPA

Functional Independence in 2015 EVT Trials Versus IV TPA		
	Endovascular Treatment	IV TPA Alone
ESCAPE	53.0%	29.3%
EXTEND-IA	71.0%	40.0%
MR CLEAN	32.6%	19.1%
REVASCAT	43.7%	28.2%
SWIFT PRIME	60.0%	35.0%

The 2015 EVT trial results led to the 2015 American Heart Association/American Stroke Association (AHA/ASA) guidelines and additional insights. These recommendations (which are neither inclusion nor exclusion criteria) include patients age ≥18, LVO, ASPECTS ≥ 6, NIHSS score ≥ 6, and treatment initiation (groin puncture) within six hours (Table 14). Subsequent research trials such as the MR WITNESS and DAWN Trials demonstrated IV TPA and EVT can be effective up to 24 hours. Despite the findings of the MR WITNESS Trial, the 2018 AHA/ASA guidelines discourage the use of neuroimaging criteria for IV TPA treatment determination in wake-up ischemic stroke patients.[1]

In addition to the DAWN Trial, the DEFUSE 3 Trial also used neuroimaging and not arbitrary time points to determine patient candidacy. Both of these titanic trials indicated that EVT for LVO AIS was effective beyond six hours for appropriate image-selected patients demonstrating adequate collateral circulation. Individual collateral circulation is determined by unique physiology and not arbitrary time points. However, this collateral circulation maintains perfusion for only a limited period of time. Thus, it is always important to perform EVT as efficiently as possible. Without timely EVT and reperfusion, LVO AIS patients will suffer large debilitating strokes. The core insights gleaned from both of these trials are summarized in Table 15. The profound results of both the DAWN and DEFUSE 3 Trials led to changes in the 2018 ASA/AHA guidelines recommendations for both imaging and mechanical thrombectomy (Tables 16 and 17).[1] The DAWN and DEFUSE 3 eligibility criteria are also summarized below (Table 18).

TABLE 14. AHA/ASA Recommendations for EVT: **ATLAS**

A	Age ≥18 Years
T	Treatment Initiated (Groin Puncture) Within 6 Hours
L	LVO (ICA or MCA M1 Segment)
A	ASPECTS ≥6
S	Score: NIHSS ≥6, Prestroke mRS 0-1

ASPECTS - Alberta Stroke Program Early CT Score, EVT - Endovascular Treatment, LVO - Large Vessel Occlusion, NIHSS - National Institutes of Health Stroke Scale, mRS - Modified Rankin Scale

TABLE 15. DAWN and DEFUSE 3 Trial Insights: **TITAN**

T	Time Window No Longer Determines Eligibility
I	Imaging Determines Eligibility
T	Thrombectomy *Recommended* Between 6-16 Hours, *Reasonable* at 6-24 Hours*
A	Always Accelerate Treatment
N	No EVT if Eligible Leads to Bad Outcomes

*EVT is *recommended* for LVO AIS patients within 6 and 16 hours of last known normal (LKN) and meet "other" DAWN or DEFUSE 3 eligibility criteria.
EVT is *reasonable* 6 to 24 hours after LKN and meet "other" DAWN criteria.

TABLE 16. Summary of 2018 AHA/ASA EVT Recommendations

Time Period	Recommendation
<6 Hours	EVT **should be** performed if the following criteria are met: **ATLAS** **(A)** Age ≥18 years, **(T)** Treatment initiated (groin puncture) within 6 hours of symptom onset, **(L)** LVO - Large Vessel Occlusion (ICA or MCA M1 segment), **(A)** ASPECTS ≥6 NIHSS score ≥6, **(S)** Score: Pre-stroke mRS score 0-1. EVT may be **reasonable** for MCA M2 or M3 segment occlusions. EVT may be **reasonable** for ACA, the vertebral artery, basilar artery or PCA occlusion. EVT may be **reasonable** for pre-stroke mRS score >1, ASPECTS <6, NIHSS score <6 and ICA or MCA M1 segment occlusion.
6-16 Hours from LKN	EVT is **recommended** for anterior circulation LVO that meet other DAWN or DEFUSE 3 eligibility criteria.
6-24 Hours from LKN	EVT is **reasonable** for anterior circulation LVO that meet other DAWN eligibility criteria.

ACA - Anterior Cerebral Artery, ASPECTS - Alberta Stroke Program Early CT Score, EVT - Endovascular Treatment, ICA - Internal Carotid Artery, LVO - Large Vessel Occlusion, MCA - Middle Cerebral Artery, mRS - Modified Rankin Scale, NIHSS - National Institutes of Health Stroke Scale, PCA - Posterior Cerebral Artery

TABLE 17. Summary of 2018 AHA/ASA Imaging Recommendations

Initial Imaging	Noncontrast brain CT within 20 minutes of arrival in the ED in at least 50% of patients who may be IV TPA and/or EVT candidates
<6 Hours From LKN EVT Eligible AIS Patients	Noninvasive intracranial vascular study should not delay IV TPA (if eligible)
	Reasonable to perform CTA for suspected LVO without serum creatinine concentration so long as no history of renal impairment
	MR or CT perfusion studies not recommended to determine EVT candidacy <6 hours from symptom onset
	Reasonable to utilize collateral flow status to determine EVT candidacy
6-24 Hours from LKN	Advanced neuroimaging (CTP, DWI - MRI or MR perfusion) to determine perfusion – core mismatch and maximum core size is recommended to help determine EVT candidacy

CT - Computerized Tomography, CTA - Computed Tomography Angiography, DWI - Diffusion-Weighted Magnetic Resonance Imaging, ED - Emergency Dept., EVT - Endovascular Treatment, LKN - Last Known Normal, LVO - Large Vessel Occlusion, TPA - Tissue Plasminogen Activator, MR - Magnetic Resonance, MRI - Magnetic Resonance Imaging

TABLE 18. Summary of the DAWN and DEFUSE 3 Eligibility Criteria

Trial Inclusion	Criteria	mRS Score	Age	NIHSS	Infarct	LVO	Exclusion Criteria
DAWN	LKN 6-24 hrs	0-1	≥80	≥10	≤20cc	ICA or MCA M1	Imaging Exclusion Criteria: MIAMI VICE***
	Clinical: Mismatch	0-1	<80	≥10	≤30cc		
		0-1	<80	≥20	31-50cc		
DEFUSE 3	Clinical: ANTMAN*	≤2	18-90	≥6	<70cc	ICA or MCA M1	A MESSI SPAGHETTI PLATE****
	Imaging: CORP**	≤2					

*ANTMAN = (A) Acute anterior circulation ischemic stroke, (N) NIHSS >6, (T) Time - EVT initiated 6-16 hours from stroke onset (groin puncture), (M) mRS ≤2 prior to qualifying stroke, (A) Age 18-90 Years, (N) Necessary Consent.

**CORP = (C) Core infarct <70cc, (O) Occlusion of ICA or MCA (M1), (R) Ratio of penumbra to a core infarct ≥1.8, (P) Penumbra ≥15cc.

***MIAMI VICE = (M) mass effect with midline shift, (I) intracranial stent in same vascular territory, (A) aortic dissection (suspected), (M) multiple vascular territory occlusions, (I) intracranial tumor, (V) vasculitis (suspected), (I) intracranial hemorrhage, (C) carotid dissection, severe stenosis or occlusion, (E) excessive tortuosity of cervical vessels

****A MESSI SPAGHETTI PLATE = (A) ASPECTS <6, (M) Multiple vascular territory occlusions, (E) Evidence of ICA dissection that is flow limiting or aortic dissection, (S) Significant mass effect with midline shift, (S) Stent that precludes safe EVT, (I) Intracranial process (hemorrhage, neoplasm or AVM), (S) Seizures at stroke onset if baseline NIHSS cannot be obtained, (P) Pregnancy, (A) Allergic to iodine, (G) Glucose <50 mg/dL or >400 mg/dL, (H) Hypertension that is severe and sustained (SBP >185 mmHg or DBP >110 mmHg, (E) Expectancy of life <6 months, severe or terminal illness, (T) TPA given 3-4.5 hours after LKN and any of the following: age >80, current anticoagulant use, history of diabetes or prior stroke, (T) TPA given >4.5 hours after LKN, (I) Interference of neurologic or functional evaluation by pre-existing disease, (P) Platelet count <50,000/µl, (L) Limited scanning, unable to obtain CTP or MRI, (A) Abnormality of labs (INR >3) or bleeding abnormality, (T) Tried EVT prior to 6 hours from stroke onset, (E) Embolus presumed septic, endocarditis - suspicion of bacterial.

ICA - Internal carotid artery, LKN - Last known normal, MCA - Middle cerebral artery, TPA - Tissue plasminogen activator

31.9 Stroke Efficiency

Stroke centers should strive to match new critical time points to improve functional outcome (Figure 19). While some research discourages the use of general anesthesia when performing EVT, the 2018 AHA/ASA guidelines state that since there is limited prospective randomized data and because only two small RCTs demonstrated no superiority of either treatment, "either method of procedural sedation is reasonable."[1] Certainly, there are many options for AIS treatment. However, whatever option is chosen, it is of paramount importance to always maintain efficiency and drive down diagnosis and treatment times. The mantra for all AIS intervention is to **find them fast and fix them fast!**

FIGURE 19. Recommended EVT Time Points

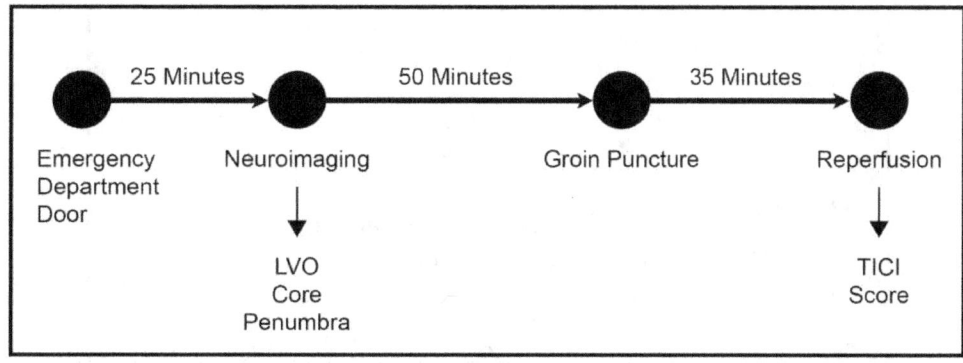

Adapted from: Saver, Jeffrey L., et al. "Time to Treatment With Endovascular Thrombectomy and Outcomes From Ischemic Stroke: A Meta-analysis." *JAMA* 316.12 (2016): 1279-1289

31.10 Prehospital Screening

The diagnosis of LVO AIS can no longer be considered a separate prehospital and hospital process. LVO AIS screening must involve emergency medical services (EMS) personnel and physicians working together to develop rapid and reliable protocols. EMS and physicians must collaborate to prioritize LVO AIS-suspected patients in the prehospital setting. LVO AIS represents only 11% of all AIS but this small fraction of stroke is responsible for all AIS related deaths, 90% of AIS cost, and 80% of significant functional disability. Thus, suspected LVO AIS patients should be transported to a comprehensive stroke center (CSC) in a timely manner (less than 30 minutes). EVT nearly doubles functional outcome and is now the new standard of care for LVO AIS. Unfortunately, 30% of LVO AIS patients transferred from a primary stroke center (PSC) to a CSC arrive too late for EVT (ischemic penumbra decays into a core infarct).

31.11 Stroke Protocols

The MANGO™ mnemonic not only increases the speed and accuracy of screening for LVO AIS; it also performs another critical function (Table 19). That is, the MANGO™ mnemonic can be effectively utilized by nonspecialist physicians and even by non-physicians so both may partake in an efficient and synchronous AIS management process. The exam on which the mnemonic is based upon was utilized by emergency department nurses with 100% correlation to their stroke physician counterparts, allowing a team approach to evaluate AIS. These emergency department nurses not only evaluated patients for LVO; they also ordered subsequent testing (CTA). Every member of a stroke center team should understand the diagnosis and treatment of AIS. At the very least, every hospital system should have the capacity to differentiate LVO from non-LVO AIS patients. This is because LVO AIS is by far the most devastating form of AIS and requires our utmost attention. For this reason, **stroke protocols must be dependent on LVO status** (Figure 20). The initial prehospital and hospital evaluation of all AIS patients should include the MANGO™ mnemonic to screen for LVO AIS status, determine hospital destination, and establish imaging protocols (Table 19, Figures 20, 21, and 22). All AIS must be diagnosed and treated quickly. This process can be simplified into five basic protocols (Figure 22). These include: (1) LVO AIS < 6 hours of symptom onset, (2) (1) LVO AIS 6-24 hours of symptom onset, (3) non-LVO mild AIS, (4) transient ischemic attack (TIA), and (5) stroke mimic or no stroke. LVO AIS imaging protocols can also be applied to those AIS patients with an NIHSS score ≥ 6 (the current AHA/ASA guideline NIHSS score recommendation for EVT candidacy). Understanding these five categories, rapid screening protocols, and neuroimaging permit any hospital to diagnose and treat most AIS. However, neurology (if available) should be consulted for the evaluation of every potential AIS patient.

TABLE 19. LVO Screening Mnemonic: **MANGO**™

M	Motor Weakness

A	Aphasia
	    Expressive (name 2 objects)
	    Receptive (follow 2 commands)

N	Neglect
	    Unable to feel both sides at the same time, or
	    Unable to identify own arm, or
	    Ignoring one side

G	Gaze Preference, Inability to Track or Double Vision
O	Optic Field Cut or New Blindness

CHAPTER 31: Summary

FIGURE 20. Prehospital Acute Ischemic Stroke (AIS) Assessment

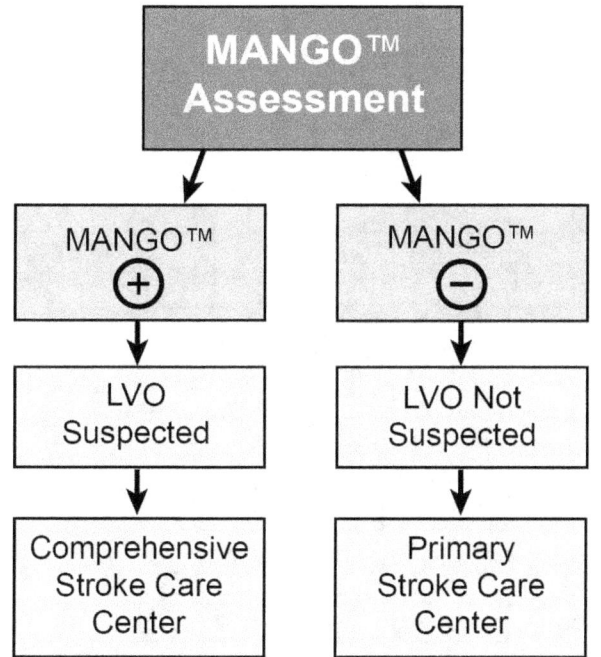

FIGURE 21. Functional and Physiologic Neuroimaging to Assess Viable Brain Tissue

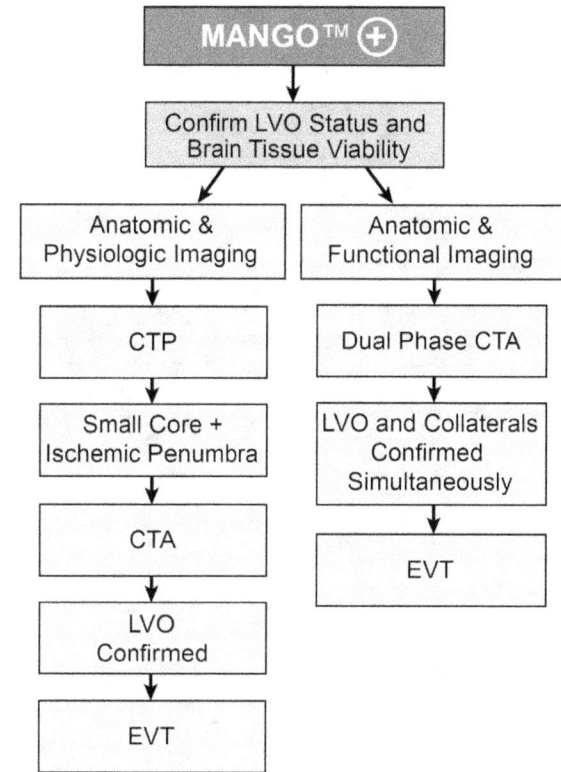

Stroke Made Simple

FIGURE 22. Acute Ischemic Stroke (AIS) Diagnosis and Treatment Protocols

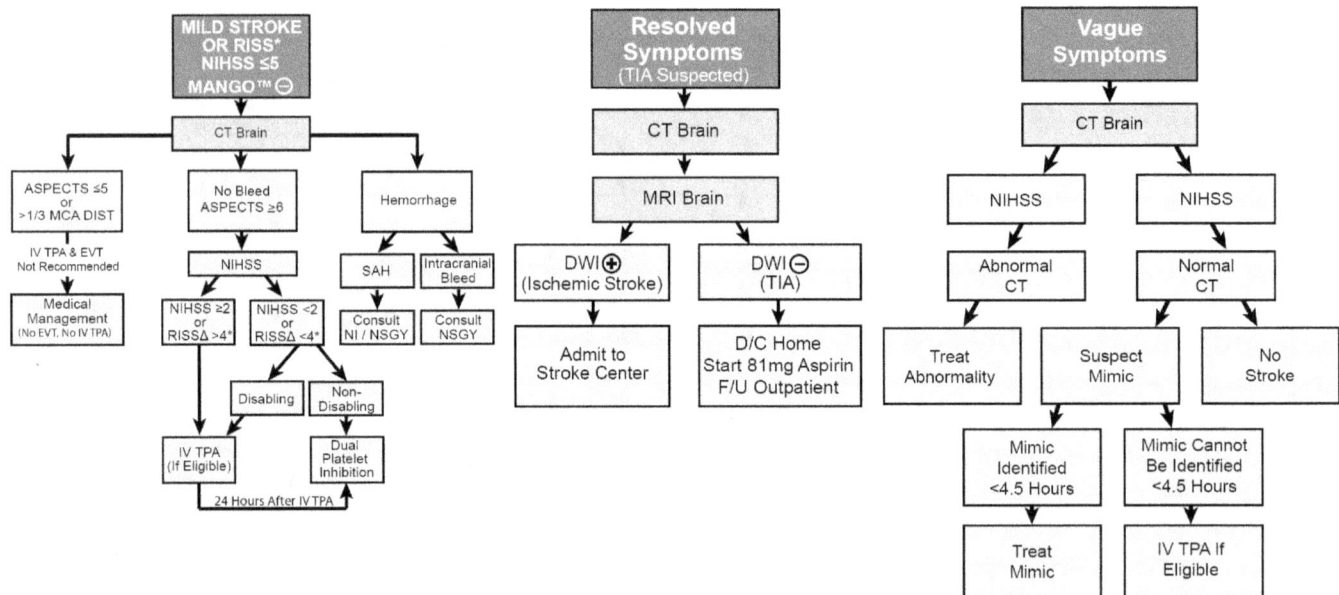

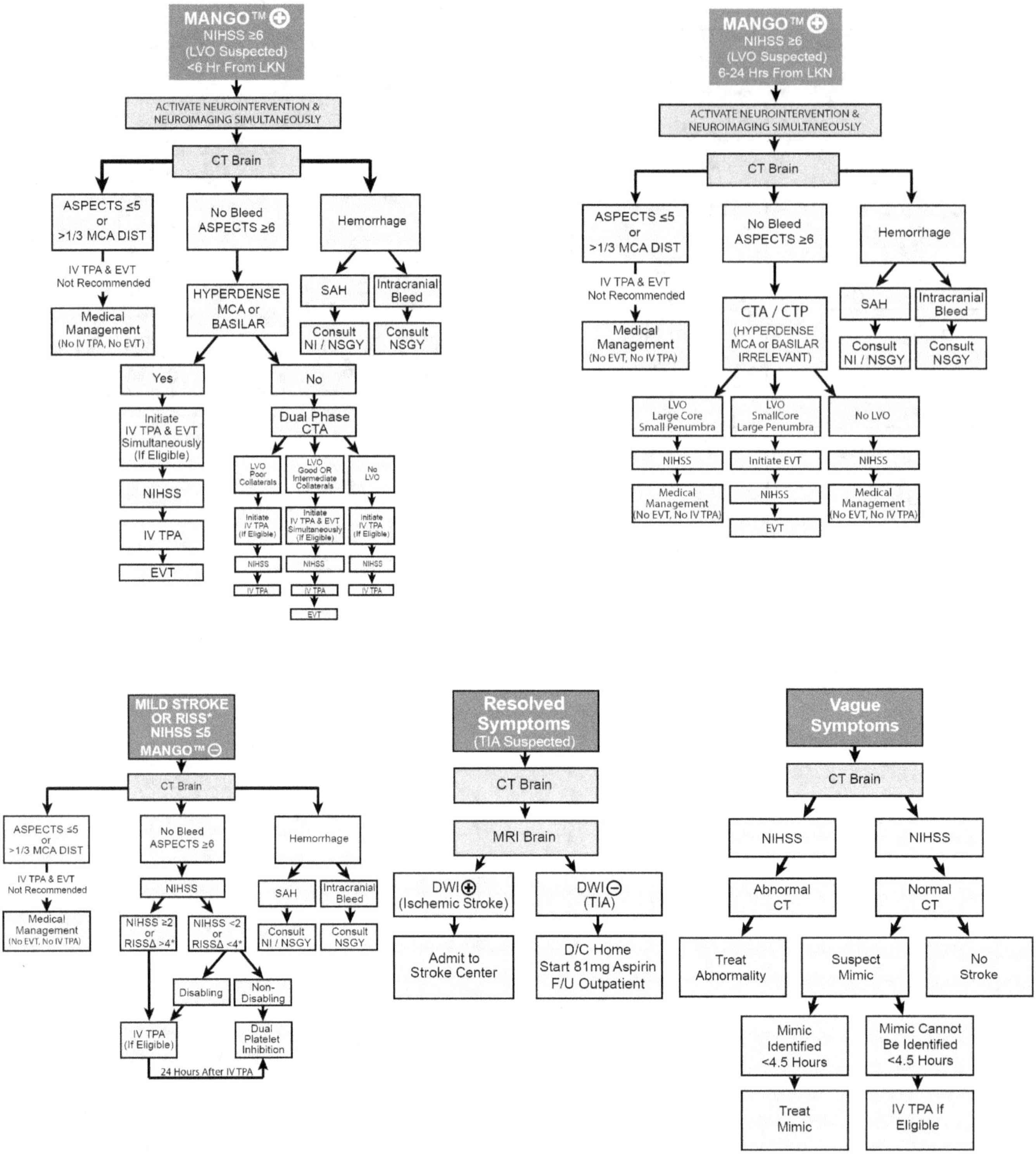

ASPECTS - Alberta Stroke Program Early CT Score, CTA - Computed Tomography Angiogram, CTP - Computed Tomography Perfusion, D/C - Discharge, Dist - Distribution, DWI - Diffusion Weighted Imaging, F/U - Follow-up, EVT - Endovascular Treatment, LKN - Last Known Normal, LVO - Large Vessel Occlusion, MCA - Middle Cerebral Artery, MRI - Magnetic Resonance Imaging, NI - Neurointervention, NIHSS - National Institutes of Health Stroke Scale, NSGY - Neurosurgery, RISSΔ >4 - Rapidly Improving Stroke Symptoms with a change in NIHSS score >4 points, SAH - Subarachnoid Hemorrhage, IV TPA - Intravenous Tissue Plasminogen Activator

31.12 Large Vessel Occlusion (LVO) or Non-LVO

The diagnosis and treatment of AIS have many overlapping concepts that can be further simplified. For example, from a purely binary standpoint, dividing all AIS diagnosis and treatment into LVO and non-LVO AIS categories is greatly beneficial. This can be done by using either the MANGO™ mnemonic or an NIHSS score ≥ 6 (based on the 2018 AHA/ASA guidelines). Using this binary approach, one can see that the diagnosis and treatment of AIS are immensely simplified (Figures 23, 24 and 25). Of course, all LVO AIS suspected patients require image confirmation prior to treatment.

FIGURE 23. Binary Approach for AIS Diagnosis and Treatment Determined by LVO Status

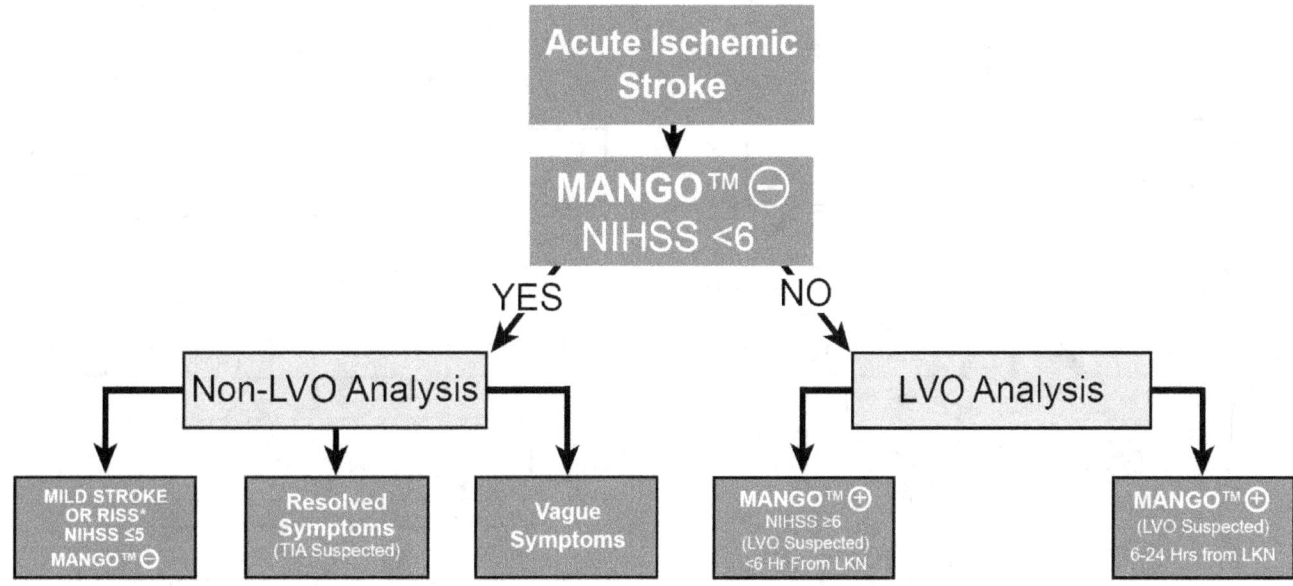

FIGURE 24. Large Vessel Occlusion Acute Ischemic Stroke (LVO AIS) Management, < 6 Hours and 6-24 Hours

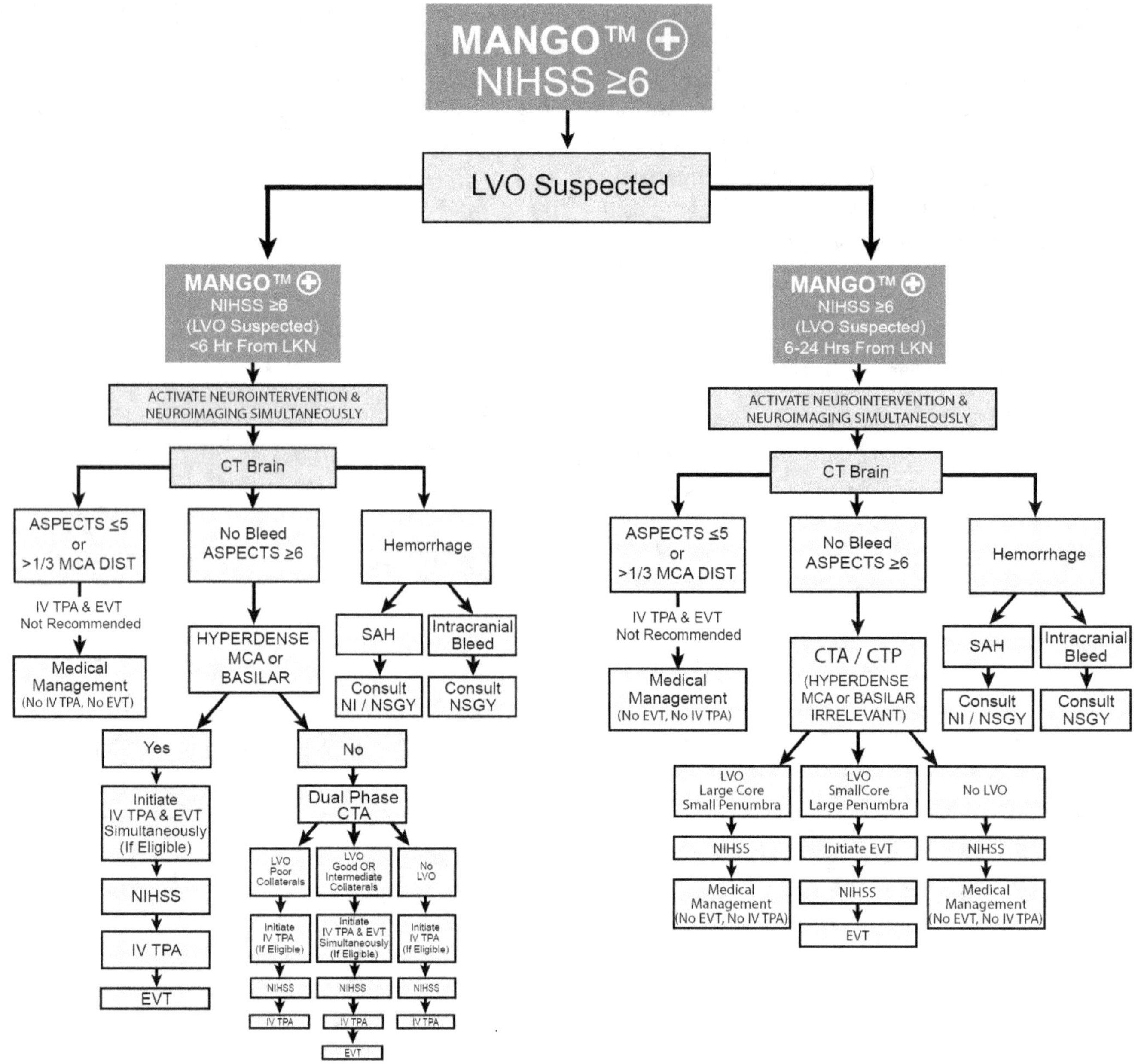

ASPECTS - Alberta Stroke Program Early CT Score, CTA - Computed Tomography Angiogram, CTP - Computed Tomography Perfusion, D/C - Discharge, Dist - Distribution, DWI - Diffusion Weighted Imaging, F/U - Follow-up, EVT - Endovascular Treatment, LKN - Last Known Normal, LVO - Large Vessel Occlusion, MCA - Middle Cerebral Artery, MRI - Magnetic Resonance Imaging, NI - Neurointervention, NIHSS - National Institutes of Health Stroke Scale, NSGY - Neurosurgery, SAH - Subarachnoid Hemorrhage, TPA - Tissue Plasminogen Activator

FIGURE 25. Non-LVO (Mild) or No Acute Ischemic Stroke

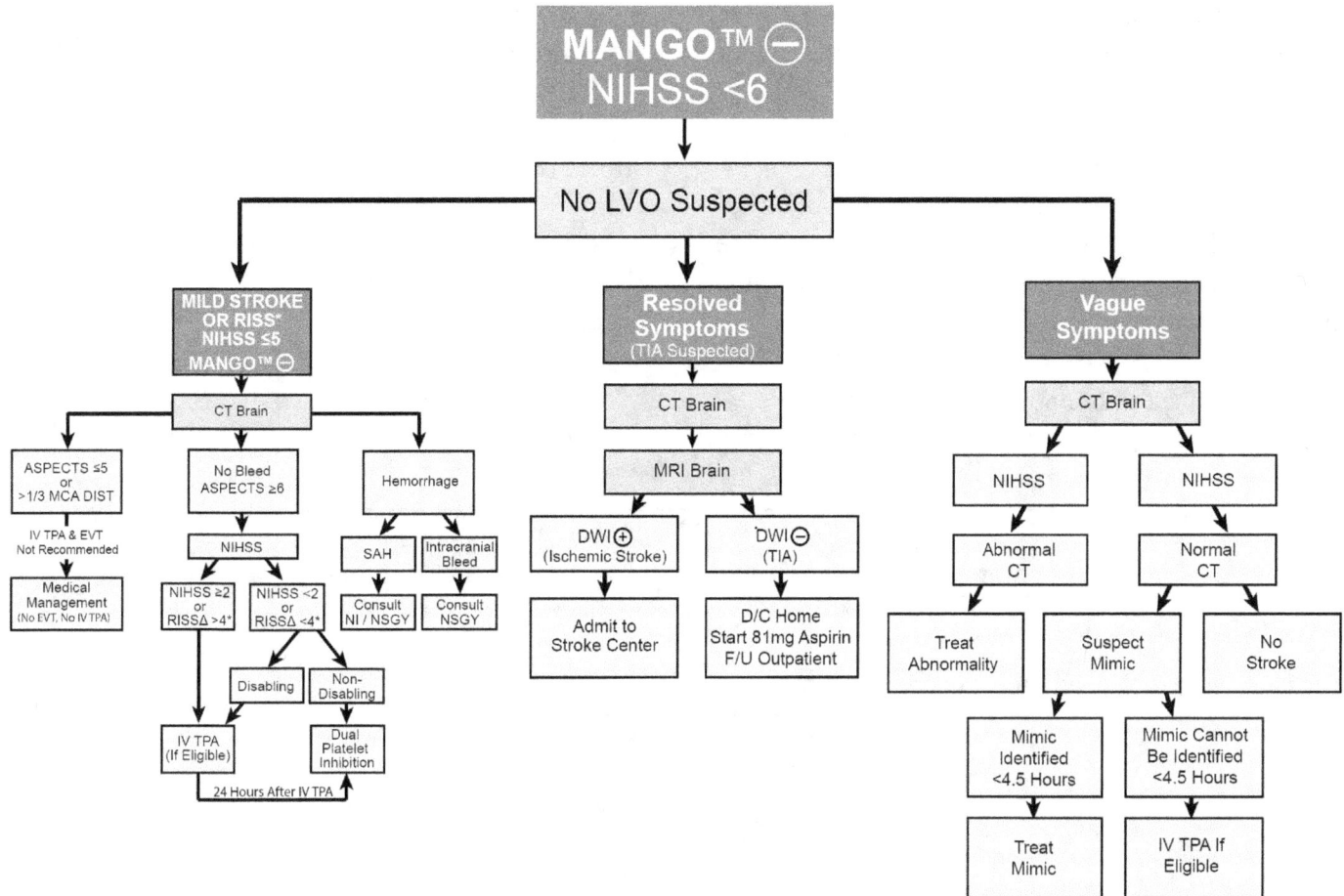

ASPECTS - Alberta Stroke Program Early CT Score, CTA - Computed Tomography Angiogram, CTP - Computed Tomography Perfusion, D/C - Discharge, Dist - Distribution, DWI - Diffusion Weighted Imaging, F/U - Follow-up, EVT - Endovascular Treatment, LKN - Last Known Normal, LVO - Large Vessel Occlusion, MCA - Middle Cerebral Artery, MRI - Magnetic Resonance Imaging, NI - Neurointervention, NIHSS - National Institutes of Health Stroke Scale, NSGY - Neurosurgery, RISSΔ >4 - Rapidly Improving Stroke Symptoms with a change in NIHSS score >4 points, SAH - Subarachnoid Hemorrhage, TIA - Transient Ischemic Attack, TPA - Tissue Plasminogen Activator

This binary approach is essential for several reasons which bear repeating. First, LVO stroke accounts for only 11% of all AIS but is responsible for nearly all AIS related deaths, 90% of societal cost, and 80% of significant functional disability. Thus, it is essential to identify and treat these patients quickly. Again, suspected LVO AIS patients can be categorized by being either MANGO™-positive or with an NIHSS score ≥ 6. Suspected non-LVO AIS patients, on the other hand, can be categorized as being either MANGO™-negative or having an NIHSS score < 6. Another way of saying this is suspected non-LVO AIS patients can be categorized as having an NIHSS score ≤ 5.

An NIHSS score ≤ 5 is one of the common descriptors of minor stroke. As discussed in Chapter 28, an operational definition of minor stroke cannot be based on an NIHSS score alone, but it is a great place to start. Conceptually, dividing LVO and non-LVO AIS is tremendously important to reduce the complexity surrounding the diagnosis and treatment of all AIS. This is because more than half of all AIS patients initially present with non-LVO or mild ischemic stroke. Furthermore, a significant number of these patients do not receive IV TPA treatment. Worse, a considerable percentage of untreated patients suffer bad outcomes. The treatment of mild or minor stroke is difficult because currently, neither an accepted definition exists nor is there an NIHSS score cut-off point to direct thrombolytic therapy.

An NIHSS score ≤ 5 is merely suggested as a consideration for the diagnosis of minor stroke. While minor stroke is commonly defined as an NIHSS score of 5 or less, this definition requires further consideration because there are no specific NIHSS criteria for the recommended use of IV TPA in mild AIS. Rather than focusing on a specific NIHSS score, it may be helpful to determine what impact current deficits will have on an AIS patient's quality of life. Based on this analysis, mild AIS can be divided into *mild but disabling* or *mild but nondisabling* categories (Figure 26). In addition to IV TPA administration, secondary stroke prevention should be considered for patients with both mild disabling and nondisabling stroke (Box 5). Recall that prior to initiating antithrombotic therapy, cardioembolic mechanisms must be excluded. Also, dual antiplatelet therapy should not be initiated within 24 hours of IV TPA administration.

BOX 5. Ischemic Dual Antiplatelet Protocol

Drug	Loading Dose	Maintenance Dose
Clopidrogel*	300mg	75mg Daily After Loading Dose
Aspirin*	81mg	81mg Daily After Loading Dose

* Must exclude cardioembolic etiology and cannot be administered within 24 hrs of IV TPA bolus

FIGURE 26. Non LVO (Mild) Acute Ischemic Stroke

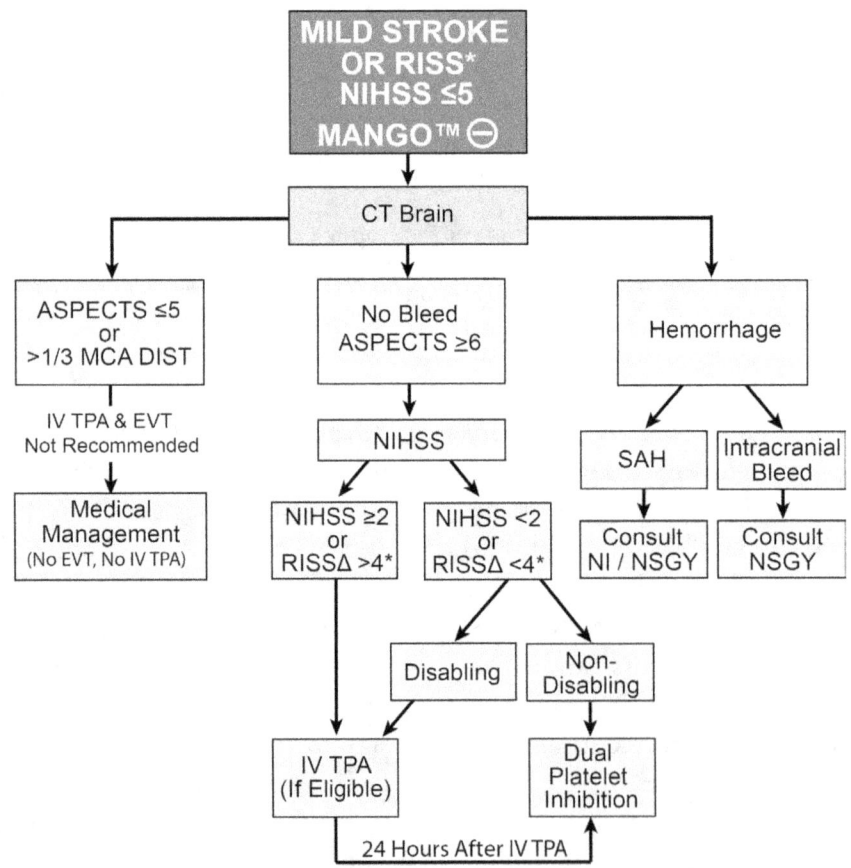

ASPECTS - Alberta Stroke Program Early CT Score, CT - Computed Tomography, Dist - Distribution,
EVT - Endovascular Treatment, LVO - Large Vessel Occlusion, MCA - Middle Cerebral Artery,
NI - Neurointervention, NIHSS - National Institutes of Health Stroke Scale, NSGY - Neurosurgery,
RISSΔ >4 - Rapidly Improving Stroke Symptoms with a change in NIHSS score >4 points,
SAH - Subarachnoid Hemorrhage, IV TPA - Intravenous Tissue Plasminogen Activator

31.13 The Power of Six

Another interesting point concerning the diagnosis and treatment of AIS is the immense significance of ASPECTS, NIHSS, and time since last known normal. Even more interesting is that all of these factors seem to revolve around a value of < 6. For example, as discussed earlier, the treatment of both non-LVO (IV TPA) and LVO AIS (IV TPA and EVT) can be based on an ASPECT score ≥6 (Figures 22 and 26). Furthermore, the distinction between a non-LVO AIS and LVO AIS can be based on an NIHSS score ≥ 6 (based on the 2018 AHA/ASA guidelines) (Figures 22, 23, and 27). Finally, EVT candidacy has different clinical and imaging eligibility in patients presenting < 6 hours since last known normal compared to those who present ≥ 6 hours since last known normal (Figures 27 and 28).

FIGURE 27. ASPECTS, NIHSS and LKN Linked to the Value of < 6

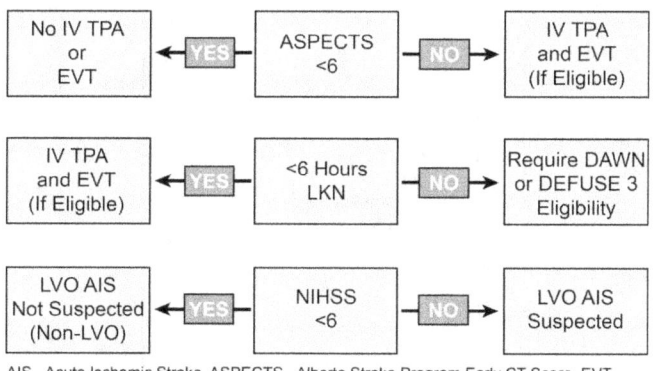

AIS - Acute Ischemic Stroke, ASPECTS - Alberta Stroke Program Early CT Score, EVT - Endovascular Treatment, LKN - Last Known Normal, LVO - Large Vessel Occlusion, NIHSS - National Institutes of Health Stroke Score, TPA - Tissue Plasminogen Activator

31.14 Stroke Efficiency and Communication

The efficient diagnosis and treatment of AIS cannot be overemphasized. There are four basic categories required for AIS diagnosis and treatment. These include **AIS screening**, **diagnosis**, **quantification**, and **treatment** (Figure 29). The more efficiently these steps can be performed, the greater the probability of having a good functional outcome. This is precisely why this book advocates obtaining an NIHSS score (quantification) prior to treatment but after imaging diagnosis (Table 20). Chapter 29 (Stroke Efficiency) outlined the step-by-step processes that allow the diagnosis and treatment of AIS to be performed more efficiently within the categories of screening, diagnosis (image confirmation), quantification, and treatment (Figure 30). These categories can be recalled using the mnemonic 'SINC' (Table 21). The importance of consistent and reliable communication in the management and treatment of AIS cannot be overemphasized (Table 22).

FIGURE 29. Acute Ischemic Stroke (AIS) Treatment Steps

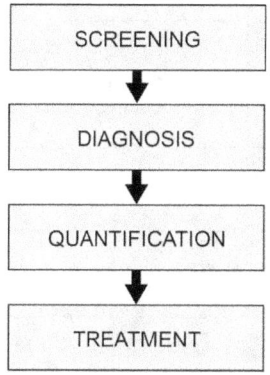

FIGURE 28. AIS Treatment Time Points

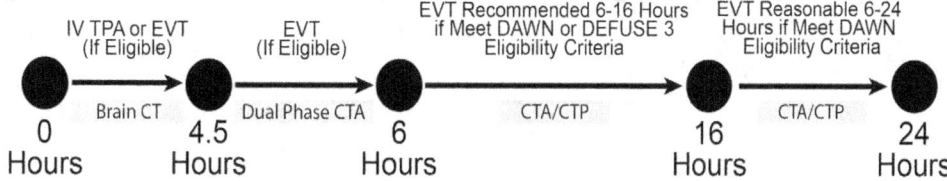

TABLE 20. NIHSS: **LEG PLEASED**™

National Institutes of Health Stroke Scale (NIHSS)			
		Item	Score
L	Level of Consciousness* *LAME	L: Level of consciousness	0 = alert (alert and responsive) 1 = not alert (arousable to minor stimulation) 2 = obtunded (arousable only to painful stimulation) 3 = unresponsive (reflex responses or unarousable)
		A: Age? M: Month?	0 = answers both correctly 1 = answers one correctly 2 = answers neither correctly
		E: Executes Commands	0 = performs both tasks correctly 1 = performs one task correctly 2 = performs neither task correctly
E	Eyes - Visual Fields	Visual fields	0 = no visual loss 1 = partial hemianopsia 2 = complete hemianopsia 3 = bilateral hemianopsia
G	Gaze	Gaze	0 = normal 1 = partial gaze palsy 2 = total gaze palsy
P	Palsy of Face	Facial palsy	0 = normal 1 = minor paralysis 2 = partial paralysis 3 = complete paralysis
L	Language	Language	0 = normal 1 = mild aphasia 2 = severe aphasia 3 = mute or global aphasia
E	Each Limb	Motor assessment each arm and each leg	0 = no drift 1 = drifts before 5 sec 2 = falls before 5 sec 3 = no effort against gravity 4 = no movement
A	Ataxia	Ataxia	0 = absent 1 = 1 limb 2 = 2 limbs
S	Sensation	Sensory	0 = normal 1 = mild loss 2 = severe loss
E	Extinction / Inattention	Extinction/inattention	0 = no neglect 1 = partial neglect 2 = complete neglect
D	Dysarthria	Dysarthria	0 = normal 1 = mild 2 = severe

TABLE 21. Stroke Efficiency Categories: **SINC**

S	Screening
I	Image Confirmation
N	NIHSS Quantification
C	Carry Out Treatment

CHAPTER 31: Summary

FIGURE 30. Stroke Efficiency and Endovascular Treatment (EVT)

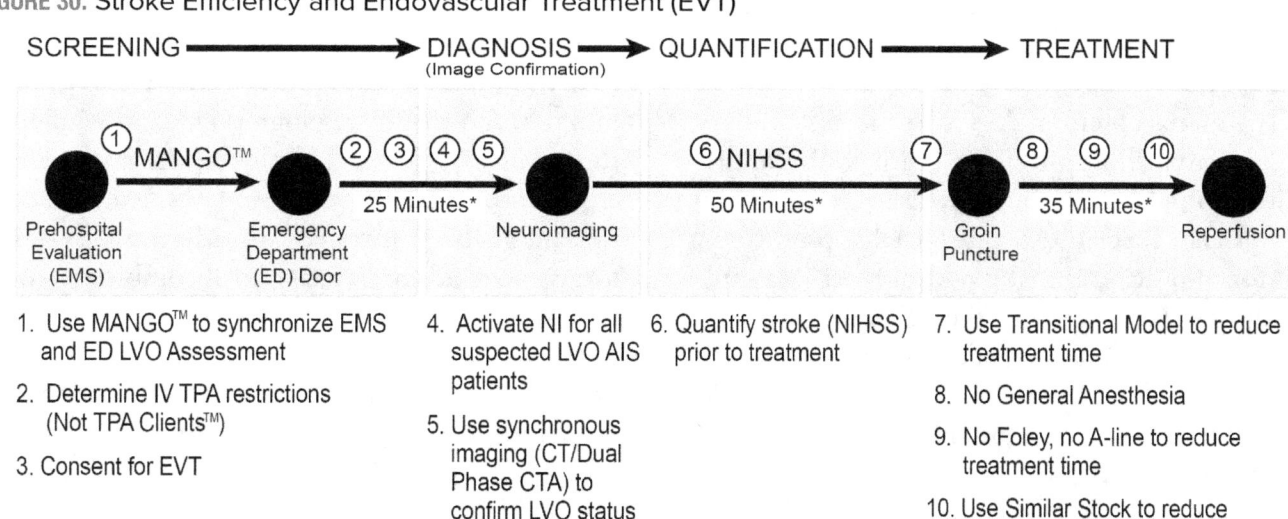

TABLE 22. Universal Stroke Vocabulary: **CHOCOLATE**

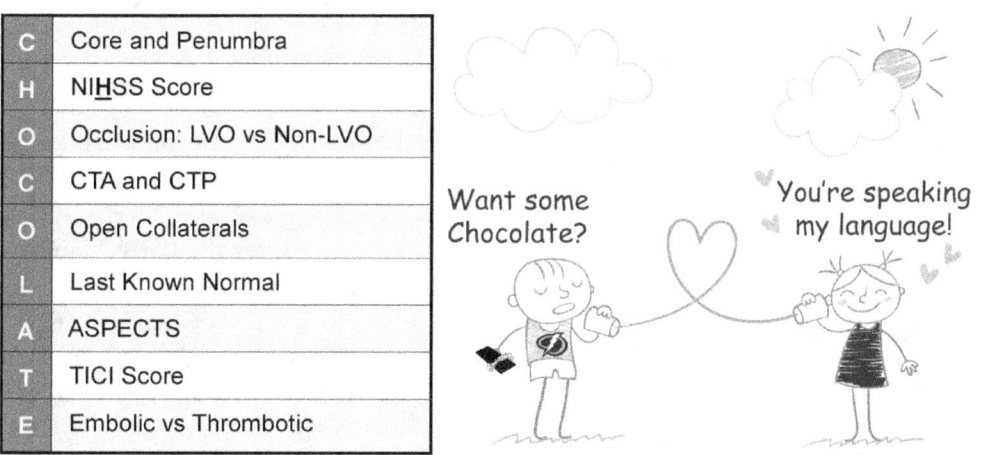

31.15 Finale

Three years ago, the publication of the MR CLEAN Trial and multiple other EVT trials marked the largest breakthrough in the history of modern stroke treatment and heralded a new stroke renaissance. These trials have consistently demonstrated that EVT in combination with IV TPA is superior to the best medical treatment alone in LVO AIS patients. Since then, the DAWN Trial has demonstrated that EVT can be performed safely and effectively as much as one day after the onset of stroke in appropriate patients. These trials also established the necessity of neuroimaging studies to detect ischemic penumbra and not yet irreparably damaged core infarct to determine EVT candidacy. Specifically, these trials emphasized that every stroke patient has a distinct collateral circulation which determines treatment, and not arbitrary time points. In the past, time windows served as surrogate markers to determine LVO AIS treatment. The DAWN and DEFUSE 3 Trials have conclusively demonstrated that many patients had been previously excluded from effective treatment due to arbitrary time points rather than imaging-based patient selection. This data continues to validate that EVT candidacy is patient-specific (based on unique collateral circulation). In this manner, each AIS patient has a unique "tissue window" which should now be the determinant of EVT candidacy, and not arbitrary time windows.

The management of AIS is a multidisciplinary endeavor requiring physicians with multiple disciplines to provide key and critical roles. However, physician specialists, non-specialist physicians, and non-physicians must work together in a multidisciplinary fashion for the efficient diagnosis and treatment of AIS. This field is now dominated by recommendations that have abruptly departed from our past treatment and understanding of cerebrovascular disease. Despite these tremendous innovations that continually occur in the AIS arena, we are only as strong as the weakest link of our multidisciplinary team. Consistent and reliable communication is key to a well-functioning acute stroke intervention team. We must continue to work together, review the latest and greatest research, and strive to improve patient outcome. This multidisciplinary team approach is perhaps the most essential element needed to achieve a successful stroke outcome. **Together, we are stronger™!**

Abbreviations list

ACA, anterior cerebral artery; AHA/ASA, American Heart Association/American Stroke Association; AILCA, anterior inferior cerebellar artery; AIS, acute ischemic stroke; aSAH, aneurysmal subarachnoid hemorrhage; BA, basilar artery; BPPV, benign paroxysmal positional vertigo; CSC, comprehensive stroke center; CTA, computed tomography angiography; CTP, CT perfusion; DWI, diffusion-weighted imaging; EMS, emergency medical services; EVT, endovascular treatment; ICA, internal carotid artery; IV TPA, intravenous administration of recombinant tissue plasminogen activator; LVO, large vessel occlusion; MCA, middle cerebral artery; MRA, magnetic resonance angiography; MRI, magnetic resonance imaging; NIHSS, National Institutes of Health Stroke Scale; PCA, posterior cerebral artery; PICA, posterior inferior cerebellar artery; PMVSAH, perimesencephalic venous subarachnoid hemorrhage; PP, pontine perforators; PSC, primary stroke center; RCTs, randomized controlled trials; SCA, superior cerebellar artery; TIA, transient ischemic attack.

References

1. Powers WJ, Rabinstein AA, Ackerson T, Adeoye OM, Bambakidis NC, Becker K, Biller J, Brown M, Demaerschalk BM, Hoh B, et al. (2018). Guidelines for the Early Management of Patients With Acute Ischemic Stroke: A Guideline for Healthcare Professionals From the American Heart Association/American Stroke Association. *Stroke*, Epub 24 Jan.

Appendix A

Mnemonics

Chapter 3

TABLE 1. The Meninges: **PAD**

P	Pia Mater
A	Arachnoid Mater
D	Dura Mater

TABLE 3. Vasogenic and Cytotoxic Edema: **VAN CAVES**

V	Vasogenic
A	Abscess
N	Neoplasm
C	Cytotoxic
A	And
V	Vasogenic
E	Edema
S	Stroke

TABLE 4. The Cerebellar Nuclei: **DEFG**

D	Dentate Nucleus
E	Emboliform Nucleus
F	Fastigial Nucleus
G	Globose Nucleus

Chapter 5

TABLE 1. Causes of Acute Ischemic Stroke: **CAUSE**

C	Cardioembolic (20%)
A	Atherosclerotic Large Vessel Disease (30%)
U	Undetermined Etiology - ESUS* (30%) (Avoid Cryptogenic Stroke Terminology)
S	Small Vessel Disease or Lacunar Infarct (15%)
E	Everything Else, or Other (5%)

*Embolic Strokes of Undetermined Source

TABLE 2. Embolic Sources: **CAP**

C	Cardiogenic (mitral or aortic valves or the left cardiac chambers)
A	Arteriogenic (proximal cerebral arteries or the aortic arch)
P	Paradoxical (venous emboli)

TABLE 3. Ischemic Stroke Plan: **S-PLAN**

S	Source (embolic or thrombotic)
P	Pathophysiology (etiology)
L	Location (of brain affected)
A	Artery (arterial territory involved)
N	Neuroimaging

Source	Pathophysiology	Location	Artery	Neuroimaging
• Embolic • Thrombotic	**C**: Cardioembolic (20%) **A**: Atherosclerotic large vessel disease (30%) **U**: Undetermined etiology - ESUS (30%) **S**: Small vessel disease or lacunar infarct (15%) **E**: Everything else or other (5%)	• Frontal • Parietal • Temporal • Occipital • Cerebellar • Thalamic • Brainstem	• ICA • MCA • ACA • Vertebral • Basilar • PICA • ACA • SCA	• CT • CTA • CTP • MRI • MRA • Angio

TABLE 4. Small Vessel Disease Risk Factors: **DASH**

D	Diabetes
A	Aging
S	Smoking
H	Hypertension or Hyperlipidemia

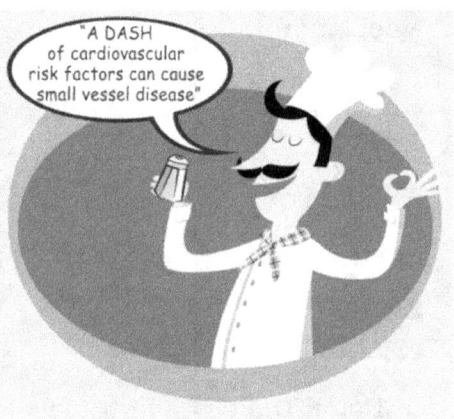

"A DASH of cardiovascular risk factors can cause small vessel disease"

TABLE 5. Lacunar Syndromes: **PADS**

P	Pure Motor or Pure Sensory Symptoms
A	Ataxic Hemiparesis
D	Dysarthria – Clumsy Hand Syndrome
S	Simple Unilateral Sensorimotor Deficits

TABLE 7. Large Vessels of the Brain: **BAMBI**

B	Basilar Artery
A	Anterior Cerebral Artery
M	Middle Cerebral Artery
B	Both Vertebral Arteries
I	Internal Carotid Artery

APPENDIX A: Mnemonics

TABLE 9. Cortical Symptoms Associated with Large Vessel Occlusion: **MANGO**™

Large Vessel Occlusion (Screening Mnemonic): "**MANGO**™"

M	Motor Weakness

A	Aphasia
	    Expressive (name 2 objects)
	    Receptive (follow 2 commands)

N	Neglect
	    Unable to feel both sides at the same time, or
	    Unable to identify own arm, or
	    Ignoring one side

G	Gaze Preference, Inability to Track or Double Vision
O	Optic Field Cut or New Blindness

TABLE 10. Features of Cardiogenic Emboli: **CARDIAC**

C	Cardiogenic Emboli
A	Anticoagulants (i.e., Coumadin®)
R	Red Thrombus (RBCs and Platelets)
D	Disrupted Heart Rhythm or Damaged Muscle
I	Infarct (Cardiac) = Stasis = Clot Formation
A	AFib Most Common
C	Cortical Distribution

TABLE 11. Major Risk Sources of Cardioembolic Stroke: **NAIL PAMELA**

N	Nonischemic Cardiomyopathies
A	Atrial Fibrillation and Flutter
I	Ischemic Heart Disease
L	Left Ventricular Thrombi Associated With Prothrombotic States
P	Prosthetic Valves
A	Acute Myocardial Infarction
M	Marantic Endocarditis
E	Endocarditis – Infective
L	Left Ventricular Akinesis or Aneurysm
A	Atrial Myxoma

Stroke Made Simple

TABLE 12. Embolic Stroke of Undetermined Source (ESUS): **NONE**

N	Non-lacunar Stroke
O	Open Arteries (Less Than 50% Stenosis)
N	No Major Risk Cardioembolic Source
E	ESUS (Embolic Stroke of Undetermined Source)

TABLE 14. Embolic Strokes of Undetermined Source (ESUS): **HAPPY MEDUSA**

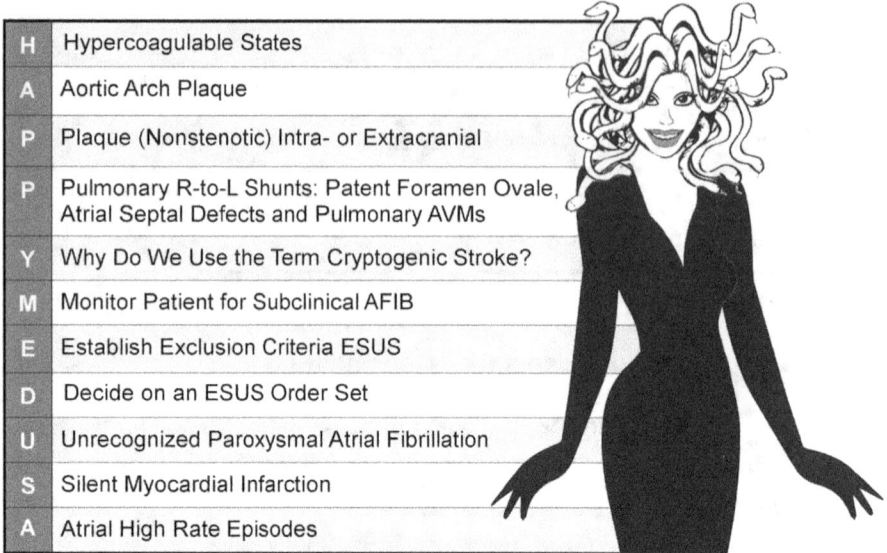

H	Hypercoagulable States
A	Aortic Arch Plaque
P	Plaque (Nonstenotic) Intra- or Extracranial
P	Pulmonary R-to-L Shunts: Patent Foramen Ovale, Atrial Septal Defects and Pulmonary AVMs
Y	Why Do We Use the Term Cryptogenic Stroke?
M	Monitor Patient for Subclinical AFIB
E	Establish Exclusion Criteria ESUS
D	Decide on an ESUS Order Set
U	Unrecognized Paroxysmal Atrial Fibrillation
S	Silent Myocardial Infarction
A	Atrial High Rate Episodes

TABLE 15. AIS Associated Blood Dyscrasias: **GREAT SHAPE**

G	Gene Mutation – Prothrombin
R	Resistance to Activated Protein C (Mutation In Factor V Leiden)
E	Erythrocyte Disorder - Sickle Cell Disease
A	Anti-Thrombin III Deficiency
T	Thrombotic Thrombocytopenic Purpura (TTP)
S	Single Lipoprotein, Lipoprotein (A)
H	Hyperhomocystinemia
A	Autoantibody Syndromes
P	Proteins C and S Deficiencies
E	Erythrocyte Disorder - Polycythemia Vera

Chapter 6

TABLE 1. Etiologies of Acute Ischemic Stroke: **CAUSE**

C	Cardioembolic (20%)
A	Atherosclerotic Large Vessel Disease (30%)
U	Undetermined Etiology - ESUS* (30%) (Avoid Cryptogenic Stroke Terminology)
S	Small Vessel Disease or Lacunar Infarct (15%)
E	Everything Else, or Other (5%)

*Embolic Strokes of Undetermined Source

Chapter 7

TABLE 5. Aneurysmal SAH Clinical Concerns: **SHAVES**

S	Seizure - No Prolonged Phenytoin Use
H	Hydrocephalus and Mass Effect
A	A Stunned Myocardium
V	Vasospasm; 4-21 Days, Use Nimodipine
E	Elevated Blood Pressure, Use Nicardipine
S	SIADH Versus CSW

Chapter 8

TABLE 1. Fibromuscular Dysplasia (FMD) Contributory Factors Related to Stroke: **SAD**

S	SAH - Intracranial Aneurysm
A	Artery-to-Artery Thromboembolism
D	Dissection

TABLE 2. Risk Factors Associated with Carotid Artery Dissection: **FEMALE**

F	FMD
E	Ehlers-Danlos Syndrome, Type IV
M	Marfan Syndrome
A	Autosomal Dominant Polycystic Kidney Disease
L	Linked to Elevated Homocysteine
E	Elevated Blood Pressure

TABLE 3. Arterial Dissection Distinguishing Characteristics: **FLAP**

F	FLAP - Subintimal
L	Luminal Stenosis or Occlusion
A	Arterial Lumen Tapering
P	Pseudoaneurysm Subadventitial

TABLE 5. Carotid Artery Dissection Symptoms: **WHAM**

W	Weakness, Contralateral
H	Headache
A	Amarousis Fugax
M	Miosis and Ptosis (Partial Horner Syndrome)

TABLE 6. The Vasculopathies: **FMD**

F	Fibromuscular Dysplasia
M	Moyamoya
D	Dissection

Consider these vasculopathies in younger patients presenting with stroke

Chapter 9

TABLE 2. Cerebrovascular Malformations: **ABCD**

A	AVMs
B	Berry-like Lesions - Cavernous Malformations
C	Capillary Telangiectasias
D	Developmental Venous Anomalies

APPENDIX A: Mnemonics

Chapter 11

TABLE 1. Cerebellar Stroke Symptoms: **DARK NIGHT DIVA**

D	Dysmetria - inability to judge distance and stop movement at a chosen point
A	Ataxia - uncoordinated movement
R	Relaxed Muscles - hypotonia (floppy and weak muscles)
K	Kinesia - Dysdiadochokinesis, inability to perform rapidly alternating movements (i.e. pronation and supination of hands) Dysrhythmokinesis, disorder of the rhythm of rapidly alternating movements
N	Nystagmus
I	Intention Tremor - during movement and not at rest
G	Gait Abnormality (one form of ataxia)
H	Headache
T	Tipsy - vertigo, falls to injured side
D	Dysphonia - slurred explosive speech
I	Ipsilateral Motor Symptoms
V	Vomiting and nausea
A	Asynergia - loss of motor coordination, jerky movements

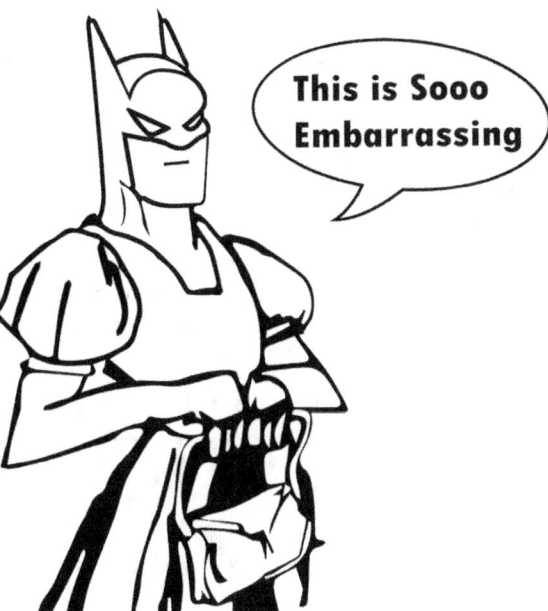

TABLE 2. The Five Principal Signs of Cerebellar Dysfunction: **GATOR**

G	Gait
A	Ataxia
T	Tremor
O	Oculomotor Abnormalities
R	Relaxed Muscles or Hypotonia

BOX 1. Cerebellar Examination: **HAL**

H: Head	Nystagmus Overshooting of eyes "Ahhh" "La, La, La"
A: Arms (Upper Extremities)	Thigh slapping Finger to nose Tap on a tune
L: Lower Extremities	Stand at rest Gait Heel-to-toe Heel-to-knee Heel-to-shin

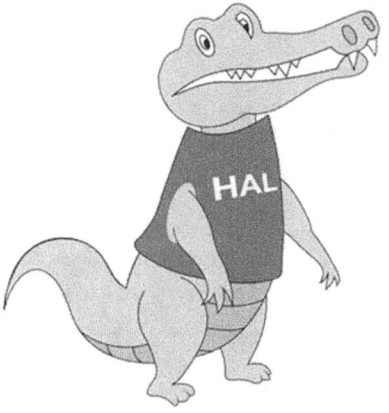

Stroke Made Simple

TABLE 4. Clues to Cerebellar Infarction: **DIVAS**

D	Direction Changing Nystagmus
I	Inability to Walk
V	Vascular Risk Factors
A	Ataxia, Severe
S	Sudden Immediate Symptoms

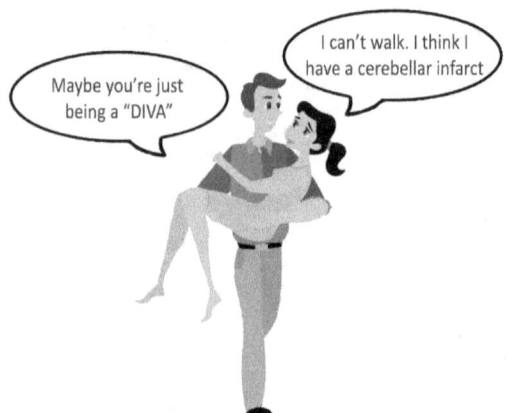

TABLE 7. The Three Components of the **HINTS** Exam

H I	**H**ead **I**mpulse Test
N	**N**ystagmus
T S	**T**est of (Vertical) **S**kew

TABLE 9. Indications for Neuroimaging for Vertigo: **IDA**

I	Inability to Walk Without Support
D	Direction-Changing Nystagmus
A	Any Focal Neurologic Deficit

Chapter 12

TABLE 1. Thalamic Stroke Symptoms: **LMAO**

	Deficit	Region	Artery	Origin
L	Language, (Dominant) and Memory	Anterior	Polar Artery (Absent in 40%)	PCoA
M	Motor and Sensory	Lateral	Thalamogeniculate Artery	P2
A	Arousal, Vigilance and Memory	Medial	Paramedian Artery	P1
O	Optic or Visual	Posterior	Posterior Choroidal Artery	P2

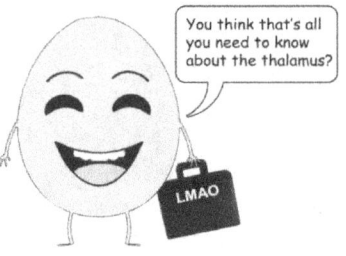

Chapter 13

TABLE 3. Brainstem Midline Structure Deficits: **MOAN**

M	Motor Weakness, Contralateral (Corticospinal Tract)
O	Ophthalmoplegia, Intranuclear, Ipsilateral (Medial Longitudinal Fasciculus)
A	Arm and Leg Numbness, Contralateral (Medial Lemniscus)
N	Neuropathy, Cranial, Ipsilateral (Motor Nucleus and Nerve)

APPENDIX A: Mnemonics

TABLE 5. Brainstem Lateral Structure Deficits: **HAND**

H	Horner's Syndrome, Ipsilateral (Sympathetic Pathway)
A	Ataxia, Hemibody Ipsilateral (Spinocerebellar)
N	Numbness, Hemibody Contralateral (Spinothalamic)
D	Distribution of CN V, Ipsilateral Facial Numbness

The hand is lateral

TABLE 6. Horner's Syndrome: **MISHAP**

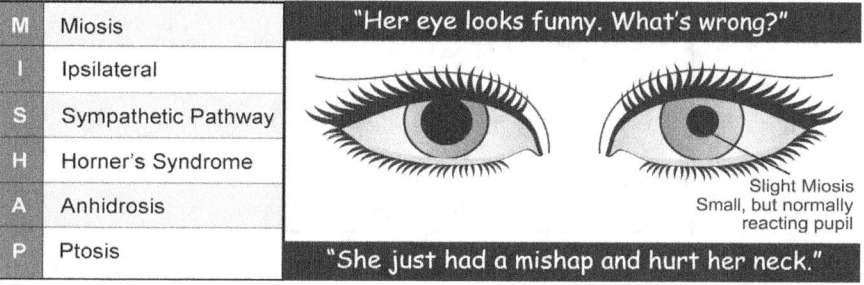

M	Miosis
I	Ipsilateral
S	Sympathetic Pathway
H	Horner's Syndrome
A	Anhidrosis
P	Ptosis

"Her eye looks funny. What's wrong?"

Slight Miosis
Small, but normally reacting pupil

"She just had a mishap and hurt her neck."

TABLE 8. Cranial Nuclei at the Level of the Medulla: **V-HAG**

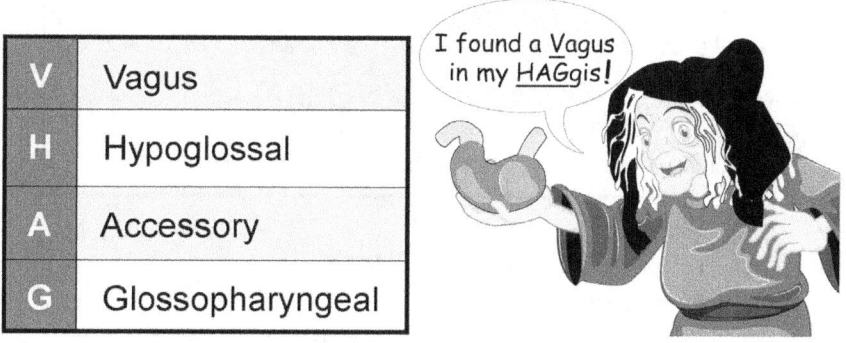

V	Vagus
H	Hypoglossal
A	Accessory
G	Glossopharyngeal

I found a Vagus in my HAGgis!

TABLE 10. Cranial Nuclei at the Level of the Pons: **V-FAT**

V	Vestibulocochlear (CN VIII)
F	Facial (CN VII)
A	Abducens (CN VI)
T	Trigeminal (CN V)

TABLE 12. Cranial Nuclei Within the Midbrain and Above: **TOO**

T	Trochlear (CN IV)
O	Oculomotor (CN III)
O	Optic and Olfactory - Above the Midbrain

TABLE 13. Brainstem Cranial Nerves: **TOOVFATVHAG**

T	Trochlear (CN IV)
O	Oculomotor (CN III)
O	Optic and Olfactory - Above the Midbrain
V	Vestibulocochlear (CN VIII)
F	Facial (CN VII)
A	Abducens (CN VI)
T	Trigeminal (CN V)
V	Vagus (CN X)
H	Hypoglossal (CN XII)
A	Accessory (CN XI)
G	Glossopharyngeal (CN IX)

TABLE 15. Deficits Associated with Medial Medullary Syndrome: **MINT**

M	Motor Weakness - Contralateral Hemibody (Corticospinal Tract)
I	Intranuclear Ophthalmoplegia, Ipsilateral (Medial Longitudinal Fasciculus)
N	Numbness - Contralateral Hemibody (Medial Lemniscus)
T	Tongue Deviation - Ipsilateral (CN XII)

TABLE 16. Deficits Caused by Lateral Brainstem Structures: **HAND**

H	Horner's Syndrome, Ipsilateral (Sympathetic Pathway)
A	Ataxia, Hemibody Ipsilateral (Spinocerebellar)
N	Numbness, Hemibody Contralateral (Spinothalamic)
D	Distribution of CN V, Ipsilateral Facial Numbness

The hand is lateral

TABLE 17. Lateral Pontine Syndrome: **7-HAND**

7	CN VII - Ipsilateral Facial Paralysis
H	Horner's Syndrome, Ipsilateral (Sympathetic Pathway)
A	Ataxia, Hemibody Ipsilateral (Spinocerebellar)
N	Numbness, Hemibody Contralateral (Spinothalamic)
D	Distribution of CN V, Ipsilateral Facial Numbness

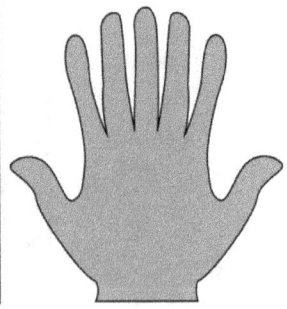

APPENDIX A: Mnemonics

TABLE 18. Brainstem Midline Structures: **MOAN**

M	Motor Weakness, Contralateral (Corticospinal Tract)
O	Ophthalmoplegia, Intranuclear, Ipsilateral (Medial Longitudinal Fasciculus)
A	Arm and Leg Numbness, Contralateral (Medial Lemniscus)
N	Neuropathy, Cranial, Ipsilateral (Motor Nucleus and Nerve)

TABLE 19. Medial Pontine Syndrome: **MOANA**

M	Motor Weakness, Contralateral (Corticospinal Tract)
O	Ophthalmoplegia, Intranuclear, Ipsilateral (Medial Longitudinal Fasciculus)
A	Arm and Leg Numbness, Contralateral (Medial Lemniscus)
N	Neuropathy, Cranial, Ipsilateral (Motor Nucleus and Nerve)
A	Abducens (CN VI) Ipsilateral Paralysis of the Lateral Rectus Muscle

TABLE 21. Medial Midbrain or Weber Syndrome: **WEB**

W	Weakness, Face and Hemibody (Corticobulbar and Corticospinal Tracts)
E	Eye "Down and Out," Unresponsive Pupil, Ipsilateral (DUI)
B	Both Face and Hemibody Weakness, Contralateral

TABLE 23. Lateral Midbrain Syndrome: **HATE**

H	Hemichorea or Hemiathetosis (Dentatorubrothalamic Tract)
A	Ataxia, Contralateral Body (Red Nucleus)
T	Tremor (Dentatorubrothalamic Tract)
E	Eye "Down and Out", Unresponsive Pupil, Ipsilateral (CNIII)

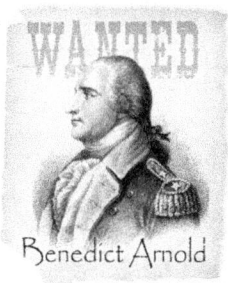
Benedict Arnold

I Hate Benedict Arnold

TABLE 24. Cranial Nerve III Deficits: **DUI**

D	Down and Out
U	Unresponsive Pupil
I	Ipsilateral

Chapter 14

FIGURE 7. Rules of Eye Movement: **LENO**

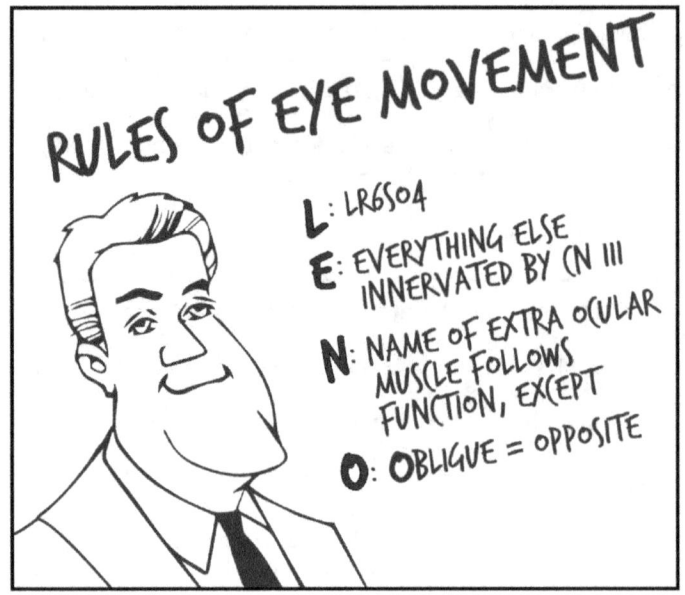

TABLE 1. Extraocular Muscles Innervated by Cranial Nerve III: **SIMI**

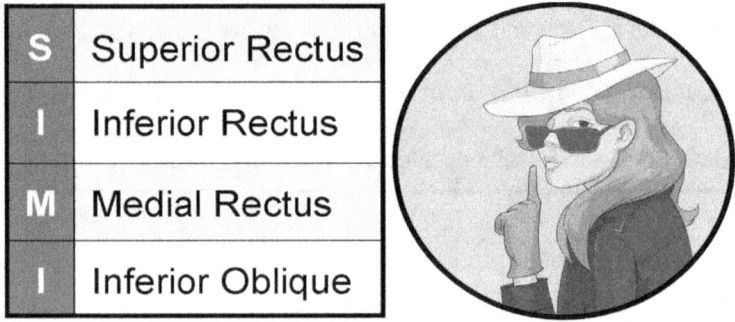

S	Superior Rectus
I	Inferior Rectus
M	Medial Rectus
I	Inferior Oblique

Chapter 15

TABLE 1. Top of the Basilar Syndrome Symptoms: **SOB**

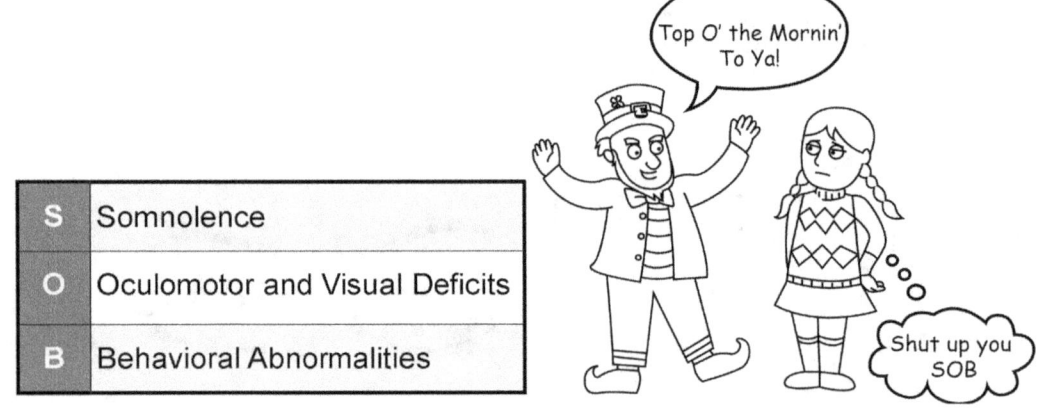

S	Somnolence
O	Oculomotor and Visual Deficits
B	Behavioral Abnormalities

APPENDIX A: Mnemonics

Chapter 16

TABLE 3. Supraclinoid ICA Segment Vessels: **OPA**

O	Ophthalmic Artery (OA)
P	Posterior Communicating Artery (PCoA)
A	Anterior Choroidal Artery (AChA)

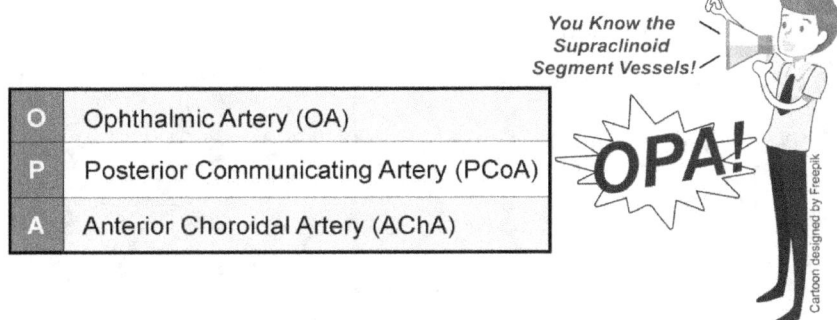

TABLE 4. The Three Vascular Components of the Anterior Circulation: **SAM**

S	Supraclinoid segment of internal carotid artery
A	Anterior cerebral artery (ACA)
M	Middle cerebral artery (MCA)

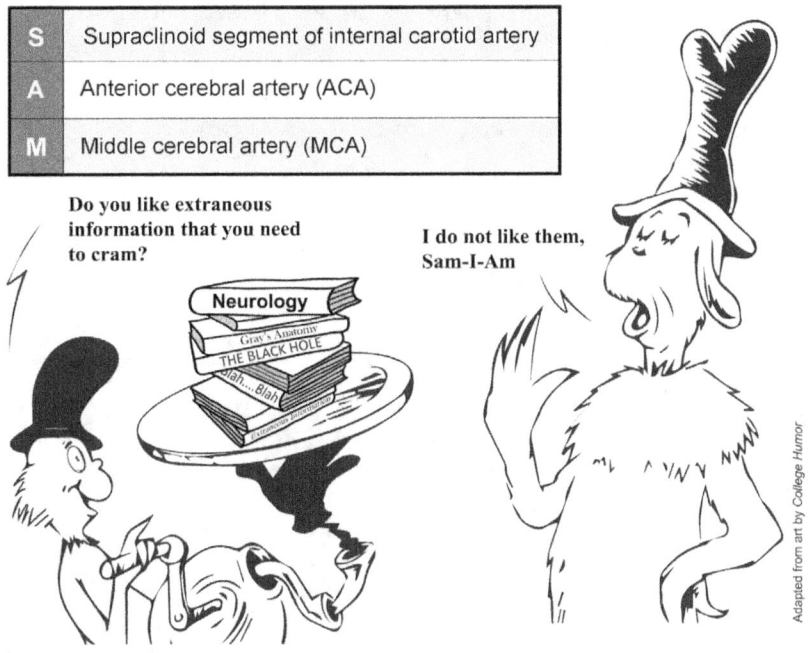

TABLE 5. AChA Distribution: **SCORING CHART**

S	Substantia Nigra
C	Choroid Plexus
O	Optic Chiasm
R	Red Nucleus
I	Internal Capsule
N	Neglect - right sided involvement
G	Globus Pallidus
C	Crus Cerebri
H	Hippocampus
A	Amygdala
R	Rear (tail) of Caudate
T	Thalamus

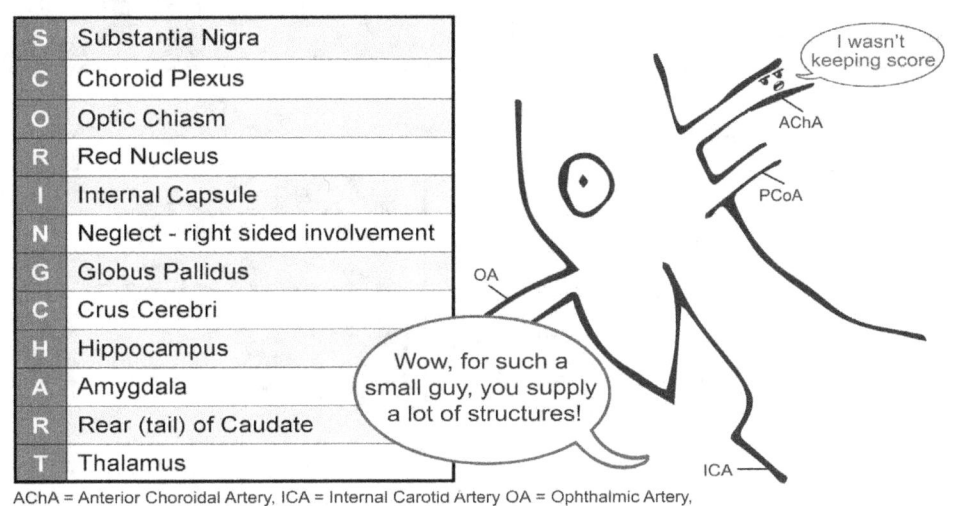

AChA = Anterior Choroidal Artery, ICA = Internal Carotid Artery OA = Ophthalmic Artery, PCoA = Posterior Communicating Artery

Stroke Made Simple

TABLE 6. AChA Symptoms: **TRIPLE H POT**

H	Hemiplegia, Contralateral
H	Homonymous Hemianopia
H	Hypo-aesthesia, Contralateral
P	Posterior Limb Internal Capsule
O	Optic Chiasm and Tract
T	Thalamus

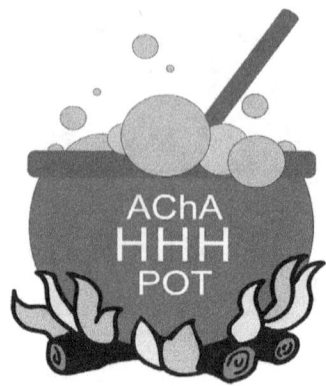

TABLE 7. Small Vessels That Can Mimic Large Vessel Occlusion (LVO): **PLAT**

P	Pontine Perforators
L	Lenticulostriates
A	Anterior Choroidal Artery (AChA)
T	Thalamic Perforator

TABLE 9. Structures Involved in Lacunar Infarcts: **SPLIT LIP**

S	Semiovale, Centrum and Corona Radiata
P	Putamen
L	Lentiform Nucleus
I	Internal Capsule - Genu
T	Thalamus
L	Lenticulostriates - Most Common
I	Internal Capsule - Posterior Limb
P	Pontine Perforators

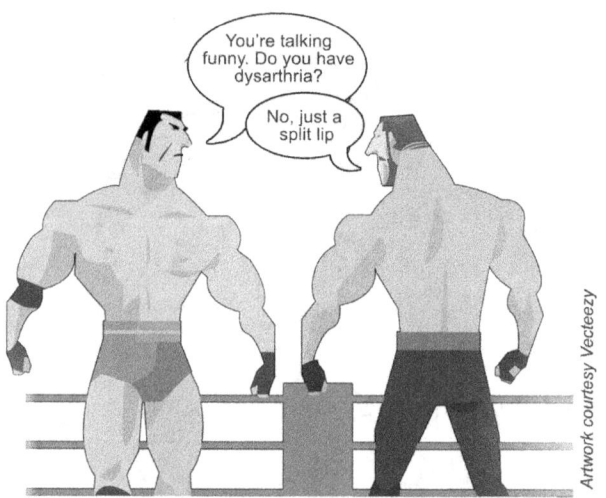

Artwork courtesy Vecteezy

TABLE 10. M1 Occlusion Symptoms: **SHAGS**

S	Sensory loss, contralateral
H	Hemiplegia, contralateral
A	Aphasia, global (dominant)
G	Gaze preference towards infarct
S	Spatial Neglect

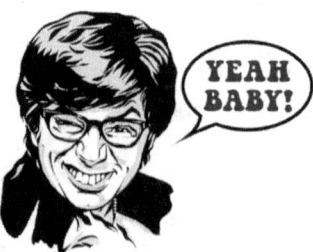

Chapter 17

TABLE 1. Antiplatelet Therapy for Recurrent Stroke Prevention: **CAT**

C	Cardioembolic Etiology Must be Excluded
A	Aspirin and Clopidogrel Therapy Initiated Early
T	TPA Precludes Treatment for 24 Hours After its Administration

TABLE 2. Transient Ischemic Attack: **TIA**

T	Tissue, not Time Definition, ↓ Risk for Stroke
I	Imaging Confirmation - DWI Preferred
A	Any DWI + Lesion = Stroke, not TIA ↑ Risk for Recurrent Stroke

Chapter 18

TABLE 1. Wingspan® Criteria: **ASS HAT**

A	Age 22 - 80
S	Strokes - Two or More Despite Aggressive Medical Management
S	Seven - Most Recent Stroke Within Seven Days Prior to Treatment
H	Have 70% - 99% Intracranial Stenosis Related to Recurrent Strokes
A	Aggressive Medical Management Failure
T	Treatment - mRS ≤ 3 Prior to Treatment

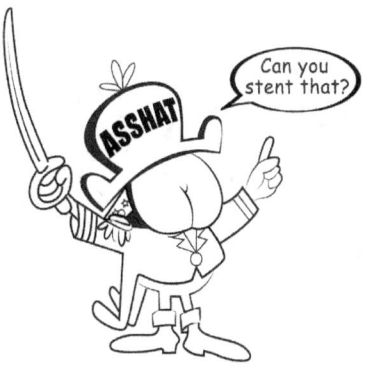

Chapter 19

TABLE 1. Stroke Mimickers: **MIMICKERS**™

M	Metabolic-Hypoglycemia or Hyperglycemia
I	Ictal-Seizures
M	Multiple Sclerosis
I	Intracranial Lesions (traumatic, infectious, hemorrhagic and neoplastic)
C	Classic and Specific Migraine Subtypes
K	Keep Balance? (Vestibular Dysfunction)
E	Encephalopathy
R	Regular Diastolic Pressure
S	Sepsis

Chapter 20

TABLE 3. NIHSS: **LEG PLEASED**

	National Institutes of Health Stroke Scale (NIHSS)		
		Item	**Score**
L	Level of Consciousness* *LAME	L: Level of consciousness	0 = alert (alert and responsive) 1 = not alert (arousable to minor stimulation) 2 = obtunded (arousable only to painful stimulation) 3 = unresponsive (reflex responses or unarousable)
		A: Age? M: Month?	0 = answers both correctly 1 = answers one correctly 2 = answers neither correctly
		E: Executes Commands	0 = performs both tasks correctly 1 = performs one task correctly 2 = performs neither task correctly
E	Eyes - Visual Fields	Visual fields	0 = no visual loss 1 = partial hemianopsia 2 = complete hemianopsia 3 = bilateral hemianopsia
G	Gaze	Gaze	0 = normal 1 = partial gaze palsy 2 = total gaze palsy
P	Palsy of Face	Facial palsy	0 = normal 1 = minor paralysis 2 = partial paralysis 3 = complete paralysis
L	Language	Language	0 = normal 1 = mild aphasia 2 = severe aphasia 3 = mute or global aphasia
E	Each Limb	Motor assessment each arm and each leg	0 = no drift 1 = drifts before 5 sec 2 = falls before 5 sec 3 = no effort against gravity 4 = no movement
A	Ataxia	Ataxia	0 = absent 1 = 1 limb 2 = 2 limbs
S	Sensation	Sensory	0 = normal 1 = mild loss 2 = severe loss
E	Extinction / Inattention	Extinction/inattention	0 = no neglect 1 = partial neglect 2 = complete neglect
D	Dysarthria	Dysarthria	0 = normal 1 = mild 2 = severe

APPENDIX A: Mnemonics

Chapter 21

TABLE 1. ASPECTS Mnemonic: **CHILI-6**™

CH	Caudate Head
I	Internal Capsule
L	Lentiform Nucleus
I	Insular Cortex
6	M1 - M6 (GL and SGL)

GL - Ganglionic Level; SGL - Supraganglionic Level

TABLE 4. Large Vessels of the Brain: **BAMBI**

B	Basilar Artery
A	Anterior Cerebral Artery
M	Middle Cerebral Artery
B	Both Vertebral Arteries
I	Internal Carotid Artery

TABLE 8. Categories of AIS Neuroimaging: **RAFT**

R	Rule Out - Bleed or >1/3 MCA ASPECTS ≤5
A	Anatomic - Arterial Territory Where is the LVO?
F	Functional - Collateral Status
T	Threatened Brain (Ischemic Penumbra) Versus Completed Infarct (Core Infarct) - Physiologic

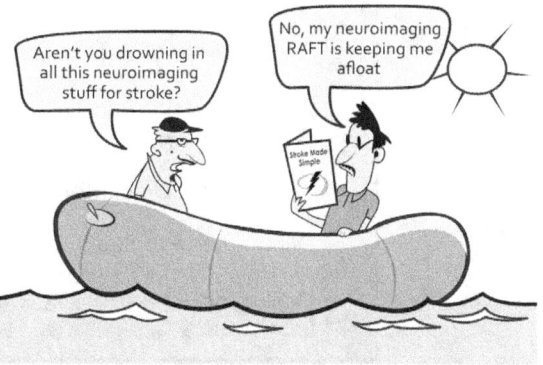

Chapter 23

TABLE 1. TPA Inclusion Criteria: **CAN**

C	Clinical Diagnosis of Ischemic Stroke (Measure Role Neurologic Deficit)
A	Age >18
N	Need to Initiate Treatment Within 3 Hours

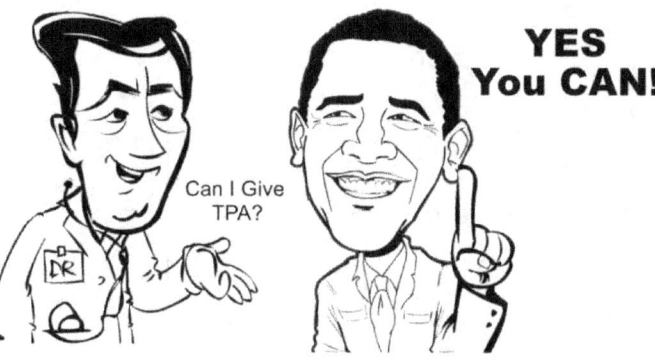

Stroke Made Simple

TABLE 2. TPA Initial Exclusion Criteria: DON'T GIVE TPA

D	Disorders of bleeding (acute bleeding diathesis)			
O	Occult SAH or SAH suspicion (even if CT negative for SAH)			
N	Not controlled HTN (SBP>185, DBP > 110)			
T	Tumor, aneurysm or AVM of brain			
G	Glucose less than 50 mg/dL (2.7mmol/L)			
I	INFARCT (>1/3 MCA) or BLEED on CT		A	aPTT elevated
V	VARIABLES for bleeding - ALPHA*		L	Labs abnormal with use of direct thrombin or direct factor Xa inhibitors (aPTT, INR, platelet count, ECT or TT or factor Xa activity assays)
E	Evidence of MAJOR SURGERY or TRAUMA within 3 months			
T	Three months - no neurosurgery, head trauma or stroke			
P	Previous intracranial hemorrhage history		P	Platelets < 100 mm3
A	Active internal bleeding w/in 22 days or arterial puncture at non-compressor site within 7 days		H	Heparin w/in 48 hours and aPTT >40
			A	Anticoagulant with INR > 1.7 or PT >15

TABLE 3. TPA Initial Relative Exclusion Criteria: MIGHT DO

M	Myocardial Infarct Within 3 Months
I	Improving (Rapidly) Stroke Symptoms or Minor Symptoms
G	G.I. or Urinary Tract Hemorrhage Within 21 Days
H	History of Major Surgery or Serious Non-Head Trauma Within 14 Days
T	Tap - Recent Spinal Tap
D	Determined Pregnant
O	Occurrence of Seizure at Onset With Postictal Neurological Impairments

TABLE 4. Different Criteria Record Related to IV TPA Administration: PLANT

P	Permissible Criteria
L	Laboratory Criteria
A	Anticoagulants
N	Not Permissible Criteria
T	Temporally Related Criteria

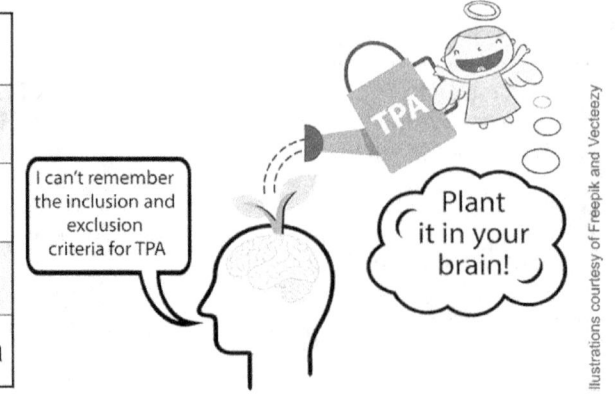

APPENDIX A: Mnemonics

TABLE 5. Permissible Criteria for IV TPA: **CAN HAPPEN**

C	Coumadin Use and INR ≤ 1.7
A	Aneurysm (< 10 mm) or AVM
N	Normalized Hyperglycemia
H	Hypertension That can be Lowered Safely (< 185/110 mmHg)
A	A Potential Bleeding Diathesis or Coagulopathy
P	Pregnant and Postpartum Patients
P	Pericarditis
E	Epilepsy/Seizure at Stroke Onset
N	Neoplasm

TABLE 6. Impermissible IV TPA Laboratory Criteria

P	PT >15
A	aPTT >40
P	Platelets <100,000/mm3
I	INR >1.7

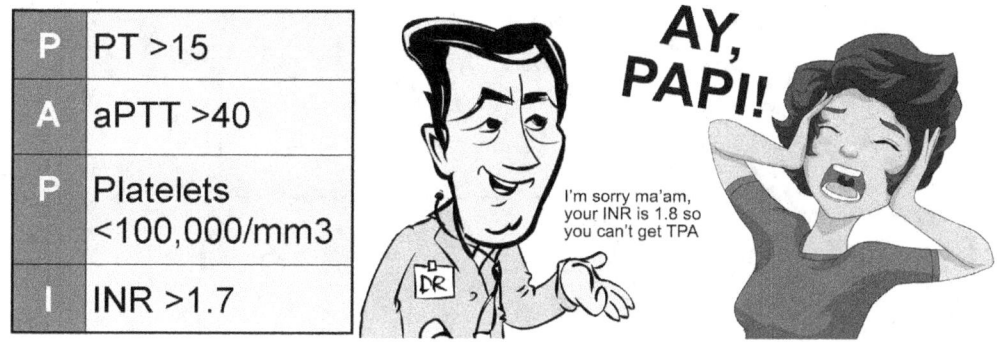

TABLE 8. Three Months CNS Events That Exclude IV TPA Administration: **SIT**

S	Surgery, Intracranial or Spinal Within Three Months
I	Ischemic or Hemorrhagic Stroke Within Three Months
T	Trauma, Severe Head Trauma Within Three Months

TABLE 9. Different Types of Intracranial Hemorrhage: **SPICES**

S	Subarachnoid Hemorrhage
P	Parenchymal Hemorrhage
I	Intraventricular Hemorrhage
C	Conversion – Hemorrhagic Conversion of Infarct
E	Epidural Hematoma
S	Subdural Hematoma

Stroke Made Simple

TABLE 10. IV TPA Restrictions: **NOT TPA CLIENTS**™

N	Non-Enhanced Contrast CT >1/3 MCA
O	Onset of Symptoms >4.5 Hrs or UNKNOWN
T	Ten, Intracranial Aneurysm ≥10mm
T	Tumor, Intra-Axial or GI (or GI Bleed <21d)
P	Prior Ischemic Stroke Within 3 Months
A	Aortic Dissection (Suspected)
C	Coagulopathy: Coumadin (if INR >1.7) and Coumadin Analogs (Direct Thrombin Inhibitors or Direct Factor Xa Inhibitors) PT >15, aPTT >40, PLTS <100,000 & INR >1.7
L	Low Molecular Weight Heparin <24 Hours (Full Treatment Dose, Not Prophylactic Dose)
I	Intracranial Hemorrhage - Acute or 3 Month History
E	Endocarditis, Infectious (Suspected)
N	Noncompressible Vessel Puncture Within 7 Days (Safety and Efficacy of IV TPA Uncertain)
T	Trauma, Severe Head Within 3 Months
S	Surgery, CNS (Intracranial or Spine) Within 3 Months

TABLE 11. Previous* Criteria for IV TPA Administered between 3 - 4.5 hours: **EXPAND**

E	Eighty, ≤80
X	X-Rays, CT ≤1/3 MCA
P	Prior Stroke and Diabetes History Excluded
A	Anticoagulant - Excluded Regardless of INR Value
N	NIHSS Score <25
D	Diabetes and Prior Stroke History Excluded

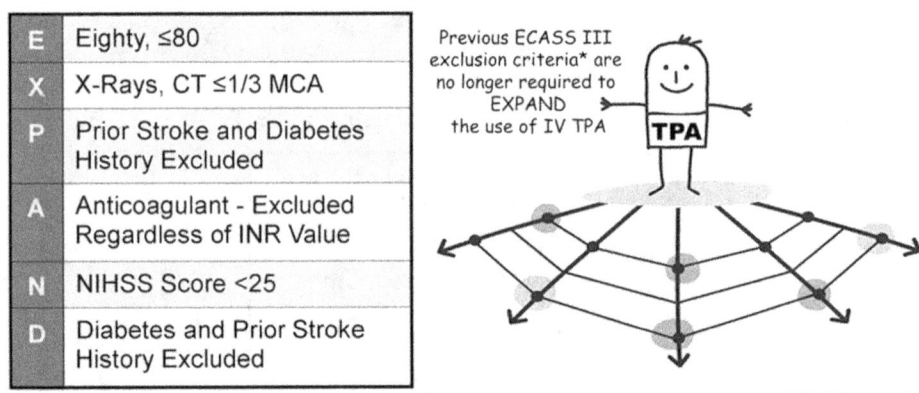

Previous ECASS III exclusion criteria* are no longer required to EXPAND the use of IV TPA

*Excluding a significant infarct (>1/3 MCA) and severe stroke symptoms (NIHSS >25), the new 2018 AHA/ASA guidelines have removed the previous ECASS III exclusion criteria for the administration of IV TPA 3 to 4.5 hours after symptom onset.

Chapter 24

TABLE 1. MR WITNESS Trial Criteria: **MINT**

M	MRI Mismatch
I	IV TPA Within 4.5 Hours of Symptom Discovery
N	No Stroke Symptoms 4.5 – 24 Hours Earlier
T	TPA Criteria Met

APPENDIX A: Mnemonics

Chapter 25

TABLE 4. Acute Ischemic Stroke (AIS) Diagnosis and Treatment Factors: **BLT**

B	Binary Process
L	LVO Status Confirmation
T	Threatened Brain Status Confirmation

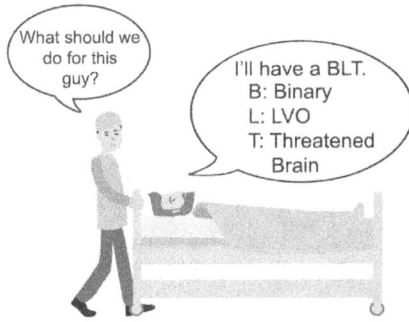

TABLE 7. AHA/ASA Recommendations for EVT: **ATLAS**

A	Age ≥18 Years
T	Treatment Initiated (Groin Puncture) Within 6 Hours
L	LVO (ICA or MCA M1 Segment)
A	ASPECTS ≥6
S	Score: NIHSS ≥6, Prestroke mRS 0-1

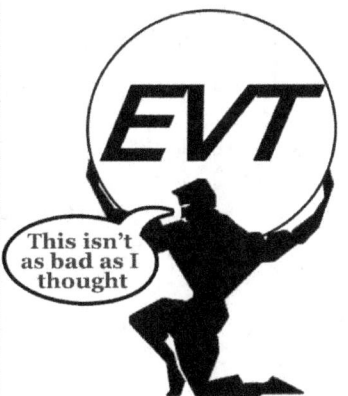

ASPECTS - Alberta Stroke Program Early CT Score, EVT - Endovascular Treatment, LVO - Large Vessel Occlusion, NIHSS - National Institutes of Health Stroke Scale, mRS - Modified Rankin Scale

TABLE 9. Large Vessels of the Brain: **BAMBI**

B	Basilar Artery
A	Anterior Cerebral Artery
M	Middle Cerebral Artery
B	Both Vertebral Arteries
I	Internal Carotid Artery

TABLE 10. General Anesthesia Recommendations for EVT Patients: **GRAPE**

G	GCS <8, Low Level of Consciousness
R	Respiratory Compromise
A	Agitation, Severe
P	Posterior Circulation Stroke
E	Endangered Airway

TABLE 11. Clinical Inclusion Criteria for DEFUSE 3 Trial: **ANTMAN**

A	Acute Anterior Circulation Ischemic Stroke
N	NIHSS ≥6
T	Time - EVT Initiated 6 -16 hours from Stroke Onset (Groin Puncture)
M	mRS ≤2 Prior to Qualifying Stroke
A	Age 18 - 90 Years
N	Necessary Consent

EVT - Endovascular Treatment, mRS - Modified Rankin Scale, NIHSS - National Institutes of Health Stroke Scale

TABLE 12. Neuroimaging Inclusion Criteria for DEFUSE 3 Trial: **CORP**

C	Core Infarct <70 cc
O	Occlusion of ICA or MCA (M1)
R	Ratio of Penumbra to a Core Infarct ≥ 1.8
P	Penumbra ≥ 15 cc

TABLE 13. Exclusion Criteria for DEFUSE 3 Trial: **A MESSI SPAGHETTI PLATE**

A	ASPECTS <6
M	Multiple Vascular Territory Occlusions
E	Evidence of ICA Dissection that is Flow Limiting or Aortic Dissection
S	Significant Mass Effect with Midline Shift
S	Stent that Precludes Safe EVT
I	Intracranial Process (Hemorrhage, Neoplasm or AVM)
S	Seizures at Stroke Onset if Baseline NIHSS Cannot be Obtained
P	Pregnancy
A	Allergic to Iodine
G	Glucose <50 mg/dL or >400 mg/dL
H	Hypertension that is Severe and Sustained (SBP >185 mmHg or DBP >110 mmHg
E	Expectancy of Life <6 Months, Severe or Terminal Illness
T	TPA Given 3-4.5 Hours After LKN and Any of the Following: Age >80, Current Anticoagulant Use, History of Diabetes or Prior Stroke
T	TPA Given >4.5 Hours After LKN
I	Interference of Neurologic or Functional Evaluation by Pre-Existing Disease
P	Platelet Count <50,000/μL
L	Limited Scanning, Unable to Obtain CTP or MRI
A	Abnormality of Labs (INR >3) or Bleeding Abnormality
T	Tried EVT Prior to 6 Hours from Stroke Onset
E	Embolus Presumed Septic, Endocarditis - Suspicion of Bacterial

ASPECTS - Alberta Stroke Program Early CT Score, AVM - Arteriovenous Malformation, CTP - Computed Tomography Perfusion, DBP - Diastolic Blood Pressure, EVT - Endovascular Treatment, ICA - Internal Carotid Artery, INR - International Normalized Ratio, LKN - Last Known Normal, MRI - Magnetic Resonance Imaging, NIHSS - National Institutes of Health Stroke Scale, SBP - Systolic Blood Pressure, TPA - Tissue Plasminogen Activator (or Alteplase IV r-tPA)

TABLE 14. DEFUSE 3 Abbreviated Exclusion Criteria: **PUMP GAS**

P	Pregnancy
U	Unable to Undergo Brain Imaging
M	Minimal Life Expectancy (< 6 Months)
P	Platelet Count < 50,000/µL
G	Glucose < 50 mg/dL or > 400 mg/dL
A	Abnormality of Bleeding
S	Seizures at Onset

TABLE 15. DAWN and DEFUSE 3 Trial Insights: **TITAN**

T	Time Window No Longer Determines Eligibility
I	Imaging Determines Eligibility
T	Thrombectomy *Recommended* Between 6-16 Hours, *Reasonable* at 6-24 Hours*
A	Always Accelerate Treatment
N	No EVT if Eligible Leads to Bad Outcomes

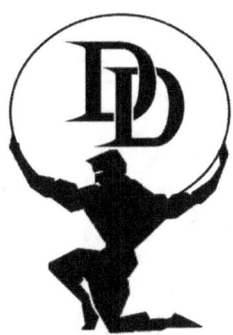

*EVT is *recommended* for LVO AIS patients within 6 and 16 hours of last known normal (LKN) and meet "other" DAWN and DEFUSE 3 eligibility criteria.
EVT is *reasonable* 6 to 24 hours after LKN and meet "other" DAWN criteria.

Chapter 26

TABLE 1. AIS Factors Associated with Collateral Circulation: **HAVE**

H	Hemorrhage Risk Increases with Poor Collaterals
A	Administration of IV TPA Better with Good Collaterals
V	Volume of Infarct Increases with Poor Collaterals
E	EVT Success Better with Good Collaterals

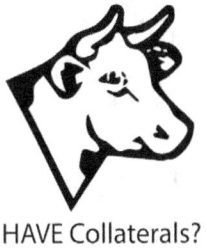

HAVE Collaterals?

TPA - Tissue Plasminogen Activator, EVT - Endovascular Treatment

Chapter 27

TABLE 1. LVO Screening Mnemonic: **MANGO**™

M	Motor Weakness

A	Aphasia
	    Expressive (name 2 objects)
	    Receptive (follow 2 commands)

N	Neglect
	    Unable to feel both sides at the same time, or
	    Unable to identify own arm, or
	    Ignoring one side

G	Gaze Preference, Inability to Track or Double Vision
O	Optic Field Cut or New Blindness

Chapter 28

TABLE 1. LVO Screening Mnemonic: **MANGO**™

M	Motor Weakness

A	Aphasia
	    Expressive (name 2 objects)
	    Receptive (follow 2 commands)

N	Neglect
	    Unable to feel both sides at the same time, or
	    Unable to identify own arm, or
	    Ignoring one side

G	Gaze Preference, Inability to Track or Double Vision
O	Optic Field Cut or New Blindness

TABLE 2. AHA/ASA Recommendations for EVT < 6 Hours From Symptom Onset: **ATLAS**

A	Age ≥18 Years
T	Treatment Initiated (Groin Puncture) Within 6 Hours
L	LVO (ICA or MCA M1 Segment)
A	ASPECTS ≥6
S	Score: NIHSS ≥6, Prestroke mRS 0-1

ASPECTS - Alberta Stroke Program Early CT Score,
EVT - Endovascular Treatment, LVO - Large Vessel Occlusion, NIHSS - National Institutes of Health Stroke Scale, mRS - Modified Rankin Scale

TABLE 3. ASPECTS Mnemonic: **CHILI-6**™

CH	Caudate Head
I	Internal Capsule
L	Lentiform Nucleus
I	Insular Cortex
6	M1 - M6 (GL and SGL)

GL - Ganglionic Level; SGL - Supraganglionic Level

APPENDIX A: Mnemonics

TABLE 4. IV TPA Restrictions: **NOT TPA CLIENTS**™

N	Non-Enhanced Contrast CT >1/3 MCA
O	Onset of Symptoms >4.5 Hrs or UNKNOWN
T	Ten, Intracranial Aneurysm ≥10mm
T	Tumor, Intra-Axial or GI (or GI Bleed <21d)
P	Prior Ischemic Stroke Within 3 Months
A	Aortic Dissection (Suspected)
C	Coagulopathy: Coumadin (if INR >1.7) and Coumadin Analogs (Direct Thrombin Inhibitors or Direct Factor Xa Inhibitors) PT >15, aPTT >40, PLTS <100,000 & INR >1.7
L	Low Molecular Weight Heparin <24 Hours (Full Treatment Dose, Not Prophylactic Dose)
I	Intracranial Hemorrhage - Acute or 3 Month History
E	Endocarditis, Infectious (Suspected)
N	Noncompressible Vessel Puncture Within 7 Days (Safety and Efficacy of IV TPA Uncertain)
T	Trauma, Severe Head Within 3 Months
S	Surgery, CNS (Intracranial or Spine) Within 3 Months

TABLE 5. AHA/ASA EVT Recommendations 6-24 Hours from Symptom Onset: **TITAN**

T	Time Window No Longer Determines Eligibility
I	Imaging Determines Eligibility
T	Thrombectomy *Recommended* Between 6-16 Hours, *Reasonable* at 6-24 Hours*
A	Always Accelerate Treatment
N	No EVT if Eligible Leads to Bad Outcomes

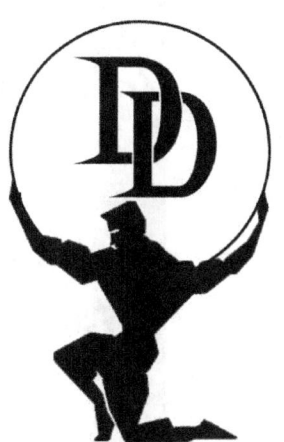

*EVT is *recommended* for LVO AIS patients within 6 and 16 hours of last known normal (LKN) and meet "other" DAWN and DEFUSE 3 eligibility criteria.
EVT is *reasonable* 6 to 24 hours after LKN and meet "other" DAWN criteria.

TABLE 8. Stroke Mimickers: **MIMICKERS**™

M	Metabolic-Hypoglycemia or Hyperglycemia
I	Ictal-Seizures
M	Multiple Sclerosis
I	Intracranial Lesions (traumatic, infectious, hemorrhagic and neoplastic)
C	Classic and Specific Migraine Subtypes
K	Keep Balance? (Vestibular Dysfunction)
E	Encephalopathy
R	Regular Diastolic Pressure
S	Sepsis

Chapter 29

TABLE 1. IV TPA Restrictions: **NOT TPA CLIENTS**™

N	Non-Enhanced Contrast CT >1/3 MCA
O	Onset of Symptoms >4.5 Hrs or UNKNOWN
T	Ten, Intracranial Aneurysm ≥10mm
T	Tumor, Intra-Axial or GI (or GI Bleed <21d)
P	Prior Ischemic Stroke Within 3 Months
A	Aortic Dissection (Suspected)
C	Coagulopathy: Coumadin (if INR >1.7) and Coumadin Analogs (Direct Thrombin Inhibitors or Direct Factor Xa Inhibitors) PT >15, aPTT >40, PLTS <100,000 & INR >1.7
L	Low Molecular Weight Heparin <24 Hours (Full Treatment Dose, Not Prophylactic Dose)
I	Intracranial Hemorrhage - Acute or 3 Month History
E	Endocarditis, Infectious (Suspected)
N	Noncompressible Vessel Puncture Within 7 Days (Safety and Efficacy of IV TPA Uncertain)
T	Trauma, Severe Head Within 3 Months
S	Surgery, CNS (Intracranial or Spine) Within 3 Months

APPENDIX A: Mnemonics

TABLE 3. EVT Accelerators: **FAST**

F	Foley Catheter, No Foley Catheter
A	A Line, No A Line
S	Stock, Use Similar Supplies
T	Tube, No Tube (Intubation)

TABLE 4. Stroke Efficiency Categories: **SINC**

S	Screening
I	Image Confirmation
N	NIHSS Quantification
C	Carry Out Treatment

Chapter 30

TABLE 1. Universal Stroke Vocabulary: **CHOCOLATE**

C	Core and Penumbra
H	Hemorrhage vs No Hemorrhage
O	Occlusion: LVO vs Non-LVO
C	CTA and CTP
O	Open Collaterals
L	Last Known Normal
A	ASPECTS
T	TICI Score
E	Embolic vs Thrombotic

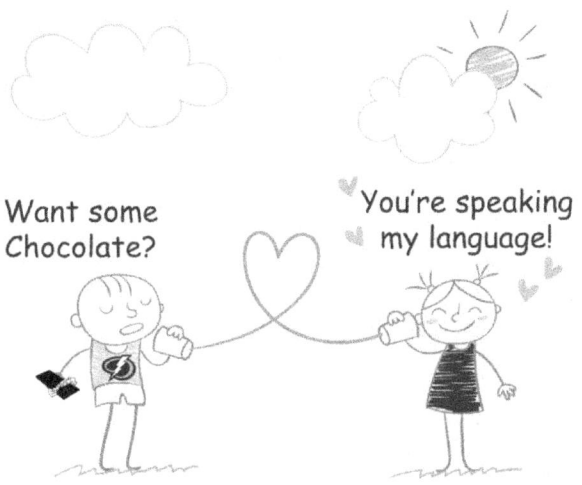

383

Chapter 31

TABLE 1. The Stroke Plan: **S-PLAN**

S	Source (embolic or thrombotic)
P	Pathophysiology (etiology)
L	Location (of brain affected)
A	Artery (arterial territory involved)
N	Neuroimaging

Source	Pathophysiology	Location	Artery	Neuroimaging
• Embolic • Thrombotic	**C**: Cardioembolic (20%) **A**: Atherosclerotic large vessel disease (30%) **U**: Undetermined etiology - ESUS (30%) **S**: Small vessel disease or lacunar infarct (15%) **E**: Everything else or other (5%)	• Frontal • Parietal • Temporal • Occipital • Cerebellar • Thalamic • Brainstem	• ICA • MCA • ACA • Vertebral • Basilar • PICA • ACA • SCA	• CT • CTA • CTP • MRI • MRA • Angio

TABLE 2. Cerebellar Stroke Symptoms: **DARK NIGHT DIVA**

D	**Dysmetria** - inability to judge distance and stop movement at a chosen point
A	**Ataxia** - uncoordinated movement
R	**Relaxed muscles**, hypotonia (floppy and weak muscles)
K	**Kinesia** - Dysdiadochokinesis, inability to perform rapidly altering movements (i.e. pronation and supination of hands). Dysrhythmokinesis, disorder of the rhythm of rapid alternating movements.
N	**Nystagmus**
I	**Intention tremor** - during movement and not at rest
G	**Gait abnormality** (one form of ataxia)
H	**Headache**
T	**Tipsy** - vertigo, falls to injured side
D	**Dysphonia** - slurred explosive speech
I	**Ipsilateral motor symptoms**
V	**Vomiting** and nausea
A	**Asynergia** - loss of motor coordination, jerky movements

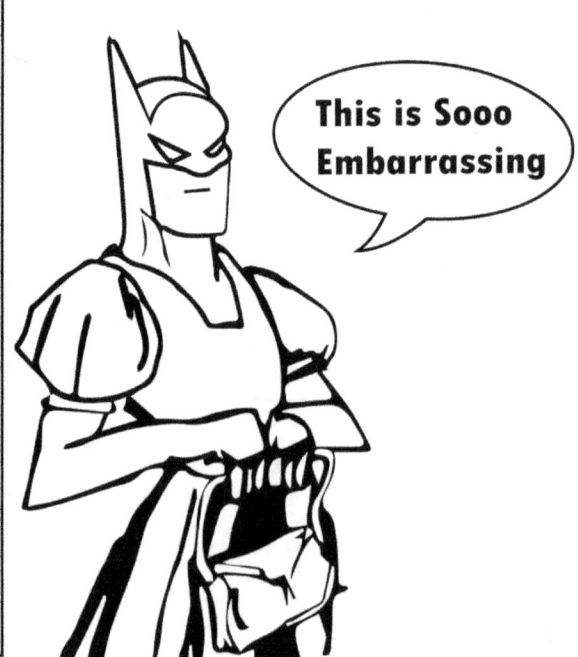

APPENDIX A: Mnemonics

TABLE 3. The Five Principal Signs of Cerebellar Dysfunction: **GATOR**

G	Gait
A	Ataxia
T	Tremor
O	Oculomotor Abnormalities
R	Relaxed Muscles or Hypotonia

BOX 1. Cerebellar Examination: **HAL**

H: Head	Nystagmus Overshooting of eyes "Ahhh" "La, La, La"
A: Arms (Upper Extremities)	Thigh slapping Finger to nose Tap on a tune
L: Lower Extremities	Stand at rest Gait Heel-to-toe Heel-to-knee Heel-to-shin

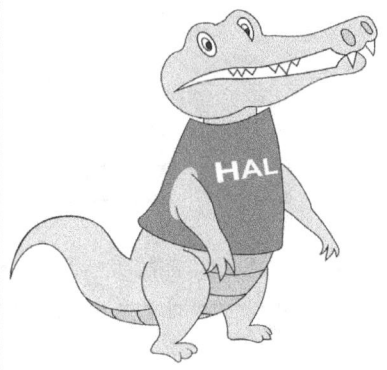

TABLE 5. Clues to Cerebellar Infarction: **DIVAS**

D	Direction Changing Nystagmus
I	Inability to Walk
V	Vascular Risk Factors
A	Ataxia, Severe
S	Sudden Immediate Symptoms

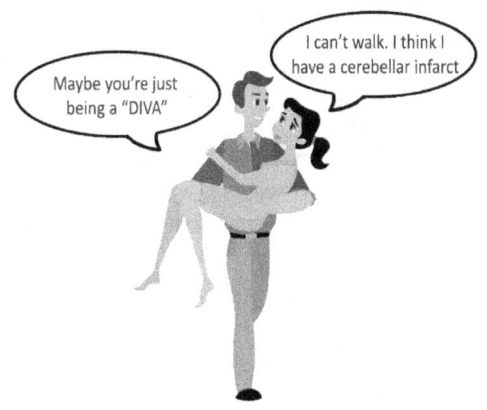

TABLE 6. Indications for Neuroimaging for Vertigo: **IDA**

I	Inability to Walk Without Support
D	Direction-Changing Nystagmus
A	Any Focal Neurologic Deficit

Stroke Made Simple

TABLE 7. Thalamic Deficits and Associated Regions: **LMAO**

	Deficit	Region	Artery	Origin
L	Language, (Dominant) and Memory	Anterior	Polar Artery (Absent in 40%)	PCoA
M	Motor and Sensory	Lateral	Thalamogeniculate Artery	P2
A	Arousal, Vigilance and Memory	Medial	Paramedian Artery	P1
O	Optic or Visual	Posterior	Posterior Choroidal Artery	P2

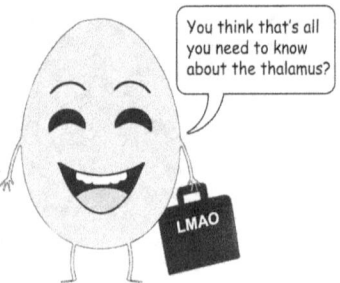

You think that's all you need to know about the thalamus?

TABLE 8. TIA

T	Tissue, not Time Definition, ↓ Risk for Stroke
I	Imaging Confirmation - DWI Preferred
A	Any DWI + Lesion = Stroke, not TIA ↑ Risk for Recurrent Stroke

TABLE 9. Stroke Mimics: **MIMICKERS**™

M	Metabolic-Hypoglycemia or Hyperglycemia
I	Ictal-Seizures
M	Multiple Sclerosis
I	Intracranial Lesions (traumatic, infectious, hemorrhagic and neoplastic)
C	Classic and Specific Migraine Subtypes
K	Keep Balance? (Vestibular Dysfunction)
E	Encephalopathy
R	Regular Diastolic Pressure
S	Sepsis

TABLE 10. IV TPA Inclusion Criteria: **CAN**

C	Clinical Diagnosis of Ischemic Stroke (Measure Role Neurologic Deficit)
A	Age > 18 (18-80 for 3-4.5 hrs)
N	Need to Initiate Treatment Within 4.5 Hours

Can I Give TPA?

YES You CAN!

APPENDIX A: Mnemonics

TABLE 11. IV TPA Restrictions: **NOT TPA CLIENTS**™

N	Non-Enhanced Contrast CT >1/3 MCA
O	Onset of Symptoms >4.5 Hrs or UNKNOWN
T	Ten, Intracranial Aneurysm ≥10mm
T	Tumor, Intra-Axial or GI (or GI Bleed <21d)
P	Prior Ischemic Stroke Within 3 Months
A	Aortic Dissection (Suspected)
C	Coagulopathy: Coumadin (if INR >1.7) and Coumadin Analogs (Direct Thrombin Inhibitors or Direct Factor Xa Inhibitors) PT >15, aPTT >40, PLTS <100,000 & INR >1.7
L	Low Molecular Weight Heparin <24 Hours (Full Treatment Dose, Not Prophylactic Dose)
I	Intracranial Hemorrhage - Acute or 3 Month History
E	Endocarditis, Infectious (Suspected)
N	Noncompressible Vessel Puncture Within 7 Days (Safety and Efficacy of IV TPA Uncertain)
T	Trauma, Severe Head Within 3 Months
S	Surgery, CNS (Intracranial or Spine) Within 3 Months

TABLE 12. Previous* Criteria for IV TPA Administered between 3 - 4.5 hours: **EXPAND**

E	Eighty, ≤80
X	X-Rays, CT ≤1/3 MCA
P	Prior Stroke and Diabetes History Excluded
A	Anticoagulant - Excluded Regardless of INR Value
N	NIHSS Score <25
D	Diabetes and Prior Stroke History Excluded

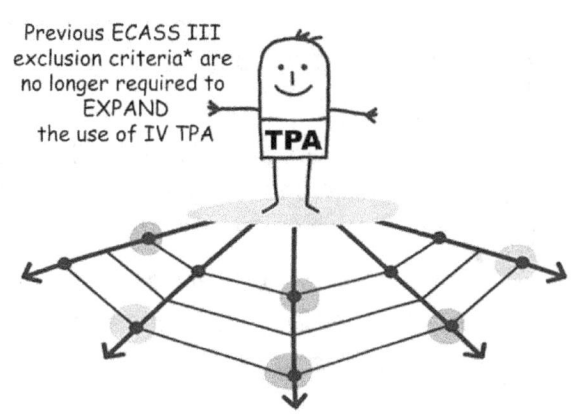

Previous ECASS III exclusion criteria* are no longer required to EXPAND the use of IV TPA

*Excluding a significant infarct (>1/3 MCA) and severe stroke symptoms (NIHSS >25), the new 2018 AHA/ASA guidelines have removed the previous ECASS III exclusion criteria for the administration of IV TPA 3 to 4.5 hours after symptom onset.

TABLE 14. AHA/ASA Recommendations for EVT: **ATLAS**

A	Age ≥18 Years
T	Treatment Initiated (Groin Puncture) Within 6 Hours
L	LVO (ICA or MCA M1 Segment)
A	ASPECTS ≥6
S	Score: NIHSS ≥6, Prestroke mRS 0-1

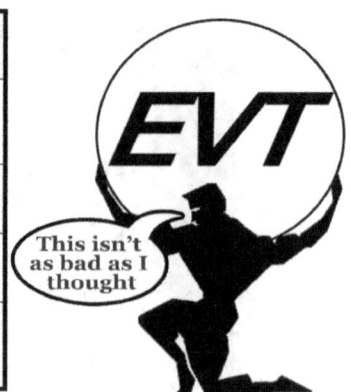

ASPECTS - Alberta Stroke Program Early CT Score,
EVT - Endovascular Treatment, LVO - Large Vessel Occlusion, NIHSS - National Institutes of Health Stroke Scale, mRS - Modified Rankin Scale

TABLE 15. DAWN and DEFUSE 3 Trial Insights: **TITAN**

T	Time Window No Longer Determines Eligibility
I	Imaging Determines Eligibility
T	Thrombectomy *Recommended* Between 6-16 Hours, *Reasonable* at 6-24 Hours*
A	Always Accelerate Treatment
N	No EVT if Eligible Leads to Bad Outcomes

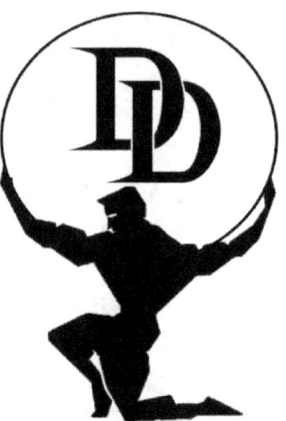

*EVT is *recommended* for LVO AIS patients within 6 and 16 hours of last known normal (LKN) and meet "other" DAWN and DEFUSE 3 eligibility criteria.
EVT is *reasonable* 6 to 24 hours after LKN and meet "other" DAWN criteria.

TABLE 19. LVO Screening Mnemonic: **MANGO**™

M	Motor Weakness

A	Aphasia
	  Expressive (name 2 objects)
	  Receptive (follow 2 commands)

N	Neglect
	  Unable to feel both sides at the same time, or
	  Unable to identify own arm, or
	  Ignoring one side

G	Gaze Preference, Inability to Track or Double Vision
O	Optic Field Cut or New Blindness

APPENDIX A: Mnemonics

TABLE 20. NIHSS: **LEG PLEASED**™

National Institutes of Health Stroke Scale (NIHSS)

L		Item	Score
L	Level of Consciousness* *LAME	L: Level of consciousness	0 = alert (alert and responsive) 1 = not alert (arousable to minor stimulation) 2 = obtunded (arousable only to painful stimulation) 3 = unresponsive (reflex responses or unarousable)
		A: Age? M: Month?	0 = answers both correctly 1 = answers one correctly 2 = answers neither correctly
		E: Executes Commands	0 = performs both tasks correctly 1 = performs one task correctly 2 = performs neither task correctly
E	Eyes - Visual Fields	Visual fields	0 = no visual loss 1 = partial hemianopsia 2 = complete hemianopsia 3 = bilateral hemianopsia
G	Gaze	Gaze	0 = normal 1 = partial gaze palsy 2 = total gaze palsy
P	Palsy of Face	Facial palsy	0 = normal 1 = minor paralysis 2 = partial paralysis 3 = complete paralysis
L	Language	Language	0 = normal 1 = mild aphasia 2 = severe aphasia 3 = mute or global aphasia
E	Each Limb	Motor assessment each arm and each leg	0 = no drift 1 = drifts before 5 sec 2 = falls before 5 sec 3 = no effort against gravity 4 = no movement
A	Ataxia	Ataxia	0 = absent 1 = 1 limb 2 = 2 limbs
S	Sensation	Sensory	0 = normal 1 = mild loss 2 = severe loss
E	Extinction / Inattention	Extinction/inattention	0 = no neglect 1 = partial neglect 2 = complete neglect
D	Dysarthria	Dysarthria	0 = normal 1 = mild 2 = severe

TABLE 21. Stroke Efficiency Categories: **SINC**

S	Screening
I	Image Confirmation
N	NIHSS Quantification
C	Carry Out Treatment

TABLE 22. Universal Stroke Vocabulary: **CHOCOLATE**

C	Core and Penumbra
H	Hemorrhage vs No Hemorrhage
O	Occlusion: LVO vs Non-LVO
C	CTA and CTP
O	Open Collaterals
L	Last Known Normal
A	ASPECTS
T	TICI Score
E	Embolic vs Thrombotic

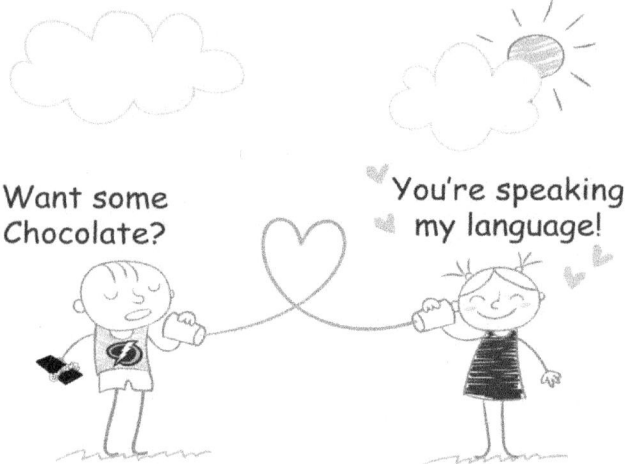

Appendix B

Abbreviations

ACA	anterior cerebral artery
AChA	anterior choroidal artery
ACoA	anterior communicating artery
AHA	American Heart Association
AHA/ASA	American Heart Association and American Stroke Association
AICA	anterior inferior cerebellar artery
AIS	acute ischemic stroke
AMM	aggressive medical management
ASA	American Stroke Association
aSAH	aneurysmal subarachnoid hemorrhage
ASL	arterial spin labeling
ASPECTS	Alberta Stroke Program Early CT Score
AVM	arteriovenous malformation
BA	basilar artery
BAO	basilar artery occlusion
BFUDD	big, fat, ugly disgusting draining vein
BNP	brain natriuretic peptide
BPPV	benign paroxysmal positional vertigo
CAA	cerebral amyloid angiopathy
CAD	carotid artery dissection
CAS	carotid artery stenting
CBF	cerebral blood flow
CBV	cerebral blood volume
CCA	common carotid artery
CEA	carotid endarterectomy
CIN	contrast-induced nephropathy
CM	cavernous malformation
CMB(s)	cerebral micro bleed(s)
CNS	central nervous system
CN III	third cranial nerve
COW	Circle of Willis
CPP	cerebral perfusion pressure
CPSSS	Cincinnati Prehospital Stroke Severity Scale
CS	conscious sedation
CSC(s)	comprehensive stroke center(s)
CSF	cerebrospinal fluid
CSW	cerebral salt wasting
CT	computed tomography
CT	capillary telangiectasias
CTA	computed tomography angiography; CT angiography
CTP	computed tomography perfusion; CT perfusion
CVM	cerebrovascular malformation
CVP	central venous pressure
CVT	cerebral venous thrombosis
dAVF	dural arteriovenous fistulas
DI	diabetes insipidus
DSA	digital subtraction angiography
DVA	developmental venous anomaly
DWI	diffusion-weighted imaging
DWI MRI	diffusion-weighted magnetic resonance imaging
ECA	external carotid artery
ED	emergency department
EICs	early ischemic changes
EKG	electrocardiogram
EMS	emergency medical service
ESUS	embolic strokes of undetermined source
EVD	external ventricular drain
EVT	endovascular treatment; endovascular therapy
FDA	Food and Drug Administration
FEF	frontal eye field
FLAIR	fluid-attenuated inversion recovery
FMD	fibromuscular dysplasia
fPCA	fetal origin of the posterior cerebral artery
GA	general anesthesia
GCS	Glasgow Coma Scale
GI	gastrointestinal

HH	hypertensive hemorrhage	PCoA	posterior communicating artery
ICA	internal carotid artery	PICA	posterior inferior cerebellar artery
ICH	intracerebral hemorrhage	PMVSAH	perimesencephalic venous subarachnoid hemorrhage
ICH	intracranial hemorrhage	PP	pontine perforators
INO	intranuclear ophthalmoplegia	PPRF	paramedian pontine reticular formation
IVH	intraventricular hemorrhage	PRES	posterior reversible encephalopathy syndrome
IV TPA	intravenous administration of recombinant tissue plasminogen activator	PSC(s)	primary stroke center(s)
		PWI	perfusion weighted imaging
LA	labyrinthine artery	RACE	Rapid Arterial Occlusion Evaluation Scale
LAMS	Los Angeles Motor Scale	RBC	red blood cell
LAPSS	Los Angeles Prehospital Stroke Screen	RCTs	randomized controlled trials
LEGS	Texas Stroke Intervention Pre-Hospital Stroke Severity Scale	RISS	rapidly improving stroke symptoms
LIS	locked-in syndrome	SAH	subarachnoid hemorrhage
LKN	last known normal	SCA	superior cerebellar artery
LMWHs	low molecular weight heparins	SIADH	syndrome of inappropriate antidiuretic hormone
LOC	level of consciousness	SO	superior oblique muscle
LR	lateral rectus muscle	S-PLAN	stroke plan
LVO	large vessel occlusion	STEMI	ST–segment–elevation myocardial infarction
LVO AIS	large vessel occlusion acute ischemic stroke		
MCA	middle cerebral artery	TCDs	transcranial Doppler studies
MI	myocardial infarction	TIA	transient ischemic attack
MLF	medial longitudinal fasciculus	TTP	thrombotic thrombocytopenic purpura
MRA	magnetic resonance angiography		
MRI	magnetic resonance imaging	VA	vertebral artery
MRP	magnetic resonance perfusion	VAD	vertebral artery dissection
mRS	modified Rankin scale	VAN	vision, aphasia, and neglect
MTT	mean transit time	VBATD	vertebrobasilar atherothrombotic disease
NCCT	noncontrast CT	VBI	vertebrobasilar insufficiency
NI	neurointerventional	VIPS	Volumetric Impedance Phase Shift Spectroscopy
NICU	neurointensive care unit		
NIHSS	National Institutes of Health Stroke Scale	VMIS	very minor ischemic stroke
NINDS	National Institute of Neurologic Disorders and Stroke	VPL	ventral posterolateral
NNT	number needed to treat	WUS	wake-up stroke
NT-proBNP	N-terminal proBNP		
OA	ophthalmic artery	3I-SS	3-Item Stroke Scale
PCA	posterior cerebral artery		

Index

A

ACT-FAST algorithm, 284, 285, 287
Acute ischemic stroke (AIS), 9, 17, 22, 35, 36, 37, 38, 39, 41, 42, 44, 45, 46, 47, 49, 59, 60, 78, 80, 81, 82, 102, 145, 146, 149, 153, 161, 162, 165, 166, 167, 168, 169, 178, 181, 183, 184, 185, 187, 194, 195, 196, 197, 198, 200, 203, 205, 206, 207, 210, 211, 212, 213, 214, 217, 218, 219, 220, 224, 228, 232, 233, 234, 237, 238, 240, 243, 244, 245, 246, 247, 248, 249, 250, 251, 252, 253, 256, 257, 258, 259, 260, 263, 265, 267, 268, 273, 274, 281, 282, 283, 285, 286, 287, 291, 292, 293, 294, 295, 298, 299, 300, 301, 302, 303, 304, 305, 306, 307, 308, 309, 310, 311, 312, 315, 316, 317, 318, 319, 320, 321, 322, 323, 324, 327, 330, 331, 337, 339, 340, 342, 343, 345, 346, 347, 348, 349, 351, 352, 353, 355, 356
Adiadochkinesia, 103
Aggressive medical management (AMM), 173, 174, 175, 179
AHA/ASA guidelines (2018), 81, 146, 167, 168, 177, 178, 184, 187, 198, 200, 203, 220, 224, 225, 226, 227, 229, 230, 231, 232, 233, 234, 238, 239, 243, 245, 246, 247, 248, 250, 251, 252, 253, 254, 256, 258, 259, 260, 267, 274, 281, 282, 283, 284, 285, 294, 295, 298, 299, 300, 301, 302, 303, 304, 305, 307, 308, 310, 311, 317, 323, 339, 340, 343, 344, 345, 346, 349, 353, 356
AIS imaging protocols, 198, 213, 217, 218, 268, 295, 311, 346
AIS screening, 286, 316, 317, 322, 323, 346, 353
AIS therapy, 35, 206, 210, 260
Alberta Stroke Program Early CT Score (ASPECTS), 198, 201, 202, 203, 212, 213, 214, 215, 247, 248, 251, 252, 253, 260, 266, 268, 269, 287, 294, 295, 297, 311, 313, 343, 353
Amaurosis fugax, 80, 151, 152
Anarthria, 133
Aneurysm, 28, 43, 53, 54, 56, 57, 61, 62, 64, 65, 66, 69, 70, 71, 72, 73, 74, 75, 76, 78, 79, 80, 82, 86, 87, 153, 164, 227, 229, 329
Aneurysmal subarachnoid hemorrhage (aSAH), 54, 56, 57, 60, 61, 62, 63, 64, 65, 66, 67, 68, 70, 73, 97, 98, 329, 356
Angiography, 23, 34, 45, 64, 65, 73, 74, 87, 91, 111, 112, 196, 206, 214, 215, 217, 220, 221, 240, 254, 257, 260, 268, 269, 270, 300, 311, 324, 356
Anosognosia, 194
Anterior cerebral artery (ACA), 31, 32, 34, 41, 124, 150, 151, 154, 155, 157, 162, 205, 248, 263, 268, 294, 332, 356
Anterior choroidal artery (AChA), 31, 34, 150, 151, 153, 154, 162
Anterior circulation, 23, 24, 28, 31, 69, 79, 115, 146, 149, 150, 151, 153, 162, 205, 239, 244, 247, 251, 253, 254, 255, 257, 259, 262, 263, 268, 301, 303, 324, 331
Anterior circulation stroke, 146, 150, 151, 153, 262, 268, 324
Anticoagulants, 44, 45, 47, 80, 81, 226, 227, 231
Anticoagulation treatment, 81, 83, 180
Antiplatelet agents, 45, 174, 176, 177
Antiplatelet therapy, 44, 45, 81, 166, 167, 169, 171, 172, 173, 174, 175, 176, 177, 178, 180, 233, 307, 339, 352
Antithrombotic therapy, 47, 166, 167, 180, 233, 307, 352
Anton's syndrome, 139
Aphasia, 115, 120, 154, 160, 161, 162, 182, 189, 193, 274, 275, 276, 281, 284, 287, 288, 307, 313, 324, 337
Apoplexy, 3
Arbitrary time points, 165, 197, 206, 208, 214, 220, 234, 237, 238, 239, 240, 250, 254, 257, 263, 265, 266, 267, 292, 315, 340, 343, 355
Arterial occlusion, 7, 156, 187, 196, 206, 212, 244, 262, 263, 288, 292, 306, 320
Arterial puncture, 228, 249, 250
Arterial spin labeling (ASL), 267, 268
Arteriovenous fistula (AVF), 85
Arteriovenous malformations (AVM), 85, 86, 87, 91, 391
Artery-to-artery embolic disease, 80
ARUBA Trial, 87
Aspirin, 45, 47, 81, 166, 167, 169, 171, 173, 174, 175, 176, 177, 180, 233, 236, 307, 339
Aspirin monotherapy, 166, 176
Asymptomatic Carotid Atherosclerosis Study (ACAS), 171
Asymptomatic Carotid Surgery Trial (ACST), 171
Asynergia, 103
Ataxia, 40, 102, 104, 105, 107, 134, 140, 191, 194, 307, 334, 335
Ataxic hemiparesis, 39
Atrial fibrillation, 42, 43, 44, 45, 181, 184, 227, 310

B

Balint syndrome, 140
Basal ganglia, 13, 17, 31, 52, 156, 201
Basilar artery occlusion (BAO), 145, 146, 251, 260
Benign paroxysmal positional vertigo (BPPV), 108, 109, 112, 335, 356
Big, fat, ugly disgusting draining vein (BFUDD), 86, 87, 91
Bilateral cerebellar disease, 104

Blindness, 80, 139, 183, 190, 191, 193, 274, 281, 285
Blood dyscrasias, 46
Blood pressure control, 65, 74, 174, 183, 225, 253
Broca's area, 150, 276
Brodmann areas, 13, 14, 138, 150

C

Capillary telangiectasias, 85, 90, 91
Cardioembolic stroke, 36, 42, 44, 47, 49
Carotid artery dissection (CAD), 78, 79, 80, 82
Carotid artery stenting (CAS), 171, 172, 174, 175, 178, 179
Carotid endarterectomy (CEA), 171, 172, 174, 175, 178, 179
Carotid Revascularization Endarterectomy versus Stenting Trial (CREST), 171, 172
Carotid stenosis, asymptomatic, 171, 172, 179
Carotid stenosis, symptomatic, 171, 172, 177, 178, 179
Carotid stenting, 81, 171, 178, 339
Carotid T occlusion, 154
Cavernous malformations (CMs), 65, 85, 88, 89, 90, 91
Central nervous system, 11, 17, 85, 185, 228
Central venous pressure (CVP), 67, 73
Cerebellar anatomy, 101
Cerebellar dysfunction, 5 principal signs of, 104, 363, 385
Cerebral amyloid angiopathy (CAA), 50, 51, 52, 59, 60, 233
Cerebral angiography, 27, 65, 68, 97, 217, 220, 266, 267
Cerebral blood flow (CBF), 7, 9, 207, 208, 209, 212, 214, 238, 240, 247
Cerebral blood volume (CBV), 7, 9, 207, 208, 209, 212, 214, 238, 240, 247, 267, 268
Cerebral microbleeds (CMBs), 50, 51, 229, 232, 233, 234
Cerebral perfusion pressure (CPP), 7, 9
Cerebral salt wasting (CSW) syndrome, 66, 67, 73
Cerebral spinal fluid (CSF) analysis, 64
Cerebral venous thrombosis (CVT), 93, 96, 97, 98
Cerebrovascular anatomy, 23, 33, 149, 162, 218, 331
Cervical Artery Dissection and Stroke Study (CADISS), 81, 83, 175, 180, 339
CHARISMA (Clopidogrel for High Atherothrombotic Risk and Ischemic, Stabilization, Management, and Avoidance) Trial, 177
Cincinnati Prehospital Stroke Severity Scale (CPSSS), 274, 277, 278
Circle of Willis (COW), 28, 34, 55, 153, 162
Clopidogrel, 81, 166, 167, 172, 173, 174, 176, 177, 180, 307, 339
Clopidogrel in High-risk patients with Acute Non-disabling Cerebrovascular Events (CHANCE) Trial, 166, 167, 176, 177, 307, 339
Clot location, 197, 218
Clumsy hand syndrome. *See* Dysarthria
Coil embolization, 71, 72, 73
Collateral circulation, 8, 35, 139, 156, 162, 197, 206, 209, 210, 211, 212, 214, 218, 234, 240, 247, 250, 251, 257, 258, 263, 265, 266, 267, 268, 269, 287, 300, 315, 318, 321, 340, 343, 355
Collateral status, 197, 210, 218, 263, 265, 266, 267, 268, 297, 300, 318
Collaterals, 9, 81, 154, 155, 206, 210, 211, 212, 214, 237, 251, 252, 257, 258, 263, 265, 266, 267, 269, 300
Coma, 19, 20
Comprehensive stroke centers (CSCs), 273, 282, 283, 285, 286, 287, 305, 311, 320
Computed tomography (CT), 22, 23, 34, 37, 45, 59, 63, 64, 65, 66, 73, 74, 87, 90, 91, 97, 111, 112, 114, 133, 145, 146, 166, 168, 183, 196, 197, 198, 199, 200, 201, 202, 203, 204, 205, 206, 207, 208, 210, 212, 213, 214, 215, 217, 218, 219, 220, 221, 229, 230, 231, 235, 240, 244, 247, 249, 250, 251, 252, 254, 257, 260, 261, 262, 266, 267, 268, 269, 270, 292, 293, 294, 295, 297, 298, 299, 300, 301, 302, 306, 308, 309, 310, 311, 313, 318, 323, 324, 356
Confusion, 162, 181, 200, 231, 292
Contralateral leg weakness, 162
Contralateral motor function, 16
Contrast-induced nephropathy (CIN), 217, 218, 219, 220
Coordination, 19, 20, 101, 110, 140, 141, 274, 279, 321
Core infarct, 1, 7, 8, 9, 35, 166, 195, 197, 198, 199, 200, 201, 203, 205, 206, 207, 208, 209, 210, 211, 212, 214, 217, 230, 237, 239, 240, 244, 246, 247, 251, 253, 255, 256, 257, 263, 267, 273, 286, 291, 292, 293, 295, 297, 298, 300, 305, 306, 316, 318, 320, 330, 340, 346, 355
Corticobulbar tract, 17, 134
Corticospinal tract, 17, 40, 128, 130, 131, 132, 133
Cranial nerve innervation, 137, 140, 141, 143
Creatinine values, 217, 219, 220, 294
CREST 2 Trial, 175
Cryptogenic stroke, 36, 44, 45, 46
CRYSTAL-AF Trial, 44
CT angiography (CTA), 23, 27, 34, 45, 56, 64, 65, 68, 73, 87, 111, 133, 195, 196, 197, 200, 206, 207, 210, 211, 212, 213, 214, 217, 218, 219, 220, 239, 240, 247, 249, 250, 251, 252, 253, 254, 257, 260, 266, 267, 268, 270, 292, 294, 295, 297, 298, 300, 301, 302, 304, 311, 318, 319, 320, 321, 323, 324, 340, 346, 356
CT perfusion (CTP), 195, 196, 197, 206, 207, 208, 209, 210, 211, 212, 213, 214, 217, 218, 219, 220, 238, 239, 240, 247, 249, 252, 253, 254, 257, 260, 266, 267, 268, 292, 294, 297, 301, 302, 311, 318, 319, 323, 324, 340, 356

D

dAVF, 87, 88, 91, 391
DAWN Trial, 239, 240, 250, 253, 254, 255, 256, 257, 258, 259, 260, 267, 284, 300, 303, 343, 344, 345, 355
D-dimer levels, 45, 96, 98
DEFUSE 3 Trial, 239, 240, 250, 253, 254, 255, 256, 257, 258, 259, 260, 267, 284, 300, 303, 343, 344, 345, 355

Celirium, 162, 183
Cevelopmental venous anomalies (DVA), 85, 89, 90, 91
Diabetes, 39, 66, 73, 75, 167, 174, 217, 231, 256
Diffusion weighted imaging (DWI), 111, 112, 119, 166, 168, 169, 238, 239, 240, 253, 254, 257, 260, 270, 301, 308, 309, 311, 335, 356
Digital subtraction angiography (DSA), 64, 73
Direction-changing nystagmus, 107, 111, 112, 335
Disability, 4, 62, 106, 205, 220, 227, 228, 239, 243, 244, 254, 282, 287, 293, 306, 323, 346, 351
Dix-Hallpike test/exam, 108, 109
Dizziness, 102, 107, 114, 182, 186
Dorsal midbrain (Parinaud's) syndrome, 135, 136
Double simultaneous stimulation, 191, 194
Dual antiplatelet therapy, 166, 167, 168, 172, 176, 177, 178, 307
Dual-phase CTA, 211, 212, 300, 318
Dysarthria, 39, 40, 102, 105, 145, 183, 186, 307
Dysdiadochokinesis, 104
Dysmetria, 103
Dysphonia, 103
Dysrhythmokinesis, 104

E

Early ischemic changes (EICs), 198, 199, 200, 214, 230, 231
Edema, 17, 67, 88, 96, 97, 106, 161, 183, 238
Embolic disease, 41, 80, 154, 171, 177
Embolic strokes of undetermined source (ESUS), 44, 45, 46, 47, 49, 60
Embolism, 41, 44, 45
Embolus, 37, 38, 41, 235
EMBRACE Trial, 44
Encephalopathy, 181, 182, 183, 185, 310
Endovascular coil embolization, 71, 72
Endovascular coiling, 66, 76
Endovascular treatment (EVT), 37, 47, 111, 112, 146, 156, 162, 197, 202, 203, 205, 206, 208, 209, 210, 212, 213, 214, 218, 220, 233, 234, 238, 239, 240, 243, 244, 245, 246, 247, 248, 249, 250, 251, 252, 253, 254, 255, 257, 258, 259, 260, 263, 265, 266, 267, 268, 273, 274, 275, 281, 283, 286, 287, 294, 295, 298, 299, 300, 301, 302, 303, 304, 305, 306, 311, 316, 317, 318, 319, 320, 321, 322, 323, 324, 340, 342, 343, 344, 345, 346, 353, 355, 356
Equilibrium, 20, 101
ESCAPE Trial, 210, 218, 244, 247, 250, 267, 269, 273, 282, 300
ESPRIT Trial, 45
European Carotid Surgery (ECS) Trial, 171
European Cooperative Acute Stroke Study (ECASS) III, 197, 231, 232, 234, 256, 340
Ever-Ready neurointerventional team model, 321, 322
EVT critical time points, 249, 250, 299, 345
EXTEND-IA Trial, 244, 247, 270, 300

Extraocular muscle function, 137
Eye movements, 14, 19, 133, 140, 141, 149, 161

F

Facial palsy, 191
Facial paralysis, 131
Familial cavernous angioma syndrome, 88
FASTER (Fast Assessment of Stroke and TIA to prevent Early Recurrence) Trial, 177, 180
Fetal origin of the posterior cerebral artery (fPCA), 153
Fibromuscular dysplasia (FMD), 77, 78, 80, 82
Fisher scale, 63, 68
Flow diversion devices, 71, 73
Fluid-attenuated inversion recovery (FLAIR), 65, 238, 239, 240
Focal swelling, 198, 230
Forced gaze deviation, 189
Four rules of the brainstem, 124, 128, 135, 136
fPCA, 115, 116, 120, 153, 155, 162
Frontal eye fields (FEF), 14, 22, 141, 143, 149, 161, 162
Functional disability, 239, 254
Functional outcome in AIS, 41, 62, 73, 145, 146, 181, 187, 198, 210, 211, 212, 218, 219, 220, 223, 234, 240, 243, 244, 245, 249, 250, 251, 252, 253, 255, 260, 266, 267, 273, 287, 295, 299, 300, 306, 308, 311, 316, 317, 318, 320, 321, 322, 323, 345, 346, 353

G

Gait abnormalities, 103, 334
Gaze preference, 141, 160, 161, 162, 275, 281
General anesthesia (GA), 47, 74, 215, 253, 260, 269, 313
Glasgow Coma Scale (GCS), 59, 60, 63, 253, 391
GOLIATH trial, 253
Greater than one third the MCA territory rule, 201, 203
Groin puncture, 146, 247, 248, 249, 250, 251, 252, 255, 274, 294, 299, 343

H

Head Impulse test, 110
Headache, 62, 64, 80, 85, 97, 98, 102, 145, 182, 307, 310
Hemianopia, 139, 153, 190, 191, 307
Hemiparesis, 40, 128, 145, 153, 157, 161, 162, 183, 276
Hemiplegia, 40, 118, 153, 154, 182, 183, 186
Hemorrhage, 35, 49, 50, 51, 53, 54, 59, 60, 61, 62, 63, 72, 73, 79, 85, 87, 88, 90, 96, 97, 98, 99, 133, 166, 167, 174, 176, 177, 178, 183, 184, 195, 197, 200, 203, 212, 213, 218, 223, 228, 229, 230, 231, 233, 237, 245, 247, 250, 265, 294, 295, 297, 304, 307, 308, 310, 318, 329, 340, 356
Hemorrhagic stroke, 3, 35, 59, 61, 62, 73, 111, 305, 329
Heparin, 42, 81, 98, 172, 227, 229, 244, 339
HINTS exam, 108, 110, 111
Homonymous hemianopia, 137, 139, 160, 161, 162
Horner's syndrome, 80, 125
Hospital-based stroke assessment, 285, 292

Hunt-Hess scale, 62
Hydrocephalus, 12, 66, 74, 106
Hypercoagulable abnormalities, 46
Hyperlipidemia, 39, 181, 184, 310
Hypertension, 39, 50, 52, 65, 68, 70, 75, 80, 167, 181, 184, 225, 227, 310
Hypertensive hemorrhage (HH), 50, 51, 52, 60, 74
Hypertonic saline administration, 67, 75
Hhypoattenuation, 198, 200, 215, 230, 235
Hypodense brain tissue, 199, 200, 217, 230, 295, 340
hypoglycemia, 181, 182, 184, 310
Hyponatremia, 66, 68, 75
Hypotonia, 103, 104, 334
Hypovolemia, 66, 67

I

ICA bifurcation. *See* Carotid terminus
IMS III Trial, 244, 269
Infundibulum, 153, 164
International Study of Unruptured Intracranial Aneurysms (ISUIA), 69, 70
Internuclear ophthalmoplegia (INO), 142, 143
Intra-aortic balloon pumps, 66
Intracerebral hemorrhage, 34, 49, 50, 59, 60, 99, 114, 195, 203, 205, 217, 223, 233, 234, 252, 260, 307
Intracerebral hemorrhage (ICH), 49, 50, 51, 53, 59, 60, 63, 64, 73, 233
Intracranial aneurysms, 28, 53, 57, 59, 61, 62, 64, 65, 66, 69, 71, 72, 73, 74, 75, 76, 153
Intracranial Hemorrhage (ICH) Score, 63, 64
Intracranial lesions, 181, 183, 310
Intracranial stenosis, 171, 173, 174, 175, 178, 179, 180
Ischemic penumbra, 1, 7, 8, 9, 35, 37, 195, 197, 198, 200, 205, 206, 207, 209, 210, 212, 214, 215, 217, 218, 230, 234, 235, 237, 238, 239, 240, 244, 246, 250, 251, 252, 253, 254, 255, 256, 257, 258, 260, 263, 265, 266, 267, 273, 286, 287, 291, 292, 293, 295, 297, 298, 300, 305, 306, 311, 315, 316, 318, 320, 321, 330, 340, 346, 355
Ischemic stroke, 3, 9, 17, 22, 35, 38, 44, 45, 46, 47, 48, 49, 60, 62, 78, 82, 96, 101, 102, 106, 111, 112, 115, 118, 146, 147, 149, 162, 164, 165, 166, 168, 169, 171, 176, 177, 178, 179, 180, 181, 182, 183, 185, 187, 195, 196, 197, 205, 210, 212, 214, 215, 216, 217, 218, 220, 221, 223, 224, 226, 229, 231, 232, 234, 235, 237, 238, 239, 240, 243, 244, 245, 252, 255, 257, 260, 261, 262, 263, 268, 269, 270, 273, 274, 286, 288, 291, 303, 306, 307, 308, 309, 310, 311, 313, 314, 315, 323, 324, 327, 343, 351, 356
Isodense brain tissue, 199, 200, 230
IV TPA, 37, 47, 111, 146, 156, 167, 177, 181, 184, 195, 197, 199, 200, 203, 204, 210, 213, 217, 218, 223, 224, 225, 226, 227, 228, 229, 230, 231, 232, 233, 234, 237, 238, 239, 240, 243, 244, 245, 246, 247, 248, 249, 252, 253, 254, 256, 260, 263, 265, 266, 267, 268, 273, 281, 282, 286, 292, 293, 295, 297, 298, 299, 300, 301, 302, 304, 305, 306, 307, 308, 310, 311, 316, 317, 318, 320, 321, 323, 324, 340, 341, 342, 343, 351, 352, 353, 355, 356, 374, 375, 376, 381, 382, 386, 387
IV TPA administration criteria, 226
IV TPA exclusion criteria, 197, 223, 224, 225, 226, 231, 232, 234, 248, 252, 255, 256, 306, 314, 340, 343
IV TPA inclusion criteria, 224, 251, 254, 255, 257
IV TPA restrictions, 200, 229, 297, 298, 317, 318, 323

L

Lacunar infarcts, 39, 41, 118, 128, 153, 158, 276
Lacunar stroke, 39, 44, 45
Lacunar syndromes, 39, 40
Language, 14, 16, 117, 161, 162, 189, 192, 193, 195, 276, 307, 327
Language assessment, 189, 193
Large vessel disease, 41, 237
Large vessel occlusion (LVO), 37, 41, 47, 111, 112, 145, 146, 153, 154, 157, 162, 195, 196, 197, 205, 206, 207, 210, 212, 213, 214, 217, 220, 232, 234, 239, 240, 244, 245, 246, 247, 248, 249, 250, 251, 252, 254, 257, 258, 259, 260, 267, 268, 273, 274, 275, 276, 277, 279, 280, 281, 282, 283, 285, 286, 287, 292, 293, 294, 295, 296, 297, 298, 299, 300, 301, 302, 303, 304, 305, 306, 311, 316, 317, 318, 319, 320, 321, 322, 323, 324, 342, 343, 346, 349, 350, 351, 352, 353, 355, 356
Large Vessel Occlusion Acute Ischemic Stroke. *See* LVO AIS
Last known normal (LKN) data, 237, 240, 311, 353
Lateral medullary (Wallenberg) syndrome, 129
Lateral midbrain (Benedikt) syndrome, 134, 135
Lateral pontine syndrome, 131
Level of consciousness (LOC), 188, 189, 196
Locked-in syndrome (LIS), 133, 135
Los Angeles Motor Scale (LAMS), 274, 277, 278
Los Angeles Prehospital Stroke Screen (LAPSS), 274
Loss of consciousness, 115, 118, 146, 337
Lumbar puncture, 64, 96, 228
LVO AIS, 37, 41, 145, 146, 157, 195, 207, 234, 244, 246, 247, 249, 254, 257, 258, 260, 273, 274, 281, 282, 283, 285, 286, 287, 292, 293, 294, 295, 296, 297, 298, 299, 300, 301, 302, 303, 304, 305, 306, 311, 316, 317, 318, 321, 322, 323, 342, 343, 346, 349, 350, 351, 353, 355
LVO, false positives, 294, 304

M

M1 occlusions, 160, 161, 252, 255, 263
M2 occlusions, 250, 251
Magnetic resonance angiography (MRA), 23, 27, 34, 65, 87, 91, 98, 111, 112, 239, 240, 252, 253, 254, 257, 260, 266, 268, 300, 335, 356
Magnetic resonance imaging (MRI), 45, 50, 52, 65, 87, 90, 97, 111, 114, 119, 166, 168, 169, 181, 185, 205, 207, 212, 214, 229, 232, 233, 234, 238, 239, 240, 254, 262, 266, 267, 268, 300, 301, 308, 309, 311, 318, 335, 356

MANGO™ mnemonic, 41, 42, 279, 281, 285, 286, 287, 293, 294, 297, 298, 299, 300, 304, 317, 322, 323, 346, 349, 351
MATCH (Management of Atherothrombosis with Clopidogrel in High-risk patients) Trial, 176, 180
Mean transit time (MTT), 207, 212, 214
Mechanical thrombectomy, 146, 147, 235, 246, 251, 252, 255, 257, 258, 259, 261, 262, 267, 270, 281, 282, 286, 300, 302, 305, 317, 343
Medial longitudinal fasciculus (MLF), 128, 135, 141, 142, 143
Medial medullary (Dejerine) syndrome, 130
Medial midbrain (Weber) syndrome, 134
Medial pontine syndrome, 132
Medusa, 89, 90
Memory, 1, 115, 117, 120
Ménière's disease, 108, 335
Metabolic disorders, 182
Micropsia, 140
Midbrain, 13, 18, 19, 20, 27, 56, 102, 115, 118, 123, 124, 127, 128, 131, 132, 134, 135, 140, 141, 143, 183, 186, 205, 337
Middle cerebral artery (MCA), 1, 31, 33, 34, 39, 41, 133, 138, 139, 140, 143, 150, 151, 154, 156, 157, 158, 159, 160, 161, 162, 195, 196, 197, 198, 199, 200, 201, 203, 204, 205, 212, 213, 214, 229, 231, 232, 234, 237, 240, 247, 248, 250, 251, 252, 255, 260, 263, 268, 269, 294, 297, 331, 340, 356
Migraine, 108, 181, 182, 183, 184, 310
Migrainous headaches, 45, 47
Migrainous vertigo, 108, 335
Mini strokes, 165
Minor stroke, 166, 167, 168, 169, 177, 180, 306, 307, 308, 313, 339, 351, 352
Mission Lifeline Severity-Based Stroke Triage Algorithm for EMS, 281
Modified Rankin scale (mRS), 178, 243, 247, 248, 249, 251, 252, 253, 255, 260, 294
Motor strength, 191, 275, 279
Motor weakness, 40, 115, 120, 194, 274, 275, 281, 293, 294, 298, 337
Moyamoya disease, 45, 47, 77, 81, 82
MR CLEAN NO-IV Trial, 260
MR CLEAN Trial, 244, 246, 253, 305, 355
MR WITNESS Trial, 238, 239, 241, 343
Multiphase CTA, 210, 212
Multiple sclerosis, 133, 181, 183, 186, 310
Mycotic aneurysms, 53, 54, 57
Myocardial infarction (MI), 43, 44, 171, 172, 176, 179, 180, 228, 234, 262, 286, 293, 311

N

National Institute of Neurologic Disorders and Stroke (NINDS) trial, 196, 197, 198, 213, 215, 218, 221, 223, 224, 234, 235, 240, 306, 307, 313
National Institutes of Health Stroke Scale (NIHSS), 156, 162, 184, 187, 188, 189, 190, 191, 192, 193, 194, 195, 196, 213, 231, 232, 239, 240, 246, 247, 248, 249, 251, 252, 253, 254, 255, 256, 257, 260, 262, 286, 294, 295, 298, 299, 301, 304, 305, 306, 307, 308, 311, 315, 318, 320, 322, 323, 324, 340, 343, 346, 349, 351, 352, 353, 354, 356
Nausea, 102, 145, 307
Neck pain, 79, 80
Necrosis, 8
Neglect, 115, 120, 161, 162, 193, 194, 274, 275, 276, 281, 288, 313, 324, 337
Neoplasms, 17, 198, 217, 227, 229, 294
Neuroanatomy, 13, 162, 197
Neurogenic stunned myocardium, 66
Neuroimaging, 37, 38, 56, 111, 112, 114, 134, 135, 145, 166, 168, 186, 187, 197, 200, 206, 212, 213, 214, 217, 219, 220, 234, 237, 238, 239, 240, 244, 246, 247, 249, 250, 252, 254, 255, 257, 260, 263, 266, 267, 285, 287, 291, 292, 293, 294, 295, 299, 300, 304, 305, 308, 313, 314, 317, 318, 320, 321, 323, 335, 343, 346, 355
Neuroimaging categories, 212, 213, 373
Neurointervention, 297, 321, 323
Neurons, 7, 9, 17, 137, 276, 286, 318
Neuropathy, 130, 132, 189
Nicardipine, 65, 74
Nimodipine, 68, 75
NINDS trial, 198, 218, 224, 234
Numbness, 40, 128, 130, 131, 132
Nystagmus, 102, 103, 104, 105, 107, 108, 109, 110, 111, 112, 128, 335

O

Ocular motor abnormalities, 104, 334
Optic field cut, 274, 281, 285

P

Palinopsia, 140
paralysis, 69, 101, 132, 135, 160, 181
paramedian pontine reticular formation (PPRF), 19, 22, 141, 143
Parenchymal hemorrhage, 50, 88, 96, 98, 229
Parenchymal hypoattenuation, 198, 215, 230
Percheron, artery of, 118
Perimesencephalic venous subarachnoid hemorrhage (PMVSAH), 53, 54, 56, 57, 59, 60, 329, 356
PHASES score, 70, 76
Pipeline® embolization, 72
Plavix, 177
POINT (Platelet-Oriented Inhibition in New TIA and minor ischemic stroke) Trial, 167, 177, 180
Posterior circulation, 13, 23, 24, 28, 39, 79, 80, 101, 109, 114, 115, 123, 135, 145, 150, 152, 179, 195, 205, 251, 253, 261, 263, 306, 331
Posterior reversible encephalopathy syndrome (PRES), 183, 185

Prehospital screening (LVO), 273, 274, 279, 281, 282, 283, 285, 287, 292
Prehospital stroke assessment, 274, 315, 316, 317, 346
Primary motor cortex, 14, 149, 157
Primary sensory cortex, 14, 149, 157
Primary stroke centers (PSCs), 273, 282, 283, 285, 286, 287
Primary visual cortex, 14, 138, 150, 275
PROACT II Trial, 244
Prosopagnosia, 140
Pseudoaneurysm, 79
Pupil abnormalities, 137, 143
Pure motor hemiplegia, 40

Q

Quadriplegia, 133

R

RACECAT Trial, 281
Rapid Arterial Occlusion Evaluation Scale (RACE), 274, 276, 277
RAPID™ (iSchemaView) software, 254
Recanalization, 9, 145, 146, 147, 210, 223, 232, 233, 234, 235, 236, 244, 245, 247, 251, 260, 263, 266, 268, 269, 270, 322, 343
Recurrent stroke, 43, 45, 47, 80, 81, 165, 166, 167, 168, 173, 176, 177, 178, 233, 307, 309, 339
Red thrombi, 42
Remote neurointerventional team model, 321, 322
Renal dysfunction or failure, 172, 217, 219, 220
Reperfusion, 8, 147, 178, 206, 209, 218, 234, 245, 246, 249, 250, 258, 262, 263, 265, 267, 269, 286, 317, 323, 343
REVASCAT Trial, 244, 247, 270, 300
Revascularization, 147, 171, 174, 175, 177, 178, 244, 245, 263, 269, 273, 288
Rule of Thirds, 62

S

SAMMPRIS, 173, 174, 175, 177, 179, 339
SAPPHIRE (Stenting and Angioplasty with Protection in Patients at High-Risk for Endarterectomy) Trial, 172
Secondary stroke, 44, 45, 47, 81, 111, 166, 167, 171, 174, 175, 176, 177, 178, 307, 308, 339, 352
Secondary stroke prevention, 45, 166, 177, 178, 307, 339
Seizures, 67, 85, 96, 141, 181, 184, 310
Sensorimotor deficits, 39, 40
Sensory loss, 153, 160, 191
Sepsis, 181, 183, 310
Simultaneous visual stimulation, 191
Small vessel disease, 36, 38, 39, 49, 158, 276
Spatial neglect, 160
Speech, 14, 145, 150, 161, 182, 183, 188, 193
Stent retrievers, 146, 147, 244, 245, 246, 251, 252, 343

Stenting, 71, 81, 171, 172, 173, 174, 175, 178, 179, 339
Stenting of SYmptomatic atherosclerotic Lesions in the Vertebral or Intracranial Arteries (SSYLVIA) Trial, 173, 179
Stenting vs. Aggressive Medical Management for Preventing Recurrent Stroke in Intracranial Stenosis (SAMMPRIS) Trial, 173, 174, 175
Stroke efficiency, 315, 322
Stroke in women, 62, 78, 93, 98
Stroke in younger patients, 77, 78, 81, 82
Stroke management, 23, 38, 106, 135, 211, 218, 220, 224, 237, 246, 251, 286, 319
Stroke mimic protocol/rule, 184, 310, 339
Stroke mimics, 181, 182, 183, 184, 185, 186, 198, 217, 284, 310, 314, 318, 339
Stroke plan (S-PLAN), 38, 47, 111, 112, 135, 149, 184, 187
Stroke severity, 184, 187, 194, 195, 235, 252, 281, 285, 288, 298, 305, 307
Stroke subtypes, 4, 329
Stroke workup, 183, 217
Stroke, diagnosis and treatment, 23, 83, 93, 145, 162, 165, 187, 197, 205, 207, 212, 213, 214, 217, 219, 246, 249, 273, 292, 294, 299, 306, 310, 311, 315, 316, 317, 318, 320, 323, 324, 327, 340, 343, 345, 346, 349, 351, 353, 356
Stroke, emergency medical services (EMS), 273, 274, 279, 285, 287, 315, 316, 317, 323, 324, 346, 356
Stroke, rapidly improving symptoms, 306, 308, 311, 313
ST–segment–elevation myocardial infarction (STEMI), 223, 228, 234, 293, 311, 342
Subadventitial dissection, 79
Subarachnoid hemorrhage (SAH), 49, 50, 53, 54, 56, 57, 58, 59, 60, 62, 63, 64, 65, 66, 68, 69, 70, 73, 74, 75, 78, 80, 81, 82, 97, 98, 229, 329
Subintimal dissection, 79
Surgical clipping, 66, 71, 72, 73
SWIFT PRIME Trial, 244, 247, 262, 270, 273, 300
SWIFT Trial, 245
Sylvian fissure, 13, 33, 150
Symptom onset, 64, 65, 111, 166, 167, 177, 197, 216, 231, 232, 237, 239, 244, 246, 247, 249, 250, 251, 252, 254, 257, 258, 260, 261, 267, 270, 292, 294, 300, 301, 302, 303, 307, 317, 339, 340, 346
Syndrome of inappropriate antidiuretic hormone (SIADH), 66, 67, 73, 392
SYNTHESIS Trial, 244

T

Test of (Vertical) Skew, 110, 111
Texas Stroke Intervention Prehospital Stroke Severity Scale (LEGS score), 276
Thalamic stroke, 115, 117, 120, 334, 337
The North American Symptomatic Carotid Endarterectomy Trial (NASCET), 171
Three-item stroke scale (3I-SS), 277, 278

Thrombolysis in Cerebral Infarction (TICI) grading system, 244, 245, 258
Thrombosis, 39, 41, 46, 65, 87, 93, 96, 98, 99, 145
Thrombus, 38, 44, 45, 80, 203, 211, 232, 236, 245, 252, 262
Tissue viability, 166, 215, 217, 218, 220, 234, 238, 239, 240, 250, 252, 258, 318
Tissue window philosophy, 254, 258, 356
TOAST Trial, 36, 44, 47
Todd's paralysis, 181
Tongue deviation, 130
Transcranial Doppler studies (TCDs), 68, 73
Transient ischemic attack (TIA), 101, 162, 165, 166, 167, 168, 169, 174, 177, 180, 215, 292, 308, 309, 311, 313, 339, 346, 356
Transitional neurointerventional team model, 321, 322
Trauma, 53, 78, 80, 87, 228, 230
Tremor, 103, 104, 134, 334
TREVO 2 Study, 245
Triple-H therapy, 68, 75
TRITON-TIMI 38 (Trial to Assess Improvement in Therapeutic Outcomes by Optimizing Platelet Inhibition with Prasugrel–Thrombolysis in Myocardial Infarction) Trial, 177

U

Unilateral cerebellar disease, 104
Unilateral sensorimotor deficits, 39, 40

V

VAN assessment (vision, aphasia, neglect), 274, 275, 276, 277, 279, 280, 287, 288, 313, 324
Vascular imaging, 45, 177, 298, 301
Vascular malformations, 65, 85, 90, 329
Vascular occlusion, 8, 181, 263, 318
Vasculitis, 57, 58
Vasculopathies, 77, 78, 82, 329
Vein of Galen malformation, 87, 94
Vein of Labbe, 94

Vein of Trolard, 94
Venous drainage, 87, 93, 94, 96
Ventral pontine syndrome. *See* Locked-in syndrome (LIS)
Vertebral artery dissections (VAD), 79, 80, 82
Vertebrobasilar atherothrombotic disease (VBATD), 101, 112
Vertebrobasilar insufficiency (VBI), 101, 112, 392
Vertigo, 102, 103, 106, 107, 108, 109, 110, 111, 112, 114, 145, 182, 183, 186, 307, 334, 335, 356
Vestibular dysfunction, 181, 310
Vestibular neuritis, 108, 110, 111, 114, 335
Vision, 14, 137, 138, 143, 145, 150, 151, 189, 191, 274, 275, 276, 281, 287, 288, 313, 324, 337, 392
Vision loss, 138
Visual abnormalities, 115, 120, 337
Visual agnosia, 140
Visual field deficits, 138, 161, 190
Visual fields, 189, 193, 194
Vitesse Intracranial Stent Study for Ischemic Stroke Therapy (VISSIT) Trial, 174, 175, 177, 179, 339
Volumetric Impedance Phase Shift Spectroscopy (VIPS), 286, 289
Voluntary movement, 14, 17, 20, 101, 149
Vomiting, 102, 145

W

Wake-up stroke (WUS), 237, 238, 239, 240, 392
Warfarin, 45, 47, 81, 175, 227, 232, 339, 340
Warfarin-Aspirin Symptomatic Intracranial Disease (WASID) Trial, 175
Warfarin vs. Aspirin for Recurrent Stroke Study (WARSS) 45
Wernicke's aphasia, 276
Wingspan stEnt system post mArket surVEillance (WEAVE) Trial, 174
Wingspan stent, 173, 175, 371

X

Xanthochromia, 64, 74